Anatomy of a Medical School

Anatomy of a Medical School

A History of Medicine at the University of Otago 1875–2000

DOROTHY PAGE

OTAGO UNIVERSITY PRESS

Published by Otago University Press
PO Box 56/Level 1, 398 Cumberland Street, Dunedin, New Zealand
Fax 64 3 479 8385
www.otago.ac.nz/press

First published 2008
Copyright © Dorothy Page 2008
ISBN 978 1 877372 24 7

Cover image:
The Operating Theatre by Russell Clark
1936 *Digest,* Otago Medical School, University of Otago

Cover and book design by Jenny Cooper
Printed through Condor Production Ltd, Hong Kong

CONTENTS

Foreword *David Skegg*   7

Acknowledgements   9

Introduction   11

Abbreviations   14

Part I.   Scott's Medical School, 1875–1914

1.   The Southernmost Medical School: An Injudicious Enterprise?   17

2.   An Outpost of Edinburgh   25

3.   The Medical School and the Dunedin Hospital, 1890s–1914   34

4.   Crisis and Expansion: Breaking out of the Financial Straitjacket, 1890s–1914   39

5.   Medical Students   46

Part II.   The Ferguson Era, 1914–1937

6.   A Statesman at the Helm   61

7.   World War I and its Aftermath   66

8.   'A Monument in Bricks and Mortar'   74

9.   Expansion and Modernisation   83

10. The Clinical Club and the Monro Collection   97

11. Medical Students Between the Wars   102

12. The Dean's Assessment   109

Part III. Research and Expansion: The Hercus Era, 1937–1958

13. World War II   115

14. Research and Expansion Under Hercus   126

15. Medical Students in the Mid-Twentieth Century   142

16. A Formidable Dean: Charles Hercus in the School and the University   151

Part IV.   The Medical School in a Changing Environment, 1959–1981

17.   From Crisis to Christie, 1959–1969   161

18.   Building a 'Three-Legged Stool': The Christchurch and Wellington Schools   181

19.   Interlude: A Year to Celebrate, 1975   199

20.   Times of Tension, 1975–1981   208

21.   Student Life: A Change of Direction   217

Part V.   Decades of Challenge and Opportunity, 1981–2000

22.   The 1980s: Economic and Political Pressures   225

23.   The 1990s: A Decade of Upheaval and Expansion   237

24.   New Ways of Teaching and Learning   254

25.   The Research Culture   264

26.   A Rich Diversity: Medical Students in the Late Twentieth Century   278

Postscript

27.   Made at Otago: Some of the Graduates   289

28.   Medical School at the Millennium   299

Afterword: Looking Forward   *Don Roberton*   303

Appendices   307

Deans of Faculty and of the Otago, Christchurch and Wellington Schools,
Assistant Vice-Chancellors (AVCs), later Pro-Vice-Chancellors (PVCs),
Health Sciences, and Professors of the School 1874–2000   307

Graduates of the Otago Medical School, 1887–2006   313
Winners of the Travelling Scholarship in Medicine, 1909–2007   345
Otago Medical Students awarded the Rhodes Scholarship, 1923–2007   346

Notes   347

Select Bibliography   383

Index   391

FOREWORD

Although New Zealand is a young country, some of its institutions seem venerable. One of these undoubtedly is the University of Otago Medical School, which has held a prominent place in education and health care for more than 130 years. Its graduates have led medical services in New Zealand for most of the past century, while many others have made their mark internationally, in both peace and war. The Otago Medical School was the first faculty of any New Zealand university to become truly research-led. Moreover, in recent years its three campuses – in Wellington, Christchurch, and Dunedin – have broadened their role from the training of doctors to embrace postgraduate education in many health disciplines.

Two earlier histories of the Otago Medical School, published in 1945 and 1964, were written by retired professors with inside knowledge. Dr Dorothy Page has not only brought the story up to the present, but has also provided the objectivity and expertise of a professional historian. As well as having an unparalleled knowledge of the University archives and records, she has made extensive use of interviews with former students and staff. These have helped her to paint a fascinating picture of the life of the Medical School and its students, and to place this in the broader context of New Zealand's social history.

Reading about the struggles of the embryonic medical school in the late nineteenth century, one marvels at how quickly it started to produce graduates who were highly regarded in all parts of the world. Moreover, by the mid-twentieth century the Otago Medical School was pouring out research of international significance. Branch faculties for the teaching of sixth-year medical students evolved into major campuses in Christchurch and Wellington, as well as a second Faculty of Medicine at the University of Auckland.

None of this could have been achieved without the flair and determination of some exceptional leaders. Dr Page chronicles their achievements, while also describing many of the other characters who have made the Otago Medical School a remarkable institution. We need to remember that the success of the medical school has depended not only on such people who are named here, but also on all the other academic, clinical, and general staff who have given loyal service – often for their whole careers.

This book will be read by people who are interested in the development of university education, the medical profession, and health services in New Zealand. For those of us who have been students or staff of the Otago Medical School, the book will hold a particular fascination. One cannot help thinking that we are fortunate to share in a great inheritance.

DAVID SKEGG
Vice-Chancellor
University of Otago

ACKNOWLEDGEMENTS

IN THE COURSE of researching and writing this book I have enjoyed the assistance of many people and it is a pleasure to acknowledge them here, although there are too many to name individually. The affection with which the Otago Medical School is regarded by those who have been associated with it, as students or staff, is striking and heart-warming.

The members of the small History Committee set up by the Faculty of Medicine and convened in turn by its Deans, Professors John Campbell and Don Roberton, have been generous in their time and expertise, both as a group and individually. Medical Emeritus Professors Graham Mortimer (for the Medical School Alumnus Association), Keith Jeffery and Ted Nye, and Head of the History Department, Professor Barbara Brookes, patiently responded to queries and commented on the manuscript. Other past and present members of the School staff allowed me oral interviews, answered questions and in some cases read all or part of the manuscript. Among them I would like to single out Vice-Chancellor David Skegg and Emeritus Professors Douglass Taylor, Lawrence Wright and David Stewart. Professor Geoffrey Rice, Head of the History Department at the University of Canterbury, made invaluable comments on the first draft of the manuscript.

Several of the group I was privileged to interview have since died and I would like to pay special tribute to them. Associate Professor John Borrie, Emeritus Professors Alan Clarke, John Hunter, James and Marion Robinson, Bill Trotter, Drs Hugh Stringer and Rex Wright-St.Clair all contributed their own distinctive viewpoint.

At times I have had the help of three excellent research assistants. I obtained the services of Dr Elaine Thomson, who had just completed a PhD in medical history from the University of Edinburgh, through a Division of Humanities Research Grant. Using the Edinburgh University archives, Dr Thomson researched the Edinburgh connection with the Otago Medical School in its early years, then spent some weeks in Dunedin working on the same period. When she had to return to Scotland earlier than expected, Mrs Leah Taylor completed the contract. More recently, the generosity of the History Department enabled me to employ Dr Austin Gee, principally to work on the appendices, and to call on the advanced computer skills of Kyle Matthews. Assistance from administrative staff in the Faculty of Medicine, especially Ellen Hendry, Bruce Smith, Barbara Lee, Glenda Stent and Ruth Brown, was also much appreciated.

Staff at the Hocken Collections, which holds most of the Medical School archives, and the Medical Library have been uniformly helpful. The quest for illustrations has also taken me to the Dunedin Office of National Archives, the *Otago Daily Times*, and the photographic sections of the Christchurch and Wellington Schools, as well as to individuals. Everywhere I have met with the utmost cooperation. I would like to acknowledge especially the generosity of

Mrs Rosalie Archer in permitting publication of a number of works (including the cover illustration) by Russell Clark.

Any history builds on what has gone before and I have been able to call on the special expertise of two histories: *Annals of the University of Otago Medical School* (1945) by D.W. Carmalt Jones, and *The Otago Medical School under the First Three Deans* (1964), by Sir Charles Hercus and Sir Gordon Bell. Both were written with inside knowledge of the Medical School and I have not tried to supersede them. My viewpoint is different, but my debt considerable.

I am also deeply indebted to the late John Hunter who, in his retirement, added another element to his contribution to the Medical School, as Head of Department, researcher and Dean.

As Honorary Archivist he persistently gathered together letters and written information from his former colleagues to make up the archive, now in the Hocken Collections, that bears his name. His energy drove the initiation of the history project. As early as 1993, he was soliciting from the Otago Medical School Alumnus Association the funds which have made this publication possible. Although I came to know John only in his last years, when his health was very poor, I benefited greatly from our long and absorbing conversations.

Finally, I would like to acknowledge publisher Wendy Harrex, copy-editor Greg Adamson, indexer Andrew Parsloe and designer Jenny Cooper, the team at the Otago University Press who have produced this book.

DOROTHY PAGE
Dunedin, February 2008

INTRODUCTION

WHAT DOES IT TAKE to create a medical school? The essential elements are easy enough to identify: teachers, buildings and a special relationship with a hospital. But that is not enough: the teachers must be academically specialised and highly qualified, the buildings must contain laboratories for research as well as rooms for teaching, and the hospital must be up-to-date and well-staffed, with enough patients to provide a variety of teaching experience for medical students. The whole must be sufficiently flexible, and well enough resourced, to be able to change over time as medical science, medical practice and society's expectations of it change. A medical school also needs students who are academically able, mature and committed to the science and art of medicine. To create a medical school is a major undertaking and, in the late nineteenth century, when the Otago Medical School was founded, it typically needed the drive of a strong and determined individual (in Otago's case, James Macandrew) as well as consistent support from the community.

A medical school operates in several contexts, one of which is academic. As it is part of the University of Otago, the fortunes of the Otago Medical School have been bound up with those of its parent institution. When the School began, a sole professor was its only full-time member of staff and its partial course was unrewarded by any degree. The dominant narrative of the School from this modest beginning is one of extraordinary, exciting, if not always steady growth, driven for much of its first century by three powerful Deans. Professor Scott, Sir Lindo Ferguson and Sir Charles Hercus were men of vision. As their records clearly show, they were also very demanding in practical matters. As soon as they achieved an immediate goal, such as a new building or additional staff, they pushed forward to the next. They could all describe in vivid detail shortcomings in facilities and staffing, to justify the need for ever more money: Ferguson said that a satisfied dean was a contradiction in terms. The Medical Faculty came to dominate the University in size and influence, but the relationship between the two altered from the mid-twentieth century, as the University grew and its governance changed. Medical Deans viewed the appointment of an executive Vice-Chancellor for the University as a challenge to their established authority and were alarmed when their direct access to government funding ceased and the School's allocation became part of the University's overall grant. The Medical School, with its capped student numbers, began to carry less weight in the ever-expanding University. Towards the end of the century, the Medical School regained status by joining with Dentistry, Pharmacy and Physiotherapy in a powerful Division of Health Sciences.

By this time, the Otago Medical School had ceased to be merely a Dunedin institution. In the 1970s, the Branch Faculties in Christchurch and Wellington which, together with Auckland, already had a track record of fifty years' teaching sixth-year students, became clinical schools of the Otago Medical School. Then they were renamed – the changes of name symbolising both their status and role in their communities and their loyalty to the Otago connection – the Christchurch and Wellington Schools of Medicine and Health Sciences and again, simply, the University of Otago, Christchurch, and the University of Otago, Wellington.

The second context in which a medical school operates is the country's health system. At its most immediate, this is likely to involve a close relationship with a public hospital. More generally, because the Government expects graduates of the school to carry out its health policies, it also assumes the right to intervene in the development of the school and determine the focus of its activities. When the Otago Medical School was founded, the Dunedin Hospital was adequate in terms of patient numbers, but would have failed every other test of suitability for a teaching hospital. Gradually, with pressure from the School's clinical teachers, it gained new buildings and facilities, and trained nursing staff. Relations between the Hospital and School at an administrative level were sometimes tense, especially when money was at issue. Nevertheless, the basic cooperation between the two culminated in 1980, with the opening of a state-of-the-art new hospital ward block incorporating Medical School facilities.

In a broader sense, government health policy has impinged directly on the Medical School, usually in a very positive way. From 1920, in the wake of the disastrous influenza pandemic, the Department of Health was charged with overseeing New Zealand's health services and determining priorities in health care. As the sole provider of medical training for much of the twentieth century, the Otago Medical School played a key role in this task. Up to the 1930s, medical care was provided on a user-pays basis, softened by some charitable care, but in 1938 the Labour Government passed the Social Security Act, which made hospital and maternity care free. Although opposition from medical practitioners prevented the introduction of free general practitioner services, the change to the health system was fundamental. While the

Social Security Act affected medical practitioners rather than medical students, another almost contemporaneous government initiative was of immediate and huge benefit to the School. The establishment of the Medical Research Council provided the framework and steady funding for a coordinated approach to research. Later, the renamed Health Research Council took a broader sweep, with an emphasis on preventive medicine. In the last two decades of the century, as the costs of new medical and surgical procedures skyrocketed, the Government modified the social security system, to the dismay of a number of Medical School staff with joint Hospital appointments. The Government's assumption of responsibility for determining the size of the country's medical workforce and, as a consequence, the number of medical students it would fund, has had a sharp impact on the School. Sudden increases or cuts in student numbers have caused staffing crises, either of understaffing or a temporary freeze on appointments. Assessing the health needs of the country, the Government has required the Medical School to focus on areas of special need, such as Maori health, women's health and rural health. It has made decisions about the allocation of health resources and which centres should receive expensive high-tech equipment. In turn pressured by a more articulate public, less overawed by doctors than was traditionally the case, the Government has demanded greater accountability from practitioners, more open communication with patients and the maintenance of agreed ethical standards. It has directed that these elements be emphasised in the medical course, and the School has responded willingly.

The growing number of Medical School buildings has both reflected and facilitated the School's key role in the health system. The move from a location within the main University complex, to a site alongside the Hospital and the accommodation embedded in it, is physical evidence of a professional journey. The location and design of the buildings, and the sophistication of their facilities have mattered greatly to staff. The determination of successive deans to build suitable housing for the School is recognised by the buildings named after them – Scott, Lindo Ferguson, Hercus, Sayers, Adams, Hunter. The internal layout and facilities reflect the changing emphases in the School's activities: more well-equipped laboratories for research, small rooms for informal classes, as well as large lecture theatres, and computers everywhere. In Christchurch and Wellington, the original 1970s buildings, which are closely connected to the teaching hospitals, have been enlarged and improved, in the new century, to meet the expanded role the Schools have assumed in teaching and research in the health sciences. At the opening of the new facilities at the Wellington School in 2007, the Dean, John Nacey, expressed the value of appropriate accommodation. 'We wanted a physical "heart" and that is what we now have …. We're part of New Zealand's top university – with excellent staff and students – and this space reflects that.'

A medical school is, of course, far more than a collection of buildings, however architecturally attractive or generously endowed with state-of-the-art equipment, computer laboratories and teaching space. It is the people who count. With its academic, research and administrative staff, technicians, support staff and students, the Otago Medical School has become a specialised community, now thousands strong. There are some wonderful people among them, past and present. Many of them appear in this narrative, but they are only a small proportion of those who might have done so. A number of former students, now themselves retired from their professional careers, have recalled, with an affection mingled with nervous respect and often tinged with hilarity, the 'characters' among their teachers. The years roll away as they remember their elation at getting into Medical School, the intense satisfaction of crossing the road to the Hospital and actually dealing with patients, the camaraderie of student life and the life-long friendships forged. The student body has changed over the life of the School, and not only in size. Medical students are no longer typically young males from comfortably-off European families. Today, they include at least equal numbers of women, a solid proportion of Maori and people from the Pacific, Asia and the Middle East. The diversity is striking and enriching.

What to teach and how to teach it are perennial concerns for a medical school. For the Otago School, far away from the traditional centres of medical education, international recognition has been of the utmost importance. Initially looking to the Edinburgh model familiar to the province's Scots migrants, the School then followed the directives of the General Medical Council of Great Britain. More recently, it has become part of an Australasian system of accreditation. Curriculum and pedagogy have been kept under constant review. The early predominance of anatomy, physiology and general surgery has given way to a wide variety of medical and surgical specialties and a greater emphasis on preventive medicine. Students are no longer required to assimilate more and more facts, but are expected to demonstrate an understanding of scientific principles. The formal lecture has given ground to small-group learning and major examinations have largely been replaced by regular tests, often self-administered by computer.

The relatively short life of the Medical School has encompassed dramatic changes in many areas. Distance has been rendered negligible by the revolution in transport and communications, which saw steamships give way to air travel, and sea-borne mail services replaced by the instant contact of the telephone, in its turn supplemented by teleconference, email and the internet. The world is an infinitely smaller place than when the first medical students enrolled at Otago. The School has participated in equally dramatic changes to the medical profession, from a time when chloroform was a novelty and amputation almost the only form of surgery, to the sophistication of organ transplants and key-hole surgery, from carbolic spray to penicillin, modern antibiotics and vaccines for diseases that had been considered incurable. It has been an exhilarating journey. The influence of the Otago Medical School extends far beyond its locality. As a centre for medical education and research, responsive to the changing demands of government and society, it forms an intrinsic part of the broader history of New Zealand. ∎

ABBREVIATIONS

ACC	Accident Compensation Corporation		MB ChB	Bachelor of Medicine and Bachelor of Surgery
ACER	Australian Council for Educational Research		MB CM	Bachelor of Medicine and Master of Surgery
AMC	Australian Medical Council		MBE	Member of the (Order of the) British Empire
AMSA	Australian Medical Students' Association		MCNZ	Medical Council of New Zealand
AVC	Assistant Vice-Chancellor		MD	Doctor of Medicine
BMedSc	Bachelor of Medical Science		MMP	Mixed Member Proportional Representation
BMLSc	Bachelor of Medical Laboratory Science		MRC	Medical Research Council
CAT scanner, or CT scanner			MRCP	Master of the Royal College of Physicians
	Computerised Tomography scanner		MRCS	Master of the Royal College of Surgeons
CEO	Chief Executive Officer		NHF	National Heart Foundation
CHE	Crown Health Enterprise		NHS	National Health Service
CMG	Companion of (the Order of) St Michael and		NZMC	New Zealand Medical Corps
	St George		*NZMJ*	*New Zealand Medical Journal*
CORSO	Council of Organisations for Relief Services		NZUSA	New Zealand Medical Students Association
	Overseas		OBE	Officer of the (Order of the) British Empire
CSM	Christchurch School of Medicine		*ODT*	*Otago Daily Times*
DHB	District Hospital Board		OHB	Otago Hospital Board
DSM	Dunedin School of Medicine		OMS	Otago Medical School
DSO	Distinguished Service Order		OSCE	Objective Structured Clinical Examination
FBBC	Faculty Board Curriculum Committee		OTC	Officer Training Corps
FCC	Faculty Curriculum Committee		OUMC	Otago University Medical Corps (or Company)
FRCS	Fellow of the Royal College of Surgeons		OUMSA	Otago University Medical Students' Association
FRCSI	Fellow of the Royal College of Surgeons,		OUSA	Otago University Students' Association
	Ireland		PBL	Problem-based Learning
GMC	General Medical Council		PhD	Doctor of Philosophy
GP	General Practitioner		POW	Prisoner of War
HEDC	Higher Education Development Centre		PVC	Pro-Vice-Chancellor
HHS	Health and Hospital Services		RAMC	Royal Army Medical Corps
HRC	Health Research Council		RHA	Regional Health Authority
HCO	Healthcare Otago		UGC	University Grants Committee
INED	Intercampus Network for Educational		UMAT	Undergraduate Medicine and Health
	Development			Sciences Admission Test
LRCP	Licentiate of the Royal College of Physicians		UMU	University Medical Unit
MBBS	Bachelor of Medicine and Bachelor of Surgery		WSM	Wellington School of Medicine

PART I

Scott's Medical School
1875–1914

CHAPTER 1

The Southernmost Medical School:
An Injudicious Enterprise?

TO FOUND a medical school in a small settlement halfway round the world from its British homeland and little more than a quarter of a century after the arrival of the first colonists seems, on the face of it, to be a foolhardy undertaking. Certainly the word 'premature' was often on the lips of opponents of the idea. On the other hand, Dunedin could be said to have had the principal requirements for a colonial medical school: a powerful individual to push the scheme through, plenty of money and a hospital with enough beds to provide clinical training for students.

There are two ways of looking at the foundation of the Otago Medical School, one very narrow, the other broad. They are not mutually exclusive. From a broad historical perspective, the found-ation of the School can be set in the context of the spectacular advances in medical science and medical education that occurred during the nineteenth century: 'Modern times dawned with the nineteenth century', notes medical historian Roy Porter. While the social changes brought about by the industrial revolution made pressing demands upon medicine, at the same time medicine itself was being radically transformed by science. In Britain, Simpson's discovery of the anaesthetic value of chloroform in 1847 and Lister's findings on the antiseptic principle, which were published in *The Lancet* in 1867, revolutionised the whole outlook of surgery. Other advances in medical science permitted more accurate diagnosis and treatment of disease. In the meantime, the

practice of medicine was becoming increasingly professionalised as nursing was transformed by the Nightingale movement and, from 1858, doctors had to be admitted to a medical register.[1] All this led to a flurry of founding new medical schools in Britain and its colonies. By the time the Otago Medical School opened in 1875 there were several schools in Canada and one in Melbourne, Australia. In these circumstances, it appears almost inevitable that a medical school would be founded in Dunedin, New Zealand's premier centre in size and wealth following the discovery of gold in Otago in 1861. The consequent gold rush also enabled plans for higher education to take shape, with the University of Otago being established in Dunedin in 1869.

From a narrow perspective, the foundation of both the University of Otago and the Medical School are clearly influenced by the actions of one man, James Macandrew. By the late 1860s, debate was well under way as to whether a colonial university should be established in New Zealand or scholarships provided to able lads for study in Britain. Macandrew, the confident, ebullient Otago Provincial Superintendent, had no doubts New Zealand needed its own university nor where it should be. As historian Jim Gardner argues, it is likely that he was looking to higher education to stem Dunedin's decline as the gold rush waned. The population, which had been 16,000 in 1864, dropped to 13,000 by the end of the decade.[2] In April 1868, with support from the local Presbyterian Church, he proposed that a 'New Zealand University' be set up in Dunedin, with an endowment of 100,000 acres of pastoral land.[3] Formal agreement was completed a year later and Macandrew signed the University of Otago Ordinance on 3 June 1869. This gave the Council of the proposed University the right to confer the degrees of 'Bachelor of Arts, Master of Arts, Bachelor of Medicine, Doctor of Medicine, Bachelor of Laws, Master of Laws, Bachelor of Music, Doctor of Music'.[4]

To Macandrew, tertiary education was about careers. He made this clear in a letter to the very first meeting of the University Council in November 1869, in which he urged that prominence be given to practical training of benefit to the colony and advocated the establishment of schools of mines and of agricultural chemistry.[5] Macandrew also

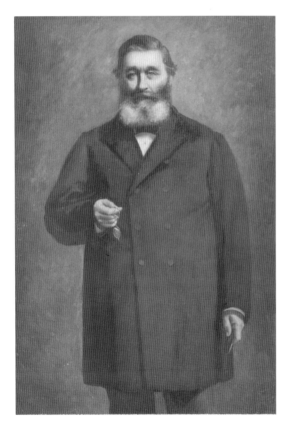

Hon. James Macandrew (1819?–87), Superintendent of Otago Province from 1867 to 1876, played a key role in the establishment of the Otago Medical School.

From a portrait by Eleanor Kate Sperry in the Clocktower Building, University of Otago. Hocken Collections, Uare Taoka o Hakena, University of Otago, Acc. No. c/n F100A/1NZ h.

initiated the move towards setting up the Medical School. Just days after the foundation professors met their classes in July 1871, the Provincial Council requested the Colonial Secretary to reserve the 100,000 acres in Southland, set aside for University purposes under the New Zealand University Endowment Act of 1868, to fund a fifth Chair at the University, 'most likely a chair of Medicine and Anatomy [which] would permit of the establishment of a medical school in connexion with the Dunedin Hospital'. This was the first specific mention of establishing a medical school at Otago.[6]

The timing of Macandrew's proposal might have appeared inauspicious, as the initiation of classes had already left the infant university in straitened circumstances. As early as May 1872, the Provincial Council was informed by the University Council that it was facing an annual deficit of £600. The Provincial Council responded immediately by setting aside another reserve of 100,000 acres for University purposes.[7] It also deputed a Select Committee to confer with the University Council on the state of its finances and on the advisability of starting classes in law and medicine. Presumably, the Council expected these would draw in students to offset the declining roll, which had fallen from eighty-one in 1871 to only seventy in 1872. The Committee could see no difficulties in establishing law classes, since at the time there were thirty-two young men in Dunedin already articled to solicitors and studying for examinations.[8] Its report was equally enthusiastic in recommending the setting up of medical classes. 'Provided the Hospital were made available for the instruction of students and a competent Professor of Anatomy and Physiology were obtained from Home', it advised, 'there would be no difficulty in affording a good and sound medical education and in fitting students properly for the practice of their profession here' and it saw 'no reason to believe that local degrees would be of an inferior character' to those granted elsewhere.[9] No doubt they believed it would be a long time before the country's population would justify having more than one medical school, so locating one in Dunedin would secure numbers of students from other parts of the Colony.[10]

In this case, however, it appears that the Select Committee was going against the advice of those it consulted on the matter. Of the eight medical experts it approached, either in person or in writing, only two recommended the project as a whole. Dr Webster, who chaired the committee, was in favour of setting up a medical school, although he warned that considerable expense would have to be faced in bringing in a Professor of Anatomy and Physiology and perhaps other specialists to teach advanced classes. Professor Black, who believed, rightly, that his lectures in chemistry would be recognised by the British authorities, also favoured a full medical school, or at least a preliminary two-year course. Professor MacGregor, of Mental and Moral Philosophy, who held a medical degree from Edinburgh, was more cautious. He emphasised the need for British recognition of any courses offered, and was strongly of the opinion that two *anni medici* were all that should be attempted. Dr Hulme, the Superintendent of the Dunedin Hospital, and Drs Burns, Hocken, Deck and Alexander, who were all in general practice, answered a questionnaire on such topics as the adequacy of the Dunedin Hospital for clinical training of students and the possibility of local practitioners contributing to teaching. In response to a general question on the advisability of setting up a school, Dr Burns thought this 'injudicious' and the others 'premature'.[11] The *Otago Daily Times* expressed the view that the project should be indefinitely postponed.[12]

Despite the Select Committee's optimism, the University Council approached the project with caution. Debate came to centre on what sort of course should be established and the University Council entered into a round of consultations. Looking across the Tasman to Melbourne University, which boasted the only medical school in Australasia, Macandrew could already see the 'matchless academic leverage' a medical school could exert.[13] Being a colonial outpost on the other side of the world from 'Home', the experience of Melbourne was obviously relevant. Early in 1873, the Vice-Chancellor sent seven questions to the Chancellor of the University of Melbourne. In his comparative study of early Australian and New Zealand universities, Gardner calls the exchange 'the most important academic link between Australia and New Zealand in mid-Victorian times', although Melbourne's replies were too tardy to affect Otago's course of action.[14] In response to the key question, whether the lectures in the Melbourne school were recognised by British examining bodies, the Chancellor appended resolutions from those that recognised the course. It was a most satisfactory list: The Royal College of Surgeons, London, King's and Queen's Colleges Dublin, the Royal College of Surgeons, England, the Royal College of Surgeons of Edinburgh. Other questions covered the equivalency of the Melbourne course to British ones, whether medical professors should be permitted posts outside the University and the availability of hospitals to students for clinical training.[15]

'The Provincial Government is exceedingly desirous that there should be a medical school in Dunedin.'

Macandrew to Chancellor, Otago University, 20 November 1873

Meantime, in November 1873, Macandrew pushed matters along by writing to the University Council and, on 9 December, the Council voted to proceed with the selection of a Professor of Anatomy and Physiology.[16] As in the choice of its first four professors, the University Council worked through its agents in Edinburgh, Andrew and Auld. No doubt they were expected to follow their former instructions, to take expert advice and recommend a man of impeccable personal character, energy, scholastic achievements and an 'aptness to teach'. Youth was also an important factor. 'Many years of colonial experience cause us to feel particularly anxious,' the Council had written Auld in 1869, 'that our Professors should not be men who are willing to leave the old country merely because after numerous trials they have in large measure been unsuccessful at "home". They should rather be comparatively young men who have been highly successful in similar, though perhaps humbler spheres...'[17] Like the other professors, the Professor of

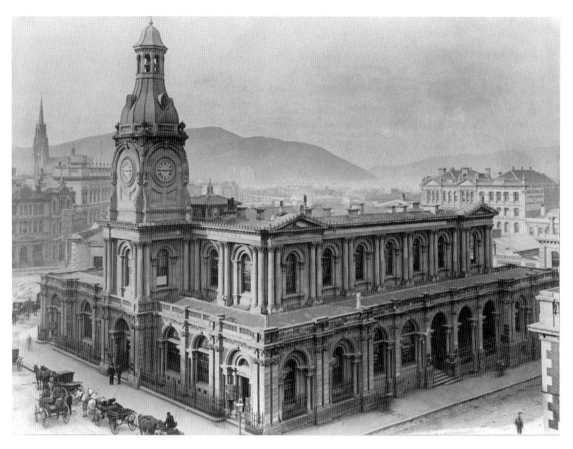

Dunedin Stock Exchange Building in the 1890s. This building, intended as a Post Office and later used as the Stock Exchange, housed the first students of the University, including medical students.
Hocken Collections, Uare Taoka o Hakena, University of Otago, Acc. No. c/n E 760/5; SO3-244.

Anatomy and Physiology was to receive £600 a year with class fees, but would not be permitted to conduct private practice. 'He must be someone,' Auld was instructed, 'of whom the Universities at home would be willing to approve as a teacher of medicine ... an arts degree [would be] a recommendation, but a medical degree indispensable. Age should not exceed thirty.'[18]

The University of Melbourne's gamble in appointing staff to its Medical School and providing a full five-year medical course (longer than the norm in Britain) from its inception in 1862 had paid off, with the School gaining British recognition in 1867.[19] Otago, however, decided to proceed more cautiously. Initially, it aimed to teach a partial course that would be completed in Britain, probably at the University of Edinburgh, which had a splendid reputation and an

established practice of taking colonial students.[20] In order to prepare the curriculum, the Council needed to know the requirements for a two-year course that would count towards a medical degree from Edinburgh. At the beginning of 1874, the Vice-Chancellor wrote to the Principal of Edinburgh University assuring him that no one would be appointed to the Chair of Anatomy and Physiology at Otago who had not previously been approved by the Senate at Edinburgh, 'for our objective is to avail ourselves of the provision made in your Calendar for a two-year course of medical study which shall be the equivalent of two *anni medici* in your curriculum.' He went on to describe the proposed lecture courses in chemistry to be delivered by Professor Black, and natural history by Captain Hutton of the Otago Museum; and the facilities of the Dunedin

Hospital, under the charge of Dr Hulme, the Provincial Surgeon, which had an average of 150 patients and from which anatomical subjects could be 'procured with unusual facility'.[21] The letter was submitted to the Medical Faculty at Edinburgh on 24 March – it is summarised in the Minutes and was cordially received. Faculty agreed to assist in 'looking out for a good Professor of Anatomy' and thought that if this were accomplished there would be no difficulty teaching two *anni medici* at Otago. The Medical Faculty sent a report to the Senate outlining the requirements that would allow an Otago medical student to proceed to Edinburgh to complete his medical degree in a further two years. Faculty believed it could accept the Otago entrance examination; it required that an academic year at Otago consist of at least a hundred lectures in each of chemistry and anatomy; that the second year include a six-month course in practical anatomy and attendance at a hospital of at least a hundred beds, with a staff of physicians and surgeons and, finally, that professors be permitted to teach one subject only.[22]

In May 1874, Andrew and Auld forwarded the testimonials of eighteen applicants, some of them well qualified for the post, to the University Council.[23] The Council had already received a direct application from a Dr Millen Coughtrey, an Edinburgh graduate of 1871, who had recently arrived in Auckland as a ship's surgeon. The tone of Coughtrey's letter, written from Auckland in January 1874, illustrates well his confident, energetic style. 'Tis quite possible', he began, 'I may be quite unknown to you and as possible that you do know something of me.' He proceeded to fill in some detail of his life and career. Since his graduation with honours in MB CM in 1871 he had been a junior demonstrator in the Anatomy Department at Edinburgh University and 'pleased [his] students so much as to receive a testimonial from them.' Travelling for his health, he had then visited a number of universities and museums in the United States before returning to the Liverpool Medical School, where he had 'obtained during the summer the largest class that had yet been there'. Following this, a combination of 'ill-health and impatient ambition' had brought him to New Zealand in 1873. Coughtrey presented himself as an all-rounder who had written articles on Anatomy, Zoology and Archaeology and could claim, 'without stretching due modesty', that he could 'not only use [the] scalpel, but the pencil and modeller's tool'. He mentioned that he had already been offered the Chair of Anatomy in the new University of the State of Louisiana.[24] Overall, there is nothing in Coughtrey's letter of application that contradicts the impression Carmalt Jones gained of him, after talking with people who had known him, that he was a 'bluff personality, not without vanity and fond of display … with something of a "waltzing gait" and full of chaff'.[25] On the other hand, this assessment does less than justice to his professional skill and breadth of ideas. His impressive inaugural lecture, for instance, which runs to forty-one printed pages, ranged over recent and probable future developments in medicine and medical training and made a plea for the role of research for medical staff.[26]

The Council appointed Coughtrey in August and advertised medical classes to commence in 1875. In the meantime, Coughtrey was granted six months' salary, plus a further £200 to buy equipment, and was sent to Britain to negotiate recognition for the course from the relevant authorities. Before he left he advised the Council on the necessary preliminaries that needed to be gone through at the New Zealand end before a two-year medical course could get under way. An Anatomy Act would have to be passed so that subjects could be made available for dissection. The general Matriculation entry examination to the University would have to be replaced by a more stringent test for medical students. Changes to the Dunedin Hospital and its staff were required before it could be opened to students and courses in dispensary practice and pharmacy would have to be developed.[27]

As Coughtrey reported to the University Council on his return to Dunedin in mid-1875, the face-to-face negotiations for recognition of the proposed medical course in Britain proved a total frustration. While his own lectures would be recognised by Edinburgh, Glasgow and Trinity College Dublin and those of Professor Black had already been recognised by Edinburgh, the Medical School as an entity could not be recognised, because the entry requirement was too low and no clinical teaching had been established. There was a hasty attempt to meet the requirements. On 2 August, the Vice-Chancellor reported to the Dean of the Faculty of Medicine at Edinburgh that the Matriculation examination had been replaced by a special medical preliminary examination and that the Dunedin Hospital, now a government institution, had been separated into surgical and medical wards and averaged a hundred medical and seventy surgical cases a year. In his report the Vice-Chancellor also gave details of the accommodation and staff at the Hospital, appended regulations for the preliminary exam and a synopsis of the medical classes, and asked what Edinburgh would want taught in each year before it would recognise the two-year course.[28]

These protracted negotiations did nothing to improve relations between Coughtrey and the University Council and administrative delays exacerbated the problem. It took until 1876 to institute the entry examination and for the Medical School to be recognised under the new Anatomy Act, as a School of Anatomy cleared to carry out human dissection. Coughtrey chafed at the delays, for which he blamed the Council. The Council, in turn, felt he had let them down. Despite their best efforts, the replies from the various British medical authorities, which were at last received in March 1876, were less than satisfactory. The British General Medical Council accepted the preliminary examination and Glasgow would accept the two-year course, if it considered individual lecturers were up to standard. Edinburgh, however, objected to the fact that Otago was a provincial rather than a colonial university and it would not recognise the School without a Royal Charter (for which the University of New Zealand was then negotiating). Other institutions maintained that the School was too immature for recognition. It was Catch 22: the Medical School needed to demonstrate it merited official recognition, but until it gained that recognition it could not function. In his report for 1875–6 to the Superintendent of the Province,

the Chancellor had to admit 'the Council had met with greater difficulty in placing the Medical School on a satisfactory basis than had been anticipated.'[29]

Coughtrey had given a well-received inaugural lecture in May 1875, but until the preliminary examination or the School of Anatomy were given official recognition, little could be achieved in medical training. Two students, both scholarship holders, passed the Preliminary Examination in 1876, but one changed almost at once to study law and Coughtrey was left with a single student, Charles Low. In 1876, the outcome of the ambitious plans for a Medical School consisted of one professor, one student, one classroom and one cadaver. In these circumstances, it is remarkable that the University continued planning for a full medical course, which the Council thought would require five to seven additional staff to bring it up to the level of Melbourne. It discussed introducing more specialised teaching and increasing the roll to a hundred medical students by 1877. It is even more remarkable in that the University as a whole was in dire straits. In 1876, there were only fifty-five students, down from sixty-nine the previous year.[30]

'Anatomy is now beyond the days in which the various organs and structures of the human body were displayed as part of a pleasant landscape ... [its study is] one of the most powerful media for mental culture exacted of the student.'

From the Introductory Address in the Faculty of Medicine, by Millen Coughtrey, MB CM with Hons, Edin., delivered at Dunedin on 31 May, 1875, in the large hall of the University Building.

Coughtrey must have had time on his hands, and he used it in a series of lively public lectures on anatomy and physiology. He contacted medical practitioners throughout New Zealand to form a New Zealand Medical Association. Although Coughtrey aimed to have branches in each main centre, the only branch to be set up was in Dunedin, with himself as Secretary.[31] He also began seeing patients, which was against the terms of his contract. In October 1875, the

Dr Millen Coughtrey, 1848–1908
Professor of Anatomy and Physiology 1874–76

MILLEN COUGHTREY was born in Lancashire, attended University in Edinburgh, and is said to have served as a medical volunteer in the Franco-Prussian War of 1870–71. While in Britain during 1874–75 he married Elizabeth Sarah Hamilton Magill. After he resigned his professorship at Otago, however, neither any ties with Britain nor the bitterness of his breach with the University affected his decision to remain in Dunedin. He and his wife raised four children, he built a thriving practice and threw himself into community activities of all kinds. Relations with the University were eventually mended to the extent that he gave the graduation address when the first MB was conferred by the University in 1887. Coughtrey used the occasion to revisit his aims in 1875. He had been determined, he said, 'that each lad and girl should, so far as medical education is concerned, be as soundly and thoroughly equipped … as those born and reared in other parts of the world' and so had fought tenaciously against a training useful in the colony alone, referring to this as a 'doctrine of partial expediency'. He also looked to the future, urging the separation of the disciplines of Anatomy and Physiology, better library resources, better clinical training for medical students, and the fostering of original research.[32] In 1891, through his position as Chairman of the Honorary Staff at Dunedin Hospital, Coughtrey became Sub-Dean of the newly established Medical Faculty.

In 1894, Coughtrey built a large private hospital and sanatorium in the Dunedin suburb of St Clair. Described in a booklet on leading business establishments of Dunedin as the most modern and extensive of its kind in the Southern Hemisphere, it was architecturally striking, beautifully furnished and set in attractive grounds. In addition to two large wards, for male and female patients, with nurses' rooms attached, it boasted fourteen other private wards, an operating room and Turkish, steam, plunge and spray bathrooms. There was electric lighting, with gas available in case of a breakdown, and gas stoves, which could readily be converted to burn coal. The property included a model dairy, 'quite a miniature gasworks', stables and glass conservatories.[33]

A man of many interests, especially outdoor ones, Coughtrey was knowledgeable about horses and, for a time, ran his own racehorses, under a pseudonym. He served from 1883 to 1892 on the committee of the Otago Rugby Union, including three years as President and was a Vice-President of the Philharmonic Society. When the South African War began, he undertook the task of equipping the Fourth Contingent of troopers for active service, apparently at considerable cost to his private and professional interests. He was Medical Officer of the Otago Mounted Rifles, with the rank of Surgeon-Major, surgeon to the gaol, Vice-Chairman of the Drainage Board and a Councillor of the Borough of St Kilda.[34] Coughtrey's employment by the University might have been brief and turbulent, but his contribution to his adopted community was generous.

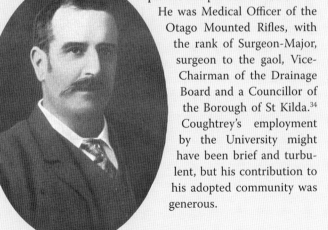

Professor Millen Coughtrey, Otago Medical School.

University Council received a complaint that Coughtrey was engaging in private practice, but he defended himself by stating that he was only consulting. Six months later there was a second complaint, ironically enough from the New Zealand Medical Association, to which Coughtrey responded angrily. He accused the Council of thwarting his efforts and threatened to resign. At a special meeting, just before Christmas 1876, the Council accepted his immediate resignation.[35]

At the end of 1876, the affairs of the Medical School thus reached a nadir. After five years of strenuous effort, British recognition of the School seemed as far away as ever. Earlier in the year the University Council's plans to appoint two clinical staff to teach second-year students – Dr Hocken as Lecturer in Surgery and Dr Gillies in Medicine – had foundered on the question of recognition, and the appointments had to be cancelled.[36] When the *Otago Daily Times* became aware of Coughtrey's resignation it lambasted the University authorities for permitting an enterprise which, it claimed, was costing £2000 a year for a single student. It was, in the opinion of the *Otago Daily Times*, nothing short of a fiasco.[37]

Changes that potentially threatened the future of the Medical School were also occurring in the wider community. On the last day of 1876, the New Zealand Provinces were abolished. As a result, the University lost the strong support of the Otago Provincial Council, Macandrew's power base. There was no reason to believe that the national government in Wellington would show the same commitment. Thompson claims that the University was 'left to fight for itself, to struggle year by year with increasing demands, starved faculties and cramped development'.[38] At the same time, a new regime was set in place at Dunedin Hospital after the Superintendent, Dr Hulme, a long-time University Council member and Medical School supporter, died suddenly at the end of 1876. Following his death, the post of Provincial Surgeon was disestablished and the Hospital came under the administration of a government-appointed committee.[39] The membership of the University Council also changed, with the departure of two influential members, Sir John Richardson and Robert Stout, and the arrival of James Macandrew.[40]

In this very uncertain atmosphere, some Council members wanted to abandon the whole scheme of teaching medicine at Otago. That this did not happen was due to the 'energy and inexhaustible enthusiasm' of Macandrew, who was surely uneasy that Canterbury College was making plans to set up its own medical school.[41] On 13 February 1877, Macandrew carried through the University Council motion that, 'While regretting that efforts to establish a medical school have not proved so successful as had been anticipated, this Council is of opinion that it is desirable to proceed to the establishment of such a school.' Even though the Medical School might not at the outset be able to offer the complete professional training that would be recognised by medical schools in Britain, the fact of its continued existence would contribute towards achieving that aim and would provide an opportunity for those who wished to pursue a medical career in the Colony. The motion concluded with a resolution to set up a committee to effect the changes necessary to continue the project.[42] Against all probability, the financial and academic frustrations of this 'injudicious' enterprise did not lead to its abandonment. The Otago Medical School was to have a second chance.

CHAPTER 2

An Outpost of Edinburgh

I F RECOGNITION of its courses by the University of Edinburgh had been a fixed, if unattainable, objective of the Otago Medical School in its preliminary phase from 1874 to 1876, the Edinburgh connection also dominated its establishment phase, right through until 1914. The close relationship between Edinburgh and Otago affected the School in a number of ways. It was immensely valuable in aiding staff recruitment, developing the curriculum and determining teaching methods. However, even after a complete course became available at Otago, students continued to transfer to Edinburgh to complete their undergraduate years, and this proved to be a serious drain on the School.

The first task of the University Council was to find a replacement for Professor Coughtrey. Only two days after Macandrew's resolution Andrew and Auld were instructed by cable to engage a Professor of Anatomy, on the same terms as before, to commence work on 1 May.[1] They received testimonials from twenty-five candidates. (Carmalt Jones believed the size of the field of applicants must have been due to their ignorance of the Otago situation.) On the advice of the Professor of Anatomy at Edinburgh and the Professor of Physiology at Glasgow, the agents recommended John Halliday Scott, a Demonstrator in Anatomy at Edinburgh. An energetic young man of twenty-six, the new professor had been selected for his distinguished career as a student, the practical experience he had acquired since graduation and the high testimony

borne to his personal character. He was allowed to delay his departure until the end of May to give him time to complete his MD thesis and he arrived in New Zealand on 31 July.[2]

There can be no doubt about the significance of Professor Scott's contribution to the School. From his arrival in 1877 until his death in 1914, he guided the Otago Medical School with a clear sense of direction. The impression can be given, however, that from the moment he took over, all the School's problems melted away and its progress towards becoming a functioning, flourishing institution was steady and almost inevitable. The earliest account of the School's history, by former student and staff member, Sir Louis Barnett, exemplifies this: 'The University Council in 1877 appointed Dr J.H. Scott as Professor of Anatomy and Lecturer in Physiology, and from that time the Medical School began to find its feet, and in a few years, under Scott's wise leadership, became firmly established.'[3] The first decades of Scott's regime were in fact much less secure than this suggests.

The Years of Constraint, 1877–1902

The Two-Year Course, 1877–1885

With the commencement of a two-year medical course that could be completed in the United Kingdom, the year 1877 can be said to mark the real beginning of the Otago Medical School. One major problem solved by Professor Scott's appointment was that of recognition by the

University of Edinburgh. The University that had nurtured, honoured and employed him had no problem in recognising his qualifications to teach at Otago. The 1878 Edinburgh Calendar lists Otago, together with a remarkably diverse collection of institutions which included various colonial and Indian universities and one in Russia, as one whose entry examination is accepted. In the list of extra-academic lecturers recognised by the University, Professors Scott (Anatomy), Black (Chemistry) and Hutton (Natural History) feature along with individuals from Dublin, Edinburgh, Glasgow, Leeds Liverpool, London, Manchester and Sheffield. Otago is the only institution in this list outside the British Isles.[4] In its prospectus of 1877, the University of Otago was able to claim not only that the Medical School provided lectures in chemistry, biology and anatomy by professors of those subjects, but that arrangements had been made to cover the whole of the first two years of the medical curriculum. 'Students of medicine will thus have the privilege of attending classes here for two years, and then, if they desire

it, of proceeding to complete the course and to graduate at one of the schools of the United Kingdom.'[5] It was assumed that, after their two years at Otago, most students would transfer to Edinburgh to finish their medical degrees.

Scott was also fortunate in that he arrived as new university buildings were in the final stages of planning. The Council approved the plans a fortnight after he arrived, and he was able to make recommendations on the layout of the space allocated to medical classes. In 1877, all university classes were held in the elaborate but basically unsuitable 'Old University', originally built as a Post Office and situated in Dunedin's busy Exchange area. In mid-1876, the Professorial Board had made a detailed submission outlining the Medical School's requirements for space in the proposed new building, which included extensive facilities for teaching anatomy and physiology.[6] However, the new buildings cost the University far more than anticipated and the Council adopted Scott's more modest recommendations. He based his estimates on an annual intake of

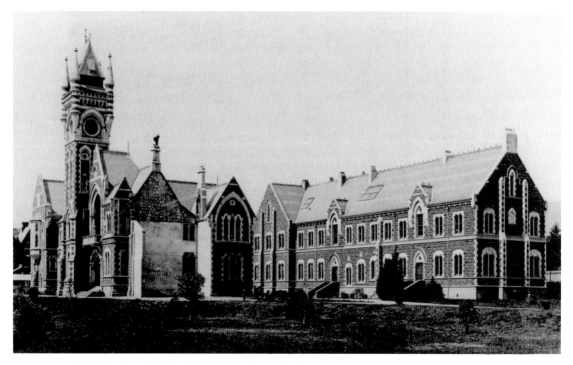

The University, 1879. The Medical School occupied the wing to the right of the picture until 1917.
Hocken Collections, Uare Taoka o Hakena, University of Otago, Acc. No. c/n E 4909/4.i; SO3244.

fifteen students and asked for a dissection room to accommodate thirty students, a preparation room and a morgue, a lecture room, an anatomy room, a laboratory to seat fifteen for histology lectures and a small office for the Professor. The chemical and anatomical buildings were ready in 1878, in which year the Medical School could be said to be fully operational.[7]

There were five students in the first class: W.J. Will, J. Closs, H. Macandrew, J.A. Murray and F.G. Westenra.

Their first year consisted of:

Anatomy: lectures and demonstrations from dissections five days a week, with Professor Scott.

Practical Anatomy: the dissecting room was open from 9 to 4 daily, with the Professor in attendance four hours daily.

Chemistry, Zoology, Botany: medical students attended the Arts course given by Professors Black and Hutton.[8]

In their second year, the Dunedin Hospital admitted the students for clinical training.

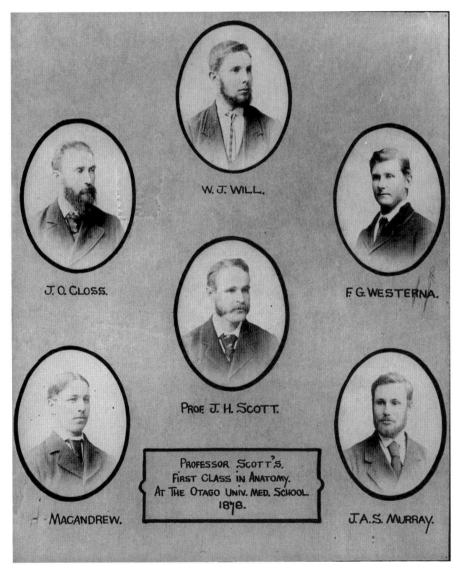

Scott's first Anatomy class, 1878: W.J. Will, J. Closs, F.G. Westenra, H. Macandrew, J.A. Murray.
Hocken Collections, Uare Taoka o Hakena, University of Otago, Acc. No. c/n F 3117/12 f.

Honorary staff gave lectures twice a week and provided bedside instruction during visiting hours. A local physician, Dr William Brown, a contemporary of Scott at Edinburgh and with experience as a missionary in China, gained the necessary recognition from his old university and settled in as sole teacher of surgery for the next twelve years, until 1889. He lectured five days a week, demonstrating 'operations on the cadaver, bandaging, surgical appliances, with the use of pathological specimens, diagrams, preparations and casts.'[9]

On finishing their two-year course at Otago, Will, Closs, Murray and Macandrew left to complete their medical degrees in Edinburgh. They were the first of successive waves of Otago medical students to do so up until World War I. The Edinburgh experience was a great adventure, which also required considerable financial outlay and a long separation from family and friends. In a memorandum written for his twenty-year-old son Herbert, just before his departure in February 1880, James Macandrew covers both financial and spiritual issues. Herbert would receive a bank draft for £25 every three months for the next two years, or three if necessary. If his father died during this time, the money was to come from his life policy, to be paid back to the family should they ever stand in need. If Herbert found he could make do with £20 or less, he was to advise his father. 'My own impression', wrote Macandrew, 'is that £45 a year will be sufficient for plain board and lodging in Edinburgh, in which case your other expenses should not exceed £30 or £40.' In no case was he to exceed £100 and should indeed aim to limit his total expenditure for the two years to £120. 'Many a distinguished man', his father advised, 'has got on with less than half this amount.' That would enable Herbert to spend his third and fourth years, if it was deemed advisable, at the University of Paris and to visit Europe. 'Whatever you do' (Macandrew underlined this sentence) 'keep clear of debt, make it a point to pay for everything as you go – have no credit for tailors' bills or anything else.' Herbert was also enjoined to be careful of his companions, to become intimate with no one until he was thoroughly assured of his character for truthfulness, honour and integrity

and to beware of wolves in sheep's clothing. 'Have no dealings with those who scoff at religion', Macandrew wrote. 'Above and beyond all, never omit to closet yourself with God every morning and every evening praying for His guidance and that He may direct your steps.'[10] One can imagine similar advice being given by other fathers over the years.

There is scattered information about the New Zealand students' impressions of Edinburgh. One of the first group, William Will, left a diary which makes it clear that he felt very much at home and had a satisfying social life, linking up with his own relatives and those of fellow Otago students. We also have his notebook for Clinical Medicine, which contains careful notes on cases he took in 1881–82 with Professor Grainger Stewart. From the Edinburgh Calendar we learn that he was Treasurer of the Edinburgh University Total Abstinence Society. No doubt his father, the Reverend Will, would have been proud of him.[11] When the student periodical the *Otago University Review* began in 1888, it included regular items on the achievements of Otago medical students at Edinburgh. In an article published in 1889, classes at Edinburgh are described as being so rowdy, even at fourth year, that the professors sometimes had to shout to be heard. A favourite amusement before a lecture began was whistling, which was done to great effect and, accompanied by stamping on the floor, gave a very fair imitation of a drum and fife band. 'I have heard the Old Hundredth', the writer affirmed, 'rolled out by three or four hundred mouths and feet with an electrifying effect.'[12] The awe James Elliott, a student in the late 1890s, felt when he entered the precincts of the University was no doubt typical. When he went to see the Old University on the site of the ancient Kirk o' Fields, he felt 'overawed with the thought of the succession of great men who had passed through its portals for generation after generation … there the great building stood with its huge cathedral dome and on the top of the dome the figure of a man holding high above the city the golden torch of learning.'[13] It was not surprising that even after the full course was established at Otago, the majority of students opted for the reputation, glamour and opportunities Edinburgh offered.

Solid pedagogical traditions were established at the Otago Medical School in Scott's day, with his own courses in anatomy being at the core of the curriculum. A feature of Scott's teaching was his skill in producing beautifully drawn and painted anatomical diagrams. Works of art in themselves, they were used for many years after his death and are still treasured. Sir Louis Barnett claimed Scott was unequalled for the speed, strength and clarity of his blackboard diagrams. He described his style as meticulous in the presentation of anatomical knowledge, as acquired and taught in Edinburgh. Every detail Scott knew was expounded on and students were expected to take in everything he taught. Woe betide those who did not. 'Most of us',

John Halliday Scott, 1851–1914

MB CM (Edin) MRCS and MD (Edin)
Professor of Anatomy 1877–1914 and of Physiology 1877–1904,
Dean of the Otago Medical School 1891–1914

'NO MAN ever made less fuss or parade about his duties', wrote Colquhoun of his colleague of many years, 'and no one ever attended to them better.' He thought he had 'a genius for order and method'. Hercus and Bell commented that Scott 'controlled the Medical School in every particular' and concluded that he 'was the Medical School'. His students regarded him with a real, if wary affection, appreciating that in his dealings with them he was 'absolutely just'.[14]

Born and educated in Edinburgh, the son of a Writer to the Signet, Scott was an outstanding student, who also had experience as a house surgeon and a demonstrator in anatomy at Edinburgh before he came to New Zealand. Sole professor in the Otago Medical School for the first twenty-seven years of his tenure, Scott 'did everything himself', both for reasons of economy and of temperament. He appeared reluctant to delegate and never had a secretary, his correspondence and Faculty Minutes surviving in his own strong hand. He ran the Faculty with what Barnett calls 'rigid adherence to cast-iron procedure and method'. Although he gave full measure of himself and expected the same of everyone else, he looked askance at new ideas.[15]

Living, as he did at first, in one of the four professorial houses adjacent to the University, Scott's academic and family life almost merged. He was a devoted family man. He met his wife, Helen Bealey, when she was visiting New Zealand from England and the couple married in England in 1883. They had five children. Artist Frances Hodgkins, who knew them well, believed that 'his sun really set' when Helen died in 1899.[16]

Scott made his closest friends and found his chief pleasure in the Dunedin art community. A talented water-colourist, careful and painstaking in style, specialising in landscape, he went on painting expeditions to North Otago, Milford Sound and even Macquarie Island. He exhibited regularly with the Otago Art Society and was its Secretary for over thirty years, from 1881 until his death. Influential in setting up the Dunedin Public Art Gallery, he served on its selection committee and sometimes selected works for the Gallery when he travelled to England. He was an astute critic. Frances Hodgkins said she cared 'dreadfully' for his good opinion and that 'one's ideas have to be of the first water before one submits them to his critical judgement'.[17]

As the years passed, Scott became more conservative and his teaching failed to keep up with new developments in his field. In his last years he suffered a series of small strokes, and died on 25 February 1914. He is remembered for his teaching skill, business ability, devotion to duty and personal integrity.[18]

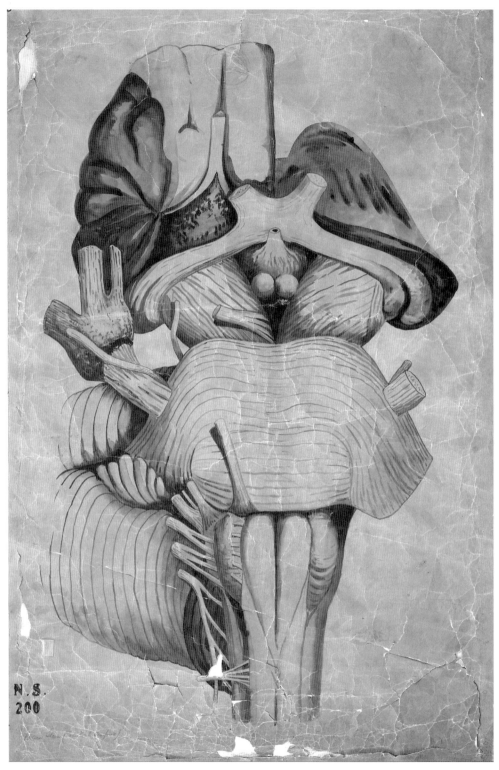

N.S.
200

John Halliday Scott, *Brainstem Ventral Surface* n.d. Nervous System Anatomical Drawing, Otago Medical
School series, is one of almost three hundred anatomical drawings by Scott in the Hocken Collections.
Hocken Collections, Uare Taoka o Hakena, University of Otago, Acc. No. 03-264.

wrote Barnett, 'writhed at times under his sarcastic criticism.' In addition to the lectures and demonstrations, Scott held Saturday morning question and answer quiz sessions, in which he was 'scathing on slackers and nitwits'.[19] A tradition of searing sarcasm was established early in the School's history.

Although, in these early years, staff were provided with minimal technical assistance, Scott came to rely on the services of Alfred Jefferson. At first employed as an untrained handyman, Jefferson was discharged at the end of each session, leaving him without regular employment for four months each year. When Scott requested his services for the whole year, he got instead the doubtful concession that Jefferson might do cleaning in other departments over the summer. Over time, Jefferson became more and more valuable. Finally, about the turn of the century, his job became full-time. In the *Annals of the University of Otago Medical School*, Barnett describes his multitude of roles, which included dissecting room porter, embalmer, plaster cast maker, carpenter and diagram hanger. He found Jefferson very capable and obliging, but rather morose; the students called him 'the corpses' friend'.[20] The setting up of the Medical School Anatomy Museum was a collaborative project of Scott and Jefferson, made possible by an initial grant of £20 in 1881. A large group of models in the present-day Museum, many imported from Germany, date from this period. Jefferson prepared specimens for storage in museum jars and made plaster casts of dissections and other models. Some 130 models and wet preparations in the present Museum were made a century ago, by Scott and his assistant.[21]

The Full Medical Course

By October 1881 Scott was ready to give specific form to the University's intention to offer a full medical degree and he set out his plans for the course in a letter to the Council. Typically low-key in tone, Scott's proposal was well-reasoned, cautious and with an eye to frugality, just the kind of tone the Council approved of and entirely in keeping with the stringent economic conditions then prevailing. His plan, he said, would meet present requirements but 'not involve the University in excessive expenditure' and could easily be added to when the time came. At that time, anatomy and physiology, chemistry and surgery were already provided for, and Scott recommended adding five more subjects to the curriculum: the practice of medicine, including insanity, pathology, midwifery and the diseases of women and children, medical jurisprudence and public health, materia medica and dispensing. Although nearly all of these would require separate teachers, he believed that, in the meantime, lecturers could be selected from practitioners in the colony. He recommended that clinical training be left in the hands of the honorary physicians and surgeons attached to the Hospital, where dispensing could also be taught. Scott requested that a botanic garden be established and that natural history and botany be removed from the medical course and made compulsory subjects of the preliminary examination. Finally, he recommended deferring the separation of the two elements of his own teaching responsibility, anatomy and physiology, and making short-term appointments in the areas of pathology, public health and insanity.[22] The plans were approved by the Otago University Council and the Senate of the University of New Zealand in 1882 and by September Scott was filling in the detail. For the five areas that needed additional teaching staff he advised advertising 'throughout Otago or even through a larger area'. The appointments should be for three years and the salaries of the lecturers in practice of medicine and medical jurisprudence, and pathology should be in line with that of the lecturer in surgery, £200 a year; for the shorter courses in materia medica and midwifery, half that amount would suffice. Early in 1883, the Senate of the University of New Zealand duly recognised the University of Otago as a full medical school.[23]

The proposed four-year degree followed the recommendations of the General Medical Council of Great Britain. The courses were focused on examinations, which were listed in the calendar as follows:

Intermediate: biology, physics, chemistry (inorganic and organic), practical chemistry.

First Professional: anatomy and physiology.

Second Professional: materia medica, pathology, medical jurisprudence.

Third professional: surgery, clinical surgery, medicine, clinical medicine, surgical and medical anatomy, midwifery, diseases of women.[24]

In November 1883, three part-time lecturers were appointed, in each case from a field of two or three applicants:

Dr Daniel Colquhoun, lecturer in the practice of medicine.

Dr Ferdinand Batchelor, lecturer in midwifery and gynaecology.

Dr John Macdonald, lecturer in materia medica.

All three gave long and loyal service to the School, with Drs Colquhoun and Batchelor, especially, wielding great influence over many years. Colquhoun, who was born in Glasgow in 1849, had gained his MD and MRCP in London. That he was highly qualified and experienced is evidenced by the eighteen glowing testimonials he produced for his application. Although Colquhoun applied for the position from Melbourne, where he was visiting his brother, he held the position of Senior Assistant Physician at Charing Cross Hospital in London.

Dr Colquhoun quickly adjusted to colonial conditions and became a firm friend of Professor Scott, replacing him on the hospital board in 1884. In the lecture room, Colquhoun was courteous, dignified and rather remote. He read his lectures, which were couched in impeccable English and drew on his wide reading of medical journals and textbooks. At his popular Saturday morning clinics, he would stand, one foot on a chair, and deliver a lengthy dissertation full of literary and philosophical allusions. By this time, the Practice of Medicine covered several subject areas, and Colquhoun was assisted in his teaching by an able group of general practitioners on honorary appointments. He took a lead in pressing for new microscopes, library books and periodicals for the School. He brought his experience as a member of the editorial staff of the *Medical Times and Gazette* in Britain, to the task of editing the *New Zealand Medical Journal* for its first six years, from 1887. Carmalt Jones, who had the advantage of speaking with Colquhoun's

former colleagues and students, describes him as having 'something of the gold-headed cane about him'. He was conservative, kind and generous, but in committee work 'rather remarkable for his fondness of figuring in a minority of one'. Jones considered Colquhoun to be a man who would be 'in the running for the highest positions open to a physician anywhere in the British Empire' and 'a great find for a young school with a dozen or so students on the other side of the world'.[25]

Dr Ferdinand Batchelor had less formal training. He held various diplomas – LSA and MRCS (Eng), LRCP and LM (Edin) – and took a practitioner's MD at Durham when he was thirty-five. He had worked at Guy's Hospital in London. A forceful, even abrasive personality, he was already settled in Dunedin when he took up his position, having come to New Zealand for health reasons in 1874. In Dunedin, Batchelor had built up a large practice in midwifery and gynaecology and had been a member of the honorary staff of the Hospital since 1877. He was always at the forefront of both controversy and fund-raising. He was largely responsible for the building of a modern hospital block in the 1890s and was a pioneer in X-ray work.[26]

Dr John Macdonald was an Edinburgh graduate, with experience in medical practice in Britain and on Trans-Atlantic mail steamers. Few records of his work in the School have survived, although he is said to have taught 'in the Edinburgh tradition'.[27] In 1885, Dr W.S. Roberts, an English-trained local physician, was appointed to a part-time post in pathology, on the basis of his experience in conducting post-mortems in the Hospital. While his formal training in pathology might have been slight, students were impressed by the fact he had represented England at rugby and surgeons admired his skill as an anaesthetist.[28]

Further positions were established over the next few years. The part-time position in medical jurisprudence and public health was unable to be filled locally in 1883, as the field was new and still not well taught in most British medical schools. However, the Dunedin City Council added a part-time position as Public Health Officer to the University's part-time lectureship, so that a full position could be advertised. Dr Frank

Ogston, Associate Professor at the University of Aberdeen, was appointed from a field of twenty-eight candidates and arrived in 1886 to take up the dual post. The same year Dr Lindo Ferguson, trained at Trinity College Dublin, began his long association with the Medical School as honorary part-time lecturer in diseases of the eye. Ferguson had already settled in Dunedin and was rapidly developing a profitable practice as an ophthalmic surgeon. In 1889, Dr Truby King was appointed Superintendent of Seacliff Lunatic Asylum and lecturer in mental diseases at the School and Dr Isaiah de Zouche, lecturer in Diseases of Children.[29]

In 1894, Louis Barnett began his outstanding thirty-year contribution to teaching at the Medical School. Barnett was the first of a line of high-achieving Otago students who pursued postgraduate study in Britain and returned to teach in the Medical School. After completing the two-year course at Otago, he transferred to Edinburgh and gained his MB CM with first class honours in 1888. Two years later, he became the first New Zealander to be made a Fellow of the Royal College of Surgeons of England. He was Professor of Surgery from 1909 to 1924, except for a period of service overseas during World War I. Methodical, dignified yet friendly, Barnett was much admired by his students. He was committed to the aseptic principle and is remembered as the first surgeon in New Zealand to use rubber gloves and gauze mask while operating. He travelled from time to time to important centres in the United States in order to keep in touch with developments in surgery overseas. A number of his students later excelled in surgical and academic careers. When he retired, Barnett gave £8000 to the Medical School to endow a chair of surgery in the name of his son Ralph, who was killed at Gallipoli.[30]

As the full course at the Medical School was introduced with the utmost frugality, the University was most fortunate that the calibre of the new staff was very high and that many of them chose to serve the School for the length of their professional careers.

CHAPTER 3

The Medical School and the Dunedin Hospital
1890s–1914

I F WELL-QUALIFIED staff, adequate lecture rooms and well-equipped laboratories were essential elements in the development of a modern Medical School at Otago, an up-to-date teaching hospital was equally important. The history of the fabric of Dunedin Hospital to 1914 is one of inadequacy, generally serious, and often shocking, and of piecemeal replacements and additions, always constrained by lack of finance and often by the grudging attitude of the hospital authorities. As early as the 1860s, the original hospital in Moray Place had been acknowledged to be quite inadequate to serve Dunedin's increased population and, in 1863, the Provincial Council had held a competition to design a replacement. However, instead of proceeding with this plan, the Council purchased a building in Great King Street, erected to house the 1865 Grand Exhibition, to convert into a hospital. In August 1866, the Provincial Surgeon, Dr Hulme, supervised the transfer of more than a hundred male and twenty-three female patients from Moray Place to the new premises in Great King Street. In 1878, the first class of Otago medical students began their clinical training. The following year part of the student fees was given to the hospital administrators to help provide lecture rooms and facilities. Because Medical School staff were reliant on patients for teaching purposes, relations between the School and the Hospital were inevitably close and often became acrimonious. In the 1890s the continually simmering disputes flared into full-scale crisis.[1]

While the old Moray Place hospital may have been considered a disgrace, its replacement also fell far short of what was required in a teaching hospital. In an article in the first issue of the medical students' annual *Digest*, published in 1934, just as the last of the hospital was being demolished, Sir Lindo Ferguson described the buildings as he had first seen them in 1883. At that time, there were eight wards, each containing seventeen beds, and two with six beds, for cases that needed to be confined to locked quarters. At the back of the main building, a flight of dangerously slippery steps led down to two maternity wards, 'one-storey wooden erections of a very flimsy character.' On Cumberland Street there was a 'huge hangar of corrugated iron like a coaching stable', off which ran a ward for chronic male patients, the hospital laundry, outpatients and dispensary. The main area was used for drying clothes and Ferguson describes how he had had to grope his way, in the dim late afternoon, through barriers of wet sheets. The wards had walls of unplastered, lime-washed brick and rough floors, and were heated by a large fireplace, which created intense draughts. Until 1882, refuse and old poultices were simply disposed of through a trapdoor in the floor. Each ward was emptied for six weeks of the year for disinfection and lime-washing. Gas burners were used for lighting and, on one occasion, Batchelor had to open up a patient's abdomen to treat a secondary haemorrhage by the light of the night wardsman's acetylene bicycle lamp.[2] 'It is hard to realise the conditions under which we worked',

Ferguson wrote years later. Not all operations took place at the hospital. 'There were no private hospitals or nurses and one had to operate in hotels or lodging houses.' On one occasion, Ferguson operated on a child of about three years, with an acute mastoid, on his own kitchen table. 'I rang up Batchelor [who] gave the anaesthetic while I opened the mastoid, and let out a drachm of pus, with the father watching and looking worse than the child.'[3] Despite the 'medieval' conditions, however, Ferguson believed that, during this time, the standard of surgical work performed by hospital staff was very high and that patient outcomes were generally good.[4]

In the 1880s, the part-time clinical lecturers at the Medical School, who were also honorary medical staff at the hospital, joined in a vociferous demand for better conditions. Led by Batchelor, Ferguson and Colquhoun, they complained publicly about the insanitary state of the hospital and its poor ventilation. They agitated for special wards for ophthalmic cases and women's diseases, a new operating theatre and modern equipment. They decried the lack of trained female nurses, who at this time were beginning to replace untrained domestics and wardsmen in caring for hospital patients. In Dunedin this was a slow and contested process. At a well attended public meeting in 1885, an English nurse gave an account of her training and urged the hospital to employ trained nurses. The Hospital Trustees refused, deterred by the cost of building a nurses' home.[5]

In *A History of the Otago Hospital Board and its Predecessors*, John Angus carefully details the changes in staff and buildings at the Dunedin Hospital, from the opening of the Medical School to the last years of Professor Scott's deanship. He divides the era into two parts – calling the period from 1877 to 1890 'The Struggle for Reform', and

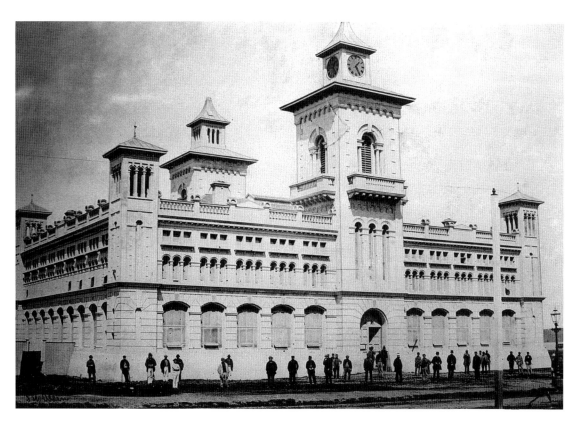

The Second Dunedin Hospital in 1865.
Archives New Zealand, Te Rua Mahara o te Kāwanatanga, Dunedin Regional Office –DAHI/D274/191a.

that from 1891 to 1910, 'Reforms Accomplished'. Angus shows that, during the first period, the honorary medical staff had some limited success: the hospital basement was cleared and cemented over, in 1886 a special ophthalmic ward was built for Ferguson and the following year a new operating theatre opened. The latter included a chloroform room, surgeons' consulting room and, in recognition of its use for teaching, facilities for twenty-three students. Although the University bore part of the cost of these improvements, the staff at the Medical School found the Dunedin Hospital Trustees to be generally uncooperative.[6]

In July 1890 a major row erupted. After one of Batchelor's patients died from post-operative infection and another became seriously ill, he withdrew all his patients and threw himself into a campaign for reform, claiming the Hospital was unsafe. He contended that his patient's death had been entirely due to unhealthy hospital influences and that if she had been operated on in a clean ward, with healthy surroundings, she would have been alive and well. Colquhoun supported him fully, commenting years later, 'We could not say to students, "Here in the hospital you see how things should be done." We had to say, "Here you see how typhoid and pneumonia cases should not be treated, conditions under which operations should not be performed."' Operations at the Hospital were suspended and both Batchelor and the Trustees engaged lawyers. In August–September 1890, a two-man Royal Commission was set up to investigate the conditions at Dunedin Hospital. They took exhaustive evidence from thirty-five people over nineteen days. Their report was a thoroughgoing condemnation of the whole hospital, from its plan of construction, through ventilation, heating and drainage to kitchen facilities. The Commission recommended building an entirely new hospital, and insisted that, in the interim, the Hospital provide a separate ward for infectious diseases, a new kitchen, improved toilet facilities, new walls, floors and ceilings in the wards, better drains, a proper heating system, a nurses' home, new male and female surgical wards, special wards for gynaecological and ophthalmic cases and two convalescent wards. Although Batchelor

had told the Commission that the Trustees 'did not take suggestions or complaints very well', and they were still hampered by a lack of finance and suspicious of the intentions of the honorary medical staff, after 1890 the Trustees finally began to accept the need for extensive modernisation of the Hospital. This marked a turning point, the start of the period Angus terms 'reforms accomplished', in which two decades of renovation and building occurred. While this was certainly a victory for the reformers, it was also an acknowledgment of the changing role of the hospital in Western society, from a charitable institution for the indigent to a centre of clinical technology for the whole community.[7]

The first new building, a nurses' home, signalled this change. Opened in 1892, the two-storeyed building in brick and stone had twenty-five bedrooms, accommodation for a matron, a lecture theatre and a library. It was extended to accommodate fourteen more nurses in 1903 and renovated and extended again in 1908. Trained female nursing staff, so long advocated by the honorary medical staff, had come to stay.[8]

With so much building and renovation required, the question arose over whether to replace the old hospital piecemeal on the same site or to build a completely new hospital at a different location. The Trustees, supported by the honorary medical staff and the Medical School, chose to remain. Their decision had far-reaching consequences, for it determined the location of future Medical School development. The next addition to the Hospital, completed in 1893, was a two-storeyed ward block, named the Campbell Pavilion, running parallel to Great King Street. Considered at the time to be the first modern hospital facility in New Zealand, it included separate twenty-four bed wards for men and women, up-to-date features such as smooth cement interior walls and effective heating and ventilation. Ferguson contributed substantially to the design of the pavilion, including the suggestion of setting its foundation on arches, on account of the swampy soil.[9] The older part of the original building was gradually taken over for non-nursing functions, such as administration and outpatients. Following the completion of the Campbell Pavilion, a new,

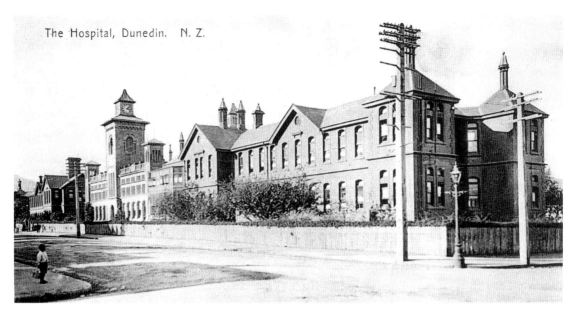

The Hospital, Dunedin. N. Z.

Dunedin Hospital, Campbell Pavilion, erected in 1893.
Archives New Zealand, Te Rua Mahara o te Kāwanatanga, Dunedin Regional Office – DAHI/D272/140.

well-appointed operating theatre, suitable for teaching, opened in 1897. It had a marble floor, gas lighting and heating, a gallery to hold sixty students, an anaesthetists' room, instrument room and surgeons' consulting room. Two years later, a two-storeyed building, the well-appointed Victoria Jubilee Pavilion, with two wards each of twenty-two beds, was opened and, in 1900 and 1901, in conjunction with the University, a new morgue and post-mortem room were built. It all added up to a very creditable record in a period of financial strain.

As the Dunedin Hospital developed, the University clinical staff pressed not only for the renovation and rebuilding of the Hospital itself and more specialised wards run by trained nurses, but also for more highly qualified doctors and more advanced equipment. They persuaded the Hospital to purchase a range of surgical instruments in 1890 and a microscope in 1896. Their major achievement was an up-to-date laboratory, to enable more rapid and accurate diagnosis of patients' illnesses. Opened in 1904, it was partly funded by student fees and was equipped and serviced by the Hospital in conjunction with the University. The University staff also insisted on modern procedures. The

new operating theatre had foot-operated taps and a glass and iron operating table. The use of rubber gloves became standard and a steam sterilising apparatus was installed in 1904. The expertise of Medical School staff was called upon whenever major purchases were being considered. When he was overseas in 1901, for instance, Ferguson looked at an x-ray plant, which Barnett purchased on behalf of the Hospital when he was overseas in 1903–04. At first housed in a temporary location, in 1910 it was installed in its own specialised facility, with x-ray set, dark room and waiting room.[10]

One subject of particular tension between the Hospital and the Medical School related to outpatients. In the depressed 1890s their number rose dramatically. The service was intended for those who could not afford to go to a doctor, and the Hospital Trustees believed the privilege was being abused. They were also concerned about the number of out-of-town patients seeking specialised services. The Trustees tried to make all those who could afford to pay fees do so, while the honorary medical staff welcomed outpatients for the number and variety of cases they provided for teaching purposes. The tension between the two continued throughout the 1890s. After the

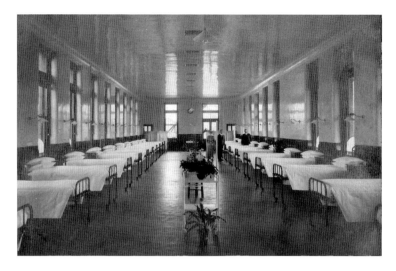

Dunedin Hospital, Nightingale Ward, King Edward VII Memorial Block, erected 1914.

Archives New Zealand, Te Rua Mahara o te Kāwanatanga, Dunedin Regional Office – DAHI/D274/191a.

markedly. This was largely due to the arrival of more powerful and better qualified resident medical staff, led by the impressive Dr A.R. Falconer, who had the title of Resident Medical Officer and a higher salary. Around this time, the composition of the Trustees also altered, with Drs Riley and Batchelor joining the board, and the new Department of Health began to take an active interest in hospital reform.[11]

At the beginning of the twentieth century, the hospital authorities engaged public support to help finance their building programme. In 1905 the Governor General, Lord Plunket, launched an appeal for another two-storeyed pavilion. The Ward Pavilion, with sixty-four beds in its two wards, electric lighting and its own heating plant, opened in 1908, enabling the old male ward, condemned eighteen years before, to be closed at last. Over the next two years, with the aid of further local generosity, a second operating theatre and a new outpatients department were added to the Hospital.[12]

While the building programme began to slow after 1910, at the same time the pressure of student numbers caused a demand for more hospital beds for teaching. Local fund-raising demonstrated a heartening degree of popular support for the hospital. More than £5000 was raised through street theatre, charity rugby matches and concerts by medical students and nurses, excursions on the harbour and street collections, as well as public subscriptions. This enabled the construction of the new sixty-bed King Edward VII Memorial Block, containing Batchelor and Nightingale wards, a clinical room for students, an operating theatre, sunrooms and balconies, which opened in December 1914. The expanded hospital needed more nursing staff and, in 1914, work began on a large new nurses' home. Situated near the hospital, in Cumberland Street, the building opened two years later. By this time, the Dunedin Hospital had been transformed from a charitable institution to a centre of medical technology, where those who were acutely ill could be treated and those requiring surgery could obtain it. With its new buildings, new equipment and trained nurses it was also well-equipped to provide clinical training for students from the Medical School, newly established just across the road.[13]

CHAPTER 4

Crisis and Expansion: Breaking out of the Financial Straitjacket 1890s-1914

IF THE LURE of Edinburgh for New Zealand medical students was one threat to the viability of the Otago Medical School in the 1890s, there were also others closer to home. Although a number of significant achievements were made during this time, low student numbers, an attack on the standard of clinical teaching and extreme financial pressures on the University as a whole made it a troubled decade for the Medical School. Early in the new century, however, secure government funding and local generosity permitted an increase in both staff and students and enabled the School to enter into a new phase of development.

The establishment of the Faculty of Medicine, in 1891, was an administrative change that would have long-term importance. The Faculty consisted of the medical professor and those members of the University and Hospital staff who

gave lectures to medical students. The Dean, in this case Scott, was appointed by Council and the Chairman of the Hospital staff was made Sub-Dean. The role of Faculty was to regulate matters concerned with teaching and the primary motivation for its establishment appears to have been the desultory attendance of students and lecturers at the Hospital. Although the Faculty formally objected to having its Dean imposed on them rather than being elected, it posed little challenge to Scott's authority.[1]

No sooner had the furore over conditions at Dunedin Hospital been resolved than another crisis arose, this time over the final examination of the six candidates in surgery. In 1893, a Dr Cahill of Wellington was brought in at the last moment to act as the external examiner. He refused to pass three students who had already satisfied the School's internal examiner. To resolve the problem, the University of New Zealand held another searching examination in Wellington, with a different team of examiners. Although all three candidates passed, this did not resolve the issue. The Wellington Branch of the New Zealand Medical Association spearheaded an attack on the teaching standards at the Otago School and heated debate on the Otago course dominated the 1894 meeting of the Association. A Committee of Enquiry, set up to investigate both the Medical School and the Dunedin Hospital, concluded, on the basis of extensive evidence, that the views of the Wellington group were out of step with those generally held in the

'It is certainly hard that [salaries] should have been reduced twice in the seven years that the School has been in existence. Two of us came out from Home to appointments advertised by you in England as worth £200 a year. In three years this was reduced by one quarter and now you have resolved on a second reduction.'

Letter to Otago University Council on 18 June 1892, signed by John H. Scott, D. Colquhoun, William Brown, W.S. Roberts, Frank Ogston, John Macdonald and F. Truby King.

country. The Committee reported that recent improvements at the Hospital had brought it up to an appropriate standard, that it provided enough clinical material to train medical students, and that the Otago course provided an excellent training, which fitted its graduates well for higher degrees overseas.[2]

Although cleared by the investigating committee, the Medical School remained in a precarious situation. By 1894 the financial position of the University had reached a point of crisis and this inevitably affected the School. The crisis was the result of a long-standing problem. As early as 1877, the fluctuating rentals from the pastoral runs, which were the sole permanent source of income for the University, were proving insufficient. Two years later, when the University was in the process of occupying its new buildings, the country began to sink into a twenty-year depression. A sharp fall in wool prices, the reduction of income from gold, the ravages of rabbits and the collapse of a land boom all combined to cause the most serious financial problems New Zealand had ever faced. The cost of the University buildings proved to be far in excess of expectations and saddled the institution for decades with a crippling debt. It was probably a temporary rise in the rental from one run in 1881 that had enabled Scott to inaugurate the full medical course. From then on, however, rentals continued to fall and, in 1894, the University Council was informed that over the previous two years it had lost £2000 in total income from the pastoral runs.[3] A specially reinforced Finance Committee recommended a series of measures the University would have to adopt to improve its financial situation. These included raising student fees, requiring the four professors (including Scott) each to pay £60 a year rent for their houses, which had previously been free, and reducing the salaries of the medical lecturers, for the second time. These were considered less drastic options than disestablishing the School of Mines and cutting the medical course back to two years. Nevertheless, they were still not enough and, in 1895, the University Council was forced to close the Law School. It was not without reason that, in his centennial history of the University, W.P.

Morrell called the period from 1879 to 1900 'The University in a Financial Straitjacket'.[4]

Professor Scott's reports to Council on the Medical School underlined the urgency of the University's financial crisis. Starved of funds, the Medical School (which Scott called 'old-fashioned' and out of date) was clearly unable to keep up with modern requirements. In June 1898, Scott stressed the immediate need to separate anatomy and physiology, to employ more staff and upgrade lecture rooms, laboratories and equipment, but money was lacking to make these changes. In May 1901, he complained that the School's inadequacies were affecting student numbers. He reported that the anatomy class had shrunk from forty-three in 1898 to twenty-two in 1901. Increasingly, young men were choosing to train in Britain.[5] The Council referred Scott's report to a committee, which agreed that there was an urgent need to appoint a professor of physiology and a number of ancillary staff. These changes would entail expenditure of over £2000 to build and equip a physiology laboratory (even in wood) and an annual outlay of £860 for salaries. As the University had no funds, the committee recommended that the Council approach the Government for help.[6]

At the 1902 graduation ceremony, the Vice-Chancellor put the University's financial situation squarely in the public arena. This marked the beginning of a concerted effort to set the University on a more secure footing. Local Members of Parliament approached the Government and Sir Joseph Ward, the Acting Premier, promised a 2:1 subsidy on any monies raised locally. Led by the press, the public responded wsith extraordinary speed and generosity. The *Evening Star* opened a subscription list which, within a matter of days, raised £820, on which the Government duly paid £1650. The *Otago Daily Times* donated £100 to another fund, which was set up to help clear the £16,000 debt the University had incurred in building expenses. Although this fund reached £2120, it was still not enough to pay off the University's overdraft if it continued to run at its current loss of £150 a year. The Registrar called a general meeting of Council and staff where it was decided, on the motion of Dr Colquhoun, to appeal to the people of Dunedin. At a large public meeting in August 1902, a 'Citizens' Fund' was established which raised another £2000. A further £6500 was donated by the trustees of the Dunedin Savings Bank, after the law was altered to enable it to donate a portion of its profits to local institutions.[7]

Thus far, the funds raised had been for the benefit of the University as a whole. In 1903, however, a local businessman, Mr Wolff Harris, donated £2000 towards the establishment of a chair in physiology, the first endowed chair in the School. As there was a time limit of three years on the gift, the Council had a strong incentive to move quickly. They decided to extend the existing University buildings, in matching stone, to provide facilities for the new physiology professor. The extensions were estimated to cost £5000, which was covered by a £2000 grant from the Government and a donation of £3000 from the Citizens' Fund.[8] Further, the Government committed itself to an annual grant of £1500 for the Medical School. As Carmalt Jones points out, this was the first time that the 'national' character of the School had received practical recognition. At the end of 1903, Premier Seddon was quoted as saying he 'liked to see the University going in for specialties and he was quite prepared to assist the Council in the work they had outlined.' In 1904, a University Reserves Act ended the uncertainties of income from the pastoral runs, by guaranteeing the University an amount equal to the revenue at that date.[9] The way was cleared for expansion and modernisation.

Expansion of the School: Staff, Teaching and Research in the New Century

In the early history of the Otago Medical School, neither what to teach nor how to teach it were matters of dispute. The need for recognition by medical schools in the United Kingdom meant that the two-year course taught during the first decade was explicitly devised as a preliminary to completing the degree there. Once the full course was established, the Otago Medical School carefully adhered to the curricular requirements of the General Medical Council of Great Britain.

Theoretical instruction was imparted through lectures and demonstrations, practical skills were acquired by dissection and students gained their bedside clinical teaching at the Hospital. Pedagogy was largely a matter of personality, and teachers were judged on the clarity of their exposition and on their wit. How effectively the students absorbed the teaching was tested by regular examinations. Even when the School entered into a period of expansion after 1905, with the appointment of a second professor and a number of part-time clinical tutors, and the promotion of several lecturers to chairs, the basic shape of the course and the style of teaching remained unaltered.

The subdivision of disciplines, and later departments, as specialisation developed, has always been the principal method of expansion at the Otago Medical School. In 1905, as the School's position was stabilised by a guaranteed government income and higher student numbers, this process began with the long-foreshadowed separation of Physiology from Anatomy. In April, Dr John Malcolm, another Edinburgh graduate, took up the new Chair of Physiology. Malcolm was from Caithness, in the far north of Scotland, and had spent four years as a pupil teacher before studying medicine at Edinburgh University. A brilliant student, he gained first class honours in almost all his university classes and picked up a collection of medals and awards along the way. On graduating MB ChB with Honours in 1897, Malcolm was awarded the prestigious Vans Dunlop scholarship which enabled him to carry out research under the Professor of Physiology at Edinburgh. He gained his MD two years later, winning a gold medal for his thesis and became an assistant to the new Professor of Physiology, Professor Schafer. Following this, he lectured in chemical physiology at Edinburgh and also did some postgraduate work in Berlin. Malcolm was selected for the Otago chair from a field of eleven applicants. In addition to his teaching experience, when he took up the position at the age of thirty-one, Malcolm already had a series of publications to his name.

On arrival, the new professor made a number of simple requests – additional apparatus, a

Dr John Malcolm, 1873–1954
Professor of Physiology, 1905–43

WHEN JOHN MALCOLM met his first class as Professor of Physiology on 1 May 1905 the thirty or so students greeted him with a rousing haka. It must have been a shock to the diffident young man newly arrived from Scotland, but he responded by promising to 'do the best he could in the way of teaching them physiology', and then they set to work.[10] At the 1905 Capping, Malcolm received another Otago student welcome, a song in his honour, to the tune of Gilbert and Sullivan's 'Tit Willow'. It began:

A doctor came sailing from over the sea,
Sing Johnny boy, Johnny boy, Johnny.
A clever wee braw little doctor was he,
And bonny sae bonny, sae bonny.
He came from the land where the porridge tree grows,
And the braw brawling' pibroch incessantly flows,
And hoots mon! I tell ye the Scottie man's clothes
Is fonny, aye fonny, aye fonny.[11]

From the start, the kindly Malcolm got on well with his students. Patrick Moore, who knew him towards the end of his career, in the late 1930s, expressed the respectful affection generations felt for him throughout his thirty-eight years as Professor of Physiology. 'He was a delightful man and all of us, brash and uncouth as we were, knew his worth and appreciated it.' Hercus and Bell describe him as being 'an altogether delightful character, soft spoken, modest and ever helpful'.[12]

Douglass Taylor, who has studied Malcolm's letters in depth, thought him greatly overworked in his early years, but all in all satisfied with his lot. By 1910, he had a satisfactory assistant, his research was under way and he felt his opinion was appreciated by the University. He married a young Dunedin woman, Vicky Simpson, in 1912 and settled down to a happy family life. The couple had three children. Malcolm took a full part in University affairs, commanding the University Medical Corps from 1909 till 1919 and chairing the Professorial Board from 1913 to 1916. For most of his working life, he taught the preclinical curriculum in tandem with Gowland. The two men were strikingly different. Patrick Moore, who captured their physical differences in a memorable cartoon in 1940, commented that the contrast between the robust, charismatic Gowland and the undemonstrative 'wee Johnnie Malcolm' was a constant source of fascination to students. When they both resigned in 1943 it truly was the end of an era.[13]

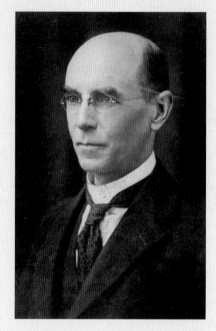

John Malcolm.
Hocken Collections, Uare Taoka o Hakena,
University of Otago, Ph74-65, sheet 208 f.

Malcolm was a foundation member of the Council of Scientific and Industrial Research in 1926 and chaired the Nutrition Committee of the New Zealand Medical Research Council from 1937 until 1949. He was a member of Knox Church and served on the governing bodies of Knox College and Columba College. He was made a Fellow of the Royal Society of Edinburgh in 1933 and CMG in 1947.[14]

trained mechanic, to be shared with physics, and electricity in his laboratory as soon as this was available. However, even these modest demands could not be met and his first impressions of the Medical School were shot through with dismay. 'They are the most poverty-stricken set of University people possible to imagine', Malcolm wrote home to his family after the first week. He made the same complaint a little later to his former chief at Edinburgh, Professor Schafer. There was no library worth the name and virtually no journals or even textbooks. The new building was incomplete and apparatus lacking. His first class in chemical physiology was held in a room without a tap, so he 'rigged up an old kerosene tin with a syphon and tubing along the bench with T-tubes'. Granted only £200 for equipment, Malcolm paid for a number of necessary instruments, such as syringes from a doctor's sale, from his own pocket. He once ordered a bomb calorimeter from Berlin, which cost him £30, half his monthly salary. He even had to buy a chair. Although Malcolm's thrift was exemplary, he was still called on to explain to the Council why it took him £65 a year to run his department, when other professors were supposedly capable of doing it for half that amount. In spite of all this, and his consciousness of isolation from cutting edge research in his discipline, Malcolm worked amicably with Scott and later Gowland. Overall, one gets the impression that he found the challenge of setting up a department from nothing deeply satisfying.[15]

In 1910 Malcolm brought in his own technical assistant, Harry Manson, who had worked in his laboratory in Edinburgh. 'His ingenuity, technical skill and devotion to duty', writes Carmalt Jones, 'must have saved the department many times his salary' and his 'pawky humour' became legendary. His apprenticeship to a demanding Edinburgh instrument-maker served him well in caring for the classes of fifty-odd students in histology, embryology, chemical physiology and 'experimental' physiology and, from the 1920s, carefully maintaining the department's first electrocardiograph machine. When he retired in 1947, the students paid him an affectionate tribute in the *Digest*. Manson was first of a line of

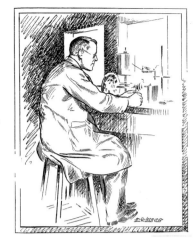

Harry Manson, from *Digest* 1947, opp. p. 20.

very able and often long-serving senior technical assistants in the Physiology Department.[16]

The first part-time clinical tutors were appointed to the Medical School the year Malcolm arrived. Dr W. Marshall Macdonald, a distinguished French scholar, later MD (Edin) and MRCP (Lond), became tutor in medicine and Dr Ratcliffe Riley tutor in surgery. Both were on the staff of the Dunedin Hospital. Riley was one of the most fondly remembered 'characters' on the School staff. As tutor in surgery from 1905 to 1907, his responsibilities were teaching of bandaging, appliances, instruments, dressings, aseptic technique and supervision of case-taking. He became lecturer in obstetrics and gynaecology in 1910 and was promoted to Professor in 1920, just two years before he retired. Affectionately known as Father Riley, he was kind and hospitable. Each year, in the first week of June, he entertained staff at his sheep run at Lake Hawea. Travelling in leisurely style, the journey took three days, with the final stage being a launch trip up the lake. Hercus and Bell describe the occasion with a rare cluster of exclamation marks: the happy times, the halcyon early winter days, the perishingly freezing nights in a corrugated iron hut and the charm of their host. A lover of the beauty of the Central Otago landscape, Riley once persuaded his guests to take axes and crowbars to unsightly advertising hoardings alongside the railway line. The police caught up with them and when the case came to trial, the Dunedin Magistrate's Court was packed with supportive students.[17]

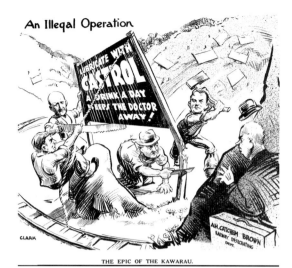

An Illegal Operation

THE EPIC OF THE KAWARAU.

CLARK

'An Illegal Operation.' Russell Clark's cartoon recalls the occasion when Drs Riley, Borrie, Thomson and Focken faced police charges after cutting down a hoarding in the Cromwell Gorge. They were each fined £5, but achieved their aim in that limitations were placed on the erection of hoardings.

Exhibition Sketcher, Dunedin Manufacturers' Association, 1930. Hocken Collections, Uare Taoka o Hakena, University of Otago. VO-DE.

Secure government funding also enabled the University to offer salaries to Dr Lindo Ferguson and Dr Truby King, both of whom had been working unpaid for some years, and to restore the salaries of the part-time lecturers in practice of medicine, surgery, pathology, public health, midwifery and materia medica to their original level. In 1909, the Council rewarded a group of these lecturers with part-time Chairs, Colquhoun in Medicine, Barnett in Surgery, Batchelor in Obstetrics and Gynaecology (until he resigned to contest a seat on the University Council at the end of the year), Ferguson in Ophthalmology, Roberts in Pathology and Ogston in Medical Jurisprudence. The title was no doubt welcome to the recipients, but it brought them no increase in salary, staff or accommodation.[18]

Frank Fitchett, one of the School's larger-than-life characters, joined the staff in 1910 as lecturer in materia medica. Dunedin-born, son of the Dean of St Paul's Cathedral, Fitchett began his medical course at Otago, completed in Edinburgh and returned to practise in his home town in 1902, before joining the teaching staff of the Hospital

two years later. He was a popular lecturer who could keep even an 8 a.m. class engrossed and expected to provoke at least three hearty laughs during each lecture.[19]

In 1910–11, the process of separating out the distinctive elements combined in certain positions was applied to the fields of pathology and bacteriology, taught since 1884 and 1891 respectively by Roberts, and medical jurisprudence and public health, taught since 1886 by Ogston. In 1891, Roberts asked the University Council for £17 or £18 to purchase equipment for teaching practical bacteriology and added a short course in the subject to the curriculum, which he taught until 1909. By this time, it was generally accepted that the Medical School needed a specialist bacteriologist. Various options were canvassed for reorganising the combinations of pathology, bacteriology, public health and medical jurisprudence. After a meeting with the Minister of Public Health, the Faculty decided to appoint a lecturer in public health and bacteriology who would also serve as Government Bacteriologist and Public Health Officer. At the same time, Roberts was promoted to a Chair in Pathology and Ogston to a Chair in Medical Jurisprudence. In 1910, the youthful Edinburgh-trained New Zealander Sydney Champtaloup was appointed as the first lecturer in Bacteriology and Public Health. Promoted to a chair the following year, Champtaloup proved a fine administrator and a gifted researcher and teacher. The reorganisation of these subjects was completed in 1916, when the brilliant young Murray Drennan arrived from Britain to take up a full-time Chair in Pathology.[20]

The Beginnings of Research

In the hand-to-mouth days of the early Medical School, research was not a priority. However, a number of individual staff, typically those who were Edinburgh-trained and who brought the aims and practices of their alma mater with them to Otago, fitted some research round their heavy teaching loads. In 1877, the same year he began teaching, Scott began to publish a series of papers in the *Journal of Anatomy and Physiology*. He was a long-time member and one-time President of the Otago Institute and his classic work on the osteology of the Maori and Moriori, which was based on an exhaustive examination of eighty skulls, appeared in the *Transactions and Proceedings of the New Zealand Institute* in 1893.[21] Malcolm was also deeply committed to research and encouraged his assistants and students to follow his example. He introduced experimental methods into his teaching, using wild rabbits to test blood pressure and frogs to study the physiology of muscles. One of his students, Emily Siedeberg, presented a paper to the Medical Society in 1907, which was said to be the first piece of real research reported at its meetings. Malcolm collaborated with Frank Fitchett in a study of tutin, a poisonous substance derived from a New Zealand plant. Their findings gained Fitchett an MD from Edinburgh in 1908 and were published the next year as an authoritative eighty-page monograph, *The Physiological Action of Tutin*. Malcolm's own research focused on the analysis of foods. Soon after he arrived at Otago, he began investigating the nutritive value of New Zealand fish and regional produce and, in 1912, he published the first of a series of articles on metabolism and nutrition in the *Transactions of the New Zealand Institute*. A later Professor of Physiology at Otago, James Robinson, describes Malcolm's work as 'the first significant breakthrough in the development of biochemistry in New Zealand'.[22]

One of the first research topics at Otago was thyroid disease. In 1894, Colquhoun published the first account of the distribution of goitre in New Zealand and went on to publish further works of prime importance in the field. As soon as he arrived at Otago, Drennan began research into the pathology of the thyroid gland, identifying the exact changes which developed in thyroid glands deprived of an adequate amount of iodine. In 1945, Carmalt Jones could still describe it as 'the subject which has provided the most fruitful research ... undertaken in this country'.[23] Research into another serious public health issue during this time, human hydatid disease, also began early and proved long-running. It was frustrating, in that although the disease and how to control it were understood, implementation of the necessary measures proved almost impossible. Sir Louis Barnett began a lifetime of research on hydatids when he performed the first surgical removal of a hydatid cyst in 1891. Between 1895 and 1946 he published over fifty articles on the disease and created the Australasian Hydatids Register. This research, and its attendant public education campaign, became a major focus of the Medical School's research programme.[24]

Champtaloup introduced the techniques of lumbar puncture and blood culture into New Zealand and made important contributions to the study of influenza during the 1918–19 epidemic. He also carried out research into tuberculosis, the disease that would be responsible for his premature death.[25] Truby King's studies in infant nutrition led to the foundation of the Plunket Society.[26]

• • •

Government support for the Medical School not only enabled the Faculty to hire additional staff and stimulated research, but also helped attract other special schools, with allied interests, to the University of Otago: a Dental School in 1907, a School of Home Science in 1911, and a Physiotherapy School (then called a School of Massage) in 1913. Their presence bolstered the security of the Medical School. Relations with the Dental School were especially close, with Colquhoun and Barnett appointed as consultants and other staff holding positions there. After 1905, the number of medical students gradually rose, to a school population of 133 by 1913, a substantial proportion of the total University population of 566. As a result of these developments, the Government accepted the need for a new, purpose-built Medical School. Although Scott did not live to see the building that was later named after him, it was an appropriate tribute to his patient determination. His death, in 1914, marks the end of the first phase of the Medical School, no longer an outpost of Edinburgh, but an established, national institution.[27]

CHAPTER 5

Medical Students

FROM the late 1870s until World War I, the Medical School occupied one side of the University quadrangle, opposite the clock tower. During this time, medical students were integrated into the general student population, although there were increasing indications of a sense of separate identity. They were few in number: two in each of 1877 and 1878, three the next year and four in 1880, two in 1881, seven in 1882 and 1883 and eight in 1884.[1] Even after the full course became available, student numbers remained low enough to put the survival of the School in jeopardy and must have made it hard to justify the new level of staffing.

The medical students' timetable was demanding. Typically their day began with biology or hospital attendance at 9.30 a.m. and then, apart from a lunch break, consisted of classes until 7.30 p.m. In spite of the pressure of work, however, medical students took a full part in general student activities. They also began to unite to further their own interests. As early as 1888, pressing for medical books for the library, two examinations a year and the improvement of the overseas value of their degree by the addition of a surgery qualification, they formed the Otago University Medical Students' Association (OUMSA).[2] When the Otago University Students' Association (OUSA) was founded in 1890, medical students played a leading part. One of them, Alexander Hendry, became the second president in 1891 and six more took on the role before 1914. During this time, the student body as a whole was struggling

to achieve what it called an 'esprit de corps' through Capping celebrations, the debating society, sporting activities and the fortnightly *Otago University Review*.[3] Medical students featured strongly in the *Review*, with reports of meetings, letters to the editor and items about former students completing at Edinburgh, where high fliers from New Zealand were doing very well indeed.[4] In 1885, for instance, Truby King – from New Zealand but not Otago – won the Ettles scholarship, the highest academic distinction for a medical student at Edinburgh. Jeffcoat from Otago was second and Lindsay, also from Otago, third.[5]

The first student to take the full Otago medical course, William Ledingham Christie, graduated in 1887. The son of a struggling farming family from South Otago, Christie was just the sort of person for whom the course was intended, as there was no way his family could have found the money to send him to Britain. They were, however, able to contribute to his support during his student days in Dunedin, where he rented a small room, by providing practical gifts such as sides of bacon. He dropped out of the medical course for a time and taught at a local school to earn the money to continue. He was twenty-seven when he graduated MB and went on to gain the first MD from Otago in 1890. In 1894, after practising for a couple of years in South Otago, Christie went to England to take his FRCS. He settled in Britain and made a fine career in Bristol. As a doctor, Christie became known as a champion

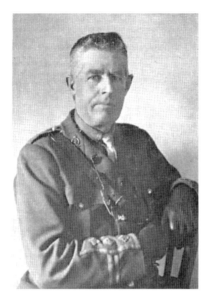

Dr William Ledingham Christie,
NZMJ vol 60 No 341, January 1961, p. 1.

of impoverished women and children and, as a city councillor, for his implacable opposition to vested interests in the public health sphere. He later worked in Sarawak, on the island of Borneo, and did not return to New Zealand.[6]

After Christie's graduation, it might have been expected that the number of local graduates would increase and the Edinburgh connection gradually dissolve. This did not happen and perhaps the most notable fact about the medical graduates listed in the Otago University calendars in the decade from 1887 to 1897 is their small number. There are twenty-nine in all, an average of fewer than three a year, and some years there was a single graduate. The majority continued to complete their degrees elsewhere. By 1893, eighty-three Otago students had completed in Britain, sixty-five after the full medical curriculum was approved in 1883. In the

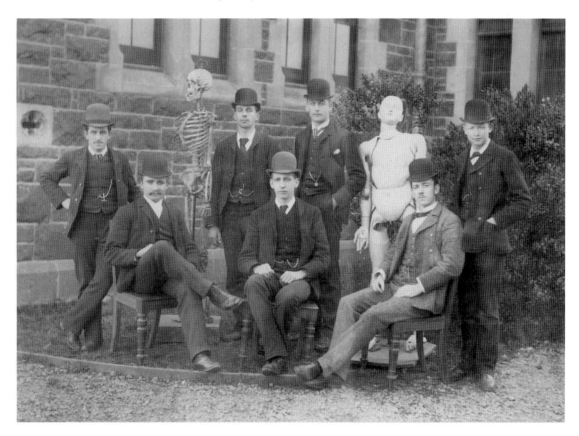

Medical Students, 1892. Back, left to right: W. McAra (Gore), J.A.T Bell (Christchurch), J.W. McBrearty (Greymouth), J.W. Anderson (Clinton and Wanganui). Front: J.L. Gregg (Wanganui), W.H. Borrie (Port Chalmers and Dunedin), and non-medical student David Black, son of Professor Black.

Hocken Collections, Uare Taoka o Hakena, University of Otago, MS-1537/306.

same period, only twenty-one students took the Otago MB. By the end of the century, fifty-six students had completed the full medical course at Otago, whereas ninety had finished their degrees in Britain.[7]

The First Women and Maori Students

By the turn of the century the homogeneity of Scott's first classes, which were made up of lads of British stock whose parents could afford to send them to the Old Country, had been breached. While the establishment of a full course at Otago made a medical degree accessible to young men such as Christie, who did not have such financial backing, it also opened the way for women and Maori students.

Women had been admitted to Otago University from the outset, with the first graduating in Arts in 1885. The speaker at her graduation ceremony, Dr William Brown, made an eloquent plea for the entry of women to higher education, including medicine. The question of women entering Medical School had already come before the Council in 1881, but no decision had been thought necessary, because women were not eligible to complete at Edinburgh. It was a different matter once the full course was established. In 1891, just four years after Christie's graduation, Emily Siedeberg entered the medical course, followed the next year by Margaret Cruickshank. The year 1891 was far from a high point for the Otago Medical School. There were two debates in the June edition of the *Review* that year, one on whether women should be admitted to the School and the other on whether the School itself should close.[8]

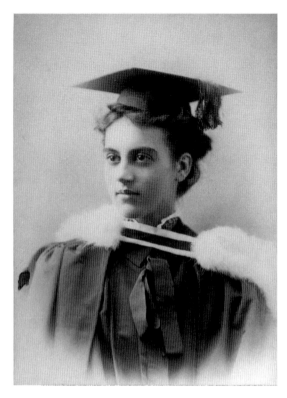

After her graduation in 1896 Emily Siedeberg studied obstetrics in Dublin and women's and children's diseases in Berlin. She returned to practise in Dunedin. From its opening in 1905 to its closure in 1938 she was also Superintendent of St Helen's Maternity Hospital.
Hocken Collections, Uare Taoka o Hakena, University of Otago, Acc. No. S 07-049a.

And soon on brass plates you shall see
Miss S— MB;
While liniments and lotions,
Strong purgatives and potions
Shall be prescribed to all,
At two-and-six a call.

Song for Capping 1892, quoted by Emily Siedeberg in an interview with the *New Zealand Free Lance*, 12 October, 1960.

There is no reason to believe that Scott wanted to keep women out of medicine. He had been a student at Edinburgh in 1870 at the peak of the controversy and violence surrounding the admission of women medical students there. He would also have been aware that, in 1891, there were twenty-five women on the British medical register and that the medical schools in Melbourne and Sydney both admitted women; indeed the first two women graduated from Melbourne in 1891. Furthermore, apart from the University's long-established policy of admitting women, the serious shortage of medical students provided a compelling reason to admit them to the Otago course. There had been only three graduates in 1890 and a mere dozen since 1887. Nevertheless, Scott's attitude to women in his

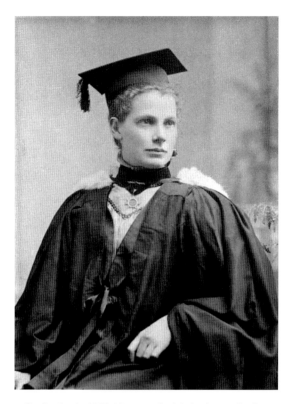

Graduating in 1897, Margaret Cruickshank was the first New Zealand woman to register as a medical practitioner and six years later the first to gain an MD. She spent her life as assistant, then partner of Dr Barclay at Waimate, except for a year (1913) when she took postgraduate courses in Edinburgh and Dublin.

Hocken Collections, Uare Taoka o Hakena, University of Otago, Acc. No. Sheet 66/3/a.

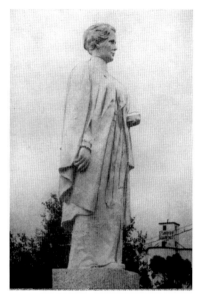

The respect and affection the Waimate community felt for Dr Cruickshank was deepened during World War I when she ran the practice single-handed. After her death in the 1918 influenza epidemic, they erected a statue to her with the inscription: 'The Beloved Physician, Faithful unto Death.'

Photo, Elizabeth Morrison, *In Memory. Dr Margaret Cruickshank.*

classes gives an impression of forbearance rather than enthusiasm. Fourteen women graduated while he was Dean of the School. This was a small proportion of a small number of students and within it the pattern of graduations was very uneven. Siedeberg graduated in 1896 and Cruickshank in 1897, then there was a gap until 1900, when four more women graduated, the biggest group in the period. Another three graduated together in 1904, but only one woman was included among the graduates in 1902, 1903, 1906, 1910 and 1911. There were none at all in the other eleven years. A graduate of 1916 could justifiably describe the five women in her first-year class as having 'appeared at the college just as the authorities thought the craze for women studying medicine had gone'.[9]

The admission of women to the School was not generally welcomed by staff, students or the local medical fraternity. In the June 1891 issue of the *Review*, 'Dunedin medico' asked indignantly, 'Why should a woman unsex herself by giving way to a morbid craving which ... can only be likened to an epidemic of insanity?'[10] While the early women students may not have had to face the overt hostility that had greeted women at Edinburgh twenty years earlier, the atmosphere in the School was chill. The main concern of staff seems to have been how to combine teaching with decorum, but there were also episodes of ill-will. At first, Professor Scott asked Emily Siedeberg to absent herself from two of his anatomy classes. However, after teaching her separately, he soon moved to inclusive classes. Eleanor Baker (later Baker McLaglan) who graduated in 1903, describes how the lecturer on public health and medical jurisprudence once stopped in the middle of a class and said to the two women present, 'I now come to the part of my lecture that I refuse to give before women. Therefore the women leave the room or I will leave it.' Covered with confusion, and accompanied by the hoots and jeers of their fellow students, the women left the class. On another occasion, the same lecturer brusquely informed Baker that she had not done well enough in her year's work to sit finals. In fact, she had come top of her class and he had mistaken her for the only other woman in the class.[11]

The dissection room posed the greatest challenge for the early women students. The most famous anecdote comes from a former laboratory assistant 'Wullie' Goodlet. After describing the unruly behaviour of the male students, which included running down the stairs brandishing an arm or a leg, and chasing him round the laboratory (which he said was good fun for them and he got used to it), Goodlet commented that Emily Siedeberg had 'a very unpleasant time'

with her class mates. 'They did not want lady doctors … and the lady students have to thank Miss Siedeberg for her pluck in making way for them …. The young men would throw the flesh at her every chance they got.' Siedeberg herself gave a much less dramatic account of the events, simply saying that on one trifling occasion 'a few pieces from another dissecting table came in my direction.'[12] It appears that throwing flesh was not uncommon, however. In her autobiography, Doris Jolly (later Gordon), who graduated in 1916, describes how students would 'let off steam in a meat fight, when hundreds of lumps of dark flesh, skin and scalp went hurtling across the dissection room.' The practice was also confirmed by Bill Anderson, a 1920 graduate, who said that because he was older than the other students, he could never join in throwing lumps of dissected meat about.[13]

In the first years of the twentieth century, there were powerful elements in society hostile to women becoming doctors. An influential group of senior staff from the Medical School, led by Truby King and Ferdinand Batchelor,

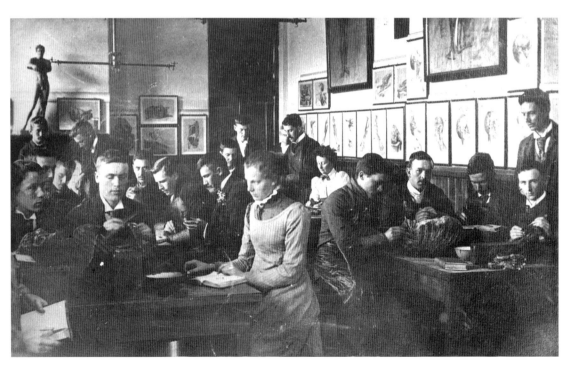

The Anatomy dissection room, 1890s. Margaret Cruickshank is centre front.
Hocken Collections, Uare Taoka o Hakena, University of Otago, Archives and Manuscripts, MS-1537/461; S06 458 d.

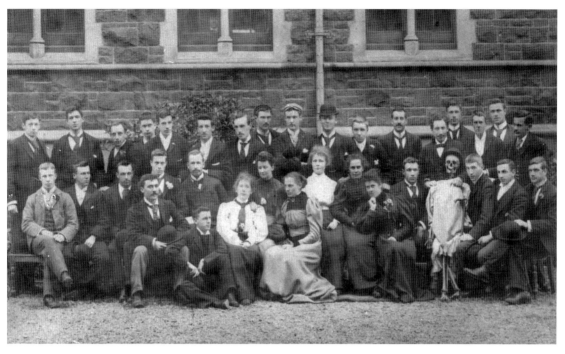

Students of the Otago Medical School in 1896.
Hocken Collections, Uare Taoka o Hakena, University of Otago, Acc. No. S 03-316a.

11

Name - Catherine Bayley
Age - 53 years - married
Residence - Macraes.
Occupation - Char - woman.
Admitted - Jan 14/97
Diagnosis - Alcoholism
Discharged

History - Last Tuesday while carrying a bundle patient felt shivery and her legs gave way and so, leaving her bundle, she made her way home as well as she could.
Patient went to bed - together with the weakness patient lost her appetite.
Patient has good family history. She is a hard worked little woman but she manages to maintain herself comfortably & has all that she requires
Excepting for a miscarriage patient has had no sickness or illness during her life - time

Besides her inability to walk patient complains of nothing - She says that her digestion is always good & that she rarely feels unwell.
On Admission Patient is a worn out hard worked little woman. She thinks that she has fallen greatly in

12

weight the last few days - She is a poorly developed creature
Examination shows a fatty tumour on the inner side of the front of the right leg just below the patella. Patient wishes this to be removed for it troubles her while walking & she thinks that it has grown lately. It is about the size of a hen's egg.
Treatment Dr Roberts prescribes.

℞
Ammon Carb.   ℨi
Spir Am Arom. ℨii
Tr Rhei   ℨv
Tr Zingib   ℨvi
Infus Quass aɖ ℨviii

℥ss ex aq t.d.s. ante cib

Catherine Bayley notes from case book 1896–97
Hocken Collections, Uare Taoka o Hakena,
University of Otago, 95-157/26.

campaigned against higher education for women in general. They argued that it placed too great a strain on them at the 'most momentous period of their lives' and was thus detrimental to the 'vitality of the race'. In 1909, Batchelor gave a lecture along these lines to an audience which included churchmen, members of parliament and doctors. He was strongly supported by King, then at the height of his influence as an expert on infant welfare. Although women doctors, including Siedeberg, sprang to the defence of higher education for women, the influence of the respected experts may well have helped account for the low number of women medical students in these years.[14] On the other hand, some of the Medical School staff who were hostile to higher education for women in theory, could be kind and helpful in practice. Eleanor Baker, for example, had reason to be grateful to Truby King, who found a position for her at Seacliff Hospital, with accommodation and a good salary, when she was newly graduated and desperately needed employment. Reflecting on this in old age, she commented, 'It was Sir Truby who probably helped me more than anyone else in my life', adding, 'Illogical animals, men.'[15]

The arrival of the first Maori medical students, Peter Buck (Te Rangi Hiroa) and Tutere Wi Repa, brought an important new element to student culture at Otago. Fellow students at Te Aute College, both young men had responded to the challenge of Apirana Ngata at the inaugural conference of the Young Maori Party, to study medicine and work to improve Maori health. Both qualified for a government scholarship of £600 a year and entered Medical School in 1899. Peter Buck, a brilliant student and a superb sportsman, with outstanding leadership qualities, was destined from the start for a stellar career. He participated fully in student affairs, serving as president of the Medical Students' Association in 1902 and of OUSA in 1903. On one occasion he took part in a mock hunt for a stuffed moa, captured from the Otago Museum. He played rugby for the University's A team from 1899 to 1903, and is credited with introducing the haka as a pre-match ceremony. He won the New Zealand long jump title twice. Buck graduated in 1904

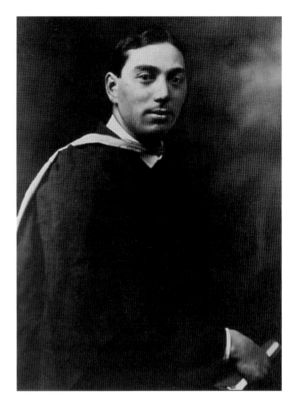

Te Rangi Hiroa (Sir Peter Buck).
Otago Medical School.

and gained his MD, with a thesis on 'Medicine among the Maoris in Ancient and Modern Times', in 1910. By this time, he was the Member of Parliament for Northern Maori. During World War I, he served as a medical officer, was awarded a DSO after Gallipoli, and rose to the rank of major and second-in-command of the New Zealand Pioneer (Maori) Battalion in France. In 1921, he became director of the Maori Hygiene Division of the new Department of Health. In 1926, Buck changed direction, from medicine to a career in his long-time research interest, Pacific anthropology. As a Research Fellow and, from 1936, Director of the Bishop Museum in Hawaii, he published widely. Buck's *Vikings of the Sunrise*, a history of Polynesian migration, became a popular classic. He also won many international academic honours, including an honorary DSc from the University of New Zealand (Otago) in 1937 and a knighthood in 1946.[16]

Tutere Wi Repa also took a full role in student activities. He represented the Medical Faculty on the OUSA executive, captained the University rugby team on occasion and played two seasons for Otago, as well as playing cricket and tennis. Wi Repa graduated in 1907 – making an impression with his polished oratory at the final-year dinner – and spent his working life serving Maori on the East Coast, often in difficult conditions. Towards the end of his life, he wrote to Carmalt Jones about his days at Otago. He had appreciated, he said, the 'kindness, courtesy and friendliness amounting almost to kinsmanship', not only of students of his own faculty, but also of the Medical School and Hospital staff, local doctors and professors of other faculties. He recalled that the hospitality extended to himself and Peter Buck during their time at Otago made them feel that Dunedin was home, adding, 'Truly, class and colour distinction have no place in university life.'[17]

Tutere Wi Repa: 'He was a Maori of the Maori. He loved his race and was proud of it.'

Obituary, *NZMJ*, 1946, p. 62.

Team Sports

Sport was an important extra-curricular activity for male students, and some staff, at the Medical School. Students began playing rugby and cricket almost as soon as classes commenced at the University in 1871. Although rugby was still in a formative phase, as this was before the advent of the Rugby Football Union, a match between University students and a team of past and present pupils of Otago Boys' High School took place in September of that year. The teams were twenty-two strong and the match apparently stretched for six hours over two days, before it was declared a draw. In October, a cricket team from the University was beaten by a team from the Citizens' Cricket Club on the Southern Recreation Ground (now the Oval).[18]

The first University cricket club was formed in 1876. Dr Coughtrey's sole student, Low, and two students, Will and Closs, from Professor Scott's first class were among its earliest members.

When the University moved from the Exchange building, which had been conveniently close to the Southern Ground, to its Leith site in 1879, the club faded away. Interest in summer sport was also hampered by the fact the University term ran from May to October and out-of-town students departed over the summer. However, medical students were instrumental in the revival of the club in 1895. In a letter to the *Review* the previous year, 'Knight of the Willow Wand', who was probably medical student James Hardie Neil, pointed out that the summer session of the Medical School now kept many students in Dunedin. The daily anatomy class ended at 4 p.m. and what better way to end the afternoon than playing cricket? When the Otago University Cricket Club formed, Professor Scott was elected president, a position he held for the next five years. Neil was a very competent secretary and a Ladies' Committee (which included medical students Helena Baxter and Alice Woodward) provided support and tea. As well as Neil, notable players of the day were medical students R.N. Adams and A.R. Falconer. Nevertheless, the golden days did not last for long. Player numbers diminished as interest in tennis grew and new sports were introduced, such as yachting and golf. In 1900, after Neil departed and the rest of the medical students who had provided the energy behind the club dispersed, the club was disbanded – this time, for twenty years.[19]

There was still inter-college cricket. Sport among the university colleges received a boost when the Easter Tournament was introduced in 1902. At first, teams competed in tennis and athletics and, by 1912, the tournament had grown to include rugby, hockey and boxing. Cricket was not part of the tournament during this time, but matches between the colleges were popular, with ten being played before World War I halted university cricket.[20]

While rugby was played at the University in the late 1870s, a formal club did not come into being until 1884, three years after the establishment of the Otago Rugby Football Union. Professor Sale of Classics, the 'great pioneer of rugby in Dunedin', was elected president and Dr William Brown, lecturer in surgery, vice-president. Brown played

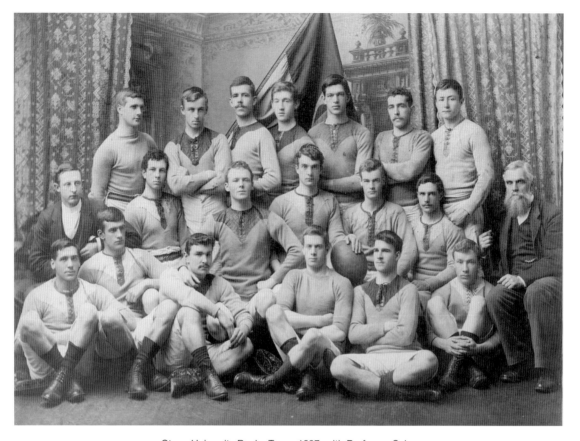

Otago University Rugby Team, 1897, with Professor Sale.
Hocken Collections, Uare Taoka o Hakena, University of Otago, Archives and Manuscripts, MS-1537/694 j.

for the team, together with some of his students, including Louis Barnett, Ninian Trotter, Thomas Burns, Sidney Gibbs and J. and W. Fitzgerald. The club was permitted to use the North Ground, near the University, during the week, but not on Saturday, when it had to make do with vacant land around the University itself, which was unsuitable for match play. In 1887, the club finally obtained its own ground, Tahuna Park, although it was some distance from the University. The club's pool of experienced players was boosted by senior medical students who could now complete their degrees locally. Otago lost their first match against Canterbury College, played on Christ's College grounds in 1886, but they won the second in Dunedin in 1887, with medical students making up more than half the team.[21]

It has been claimed that the 'critical turning point' for the club came in 1904, when Dr Irwin Hunter, a former University player and Otago representative, began coaching the University A team. Hunter, who lectured at the Medical School, coached the team until 1911, when he took over as club president. Under his guidance, University A won the Dunedin senior competition three times. Regarded as 'one of the great rugby thinkers', he wrote *New Zealand Rugby Football – Some Hints and Criticisms*, in which he analysed every field position and the best strategies for playing the game. In 1905, he sent a University touring team of eighteen players to Sydney, the first New Zealand club team to tour overseas, and in 1908 he managed the first University team to tour Australia. Rugby declined in Dunedin during World War I, with many players absent on military service. Even so, the University was still able to field three teams in the senior grade, mostly made up of medical students.[22]

A Home Away from Home

A new stage in the medical student experience began in 1909, when Knox College opened its doors for the first time and Selwyn College became a full-scale residential institution. Before this, private board had been the norm for out-of-town students. It was not always a comfortable experience. In his one year at Otago, in the late 1890s, James Elliott boarded in four different establishments. The first was with a married student, whose treatment of his wife – 'he worked her with a whistle, navy-style' – roused him to her defence; the couple then united against him and turned him out. His next landlady, a 'predatory widow dressed in black with white trimmings', gave him short shrift when she returned home to find him using her kitchen, trying to boil clean a meaty human skull he had been tricked into buying. After one more unsatisfactory set of digs, he settled into a private hotel for the rest of the year.[23] Stories of odd landladies, and student boarders with a taste for bizarre practical jokes, abound for this era, as later.

Knox and Selwyn Colleges quickly became the special preserve of male medical students, as St Margaret's College would become for the women students a year or so later. Of the forty-two foundation residents of Knox in 1909, thirteen were doing medicine, while the sole dental student, Charles Hercus, would spend the greater part of his working life at the Medical School. Additions to Selwyn College, which had begun as a very small-scale operation in 1893, enabled it to take thirty-seven students in 1910, of whom eighteen were medical students. By 1914 more than a quarter of the 618 students at Otago, a high proportion of them medical students from beyond Dunedin, lived in colleges. The war caused a temporary slump in numbers, Knox dropped from ninety-three students at the beginning of 1914 to a low point of fifty-seven in 1915 and Selwyn was forced to close for a time in 1918–19. The Medical Faculty correspondent to the *Review* regretted the closure, because Selwyn 'was always a favourite institution with everyone, not only as an afternoon tea resort,

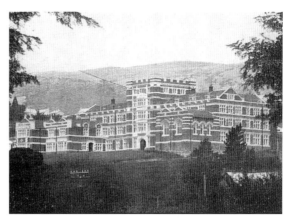

Knox College.
from *Descriptive Syllabus of the Medical School*, 1916, p. 29.

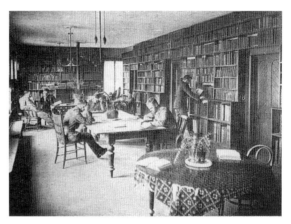

Selwyn College library.
Descriptive Syllabus, 1916, p. 29.

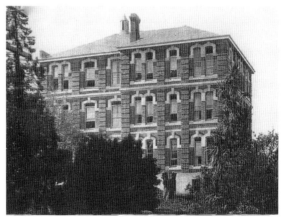

St Margaret's College.
Descriptive Syllabus, 1916, p. 40.
The Residential Colleges provided an ideal base for medical students from other parts of New Zealand.
Medical Library, University of Otago.

but also as a home for drunken students, who always found it a welcome resting place on the long and weary trudge home to Knox'.[24]

From 1912, women medical students settled in at St Margaret's College, which had opened with a handful of students the previous year. There were four studying medicine among the twelve students in 1912 and the proportion of medical students remained high as the college grew. In 1917, they numbered twenty-two out of a total of sixty. Typically, they stayed throughout their course. When the first graduated in 1916, the college held a 'corroboree' in their honour. The college played an important part in the university life of the women students, the more so because their role in general student activities was limited. The Otago Medical Students' Association and the Otago University Students' Association both excluded women from their committees, on which they were represented by male delegates. They were called on to provide supper for socials, but women students did not take part in Capping festivities and women medical students were not invited to the fifth-year dinners.[25]

The Otago University Medical Students' Association

Although it has scarcely been mentioned in histories of the Medical School, the Otago Medical Students' Association has loyally served the student body from 1888 to the present. The earliest surviving set of minutes begins in 1905, but it is evident that medical students had begun to see themselves as different from other undergraduates before this date.[26] The turn of the century was a boisterous period in student affairs. In his social history of students at the University of Otago, Sam Elworthy depicts the divisions among the faculties at this time as assuming 'almost fanatical proportions'. He adds, in a statement that suggests the later stereotype of the medical student was already in place, 'If you were a serious arts student studying to be a minister of religion, then you were going to fight the irreligious, arrogant, medical pranksters for all you were worth.'[27]

In 1902, matters came to a head in a dramatic confrontation, referred to as the 'Grand Schism', between the medical students and OUSA. When OUSA refused to defer their elections for two weeks, until the Medical School was in session, the medical students, led by their president Peter Buck, responded by threatening to secede. A general student meeting was called to settle the dispute. Although it was agreed that the date of the elections should be changed, the meeting was a scene of such disorder it left much ill-feeling. It was the first, but would by no means be the last, time that medical students believed OUSA had treated them unfairly.[28]

The first volume of the OUMSA Minutes includes the 'Rules of the Association,' which had a broad mandate to 'conserve the interests of medical students generally'. According to the 'Rules,' the Association required a president (in the early years an invited senior member of the Medical School staff), a vice-president (the senior house surgeon), and a committee of seven, made up of representatives from all the years of the course. The annual general meeting was to be held in May, prior to that of OUSA.[29]

The first volume of the Minutes show the day-to-day activities of the Association over the decade. It is generally small-scale stuff, administrative, social or sporting, and gives a clear impression that the Association lacked clout. To take some examples: at a meeting in 1905, attended by about forty members in the students' room in the hospital, Dr Batchelor was elected president. At this meeting it was also agreed that the Association would send a letter to Dr Truby King explaining why junior students had left a lecture he had given at specific student request. The OUMSA executive was unsuccessful when it asked the University Council for a special room to be set aside for medical students. It was equally unsuccessful when it wrote to the Hospital Trustees asking for an increase in the salary of junior house surgeons from £75 to £100 and to the University Council protesting the imposition of extra fees for clinical medicine and surgery. The Medical School staff did agree to OUMSA's request to donate periodicals to a student library, on condition that the Association also contribute, but it was unable to do so, because it had not collected any subscriptions.

The Association had greater success organising medical dinners. The one in 1905, described at the time as the largest yet, was attended by fifty students and seventeen doctors. The numbers attending the dinners continued to grow over subsequent years. The role of alcohol in the social life of medical students surfaced early. In 1908, at a general meeting of OUMSA, sixty-two students defeated a motion that alcohol at medical dinners should be restricted to wine and there was an even more emphatic defeat of an amendment that no alcohol at all should be served. The Association sent a deputation to Professor Scott supporting the introduction of special examinations for those who failed their finals. OUMSA presented him with a gold-mounted pocket book when he went on leave at the end of 1908 and thanked Dr Hocken for a generous gift of books for the library.

This set of minutes ends on a sober note. In 1914, the students recorded a motion of sympathy on the death of Professor Scott. The next year, they noted that a cup in memory of student Rutherford Nichol, who had been killed in an accident at Knox College, had been presented to the School, to be competed for annually by rugby teams representing the various years of the medical course. There were broader concerns, too. The report of the 1915 Annual General Meeting includes a list of the names of students and Hospital staff serving overseas. Five of those listed are staff, seven are students from the first year, five are from second year, twelve are from third year, one is from fourth year and eleven are from fifth year.[30] Otago medical students were entering a new, less carefree, world.

PART II

The Ferguson Era
1914–1937

CHAPTER 6

A Statesman at the Helm

IN 1914, the University of Otago was, in Morrell's words, 'rejuvenated and reinvigorated … full of energy and promise'.[1] The Medical School was establishing itself firmly. There were 155 students in 1914, up from 96 in 1910. The School had recently appointed additional staff, was planning to reorganise its curriculum and was looking forward to more spacious accommodation.[2] Professor (later Sir) Lindo Ferguson, Dean from 1914 to 1937, set his stamp on an era of expansion and modernisation. The careful, small-scale, economical build-up of the School in the Scott period gave way to a broader, more cosmopolitan outlook. Staff began to travel more and there was increased contact with overseas institutions, in America as well as in Britain. In addition to funding an extensive building programme, the Government trebled its financial support over the period, and this public money was supplemented by substantial private donations. Student numbers increased strongly and young and talented staff were employed. The curriculum evolved, the course was extended to six years and hospitals in Christchurch, Wellington and Auckland were drawn into the training of final-year students.

Two serendipitous developments provide evidence of the growing maturity of the Medical School during the Ferguson period. The first demonstrates the enthusiasm and collegiality of the staff, a dynamic group of whom met regularly over many years in the 'Clinical Club' to socialise, discuss their research and report on advances in their disciplines. The other affirms the standing of the School, which made it an appropriate repository for a gift of bibliographic treasures, the Monro Collection. Ferguson's annual reports provide an invaluable commentary on the development of the School over the whole period. His final report, in 1936, sums up the achievements of the past and lays down some guidelines for the future. But before all of this could take place, the School had to endure the four-year-long crisis of World War I.

The Dean in Person

Of all the personal anecdotes that go to make up the folklore of the Otago Medical School, none is more fondly or frequently recalled than Sir Lindo Ferguson's majestic response to a traffic inspector who asked him to reverse his car during a driving test: 'I *never* reverse', he said, 'I go round the block'.[3] Those who worked with Ferguson and knew him personally, were unstinting in their praise of the forward thrust he maintained at the Medical School throughout his long deanship. Gordon Bell, who arrived in Dunedin in 1925 to take up the Chair of Surgery, was awed by the paradox of 'a Victorian and all that implies in class distinction, a perfect specimen of a past age and a passing class, living in a leisurely, dignified elegance and secure in an ample affluence' but dedicated to creating a modern medical school.[4] In a tribute written when Ferguson retired, Carmalt Jones wrote that, 'Without question,

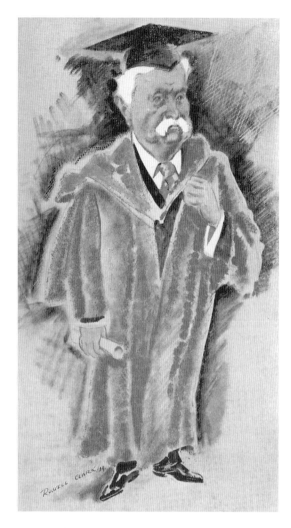

Ferguson, caricature by Russell Clark,
Digest 1.1, 1934, p. 10.
Medical Library, University of Otago.

The jaunty theatricality of this depiction of
Sir Lindo was matched by a Gilbertian verse
celebrating his career. 'Song, Sir Lindo' began

When I was a lad I served my time
At a Medical School in the Irish clime;
In the first year subjects I swept the floor,
And I polished off Anatomy in one year more.
But I polished off my Optics most carefulee,
For I had my eye on the top of some tree.

Digest, Vol 1 no 1, October 1934, p. 10.
Medical Library, University of Otago.

and acknowledging the loyal support he has received, he has been the centre round which the medical school has revolved.' According to Jones, his colleagues appreciated his 'single-minded devotion to the School, his vision of its needs, his quiet pertinacity in attaining its objects, his generous hospitality and his unfailing and unvarying kindness to themselves.'[5] Hercus and Bell, the one his Sub-Dean for thirteen years, the other his long-term colleague, affectionately describe the trim, erect figure in the invariable white pique tie, as being as much a feature of Dunedin life as the Burns monument. Ferguson was a generous and discriminating patron of the arts who contributed to the social life of the city for sixty years and, in the words of Hercus and Bell, 'radiated a captivating old-world charm recalling that past, more gracious, cultivated and leisured age of which he was a perfect exemplar.'[6]

That Ferguson's reforms sometimes evoked incomprehension, jealousy and even overt hostility could not shake his imperturbable calm. The Faculty of Medicine, acknowledging his retirement with 'profound regret and with a unanimous sense of irreparable loss', recognised the opposition as well as the achievement:

> His leadership has been characterised by such foresight and breadth of view that in his endeavour to place the New Zealand Medical School in the front rank of educational institutions he has encountered considerable opposition from local Governing Bodies and Government officials. But undeterred by rebuffs and lack of understanding he has single-heartedly pursued his aim, and by unflagging advocacy has overcome opposition and has surmounted difficulties that seemed insuperable.[7]

From time to time, Ferguson certainly faced opposition within the University. The 'serene urbanity' his friends describe and the privileged position he claimed for the Medical School, must at times have been intensely galling to his non-medical colleagues. At evening meetings of the Professorial Board he would customarily make a late entrance, looking as if he had enjoyed a good dinner with appropriate accompaniments. If, as happened on occasion, the Board was debating the disparity between arts and science salaries and medical ones, Ferguson would end the debate with the smiling comment, 'It is just a question of market value, gentlemen.'[8]

Henry Lindo Ferguson came from a privileged background and demonstrated a precocious intelligence. He was born in London on 7 April 1858, the son of an analytical chemist who became a brewer and was a founder of the Chemical Society. In 1866, the family moved to Dublin. Ferguson entered the Royal College of Science in 1873, aged only fifteen, and won one of two Royal Scholarships the following year. After qualifying in chemical manufacture, he went on to study medicine at Trinity College Dublin, where he was a gold medallist in arts. While at Trinity, Ferguson became interested in ophthalmology and he completed his training in this specialty in 1880. After a residence at St Mark's Ophthalmic Hospital, he became assistant to the Oculist to the Queen in Ireland, and to the Richmond Hospital and the National Eye and Ear Infirmary. In 1883, Ferguson became a Fellow of the Royal College of Surgeons of Ireland (FRCSI).[9]

As assistant, then partner, in the largest ophthalmic practice in Dublin, Ferguson was launched on a fine medical career in Britain, when this was jeopardised by a health scare. He damaged his eyes attempting to take photographs of the retina, using himself as model. On medical advice, Ferguson decided to come to New Zealand for a year or two, accompanied by his mother and brother. The voyage itself did wonders. By the time they reached Port Chalmers, on 12 October 1883, Ferguson's eyesight was so far restored that he could discard his glasses. Seeing potential in the infant Medical School, he settled in Dunedin and quickly established himself. He set up in private practice as an ophthalmologist, who also took ear, nose and throat patients and, in January 1884, he opened an ophthalmic department at the Dunedin Hospital. As the first trained ophthalmic surgeon in Australasia (Ferguson estimated that before he came to New Zealand he had handled some 10,000 to 12,000 patients) he was soon widely consulted. At the end of 1884, Ferguson married Mary Emmeline Butterworth, the English-educated daughter of a prominent Dunedin businessman. In 1886, he began his long association with the Otago Medical School as an honorary part-time lecturer in diseases of the eye.[10]

The years Ferguson spent in Dunedin prior to becoming Dean of the Medical School were professionally satisfying and personally enjoyable. He understood well the inter-relationship between a hospital and a medical school and, during the 1890s, he worked effectively with his good friend Ferdinand Batchelor to promote reforms at Dunedin Hospital. He was said to have exercised a restraining influence on his forceful and impetuous colleague, although this was something Carmalt Jones found hard to believe. When the Inter-Colonial Medical Conference was held in Dunedin in 1896, Ferguson was President of the New Zealand Medical Association and began negotiations to form a local branch of the British Medical Association. Cosmopolitan in outlook, he enjoyed travel and used it to maintain professional contacts overseas. In 1892 he went to England to 'keep in touch', sat his MB in Dublin and was awarded the MD for a thesis he wrote on the voyage. In 1901, when he went to 'renew contacts in Britain', he travelled via Sydney and also managed to include Naples, Rome, Florence, Venice and Vienna in his itinerary. He made 'a great many trips' to Australia, where he had a wide circle of friends. He spent 1908 in England. Both Ferguson and Batchelor became professors in 1909. In 1911, when they were both 'at Home', they attended a postgraduate course on diseases of the nervous system. Ferguson arrived back in Dunedin at the end of that year with the intention of returning to England, probably permanently, in 1914 or 1915.[11]

Ferguson's plans for the future were thrown into disarray when Professor Scott died early in 1914 and he was nominated Dean of the Medical School. The Medical Faculty might well have thought that they were choosing a stop-gap, a man of the past rather than of the future. Ferguson had been on the staff of the Medical School for almost thirty years and even longer on the staff of the Hospital. Most of his long-term colleagues had left the School, including Batchelor, who had resigned in 1909.[12] In the wider University, the founding professors, his colleagues for many years, had all retired by 1914 – Professor Scott was the only one to die while still in the employ of the University.[13] Ferguson was not chosen for his seniority, however. Professor Malcolm had been acting Dean during the last months of Scott's life. The most senior member of Faculty at the time was Professor Colquhoun. Colquhoun might indeed have seemed the obvious choice. He had been called on to defend the School before the Education Commission in Wellington in 1913, had been actively involved in many of the reforms relating to the Dunedin Hospital, founded the *New Zealand Medical Journal* and had worked to establish a medical library. But he was already three years older than Scott, in indifferent health and perhaps too well known for his unwillingness to compromise.

Ferguson himself attributed his selection to the Faculty's desire to avoid a contested election which, he suggested, 'would have imperilled harmonious relations among the members of staff'. His nomination as Dean was confirmed by the University Council on 16 March and he deferred his plans of retirement to London. Within five months war began in Europe, altering everything. By 1917, Ferguson had become 'so tied up with School affairs that all [his] plans for a peaceful old age were scrapped'.[14] It was at this point he sold his house in Hampstead, London. It might not have been expected, but that was the greatest good fortune for the School, for Lindo Ferguson provided twenty-three years of energetic and statesmanlike leadership before he stepped down in 1937, at the age of seventy-eight. He was Dean during the period Morrell calls 'the dominance of the special schools' at the University and was the driving force behind the expansion and development of the greatest of these, the Otago Medical School.[15]

Grand Plans in Grand Style

Lindo Ferguson had a clear concept of what his role as Dean entailed. He expressed this in a striking, if mixed, metaphor. It was to take the broadest view, to provide vision. 'Only the Dean' he wrote, 'sees the effect of the tessellated pavement, the individual tiles are all disgruntled because they think they have not sufficiently prominent places in the design or a sufficient illumination from the spot light.' As soon as the prolonged crisis of the war was over, he set his mind to shaping the Medical School into a modern institution. He pursued his aim with a combination of single-minded determination and imperturbable aplomb. Ferguson's self-confident style derived in part from his financial independence. He had no personal stake in the money he spent so much time and energy extracting from the Government and the University Council. 'I was able', he said, 'to do much for the School that a salaried whole-time man could not have done. I was absolutely independent and could say what I liked and the Council took it cheerfully.'[16]

Ferguson had made it a condition of his acceptance of the deanship that he should have a Sub-Dean to assist him at policy level. This position was filled in turn, with superb efficiency and often flair, by Professors Sydney Champtaloup, Murray Drennan and Charles Hercus, a group of 'able, self-sacrificing and progressive younger men of pre-eminently academic leanings', as the last of them put it, careful in his choice of words.[17] The day when the Dean could personally handle all his correspondence and reports, as Scott had done, was also well past. From 1920 Ferguson had the assistance of Miss Thomson. The perfect Dean's Secretary, she was never fussed by any emergency, could lay her hand on any document at a moment's notice and found nothing to be too much trouble.[18] The Dean also worked closely with the Reverend Andrew Cameron, Chancellor of the University of Otago from 1912 to 1925, who was convinced that the greatest service he could perform for the University was to advance the cause of the Medical School. The pair often visited Wellington together, to acquaint Ministers at first hand with the needs of the School. Bell recalled how much he appreciated the courtesy of an early morning shipboard visit from them, during one such visit to Wellington, to welcome him and his family to New Zealand. After Cameron's death in 1925, Ferguson referred in his annual report to the loss the School had sustained. 'Had it not been for the Rev Cameron's unflagging interest and support', he wrote, 'the progress which [had] been made during the last twelve years would have been quite impossible.'[19]

The Fergusons were leaders of Dunedin society, renowned for their gracious hospitality. Their home was filled with art treasures, including a valuable collection of paintings, several of which were later bequeathed to the Dunedin Public Art Gallery. Ferguson served on the Art Gallery Council from 1922 until his death.[20] He also served several terms as president of the Dunedin Club, where professional and business leaders gathered. Mary Ferguson also played a significant role in public life. She was one of the first two women on the Hospital Board, she served in the Red Cross and St John Ambulance and was the long-serving, strikingly successful first president of the Dunedin Women's Club. Guests at the Fergusons' home included politicians and vice-regal parties, but their hospitality also extended to medical students.[21] Dr Elaine Gurr describes being invited as a student to elegant dinner and evening parties at the Ferguson home. In 1918, when two second-year women students contracted influenza, through working as volunteers in the Dunedin Hospital, the Fergusons took them in to nurse them back to health.[22] Sir Randall Elliott, whose parents often entertained the Fergusons in Wellington, considered them to be a formidable couple. He was convinced that a great deal of Sir Lindo's fame rested with his wife, who left no stone unturned to ensure that his skill and fame were recognised and his dignity upheld, even to the point of confiscating the crossword puzzles he was addicted to. (He routinely kept a spare copy in his pocket.) Elliott found Sir Lindo a kind and very lovable man but could never quite overcome his awe of his wife's 'formidable but regal small figure.'[23]

It is ironic that, for someone who had contemplated retirement in 1914, Ferguson should still be carrying a full workload more than twenty years later, when in his late seventies. The University, which had been firm in its policy of appointing youthful professors, to get the maximum value out of them, had not looked so far ahead as to legislate an age for retirement. The Chancellor, W.P. Morrell (who had recently been obliged to relinquish his post as rector of Otago Boys' High School after reaching retirement age) raised the issue in Council in 1935. A committee deputed to consider the question recommended the normal retirement age at the University should be sixty-five, with the possibility of an extension to seventy after annual review. Sir Lindo took credit for the option of this annual extension of service. He later wrote that when the Chancellor introduced the subject of an age limit for University teachers, he 'fought to the last ditch' for his men, because they had been appointed without such a limit. Being over seventy himself at the time, he resigned, but consented to stay on for a year as Dean because he 'held lots of threads in his hands'. He gave up lecturing, however, and for the first time insisted on a Dean's salary: 'Of course the £300 went into the School to pay for things the Council would not have given me, as had every penny drawn from the School from the time I was first associated with it.' He believed it was necessary for the School to establish the principle of paying the Dean. Early in 1937 Ferguson duly stepped down, handing over to his Sub-Dean and heir apparent, Charles Hercus.[24] Honoured within the University, Ferguson also garnered honours further afield: he was made CMG in 1918, the first person in medicine to receive an honour for civilian services in New Zealand, and Knight Bachelor in 1924. Lady Ferguson died in Dunedin in 1945 and Sir Lindo in 1948.[25]

CHAPTER 7

World War I and its Aftermath

WORLD WAR I, which dominated Ferguson's first four years as Dean, erupted with startling suddenness. On 4 August 1914, the day war began, Ferguson was in Australia, on a tour of medical schools. There was a fortnight's delay before he could get back to Dunedin and he returned to what he called in his autobiographical memoir 'a state of chaos'. Batchelor, although sixty-five, had 'wangled it to get away' as an Army radiologist and was in camp in Auckland. Dr O'Neill of the Anatomy Department had already enlisted and Professor Barnett was anxious to do so as soon as possible. Professor Colquhoun had resigned for reasons of health. (He was persuaded to stay on for what proved to be the duration of the war.) Professor Roberts was working from a disused hospital ward and Professor Champtaloup from a cellar under the old Medical School building. Moreover, 'the army was demanding two men of senior house surgeon standing each month to go with the monthly reinforcements and half the women in town were plucking their hens to send white feathers to our students.'[1]

World War I placed entirely new pressures on both the staff and students of the Medical School. It was not, however, New Zealand's first involvement in an overseas conflict. Ten contingents, totalling 6500 troops, had volunteered for the South African War of 1899–1902. The force included twenty-six doctors, most of them graduates of the Otago Medical School, including some who would later have an influence on its development. One of these was Eugene O'Neill, the only staff member to serve in both the South African War and World War I. After graduating from Otago in 1899, he set off at once to fight the Boers. O'Neill has left an account of the training and equipment of the medical officers bound for the Veldt. They were given a couple of months' training in Wellington, on foot and horseback, and were then each allocated an orderly they were expected to train themselves. Their equipment included a medical and surgical pannier, some stretchers and surgical haversacks and a medical companion chest, containing fourteen numbered bottles of pills. As it emerged, the main medical problem in South Africa proved to be alimentary infections, along with lice, skin sores, and kicks from the horses. Prompt to enlist for the 1914–18 war, O'Neill served at Gallipoli and in France, where he commanded the New Zealand Stationary Hospital, earning the DSO and the CMG. His personal qualities won him the affection and respect of generations of medical students.[2]

Other Otago students who served in the South African War included Frank Fitchett, who went straight after completing his medical degree at Edinburgh. He also volunteered for active service in World War I but was kept back for teaching duties.[3] Dr A.R. Falconer, who graduated from Otago with a BA, BSc and MB ChB, went on to study in Britain after serving in South Africa. He became the first Medical Superintendent of Dunedin Hospital and later of Ashburn Hall.[4]

The medical officers who took part in the South African War did so as individuals. There was no field ambulance, hospital or other medical unit sent from New Zealand. Doctors were attached to combatant formations or to the Royal Army Medical Corps, which had field hospitals and larger medical units, hospital ships and trains.[5]

The Otago Medical School was not involved in the South African War as an institution. However, soon after the war, medical students began training at Otago to serve as wartime medical officers should the need arise. In the face of Germany's growing military power, New Zealand established its first Medical Corps in 1905 and, in 1908, all officers and other ranks connected with the medical service were formed into the New Zealand Medical Corps. The following year, the Otago Officers' Training Corps (OTC) was set up, as part of the Voluntary Defence Scheme. It included a field ambulance company, made up of medical and dental students, commanded by Captain John Malcolm, who filled the position through until 1919. Charles Hercus also began his long association with the unit at its inception, as a student with the rank of corporal. Training in infantry and stretcher drill was held on Saturday mornings and, from 1910, in annual camps. At the camps, students took part in physical training, attended lectures and sometimes worked for certificates towards promotion. The New Zealand Government brought in compulsory military training in 1910 and the OTC was disbanded. Although the Medical Unit was kept together as B Section of No 2 Field Ambulance, Hercus regretted that 'the elan of the previous Officers' Training Unit' was lost in the change.[6]

World War I greatly exacerbated administration difficulties at the Medical School. In his annual report for 1915, Ferguson wrote that at least a hundred medical students were 'wearing the King's uniform'. To help meet the demand for surgeons, the 1914 final examination had been held in August instead of at the end of the year. The change had been made at the request of a group of final-year medical students, eager to leave for the war without delay, in case it should be over by the time they got there. One of them later wrote:

The *Otago Daily Times*, which announced the war, also declared that the war could not last longer than three months. There was not enough money in the world to run a modern war longer than that. Believing this naïve statement we petitioned the authorities to let us sit our exams now [in August] instead of in January when the war would be over.

On 5 August, a document signed by twenty-one students was delivered to Major Falconer, the senior Territorial Officer, at Dunedin Hospital, stating 'that the following final-year medical students are willing, if qualified, to place themselves at the disposal of the New Zealand Government as Medical Officers for the Expeditionary Force'. The University authorities agreed, the fifth years duly passed their examinations, were commissioned and joined the Medical Corps immediately.[7] Ferguson noted in his annual report that all the new graduates of the School had either enlisted themselves or had replaced doctors who did so.[8]

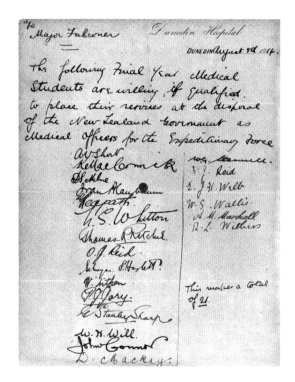

Letter to Falconer from twenty-one students, August 1914, asking to enlist. Otago Medical School.

The eagerness to enlist was not confined to final-year students. In an article written in 1942 for the medical students' *Digest,* Hercus claimed that 'practically all the first years and a large number of the second and third year medical students [had] volunteered.' A group of third-year students who enlisted were a special case. Montgomery (Montie) Spencer was one of those who could not wait to join the action. His enthusiasm was probably typical. He wrote to his parents from Knox College on 8 August 1914, 'I don't know I could stay at home and see others go out and fight for their King and country ...' Spencer took it for granted that the fight would be short. He also reasoned that because he was still 'pretty young ... to qualify a year later would not be anything of a disadvantage.' He passed an early First Professional examination on 17 August. Three days later, the Faculty gave a farewell dinner for students who had enlisted and the following day Spencer left with his section of the Field Ambulance for training in Auckland. They were first sent to Egypt, then in April 1915 to Gallipoli.

A description of their arrival at Gallipoli, written by one of the group, was printed in the 1915 *Otago University Review.*

> It seems still that we were in a dream. But a little previously, in the perfect morning hours, we had glided out of Lemnos Harbour, and now we were standing in this awful inferno, helplessly holding a stretcher in a dazed manner with shrapnel spitting all round us. But a few trenchant remarks from our officer wakened us up and we speedily assisted to look after the enormous number of wounded who covered the beach. Barge after barge was filled up and taken away to the transports and hospital ships.

In June, one of the medical students, first-year James Paterson, was killed. Another, Robert Church, also a first-year, was later awarded the Military Medal for gallantry. In July, the group of third-year medical students were ordered home to complete their studies. They took a compressed fourth-year course, under special arrangements, over the six months after their arrival in August.

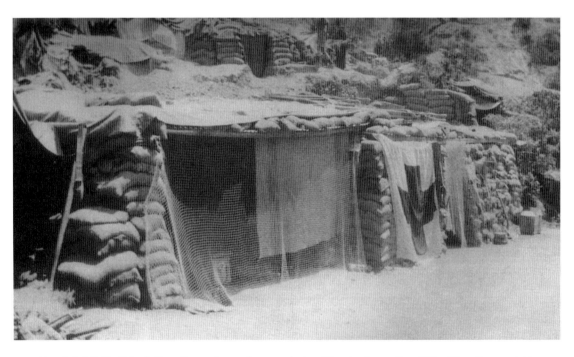

Hospital at Gallipoli: 'a shelter with sandbag walls up against a cliff and not more than 20ft x 9ft … On one night, after a bit of a battle, 97 wounded were treated here, by four doctors, each with an attendant.'
(Montgomery Spencer, cited in Christine Daniell, *A Doctor at War*, p. 5.)
Photo, Christine Daniell, Montgomery Spencer collection.

Meantime, the war was dragging on for years rather than the weeks or months they had expected. Spencer spent time as a house surgeon in Auckland and Hamilton and graduated in time to rejoin the army early in 1918. He served in England, and France in the last weeks of the war and with the Army of Occupation in Germany until 1919.[9]

In 1915 the final examination was again held early, which enabled twenty-two newly qualified doctors to take up their duties as house surgeons. But with almost one third of New Zealand's doctors diverted to military service, this acceleration was still not enough for the Minister of Public Health. He urged the University Council to increase the intake of medical students.[10] This pressure was exerted on the School while it was depleted of staff and

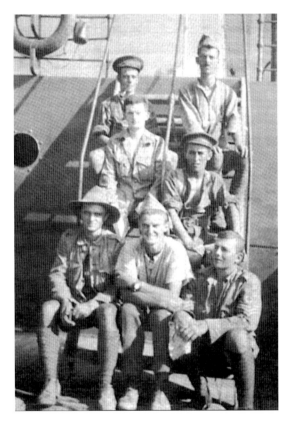

Medical students returning from Gallipoli on HMNZT *Tahiti*. Clockwise, from back left: W.T. Glasgow, L.H. Booth, S.T. Parker, G.P Fitzgerald, F.M. Spencer, R.L. Christie, A.W.T. O'Sullivan. They all graduated in 1917.
Photo, Christine Daniell, Montgomery Spencer collection.

in the throes of curriculum change, which made shortening the course problematic. As Ferguson pointed out to the Chancellor, it meant that four terms rather than three had to be fitted into a twelve-month period. The reduced staff also meant that extra administration fell on more junior members. At the same time there was a sharp rise in student numbers, which Ferguson put down to the fact students from the North Island could no longer study in Britain and had no option but to come to Otago.[11] When conscription was introduced in 1916, medical study at fourth and fifth year was classed as a reserved occupation. Third-year students were permitted to sit their examinations, but failure invalidated their exemption from service. After rumours of young men enrolling in the medical course to avoid the ballot began to circulate and cases of medical students receiving white feathers came to light, Ferguson mounted a strenuous defence of his students. He invited the new Director of Medical Services, regular Royal Army Medical Corps (RAMC) officer Surgeon-General R.S.F. Henderson, to address the School. He impressed on students that they could best serve their country by completing their studies, in order to maintain the vital supply of officers for the New Zealand Medical Corps. Henderson also recommended separating out medical and dental students into a special Officer University Training Corps and Malcolm, with the rank of Major, took over a newly energised unit, with a total strength of 113. By 1917, the Officers' Training Corps (Medical) comprised four officers and 130 other ranks. Twenty-two of its members joined the Expeditionary Force during that year.[12]

The Government was concerned not only about the shortage of doctors in New Zealand as a result of the war, but also about what it perceived to be the élitist background of medical students. The Minister of Public Health set aside £1000 to provide £100 bursaries to impoverished students. In his history of the Medical School, Carmalt Jones is dismissive of this attempt to 'democratise' the medical profession and is critical of the working of the scheme. Eventually, ten final-year bursaries, each worth £100, were taken up. However, the bursars complained that, by the time they had paid tuition fees and the high rate the Hospital Board charged for accommodation, they would have been better off as house surgeons at £2 a week. They were also bound to work for two years after graduation in public or mental hospitals. Under modified conditions, the scheme continued until 1921.[13]

Problems of staffing at the Medical School were acute and ongoing. There was a delay before Scott's replacement as Professor of Anatomy, Percy Gowland, arrived at the end of 1914. Sub-Dean Champtaloup took leave in 1915, to visit overseas medical schools. Colquhoun's health remained fragile. Early in 1915, Barnett was given leave to serve in the war. In his absence, lectures in surgery were given by Drs Stanley Batchelor, William Newlands and Sydney Allen. A new Chair in Clinical Pathology had been approved just before the outbreak of war and Dr Murray Drennan, from Edinburgh, was appointed in June 1915. However, he was serving with the Royal Army Medical Corps at the time and at once applied for leave to remain for the duration of the war. Marshall Macdonald, a highly respected teacher in the Department of Medicine, went to serve in France with the French Red Cross.[14] The point of crisis was reached in 1916. The number of students entering the Medical School had doubled from an average of thirty, to sixty a year. The Dean wrote to the Chancellor in April, informing him that Intermediate lectures had to be repeated and that the same would have to be done with anatomy and physiology at second year. Ferguson needed more room, more demonstrators and more equipment.[15] The pressure of teaching double classes, as well as his hospital and public health work, forced Champtaloup to resign the sub-deanship at the end of the year. When Stanley Batchelor became ill, Ferguson had no option but to recall Barnett and require Drennan to take up his appointment, which he did in October 1916.[16] The accommodation situation eased in 1917, when the new Pathology and Bacteriology building (now the Scott building) opened. Conscription also dramatically reduced numbers in some junior classes. While third-year students were exempt from military service, the call-up of

second years left that class reduced from some forty to a mere dozen, several of them women. Ferguson rightly predicted a shortage of male medical graduates when this class completed, in 1921.[17]

In November 1918, the very month the war ended, the great influenza pandemic struck New Zealand. Medical School staff, in practice or not, were called on to assist, and medical students were extensively employed. The seniors served as hospital residents, or in districts without doctors, and the juniors were employed as nurses. One described being sent to Waiuku, provided with a car and a list of patients, and left to cope. On one occasion, when he visited a remote Maori meeting house with the local policeman and chemist, he found the floor covered with bodies, some of them dead, and women cooking on little methylated spirit lamps.[18]

Influenza

'We had not been near the hospital (being our second year only) but were suddenly thrown in as emergency aides and "nurses" to cope with deficiencies and casualties in the regular staff. Most of the time I was on duty through the night, and the numerous fatal cases, for which seemingly little useful could be done, made a deep impression on my youthful spirit. It was a sudden and catastrophic introduction to hospital life and practice.'

Sir Douglas Robb, *Medical Odyssey. An Autobiography*, p. 27.

World War I marked a new stage in the development of the Otago Medical School. Morrell identifies the increased size and influence of the School within the University as a whole, as one of the most significant developments of the years 1914 to 1918. The war had meant crises of staffing and overcrowding but the need for medical graduates to serve with the fighting forces, or to replace doctors who were doing so, gave the Dean powerful leverage with the Government of the day. While the Medical School had its difficulties during the war, it also benefited from them.[19]

The Lessons of War and the Otago University Medical Company

World War I was a formative experience for the generation of men who became leaders of the Medical School in the interwar period. Hercus, who graduated from the Otago Medical School in 1914, was foremost in this group. After graduating, he at once enlisted in the New Zealand Medical Corps and served in a wide variety of theatres throughout the war. He assisted Colonel Ferdinand Batchelor in a venereal disease clinic in the red-light district of Cairo. He treated the sick and wounded in the misery of Gallipoli, where he saw the three-stage process for dealing with casualties – stabilisation at a field ambulance away from the front line, transfer to a casualty clearing station further back, and from there to a hospital. The hospitals were soon overwhelmed by the sheer numbers of casualties and dysentery and typhoid took hold. By August 1915, some 10 per cent of the New Zealanders were being evacuated each week. While serving with the Anzac Mounted Division in Palestine, Hercus was involved in urgent malaria control. In the first two weeks of October 1918 alone, the New Zealand Field Ambulance dealt with seven hundred cases. Hercus's military record gained him the DSO in 1917, five mentions in dispatches and an OBE in 1919. His service during the war also reinforced his commitment to preventive medicine and military medicine. He became Professor of Public Health in 1921 and began to revitalise the Otago University Medical Company in 1927.[20] Other senior Medical School staff also had wartime experience. Dudley Carmalt Jones, who came from England to take up the new Chair of Systematic Medicine in 1920, had met Hercus in the Sinai Desert when, as a consulting physician to the Egyptian Expeditionary Force, he made contact with the Anzac Mounted Division.[21] Barnett had worked in the thousand-bed New Zealand General Hospital in Cairo.[22] His successor as Professor of Surgery, Gordon Bell, spent four years as a military surgeon in Britain and France, was mentioned in dispatches and awarded the military cross for his front-line work at the Somme, movingly detailed in his autobiography, *Surgeon's Saga*. Murray Drennan came straight from service in the Royal Army Medical Corps (RAMC) to the new Chair of Pathology at Otago.[23]

These men had witnessed many of the medical advances stimulated by the war. Early in the conflict, for example, few of those who suffered abdominal wounds survived. However, by the end of the war, the survival rate increased to around fifty per cent, thanks to the practice of operating promptly on the wounds, then leaving them open to drain and irrigating them with antiseptics. Advances were made in the treatment of shock and the use of blood transfusions, which saved many lives. Bell mentions that, when the battle of Cambrai began in November 1917, his Casualty Clearing Station had forty pints of blood on hand and, although it was quickly used up, plenty more was available. The new field of plastic surgery dates from June 1917, when an Empire Centre at Sidcup in England was set up to treat the many thousands of war casualties who required prolonged reconstructive treatment. During World War I, orthopaedic surgery also developed apace.[24]

The advances do not seem to have had as significant an impact on teaching at the Otago Medical School as might have been expected. In 1923, for example, the Faculty recommended that a course of twelve lectures on the application of psychiatry to medicine should be included in the curriculum. However, this proved to be controversial and failed to eventuate.[25] On the other hand, it seemed likely that the field of plastic surgery would be established locally, as it had strong Dunedin connections. Sir Harold Gillies, the Dunedin-born and Cambridge-trained specialist in jaw and facial injuries, is regarded as the father of plastic surgery. In the thousand-bed hospital at Sidcup, Gillies and his colleagues carried out over 11,000 operations on more than 5000 war casualties. Dr Percy Pickerill, Dean of the Otago Dental School and also medically qualified, was in charge of the New Zealand section at the hospital. At the end of the war, with Red Cross support, arrangements were made for him to provide ongoing treatment in Dunedin for forty-three New Zealand patients from Sidcup.

For a time after the war, he carried on working with patients in Dunedin, at Woodside, the 'Jaw Hospital'. Pickerill's biographer, Harvey Brown, refers to him as one of a highly experienced, élite group of pioneers in the new discipline of plastic surgery. By 1920, however, most of the patients in Dunedin had been discharged and Pickerill returned to the Dental School. When he left Dunedin for Sydney in 1927, plastic surgery languished as a specialty.[26] One field that did take root at Otago after the war was orthopaedic surgery, which is associated with the wartime experience and teaching brilliance of James Renfrew White. White returned to the Medical School after treating war injuries to bones, joints, nerves and muscles at the Royal National Orthopaedic Hospital in London and with the RAMC in France. At first, he worked on wounded servicemen who had been brought home.[27]

The Otago University Medical Company

During the interwar period, a link between the Medical School and the military was maintained through the Otago University Medical Company.

This was due in large part to the foresight and energy of Hercus. No one better understood, or was more committed to, the specialised training required of medical officers. The medical section of the Officers' Training Corps came out of World War I with a fine reputation for high morale and efficiency. Its Roll of Honour includes 133 officers and seventy other ranks, of whom three officers and three other ranks lost their lives. Of the 385 New Zealand medical officers who served overseas, in locations as varied as Gallipoli, France, Sinai, Palestine, Syria, Macedonia, Egypt and Samoa, a large proportion were graduates of the School who had received their preliminary training in the Corps.[28] In recognition of their contribution to the war effort the Governor General, through Mr Allen, the Minister of Defence, offered the University money left over from the Hospital Ships Fund to erect a permanent base for training medical students in the 'medical sciences of war'. The Corps had requested such a headquarters in 1917 and the University gladly accepted the offer, contributing a site adjacent to the student union. The new hall was constructed in bluestone to match the original university buildings and

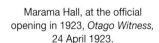

Marama Hall, at the official opening in 1923, *Otago Witness*, 24 April 1923.

Hocken Collections, Uare Taoka o Hakena, University of Otago, Acc. No. c/n E 3097/11 b.

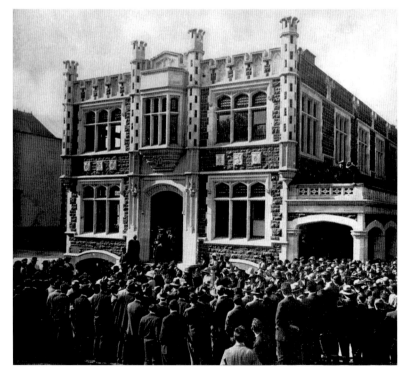

opened in 1923. At first named the Maheno and Marama Memorial Hall, after the two New Zealand hospital ships for which the money had been collected, the building later became known simply as Marama Hall.[29]

At the end of the war the medical unit of the Otago University Officers' Training Corps lost its impetus. According to Hercus, this was due to what he scathingly termed the 'inevitable reaction against all things military', that led to a strong swing towards pacifism in the University and the community. The Corps, in his view, 'fell upon evil days' with the abolition of compulsory military service and the resignations of Majors Malcolm, Ritchie and Gowland. The problem was not merely local. After the war, the New Zealand Medical Corps was left without a single full-time medical officer and the 2nd Field Ambulance ceased to function.[30] Within the Medical School it proved difficult to find a replacement for Major Malcolm and, following two brief appointments, Lt Col Hercus accepted the command in 1921. He found 'attendance at parades slack, uniforms sloppy and training for the certificates disappointing'.[31] At the end of 1921, before reforms could be put in place,

a low point was reached. The Defence Department terminated the unit as an Officers' Training Corps, turning it instead into the Medical Depot for the South Island Territorial system.

The revival of a unit for training medical students as medical officers came through the army. In August 1927, Hercus was made Assistant Director of Medical Services, Southern Command. Soon afterwards he was also appointed to the command of a reconstituted Officers' Training Corps, now named the Otago University Medical Company. Training was re-established on the lines laid down in 1916 and received an excellent response from medical and dental students. The Company continued successfully throughout the 1930s, despite the impact of the Depression. The key element was the annual camp, held over a fortnight in an isolated area. Basic military training was combined with special instruction in medical and dental military requirements. A camp library was established and the A and B certificate examinations were retained. When Hercus withdrew from the command in 1933, Lt Col R.A.H. Fulton took over and, in 1939, he was replaced by Major Iverach.[32]

CHAPTER 8

'A Monument in Bricks and Mortar'

A S FERGUSON neared retirement at the end of 1936, a Faculty minute of appreciation referred to the buildings erected during his deanship as a 'monument of bricks and mortar that [would] outlast generations.' Historians have concurred with this opinion. Carmalt Jones commented that Ferguson was not only 'always keenly interested in bricks and mortar' but possessed 'great imagination and sound judgment in everything he built in them'. Hercus and Bell surmised that a completely new medical school, envisioned as a whole and built in part – the Grand Plan – might have been the most outstanding of Ferguson's achievements.[1] The need for medical officers in World War I gave Ferguson leverage to secure government support for the Scott Building and the post-war growth in student numbers enabled him to build the New Medical School, which was later named after him. Although the most impressive, these buildings were by no means the only fruits of Ferguson's involvement in campaigns to provide an appropriate environment to teach the medical course at Otago. The object of his earliest campaign was the rebuilding of Dunedin Hospital, the last was the provision of a new maternity hospital.

The Scott Building, 1917

Well before Professor Scott's death it had become clear that there was an urgent need for increased accommodation at the Medical School. Classes were still held in the original University quadrangle building, completed in 1878 and substantially enlarged when Physiology gained its own professor in 1905. In that year, thirty-four students were enrolled in Physiology classes. By 1913, the roll had increased to sixty-one. There was not enough laboratory space and teaching was carried out under great difficulty. In 1912, the Inspector-General of Education, George Hogben, given the responsibility of reviewing the needs of the colleges of the University of New Zealand, agreed that the School needed new buildings and equipment and recommended a grant of £11,000. Early in 1913, the Medical Faculty, in consultation with the Chief Health Officer and Inspector General of Hospitals, Dr Valintine, put forward two schemes: one was to enlarge the Departments of Anatomy and Physiology on the University site; the other was to construct a completely new building, mainly for Pathology and Bacteriology, but also for a range of other subjects which were being taught in cramped conditions in the Hospital. These included materia medica, public health, medical jurisprudence, medicine, surgery, midwifery and gynaecology. The Faculty meeting of May 1913 affirmed the need for both developments. In March 1914, the Government gave a grant of £10,000 for the anatomy/physiology extensions, which duly went ahead.[2]

The pathology/bacteriology building was a larger undertaking. First of all, the site proved controversial. Ferguson, who had taken a lead in the Faculty on this issue even before he became Dean, was determined to have the building

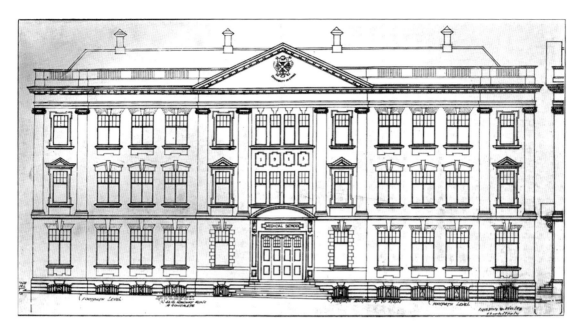

Architectural drawing of the New Medical School (Scott Building), 1916.
Descriptive Syllabus of the Medical School, 1916, p. 8. Medical Library, University of Otago.

situated on Great King Street, opposite the Hospital. He met bitter opposition from some members of the University Council, who wanted any development to be on the University site, but he had a powerful ally in the Chancellor, the Reverend Andrew Cameron. When two cottages opposite the Hospital came up for auction, Cameron used his authority to purchase the properties for the Medical School. Adjacent land was also made available by the Hospital Board, which had taken out an option on it. 'I cannot adequately express what I owed to the Chancellor for his support through many years until his death', Ferguson wrote later.[3]

To finance the proposed building, the University Council decided to raise money through a public appeal, tapping in to that local support which had been demonstrated so wholeheartedly to the University in 1903 and the Hospital in 1910. The target was £7500, which would qualify for an equal subsidy from government. In March 1914, Champtaloup produced a pamphlet which ran under the headline, 'The Otago Medical School Proposed Extensions. An Appeal to the Citizens. Wanted £7500.' The pamphlet brought together items written for the *Otago Daily Times* by some

of the most influential of the Medical School staff. The Chancellor urged contributions to 'an object worthy of the support of all classes'. Malcolm, who was Acting Dean at the time, explained the need for 'an increased area' to train medical students. Champtaloup provided specific information on the overcrowding in his own classes in public health, where in 1913 there were thirty-one students but only sixteen seats. He argued strongly against trying to solve the problem by extending existing accommodation. Batchelor was interviewed on the growing importance of bacteriology and Colquhoun added his considerable weight to emphasise the extent to which all the departments of the School were hampered by lack of space. The pamphlet was widely distributed and is likely to have contributed materially to the enthusiastic response to the appeal from the press, the city and the province. In a short time, a total of just over £10,000 was raised.[4]

As Sub-Dean, Champtaloup visited a number of overseas medical schools in 1915 to get ideas for the building. He then drew up specifications for a three-storey quadrangular building, with a basement for storage and animal houses on the roof. Most of the ground floor was to be given over to lecture rooms, student facilities, offices and the museum. The first floor would house the Department of Pathology, the library, the professor's room and laboratory and the materia medica museum. The top floor would be home to Bacteriology and would include a large laboratory and some smaller ones, the professor's room and laboratory and various service rooms. The estimated cost was £13,000. Architects Mason and Wales, who provided a sketch plan, raised the estimate to £14,200. In the event, this sum also proved too low, as trouble with the foundations eventually raised the total cost of the building to £20,000. Meantime, the number of entry-year students doubled from thirty to sixty and looked likely to stabilise near the higher figure, which meant that a scheme to economise, by leaving the third storey vacant, had to be abandoned. Despite delays due to the war, and a proposal from the Department of Education that all works should be suspended for the duration, the foundation stone was laid on 1 June 1916 and the building was completed within a year.[5]

In August 1916, Champtaloup produced a descriptive syllabus for the Medical School. Comprehensive, well illustrated and easy to read, it must have been a very good marketing tool. In addition to a brief note on the School's history, details of the medical course at all levels and information on student facilities, such as the new Union building and accommodation in the residential colleges, the syllabus contains a description of the recently extended facilities for Physiology and of the still-to-be-completed building for Bacteriology and Pathology. Champtaloup's enthusiasm for the new facilities shines through his writing. The Physiology Department now had about twenty rooms in all, arranged to serve its practical classes. They included two large and well-equipped laboratories, each capable of accommodating about fifty students, with a working space of four feet for each student at fully appointed benches. There was also an experimental room with apparatus to record the heart, pulse, respiration, muscle etc., preparation and store rooms for histological, chemical and experimental work, a workshop with an electrically driven lathe,

animal rooms and demonstration rooms.[6] The syllabus included an architect's drawing of the façade of the new pathology/bacteriology block. The Pathology Department would have ample accommodation and its classrooms would be fitted with every facility for teaching and research. The students would also have the advantage of a large museum, where specimens might be seen permanently preserved in their natural colours. The lecture rooms would be provided with lantern, cinematograph and epidiascope. There would be a new post-mortem block.[7]

The New Medical School was formally opened on 2 April 1917, in front of a very large crowd. Appropriately, it was Acting Prime Minister Sir James Allen, former Chancellor of the University of Otago and a loyal friend of the Medical School, who did the honours. Sir James spoke of the need for more junior staff for the Medical School and of the need to provide the opportunity for staff to engage in research. Ferguson then took the opportunity, as he so often did, to talk about money. He told his audience that the development of the School to date had required a great deal of money, but that demands would be even greater in the future. Laughter greeted his remark that if the School ceased to demand money, it was a sign it was moribund.[8]

As World War I drew to a close, a new Medical School and an extensively rebuilt and modernised Hospital faced each other across Great King Street, ready to enter the brave new postwar world together.

The Lindo Ferguson Building

Satisfying as the new Bacteriology and Pathology building must have been to him, Ferguson was not one to rest on his laurels. As returned servicemen swelled the postwar classes and the anatomy and physiology classes outgrew their recently enlarged accommodation, he used the pressure on resources to push for a new building. It soon became evident that siting the Scott Building opposite the Hospital had not resolved the debate over where the heart of the Medical School should lie. Strong opposition to another Medical School building in Great King Street emerged in the University Council. By mid-1919, the dispute had become heated. Despite Ferguson's advocacy of a site next to the Scott Building, the University Council voted in favour of placing the extensions in the main University area. The *Otago Daily Times*, frustrated that the Council was dealing with the matter in committee, strongly supported a Great King Street site. It described the Anatomy and Physiology Building as 'the corollary of the erection of the bacteriology and pathology block in that street' and even forecast a future link between the proposed building and the Hospital by either a subway or an overhead bridge.[9] At a special meeting of the University Council, a deputation of twenty representatives, from the Otago Branch of the British Medical Association, the Faculty of Medicine and the honorary medical staff of the Hospital, expressed their support for the Great King Street site. Barnett, their spokesman, outlined the advantages that had been gained from grouping pathology, bacteriology and public health near the Hospital. The Dunedin Hospital, he said, was 'the hub of the New Zealand medical students' scholastic universe'. The Council backed down, rescinded its previous resolution and accepted the Great King Street site. In 1920, Ferguson vetoed a proposal to build a new Dental School on the same block and secured a grant from the Director of Education to purchase the land on the northern part of the block as far as the corner. It was a clear statement of future intentions.[10]

The finance to erect a major building at this time – and Ferguson's plans were ambitious –was not easy to obtain. The Medical School sent a high-level deputation to Wellington to interview the Prime Minister and the Minister of Education and they elicited a promise of £75,000, to be given in instalments. It was the first of many such fund-raising expeditions, which were led by the Dean and took three days, most of which were spent on the train and inter-island ferry. Ferguson relished the comment that his role was to educate successive Ministers of Education on the needs of the Medical School.[11] Changes in the plans of the proposed building led to increased expenditure, which took ten years' determined effort to raise. It eventually cost £112,000, including equipment.

Carmalt Jones, who worked for many years with Ferguson and admired him greatly, wrote that he could 'approach Ministers and command attention as no other member of the staff could have done'.[12] When describing Sir Lindo's tactics in eliciting government money, Jones broke the steady pattern of his year-by-year narrative of the *Annals of the Otago Medical School* with a personal, openly gleeful comment:

> One follows with delight his successive requests, first for the site. It is of the utmost importance to secure the site, otherwise a gasworks is sure to be built upon it. The site, yes; but what is the good of a site? Let us have the shell; we ask for no more than the shell. But, after all, a shell must deteriorate rapidly unless the building is completed. And a completed building, eating its head off, so to speak, without equipment. One sees the victim, as in Leech's old *Punch* picture, at last saying wearily, 'Oh, give us the pen.'[13]

The foundation stone was laid in June 1925, with some ceremony. The University Council and staff in academic dress walked in procession from the University to Great King Street. In his address the Minister of Education, Sir James Parr, stressed the national character of the Medical School, and commented that since this building would cost at least £100,000, including equipment, another medical school was not likely at the present time. As a loyal Aucklander, he added, 'No doubt Auckland's day will come, but not yet.' Both he and Ferguson laid foundation stones and Hercus, as Sub-Dean, deposited a casket containing miscellaneous items, a history of the University, the day's newspapers and some coins. The dignity of the occasion was probably somewhat marred by a large number of students, who 'enlivened proceedings with comments and untimely applause', and by a downpour part way through.[14]

Just over a week later Ferguson presented the Chancellor with a full report on his plans, already approved by Faculty, for the future development of the Medical School. Because they either required more space or affected usage of the existing accommodation, most of the developments involved buildings. Ferguson predicted, for example, that the medicine of the future would require a deeper knowledge of biochemistry. Accordingly, when the new building was occupied, Biochemistry would need to become a sub-department of Physiology and would require more teaching staff. Preventive Medicine likewise had to expand because it was probable that much of the medicine of the future would be preventive rather than curative. Ferguson advocated encouraging senior staff into research, which would mean additional laboratories and more junior teachers, with better pay, to free up their time. He also dealt directly with immediate questions of accommodation and equipment, such as the need to transform the rooms temporarily allotted to the Professors of Medicine and Surgery into research laboratories. The report gradually led up to Ferguson's chief proposal, a series of Medical School buildings stretching right along the block of Great King Street opposite the Hospital. These included a purpose-built, staffed library, 'a very important essential for any School'. The facility, he argued, would need to be 'about as large as the present buildings' and would require a large reading room, capable of accommodating a couple of hundred students, a book stack and a reading room for members of the profession. Other buildings Ferguson thought necessary were a new post-mortem block and a building for the biological departments, on the north side of the Anatomy and Physiology Building to enable close cooperation. Another new block, to the south of the present buildings and reaching to the Albany Street corner, would house the Public Health Department and serve for the teaching of public health and preventive medicine. Eventually, a block for research work to the north of the library block would be required. A hostel for final-year students would have to be built, close to the Hospital, and accommodation was needed for students doing their maternity work. In establishing priorities for the building programme, Ferguson suggested that the post-mortem and preventive medicine blocks should probably be erected first, then the library. He was well aware of the resource implications of his plan, concluding:

[T]he School will continue to fulfil a most valuable part in the life of the community, with increasing efficiency but at increasing cost. The completion will call for further buildings which, apart from the hostel, will probably cost £100,000 or more; and in the not distant future necessary additions to the teaching and auxiliary staff and their adequate payments with the foundation and maintenance of a library and other maintenance costs will swell our annual budget from £16,000 to £25,000 a year.[15]

The new Anatomy and Physiology Building was opened in February 1927 by the Hon. Downie Stewart. It had already been the admired venue for the Triennial Australasian Congress. Designed by architect Edmund Anscombe, and built in brick with facings of Oamaru stone, it consisted of four floors and a basement. In their book on Dunedin architecture, Hardwicke Knight and Niel Wales describe its façade as 'dignified but economic' with an entrance above street level approached by steps from both sides. They admire the spacious, attractively proportioned interior, with its wide corridors and broad stairways. When it opened, even the students were impressed. The *Review* described the building as a 'massive structure, with signs of some architectural beauty'. It added, with evident satisfaction, and echoing what Parr had said when the foundation stone was laid, that with '£125,000 worth of bricks and mortar deposited in King Street', it would be many years before the Government would sanction the establishment of a second medical school.

'The impression that remains with me is one of large, empty rooms, many of which were seldom used.'

Professor Norman Edson, in 1927 a junior assistant in the Physiology Department, undated typescript, private collection.

The ground floor was given over to student facilities, with a canteen and separate common rooms for male and female students, some accommodation for Physiology, a large room, adjacent laboratory and secretarial room for the Professors of Medicine and Obstetrics

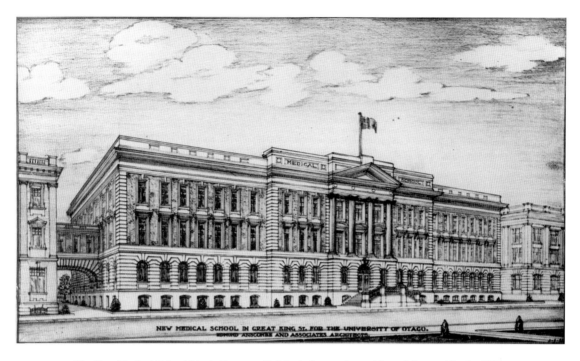

The New Medical School (Lindo Ferguson Building), Anscombe and Associates, architects, 1926.
Hocken Collections, Uare Taoka o Hakena, University of Otago, S05-177a.

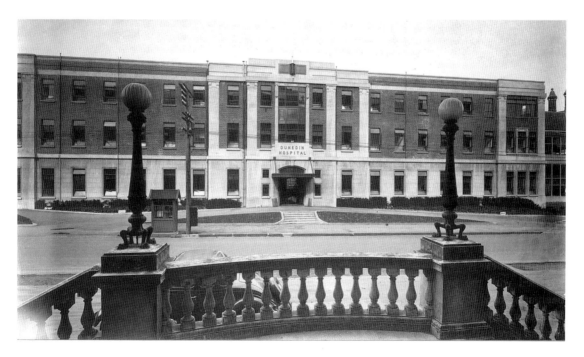

The new Dunedin Hospital Building, 1936, photographed from the steps of the Lindo Ferguson Building. By the 1930s the old hospital was seriously dilapidated and turrets had had to be removed from the towers for safety reasons. This replacement three-storey concrete building (*ground floor*: reception and casualty; *first floor*: wards; *top floor*: ear, nose and throat facilities) increased hospital beds to 330. There was further hospital building, including new lecture theatres, in 1936.
Archives New Zealand, Te Rua Mahara o te Kāwanatanga, Dunedin Regional Office – DAHI/272/140.

and Gynaecology, and a retiring room for the Professor of Surgery. The second floor contained the Department of Physiology and Biochemistry, as well as several research laboratories. The upper floors housed Anatomy and Histology and included the Anatomy Museum and a large dissecting room. The Anatomy and Physiology Building was the great achievement of Ferguson's 'master plan', permitting the development and consolidation of teaching and research at the School. It is entirely fitting that this fine building, the end result of his formidable diplomatic skills, should have been named after him.[16]

The rest of the master plan, for a self-contained, modern Medical School, which would occupy the whole of the block of Great King Street opposite the hospital, was for the future, some of it for the distant future. In 1925 Ferguson added some detail to the broad brush picture he had painted for the Chancellor. To cope with increased specialisation and subdivision in clinical subjects, for example, there would need to be private rooms and laboratories for clinical professors in midwifery and gynaecology, medicine, orthopaedics, military surgery and psychological medicine. Generally, his view was remarkably far-sighted. As it has turned out, perhaps the only major feature of Ferguson's plans that has not eventuated were the well-tended lawns in which he set his imagined future Medical School.[17]

Obstetrics and Ophthalmology

For most of the interwar period a notable exception to the provision of satisfactory facilities for medical training at Otago related to obstetrics. This was due to a serious shortage of maternity cases for student instruction, which was not a new issue. Ferdinand Batchelor had wrestled with the problem ever since he had been appointed to lecture in midwifery in 1883. In the early years of his teaching career most women gave birth at home and only the indigent were hospitalised, at the Benevolent Institute in the suburb of Caversham, well away from the Medical School. Even if the lecturer and the student could get there in time for the birth, there were not enough cases to satisfy the requirement

that each student should attend and conduct nine deliveries. In 1887, Batchelor organised a successful domiciliary scheme, paid for by the University Council and based at the Dunedin Hospital. However, when the General Medical Council (GMC) increased their demands for each student's deliveries to twelve, the School once again found itself lacking sufficient cases. The establishment of the St Helen's Maternity Hospital in 1905 did not help the situation, as the hospital was intended for the training of midwives and excluded medical students. In 1907, before his retirement, Batchelor pushed through the conversion of a female refuge in Forth Street, near the University, to a twelve (later sixteen) bed establishment, the Batchelor Hospital. Although some extra cases were provided by the Salvation Army Home, Redroofs, this was still the situation regarding student maternity training when the war broke out in 1914. After the war, pressure again mounted. On the one hand, on top of the influx of students, the GMC recommended that each student should attend twenty births. On the other hand, women began to move away from home births, instead choosing the reduction in pain offered by hospitalised childbirth.[18]

From the late 1920s until Ferguson retired, the need for a modern maternity hospital to provide the training in obstetrics for medical students required by the GMC was to the forefront of his concerns. In his 1928 annual report, he described the situation clearly and at some length. Although the Health Department had made the St Helen's Hospital available to medical students, both the St Helen's and Forth Street hospitals were also training schools for midwives, who each required twenty deliveries. As a consequence, the number of births was simply not enough to train the midwives as well as the medical students. The Health Department 'very kindly undertook to abolish the training of midwives in Dunedin' by cancelling the Batchelor Hospital as an approved training centre. While this helped increase the numbers of deliveries available to medical students, it did not meet the GMC's additional requirements that each student should spend a month in residence in a lying-in hospital, devote some time to antenatal clinics and study gynaecological conditions resulting from maternity. Ferguson argued that the two existing hospitals, which were both converted dwellings, should be replaced by one central institution where the teaching was in the hands of University staff. Since the Health Department was sympathetic, he was optimistic that they would soon see an up-to-date maternity hospital near the main Hospital. The next year, he reported with satisfaction that the Government had placed £50,000 on the estimates for a new maternity hospital.[19] Ferguson's optimism proved to be misplaced. By 1930, a row had broken out over the site of the proposed hospital and the question of medical student access. An active lobby wanted the hospital closed to medical students. Furthermore, the University Council and the Hospital Board, on the one hand, and the Faculty and hospital staff, on the other, were deadlocked over whether it should be near the hospital or some distance away, in London Street. Although a special committee recommended a site near the Hospital, the Council and Board refused to adopt its report. The Minister of Health planned to investigate for himself, but there was no provision for the building on the year's estimates and the whole scheme was 'hung up for a period one [could not] foresee'. In his annual report, Ferguson's sense of frustration is palpable. 'If a decision had been arrived at promptly twelve months ago', he wrote, 'the building would have been three parts completed.'[20]

The delays proved longer than could have been foreseen, because at this point the Depression intervened. In 1931 there was a general reduction in expenditure and, over the next two years, the 'most crying need of the School' remained in limbo. The site was no longer the issue, as it was agreed that the hospital should be adjacent to the nurses' home in Castle Street. The problem was now one of finance. Ferguson was clearly heartily sick of the long-drawn-out process and the complexity of the seemingly endless negotiations. He wrote in 1933:

> It is particularly unfortunate that in New Zealand the training of the medical profession should be influenced by the decisions of so many unrelated bodies and individuals. The question of a maternity hospital depends on the decision of the Minister for Health, while the grant for School purposes comes out of the amount controlled by the Minister for Education. The question of hospital expenditure depends on the Hospital Board, which naturally resists any tendency to increase in their expenditure attributable in any way to the presence of the School. The University Council, which is naturally the body in charge of the School, has really very little say in the matter.

He thought the Government was deliberately postponing its financial commitment and trying to shift costs on to the Hospital Board:

> To put the matter briefly, the efficiency of our teaching and training of the profession of the future is at present being prejudiced by a haggle between the Minister of Health and the Hospital Board as to whether a few thousand pounds should come out of the general revenue of the country ... or should be a charge on the ratepayers of Dunedin.[21]

Over the next two years, the division of the cost was agreed on, plans were drawn up and approved in Wellington, the site was cleared and building finally began. The foundation stone was laid in November 1936, a matter of weeks before Ferguson's retirement and it must have been with a sense of satisfaction that he could write in his last report, at the end of that year, that the construction of the maternity hospital was now far advanced.[22] In November 1937 the Minister of Health Peter Fraser opened the Queen Mary Maternity Hospital. Although students were guaranteed access, it had only twenty-six beds rather than the forty originally planned. Professor Dawson of Obstetrics and Gynaecology, who had been appalled by conditions in the Batchelor Hospital when he arrived in 1932 and had lobbied hard for a much larger, up-to-date replacement, called the reduction in size a 'short-sighted, cheese-paring policy'. He criticised the hospital as being too small, even before it was finished, but he also welcomed it as a modern hospital with living quarters for house surgeons and six students. In 1938, the St Helen's and Batchelor Hospitals

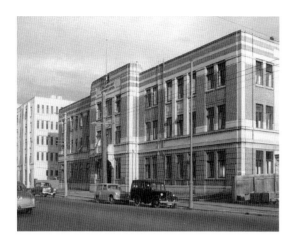

Queen Mary Maternity Hospital, 1937.
Archives New Zealand, Te Rua Mahara o te Kāwanatanga,
Dunedin Regional Office – DAHI/D274/193.

closed. Angus calls the new Queen Mary Hospital the most important development in hospital services between 1927 and 1941. He also credits Ferguson with leading the University through the tangled negotiations to bring it to pass. For the Medical School it was a satisfying conclusion to a long-standing and intractable problem.[23]

Throughout his deanship, Ferguson remained head of Ophthalmology at the Hospital, a total of fifty-two years. It is therefore fitting to end this narrative of his contribution to the fabric of the Medical School in his own department. Since 1926, the honorary medical staff had sought new facilities for the eye, ear, nose and throat department, on the grounds that at least a fifth of the operations carried out at the Hospital were ophthalmic. The provision of these facilities came as part of a major rebuilding of the last remaining section of the exhibition building. By the 1930s, the central block of the building, still used for administration, was deemed so unsafe that its turrets were removed. The Hospital Board replaced this section with a three-storey building that served as the administrative centre for the Hospital. This opened in 1936 and contained reception, offices and casualty on the ground floor, wards on the second, and facilities for eye, ear, nose and throat on the third. The eye ward was named in honour of Ferguson who, in a final gesture, performed the first operation there.[24]

It was typical of Ferguson that, on the occasion of his last University Council meeting, on 17 March 1937, instead of basking in the warmth of the praise heaped upon him, together with the new title of Emeritus Professor, he should have taken the opportunity to deliver a sharp lecture on the needs of the Medical School. Aware that it would be fully reported in the press, he said, the School had been treated as a Cinderella and those interested in its progress had worked under great difficulties. Looking back at what he had done for the School, he commented, 'It is not what has been done, but that which has not been done that has been hurting me so much.' At the forefront of his mind were the new buildings that had been deferred or denied. There had been a long delay in building the new maternity hospital and two lecture theatres in the Hospital block. And, after twelve years' lobbying, the Medical School still lacked its own library. The Council might accuse him of showing his Irish temper, he said, but he was frustrated by 'red tape'. During the long period he had been on the Council, he had differed very strongly with various members. 'In the many fights I have run foul of the prejudices of others not so interested in the Medical School as I was. I have had to fight very hard for the Medical School.' And, he added, 'There are a good many points on which I have struggled with the Council, and they will have to be fought over again by Dr Hercus.'[25]

In spite of the hectoring tone of this final address to Council, Ferguson had reason to be proud of the built heritage he left to the School. When he died in 1948, a tribute in the *New Zealand Medical Journal* affirmed that 'the great monument to his life's work stands in King Street, Dunedin.' It is likely the writer had in mind the building named after Ferguson and the adjacent Scott Building, imposing frontages along the Medical School side of the street. However, it is worth recalling the extent of his contribution to the buildings on the other side of the street as well, the block containing the Dunedin Hospital, the nurses' home and Queen Mary Maternity Hospital. The whole is indeed an impressive 'monument in bricks and mortar'.[26]

CHAPTER 9

Expansion and Modernisation

AS STUDENT numbers in the School rose during the interwar period, from 150 in 1914 to 422 in 1936, and the Medical Faculty took on the responsibility of teaching health-related courses for dental, home science and physiotherapy students, staff numbers also increased. In 1914, Ferguson had inherited several part-time professors, recently promoted from part-time lectureships. However, this did not mean that the staffing situation was static. There were replacements over subsequent years in some of these chairs, which became full-time positions. A number of subjects were also reorganised to reflect a changing emphasis in teaching. To consider the professors: after Ferdinand Batchelor resigned as Professor of Midwifery in 1909, there was no professor in that field until 1928, when Riley was promoted for the last couple of years of his working life. Champtaloup ceased his work as Government Health Officer in 1914, when he was appointed full-time Professor of Bacteriology and Public Health, and he also became Sub-Dean. New appointees, Percy Gowland in Anatomy and Murray Drennan to the new Chair of Pathology, arrived in 1915 and 1916 respectively. Drennan also took on Medical Jurisprudence after Ogston died in 1917. Although the pressures of the wartime environment obscured the extent of the changes, by around 1920 it was evident that a whole new, young and well-qualified team was in place. Most of these men served the School throughout the interwar period. From 1920, the long-established local, Frank Fitchett and the English newcomer, Dudley Carmalt Jones, shared the professoriate of Medicine. Hercus succeeded Champtaloup as Professor of Bacteriology in 1921. Barnett was the last of the older generation to retire, in 1924, and his generosity enabled the establishment of a new part-time Chair in Surgery, which was filled by Gordon Bell. Eric D'Ath replaced Drennan in Pathology in 1928. Bernard Dawson, who became Professor of Obstetrics and Gynaecology in 1931, was the last of Ferguson's professorial appointments.[1]

Even more important than professorial appointments, in Ferguson's view, was the development of 'a service of junior teachers', promising men who could be retained by the prospect of a career path with salary increases, leading to lectureships and associate-professorships. He complained that if his budget was twice as large as it was, he could spend it to immediate advantage in paying his staff adequately.[2] Most of the appointments to this second tier of staff were Otago graduates and some gave outstanding service, but they proved difficult to retain. John Cairney, Gowland's assistant in anatomy, for instance, who was made the first Associate-Professor, the only one during the Ferguson period, found the salary inadequate and moved on. Muriel Bell lectured in physiology for some years. New appointments were made in response to developing areas. In the aftermath of the war, Percy Pickerill developed plastic surgery, and James Renfrew White orthopaedics.

In 1928, Marion Whyte became the first lecturer in anaesthesia. The increase in the number of lecturers and more junior staff over the period is striking. Eight new appointments, excluding honorary hospital staff, are listed in the 1914 calendar and thirty-four in 1937.[3] In 1925, Gordon Bell noted that behind the modest brick and mortar façade of the young institution a 'new ferment was brewing which in the next thirty years was to change the whole character of the school. Its original, almost entirely vocational character gave way to a combination of teaching and research as spatial resources and more liberal staffing encouraged and facilitated original investigation.' Bell credited this change to the Dean. By the mid-1920s, Ferguson was the single active representative of the original teaching staff. He had begun practice before most of his young colleagues were born.[4]

One of the most important aspects of the more cosmopolitan outlook of the Otago Medical School under Ferguson was increased overseas travel by staff. Ferguson himself was a firm believer in the value of learning from other medical schools. He had intended following up his 1914 investigation of the methods and curricula of medical schools in Australia with a tour, the following year, of schools in Britain and America. He had also planned to use 1916 to implement the ideas gathered on these tours at Otago and to retire in 1917. Although the war upset this schedule, it did not prevent him sending Champtaloup to visit overseas medical schools to get ideas for the proposed Otago building. It was 1924 before Ferguson himself could embark on an extensive tour of American schools. He spent 1927 in Britain, where he 'did all the London and many provincial schools'. Each evening he would write to Hercus about anything he thought should be recorded. (This habit died hard: during his post-retirement year in England in 1937, he continued to visit medical schools and write to Hercus about them.) The annual reports of the interwar period routinely note the comings and goings of staff. In 1925, for example, it was recorded that Drennan and Fitchett had returned from visits to Europe, bringing with them much information which would be of value

to their departments. Ferguson believed their European perspective would supplement the extensive information he himself had brought back from America. In 1929, Gowland travelled for fifteen months on a Rockefeller Fellowship which enabled him to 'get in touch with the anatomical work in every School of importance in the world'. In 1931, before taking up his duties in Dunedin as Professor of Obstetrics, Bernard Dawson was instructed to make a six-month tour of obstetrical and gynaecological units in Britain, Europe and North America, while on full pay. In 1936, Mr Renfrew White and Dr Marjorie Barclay were recorded as having visited various overseas orthopaedic and radiological clinics respectively.[5]

If the style of the interwar Medical School was more expansive, it was also more expensive. Through Ferguson's skill in eliciting money, from government and from private donors, the School budget, £10,000 when he became Dean, had tripled to £30,000 by the time he retired, and private donations added £85,000 to this sum. New buildings in his time cost £150,000. Ferguson was, of course, not satisfied and considered the funding of the School to be meagre in comparison with similar institutions overseas. This was a recurring theme of his annual reports. In his 1928 report, for example, after his visits to British schools the previous year, he claimed the Otago Medical School was 'starved in a manner which does not indicate any very keen appreciation of its needs on the part of the Education Department.' He compared its total budget, which at the time was slightly over £19,000, with those of comparable schools in Britain, which received from £30,000 a year to a probable £100,000. In 1929, he backed up his claim by listing the names of staff who had left for better paid positions and commented that the School's salary scale throughout was below the market rate. The University of Sydney, he said, was appointing a Professor of Bacteriology at £1500 a year, compared to the £1000 paid at Otago for the joint Chairs of Bacteriology and Public Health. The situation worsened as the country moved into the Depression. In 1931, when the School, in common with the whole education system, was forced to cut expenditure, Ferguson thought retrenchment had gone 'about as far as [was] possible, consistent with efficiency'. 'It is much to be hoped', he added, 'that there will be some early improvement in the financial position of the University, as a Medical School which is not progressing is going backwards'. It cannot be too widely known that our School is run on exceedingly economical lines and that our annual budget is not more than two thirds of that of an English School of the same importance'.

To supplement government funding, Ferguson carefully nurtured a number of special funds. Three dated from 1920: the Dean's fund, which attracted an equal government subsidy, was to aid research, purchase apparatus or additions to the library or add in any way to the efficiency and satisfactory working of the School; the Sir Louis Barnett fund of £1000, also with a government subsidy, was for the general benefit of the School and the Sir John Roberts fund, of the same amount, was intended to promote research, especially in clinical medicine. In 1929, the Chamberlain and Colquhoun fund was set up, with the principal sum of £12,000 donated by Chamberlain, and a fund was established to make small loans to needy senior medical students. In 1930–31, Ferguson took immense satisfaction in the 'wonderful effort' of the Obstetrical Society, which endowed a fourth chair, to be added to those in physiology, medicine and surgery. The Society raised enough money for both a chair and a travelling scholarship in obstetrics. Nevertheless, at the same time Ferguson was quick to point out (and to repeat in his annual reports from then on) that obstetrics could only be developed if a new maternity hospital was provided.[6]

Research

Limitations on time and funding meant that research was not a strength of the Medical School under Ferguson, but it was not totally ignored. Malcolm, Barnett, Champtaloup, Drennan and Hercus all maintained research programmes and a number of research fellows were employed at the School during this time. The impact of the war, and the disastrous influenza pandemic that followed, stimulated interest in medical research. In 1920, when the Department of Public Health was replaced by a Department of Health under a Director-General, it was entrusted with promoting or carrying out research in matters concerning public health and the prevention of disease. The transfer of the School Medical Service and the School Dental Service to the Department of Health boosted research in the epidemiological field.[7] Hercus's research into goitre began before he joined the staff of the Medical School. In 1921, while he was working for the School Medical Service in Canterbury, he and Dr Eleanor Baker conducted a survey of 15,000 school children. Their results linked the varying prevalence of childhood goitre in Christchurch and Lyttelton to the low iodine content of the local soil. This greatly impressed the Director-General of Health and led to the iodisation of domestic salt in 1924 and an ongoing, expanded research programme.[8] Malcolm received modest financial assistance from the Government through the New Zealand Institute for his nutrition-related research. In 1919, he was able to use £250 from the Department of Internal Affairs to employ a researcher to investigate the nutritional value of New Zealand fish. By 1926, his department had received £650 in research funding.[9] Malcolm also introduced the use of rats and chemical methods for vitamin assays. Given special permission to import twenty Wistar rats in 1922, he had to explain how they had become forty by the time they arrived.[10]

In 1925, a Royal Commission on University Education in New Zealand recommended increased financial support for the Medical School. While most of this was absorbed by the additional staffing needed to cope with the growth in student numbers, between 1926 and 1937 a total of £10,000 was directed toward research, enabling longer-term projects.[11] Thanks to the formation of a New Zealand branch of the British Empire Cancer Campaign in 1930, Dr A. M. Begg was able to set up a cancer research laboratory in the Medical School.[12] The University's annual list of benefactions show that a number of donations were tagged for medical research. In 1920, Sir John Roberts, Sir Lindo Ferguson and Dr Louis Barnett each gave £1000 and throughout the decade there were five more donations, of amounts ranging from £100 to £1000, sometimes specifically for cancer research. During the mid-1920s, several research fellows were employed. A government grant enabled Dr Hector to work under Hercus on poliomyelitis until 1926, when the waning of the epidemic necessitated a change of direction. After studying pollens, Hector transferred to the Health Department in 1928. Other research fellows listed were Dr Steenson, who conducted research into arthritis and Dr Fulton, who did statistical work relating to cancer. Hercus and Drennan collaborated on research into tuberculosis and goitre. In the financially straitened circumstances of the early 1930s, however, mention of research disappears from the annual reports.[13]

In 1922, Carmalt Jones drew together the various published research papers from the School in the first issue of the *Proceedings of the University of Otago Medical School*. At first, the University Council refused a request for £100 to produce the volume, but when staff contributed £40, it agreed to make up the difference. Following issues were financed from Dr Barnett's fund. The first print run was just a hundred, made up of papers already published in the *New Zealand Medical Journal*, with a few from the *British Medical Journal* and *The Lancet*. Carmalt Jones continued to edit the *Proceedings* until 1940. He believed that it was particularly useful in bringing together the work done in the School on goitre and hydatids. The publication was sent to a number of British and American medical schools.[14]

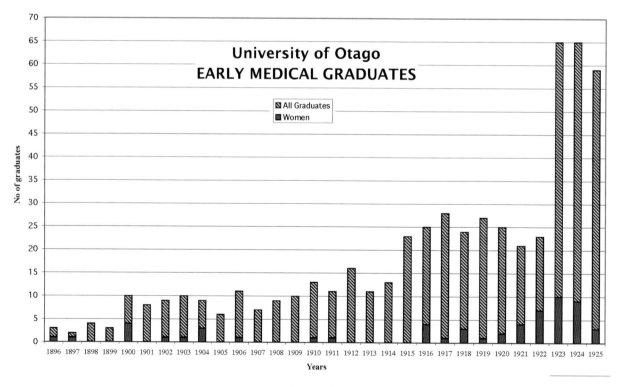

Student numbers to 1925.

Teachers and Teaching

In 1920, in the aftermath of World War I and amidst the influx of returned servicemen studying medicine, the Deans of the four Australasian medical schools met and agreed to extend the medical course in their schools to six years. The change was controversial and the New Zealand branch of the British Medical Association agreed only on condition that the final year would be spent entirely on clinical work. After approval by the Otago Medical Faculty, the University Council and the Senate of the University of New Zealand, the scheme came into operation in the Otago Medical School in 1923. The first year of the new course was a general 'intermediate' year of physics, chemistry and biology, which could lead to a medical course, to other professional courses such as dentistry, or a general science degree. The medical course proper began in second year and consisted of two pre-clinical years, with anatomy, physiology, biochemistry and pharmacology, followed by hospital-based clinical training. The curriculum proved satisfactory in that it ushered in a long period of stability, in terms of the subjects taught and the allocation of teaching and examination time, although it was constantly reviewed in detail by conferences and committees to ensure compliance with the recommendations of the General Medical Council in England.[15]

The clinical sixth year agreed to by the Deans posed a problem for the Otago School because the Dunedin Hospital did not have enough patients (referred to as 'clinical material') to cope with the increased number of students. In 1923, a crisis arose when forty-one students failed their final examination and were required to obtain more clinical experience. In response, the School adopted an innovative solution by arranging for the students to receive extra training at Christchurch Hospital until they could sit a special final examination, which most passed. Over the next few years the use of other major hospitals for final-year training was extended. The class was split and groups were sent to Auckland and Wellington as well as Christchurch. The innovation would have a remarkable future. It laid the foundation for Branch Faculties, which in time would in time evolve into the University of Otago Schools of Medicine and Health Sciences in Christchurch and Wellington, and eventually eased the establishment of a medical school in Auckland.[16]

During the interwar years, there was little experimentation in teaching methods. Theoretical instruction continued to be imparted in lectures and demonstrations, and practical skills acquired through dissection and bedside clinical teaching in the Hospital. How effectively the students absorbed the teaching continued to be tested by regular examinations. In an unpublished account of the Medical School during his student years, Russell Chisholm, who graduated in 1929 and claims to represent the views of 'a group of very successful students', shows a preference for a teaching style generally associated with more recent times. He thoroughly enjoyed his years at the Medical School and appreciated that the small number of students meant that teaching staff knew them as individuals and could take a fatherly interest in them. He greatly admired certain lecturers but thought the course as a whole was 'overcrowded' and some of the lectures 'dry'. He reserved his most trenchant criticism for the lectures in public health and medical jurisprudence, which he thought had too much detail and too little interest. In his final year, Chisholm was one of a group of six at Auckland Hospital who 'worked as a team' without real supervision. 'We had four clinics a week – no lectures', he wrote, with evident satisfaction. 'We educated ourselves'.[17] In the Depression of the early 1930s, lack of resources and pressure of student numbers meant that there was little room for innovation, and reinforced the strong tradition of didactic lectures.

Anatomy: Gowland and Cairney

The Otago Medical School's third full-time professor, Percy Gowland, was a dynamic personality, loud of voice and hearty in manner. His charismatic style was as far away from Scott's measured restraint or Malcolm's undemonstrative reticence, as his strong Lancashire accent was from their softer Scots brogue. Gowland was thirty-five when he was appointed, from a field of nine candidates, to the Chair of Anatomy at Otago. He came with varied experience, having worked as a general practitioner in Lancashire, a ship's doctor and a senior demonstrator and assistant lecturer in anatomy at the Liverpool Medical School. He was an inimitable teller of outrageous stories from his days in private practice, recounted (as one former student described it) 'with slap on thigh and 'ho-ho-ho' to emphasise the point'. Students throughout the period were unstinting in their praise of Gowland. Chisholm rated the course he ran in applied anatomy in the 1920s, with his assistant John Cairney, a highlight of his medical training. He described Gowland's style as informal and chatty, his time with students in the dissection room 'really a series of brilliant tutorials'. Gowland knew his students personally and once arranged a place at Selwyn College for a student who was struggling because he was living in unsuitable digs. Patrick Moore, who graduated in 1943, thought that students probably owed more to Gowland than to any other staff member for 'elevating what must have been an essentially

William Percy Gowland, 1879–1965

MB BS (Lond) MD (Lond) FRCS (Eng) Hon DSc (Otago)
Professor of Anatomy, Otago Medical School, 1914–43.

PERCY GOWLAND was selected in Britain to fill the Chair of Anatomy, left vacant after the death of Professor Scott in 1914 and his influence spanned the whole of the interwar period. Ironically, his career in the Anatomy Department ended during World War II as it had begun in World War I, coping with swollen student numbers in cramped accommodation.

Gowland's larger-than-life personality and robust presentation of his subject meant not only that he made a vivid impression on all his students but also that he was able to attract some of the best graduates to join his department as demonstrators. Some forty in all did so, and he encouraged them to engage in research, so that among them they published around twenty papers between 1928 and 1940. Many went on to have distinguished careers: three became professors of anatomy, and from their departments emerged six more professors of anatomy. One of the most outstanding, Derek Denny-Brown, Professor of Neurology at Harvard, warmly acknowledged his own debt to Gowland, whose department, he said, was known the world over for the calibre of its former students. He believed that Gowland's great achievement lay in his teaching, in stimulating ideas rather than in publishing them. He thought Gowland one of the best lecturers he had ever heard and claimed that hundreds who later took the English Primary Fellowship examination realised then how excellent their anatomical education had been. 'It was a brilliant three-dimensional functional anatomy', he wrote, 'that distinguished New Zealand surgeons, whether at home, in the Western desert, or in repairing facial injuries in the Battle of Britain.'[18]

For thirty years Gowland gave all the lectures in embryology and histology and participated in all the practicals in the anatomy course. He took one leave only, which he used to investigate teaching in his subject at medical schools in the United States, Canada, Britain and Europe. In London, former students travelled from all over England to see him, as one put it 'to hear again the strong familiar voice, the hearty laugh, the incredible anecdotes, told with a gusto unabated with the passing years'. After leaving the Medical School in 1943, he took a position as Director of Medical Services at Wellington Hospital, where he worked until 1949 with his former assistant John Cairney, who was its Superintendent. The estrangement from the Otago Medical School caused by his precipitate departure was ended when in 1962 the University awarded an honorary DSc degree to one of its outstanding teachers.

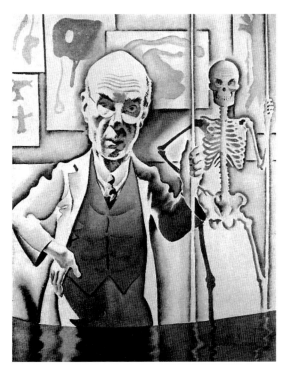

Gowland, with skeleton. Russell Clark,
Digest 1936, opp. p. 36.
Medical Library, University of Otago.

dull subject into something vividly appealing and certainly very pertinent'. Derek Denny-Brown wrote, 'How fortunate for the young to have had such an intensely vital man as their mentor!'[19]

Gowland would have been memorable for his personality alone, but he was also a dedicated and innovative teacher. When he died in 1965 Gowland had been away from the Medical School for more than twenty years, so it is fortunate for the record that the task of writing his obituary for the *New Zealand Medical Journal* fell to someone who knew his teaching well, as his student, demonstrator and finally successor in the Chair of Anatomy, Professor Bill Adams. For the first twelve years of his tenure, Adams wrote, Gowland concentrated on building up his department, which he had found in a run-down condition, without either academic or technical assistance. There were fifty-three students in his first class and the numbers increased hugely, during and just after the war, to two hundred in 1921, necessitating the duplication of classes. Gowland at once appointed the first of a long succession of

demonstrators and brought a qualified technical assistant over from Liverpool. It was not the time to make major changes in teaching, but he and his technician produced meticulous diagrams, and he used his dissection fees to add to Scott's bequest of books, forming a good anatomy library. One of Gowland's skills was his ability to choose capable staff. Outstanding among them was Cairney, who joined in 1919 while still a student, and stayed until 1927, by which time he was the School's first associate professor. He and Gowland later published two textbooks together, *Notes on Anatomy* for medical students in 1938 and *Anatomy and Physiology for Nurses* in 1941.[20]

Adams was able to detail specific innovations in Gowland's teaching. He and Cairney discarded the conventional British system, where a class would dissect different parts of the body at the same time, for the much more satisfactory and, at the time, entirely novel method of having all the students dissect the same part at the same time. In 1927, he took over the teaching of histology, and melded it into the teaching of anatomy – Otago was one of the first schools in the Commonwealth to teach histology this way. He perfected his embryological approach to the teaching of anatomy, so that it became possible to dispense with intensive memorising of a mass of factual detail. Adams claims that this approach was 'revolutionary at the time', and its value, when he wrote, was still not widely appreciated.[21]

Physiology: Malcolm and Bell

Malcolm taught physiology throughout the Ferguson years, assisted by a succession of very able graduate assistants. The first in 1914, for a year only and shared with Anatomy, was Michael Watt, who later became Director General of Health.[22] Dr Muriel Bell, a graduate of 1922, stayed longer. Malcolm supervised the thesis for her MD, which she achieved in 1926, the third woman to do so at Otago. She lectured in physiology between 1923 and 1927 and, after some time overseas, rejoined the department from 1935 to 1940 as lecturer in physiology and experimental pharmacology. People called her Professor Malcolm's 'right hand man'. Muriel Bell wrote appreciatively of Malcolm's teaching, a skill she surmised he had learned in his youth as a pupil teacher in Scotland. He presented his subject, she said, 'audibly, visually and with technical demonstration'. Forced to teach second- and third-year students without adequate assistance, he introduced a system of tutorials in which student groups discussed among themselves questions he had set, with the 'residue of unanswered questions' being handled by himself or his assistant. He introduced the experimental method into the Medical School and encouraged its application to pharmacological and clinical problems. When applied physiology became a fifth-year subject, he put a great deal of effort into giving students the physiological background of disease: Otago graduates who went overseas found themselves admirably prepared for the Primary Fellowship in England.[23] Not all his students were so admiring of his expertise in teaching, although all shared a warm affection for Malcolm. Towards the end of his academic career, wrote one student of the early 1940s, the full-class demonstrations rarely seemed to work, and when they did they elicited a round of applause. Another, in the same period, described an attempt to demonstrate how the righting reflexes of a cat would automatically come into play if the animal were to fall. To illustrate this, the professor dropped a cat from his arms; the animal landed on its back, stood up and walked off the stage with 'the aggrieved and

reproachful air that only a cat can assume'. That no one laughed was proof that the class felt for the professor more than for the cat.[24]

Muriel Bell's own teaching must have been memorable. Her 'serene influence over the practical physiology classes', a student wrote in the *Digest* in 1940, when she was leaving the department, 'has been our inspiration for the last five years. We have always found her so incredibly cool and capable in the midst of rabbits and frogs .... Most of us will remember her too for those wildly successful pharmacology demonstrations, which entailed an enormous amount of preparation and were so often received with riotous delight.'[25]

The Clinical Disciplines

Medicine

Colquhoun retired in 1919 and, for the next two decades, the Department of Medicine was headed by two part-time professors. In 1920, Mrs Mary Glendining gave £8000 to endow a chair in the Medical School. However, the sum was not considered sufficient to support a full-time position, so it was used, together with a government subsidy, to appoint two professors, with separate responsibilities, who would supplement their salary by private practice. The men appointed formed a striking contrast. Dudley Carmalt Jones, an Englishman with an Oxford background, literary and artistic gifts and recent war experience, became Professor of Systematic Medicine. Frank Fitchett was promoted Professor of Clinical Medicine and Therapeutics. Carmalt Jones, who was forty-five when he arrived in Dunedin, found conditions very different from his expectations. After a few years his wife and family returned to England and he lived alone, finding companionship in the Dunedin Club and the University Club. Carmalt Jones disliked private practice, found interaction with patients awkward and famously lost his temper with students on ward rounds, especially if they were late. Chisholm singles him out for unfavourable comment, convinced that he kept a list of all his lectures right through

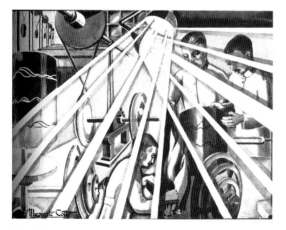

'Physiology' by Marguerite Cotton, *Digest* 1937, opp. p. 30. Medical Library, University of Otago.

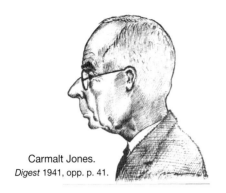

Carmalt Jones.
Digest 1941, opp. p. 41.

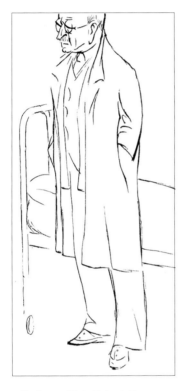

Professor Fitchett, by J. Ramsay.
Digest 1937, opp. p. 18.

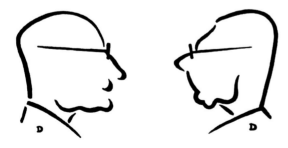

'The Professors of Clinical and Systematic Medicine':
Fitchett and Carmalt Jones as they appeared
in *Digest* 1937, p. 47.
Medical Library, University of Otago.

to retirement and crossed each off his list once he had delivered it. Nevertheless Carmalt Jones was devoted to the Medical School and its students, generously supporting athletics and rowing. His plans to return to England when he retired in 1939 were disrupted by the outbreak of war, and he spent the years from 1939 to 1945 meticulously recording the invaluable *Annals of the University of Otago Medical School*. It concludes on an unaccustomed personal note. 'I consider my election to the Chair of Systematic Medicine in the University of Otago as the greatest piece of good fortune which has ever befallen me.'[26]

Outgoing and gregarious, comfortably settled in his home town, Fitchett brought to his new post the fruits of long experience in private practice and almost a decade of service to the Medical School. He excelled in demonstrating to students the practical skills they would need as doctors, how to take a meticulous history of a patient and follow it up with a thorough physical examination. Neil Begg, who was his student in the 1930s, admired him as one of the last of those old-fashioned clinicians 'whose whole life experience had enhanced their bedside skills of observant eyes, acute and educated hearing and a sensitive and understanding touch.' Fitchett's sensitivity did not automatically extend to his students. He was intolerant of inattention, or the covering up of errors and he took a special joy in deflating an ego or dispelling complacency. Chisholm admired him greatly. 'Of all the staff,' he wrote sixty years on, 'Fitchett (Franky) was king.' He thought him a quiet and charming man, although his voice could 'drip acid.' He still remembered how Fitchett had humiliated one student by stopping him, halfway through examining a patient for his final examination, to call for a pair of nail scissors. He covered another with confusion by advising that 'you don't lift a pendulous breast by its nipple to find the apex beat.' Hercus and Bell describe him as a man of 'polished speech and immaculate attire, a lover of literature, gardens, birds and fishing.' 'There can be only one Fitchett,' they comment, 'the mould is lost.'[27] Both professors retired in 1939.

Surgery

The £8000 endowment that Professor Barnett gave to the Medical School in 1924 was sufficient, with the usual subsidy, to establish a part-time Chair of Surgery, also to be supplemented by private practice. The post was advertised in Britain, Australia and New Zealand and Gordon Bell MD, FRCS (Edin), FRCS (Eng) was appointed. Although born in Marlborough, Bell had been in Britain from the time he left to study medicine at Edinburgh in 1905. An outstanding student, he graduated in 1910, completed his FRCS in 1912 and his MD the following year, before doing postgraduate work, briefly in Berlin and for a year at the Mayo clinic in the United States. He served with the Royal Army Medical Corps from 1915 to 1918. When he was appointed, he was assistant surgeon at the Royal Infirmary, Edinburgh, and assistant in the Department of Systematic Medicine. Bell arrived in Dunedin early in 1925, with his wife and young baby, to commence a twenty-seven year tenure as Professor of Surgery. In his day, Barnett had been an innovative and inspiring teacher, but times had changed and the new professor was startled by the inadequacy of the facilities awaiting him. It must surely have been Bell who described the conditions in the history of the Medical School he and Charles Hercus wrote in their retirement. 'A Department of Surgery in the modern acceptance did not exist', the account runs. 'There were two lecture rooms available in the Pathology and Bacteriology block and the new boy was properly accorded the smaller ...' There was no surgical museum and few diagrams or clinical photographs. In the Hospital there was a small theatre for clinical lectures and demonstrations off the old entrance hall, warmed by steam pipes which interrupted proceedings with 'discordant rumbles, gurgles and crackles reminiscent of machine gun fire.' More important though, there were students, mostly eager and intelligent, nursing service of a high order, cooperative patients (he wrote elsewhere that 'no one could have wished for a nicer lot') and a blackboard. Bell also liked the smaller lecture room, because it met his taste for talking to students at close quarters. He believed that, with good textbooks available, 'the days of the systematic lecture were numbered'. The lecture should be used sparingly because 'the proper place in which to learn surgery [was] in the ward and clinical lecture theatres within the Hospital.' Bell practised what he preached. In an obituary tribute to him at a meeting of the Otago Medical School Research Society in 1970, surgeon John Heslop described him as a 'magnificent bedside teacher and diagnostician', but not at his best as a formal lecturer. All his past students, Heslop was sure, would remember that his lectures were 'usually derived from pencilled notes on the back of opened envelopes from last week's mail.' Overall he was rated an excellent clinical teacher, known for his dry wit, who gave generations of students a firm basis in the elementary principles of surgery.[28]

Bell was assisted by an increasingly numerous and specialised staff. As Professor of Surgery, he was also appointed by the Otago Hospital Board Head of the Clinical Department at the public hospital. Although the number of beds scarcely warranted it, he chose to retain all three members of the able and well qualified senior staff then in place: Drs Stanley Batchelor, who had already given thirty years' service, Eugene O'Neill, Otago graduate of 1899 and hero in two overseas wars and William Newlands, locally born and Edinburgh trained, who had worked for the Medical School and the Hospital since 1906. The Hospital staff were formally recognised, and paid, as University clinical lecturers.[29] Although he himself belonged to an era when all fields of surgery had to be practised, and was proud to call himself a general surgeon, Bell oversaw the development of specialist services within the Department of Surgery, which was characteristic of the 1920s. For a few years after the war the Dean of the Dental School, Percy Pickerill, used his skill in plastic surgery as lecturer in stomatology within the department. From 1920 orthopaedic surgeon, James Renfrew White, pioneer of the discipline in New Zealand, became one of the School's most memorable personalities. An Otago graduate of 1912, White had gained his FRCS in England and worked during the war as a house surgeon at the Royal National Orthopaedic Hospital in

London, with the RAMC in France, and on injuries to bones, joints, nerves and muscles in various military orthopaedic hospitals in England. Back in Dunedin, he attended to wounded servicemen who had been brought home. He was given the temporary rank of Major, which he used from then on. His skills were also needed to deal with a backlog of cases of children, from all over New Zealand, with deformities caused by such diseases as rickets or poliomyelitis. As well as teaching orthopaedics, White established an orthopaedic department in the Hospital and lectured to massage (later physiotherapy) students through until 1948. He promoted physical education for children and published on this and other topics. 'Eefie', as White was known, was an exuberant character. He enlivened his journey to and from the Medical School by swinging round lamp-posts and jumping over rubbish tins, and his teaching style was equally energetic.[30] A post in urological surgery also dates from the early 1920s. James Alfred Jenkins, an Otago graduate who had been Travelling Scholar in 1917, had served in the NZMC and done postgraduate work in surgery and urology in Britain, was appointed to an assistant lectureship. Like White, he had completed his FRCS in England. Both men also did a Master of Surgery when the degree was brought in at Otago in 1922. Jenkins built up a well-equipped urological department. Bell himself took on a very heavy load of teaching and clinical work, especially during World War II when Jenkins was the only other member of the surgical staff. Although Bell referred to the part-time clinical professorships as 'outmoded and unfashionable', when given the option of a full-time Chair after the war, he rejected it as coming too late for him, choosing to remain the 'last of a genus, the part-time clinical professor in Dunedin'.[31]

In the 1920s, anaesthesia developed alongside surgery. Dr A. McPhee Marshall, a graduate of 1915, who has been described as the first specialist in anaesthesia, served on the Hospital staff from 1921 to 1927, working with Pickerill in the Surgical Dental Unit and giving a few lectures in the Medical School. The appointment of Dr Marion Whyte, as the first lecturer in anaesthesia in 1928 marked a new era. A graduate of 1918, she had handled a busy general practice since 1920. The year before her appointment she visited the United States and Britain, learning detailed techniques of gas and oxygen anaesthesia, especially from Dr McKesson. She was one of the first in New Zealand to use endotracheal intubation and supportive intravenous fluids during operations and was also a pioneer of spinal anaesthesia. When the College of Surgeons of England introduced its Diploma of Anaesthesia in 1938, she was elected to a Foundation Diploma. Whyte taught fifth-year students, who affectionately dubbed her 'Maid Marion', until her retirement in 1948.[32]

New configurations: Bacteriology and Public Health; Pathology and Medical Jurisprudence

Sydney Champtaloup, who was appointed lecturer in bacteriology and public health in 1910, and later Professor, brought a new energy to Medical School affairs. It is also likely that he was responsible for persuading his Scottish friend Murray Drennan to accept the Chair of Pathology in 1915. Drennan, who had been an outstanding student at Edinburgh, where he was First Assistant to the Professor of Pathology when he was appointed to Otago, was an enthusiastic teacher. He at once introduced changes in the teaching of morbid anatomy along the lines of what was being done in Edinburgh, insisting on the study of individual cases of disease, rather than individual organs. Students were supplied with clinical notes and microscopical specimens from a particular case and, with tuition from demonstrators, were expected to write full reports that incorporated both clinical and pathological data. Drennan established the post of Clinical Pathologist, encouraged research in his department and built up a valuable teaching museum. His zest for teaching is evident in the information he provided for the 1916 'Descriptive Syllabus of the Medical School', which describes how a lecturer might use the advanced facilities in the new building. Lecture rooms with lantern, cinematograph and epidiascope would enable him to 'demonstrate on the screen first a museum specimen preserved to show the naked eye the natural colour of a diseased structure, then a lantern slide showing its microscopic anatomy, and then for contrast any plates or illustrations from books which may further elucidate the subject under discussion.' After 1917, Drennan's teaching in Medical Jurisprudence led to the development of a school of medical jurists that has served all the main centres in New Zealand. Not all his students appreciated this course. Russell Chisholm, for instance, thought it 'very, very dry'. Both Champtaloup and Drennan seemed eager to assume extra responsibilities. Each in turn served with distinction as Sub-Dean. Champtaloup was extensively involved in the design and fundraising for the new Medical School building and Drennan organised the new Medical Library. Champtaloup, whose research into tuberculosis gained him a DSc with honours from Edinburgh, inspired a number of his students to enter laboratory medicine. He was also responsible for the formation of the Clinical Club. Neither Champtaloup nor Drennan had long careers at Otago, eleven years in the one case, twelve in the other: Champtaloup died of tuberculosis in 1921, Drennan moved back to Britain in 1928, first to Dublin, then in 1931 to take up a chair in his old University, Edinburgh.

Poem by Carmalt Jones, and tribute to Champtaloup by Drennan. *Otago University Review*, XXXV, July 1922, pp. 9–11.

In Memoriam – S. T. C. (December 12, 1921)

Priests pray that through the ages they may lie
    Beneath a church dome, where the sunbeams fall
    Through carven gloom on rood and groin and stall.
And music rolls and incense rises high:
On sunny sandhills underneath the sky
    He lies, where yellow sprays of lupin tall
    Fold over all the dead their perfumed pall,
And all is silence save the seabird's cry.

'Tis a wide prospect opens to his view:
Headland on headland to the horizon's height
Thrust out to sea; that strange Pacific hue,
Beflecked this windy noon with crests of white,
Chill Northern grey through blazing Tropic blue –
Fit resting place; for he was wide of sight.
                      C.J.

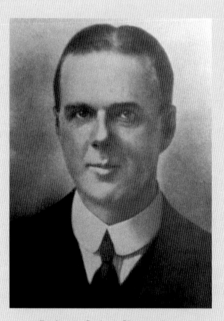

Professor Sydney Champtaloup
Hocken Collections, Uare Taoka o Hakena,
University of Otago, Acc. No. c/n E3605/23 d.

Champtaloup and Drennan renewed in Dunedin the friendship begun at the Edinburgh Medical School in 1901. After Champtaloup's death Drennan wrote in the *Review*:

'As I remembered him, always dapper, bright of eye, a little deaf in one ear, quiet of speech, orderly in mind and habit, ever kindness itself, so I still found him in December 1916. It was a great inspiration to have such a colleague and our early friendship deepened and broadened by community of thought and interest. [But] he sacrificed everything to his work ... and did not know how to indulge in a care-free holiday.'

Drennan died in 1984, one hundred years old. During their few years together at Otago from 1917, the two brilliant young friends must have relished the chance to help build up the Medical School, and especially their own departments, in their brand new building.[33]

Charles Hercus, who worked in the Department of Bacteriology and Public Health in 1921, while Champtaloup was on sick leave, was appointed to the Chair the following year. This was the beginning of a twenty-two year period of dual responsibility, until the department was divided into its two components in 1954. In the 1920s, Hercus carried out routine teaching and diagnostic work in bacteriology and devoted a great deal of attention to the development of the field of public health. While students remembered his lectures most vividly for the great armload of books he would bring to class, in 1923 he inaugurated a scheme to give his students some

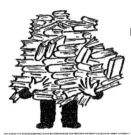

Hercus preparing to lecture: 'I shall put this book in the Museum for those who may be interested.'

Digest 1941, p. 32. Medical Library, University of Otago.

experience of research in the public health field. In a letter to the Rockefeller Foundation that year, Ferguson describes how Hercus gave his public health students the option of researching and writing a thesis rather than sitting an end-of-year examination. All but two of the sixty students chose the thesis and worked in pairs under the professor, on such diverse topics as 'housing, water supply, milk supply, goitre, hydatids, tonsils and adenoids, healthy teeth, influenza in an institution, gonococcal blood tests, buccal cancer etc.'. The Dean was impressed by the students' enthusiasm for research. 'I much doubt if ten years ago we could have got a pair of students to have voluntarily scoured the city and suburbs to collect dogs' faeces to determine the regional prevalence of tape worm', he commented, adding that he himself 'would not have the assurance to invade hundreds of homes to see the condition of life of the adenoid children.'[34]

In Pathology, Drennan was also replaced by someone familiar with his department, his former assistant, Eric D'Ath, who graduated from Otago in 1923. Thirty-two years old at his appointment and with only brief overseas experience in Sydney, D'Ath became an institution in the Medical School and the community. He held the Chair of Pathology from 1929 through the changing decades until 1961, and continued to serve as pathologist to the coroner and the police for ten years after that. He has been described as 'a serene and suave man of the world, experienced not only in his particular field but also in business and the law, making his way not only by expert knowledge but by immense personal charm'. A lecture from Professor D'Ath was a 'vivid occasion, marked by narrative flair spell-binding even to the most wayward' and the spontaneity and clinical flavour of what he said made it unforgettable. Although D'Ath did not engage in research, he chaired the Medical Research Council committee on cancer from its foundation. He successfully administered a large laboratory serving the Hospital and private practice and, as an expert medical witness in court, he was almost impossible to catch out. One famous cross-examiner was on record as saying that it would be very much easier 'to trap the greasy pig at the summer show'. D'Ath was awarded a CBE, honoured by the Police Association and was among the select group recognised by an honorary doctorate at the centenary of the Medical School in 1975.[35]

Obstetrics and Gynaecology

It was probably in obstetrics and gynaecology that the most striking teaching developments occurred during the interwar years. All three clinical departments, Medicine, Surgery, and Obstetrics and Gynaecology, lacked space, staff and laboratories. Whereas Medicine and Surgery could work under these austere conditions, the facilities for Obstetrics and Gynaecology were chaotic and completely unsatisfactory, and this at a time when the expectations of society for safe childbirth were not being met.[36] In Britain, concern that the maternal mortality rate was higher than in Continental countries had led to the establishment of full-time chairs in obstetrics and gynaecology in some medical schools. New Zealand's maternal mortality rate was also unacceptably high and brought Otago's teaching under scrutiny. In 1927, Dr Henry Jellett, an eminent Irish obstetrician who had settled in Christchurch, visited the School to report on facilities and other conditions affecting teaching in his area of expertise. He recommended the establishment of a full-time Chair in Obstetrics, the appointment of tutors in both obstetrics and gynaecology and a new maternity hospital with a resident medical officer. He was preaching to the converted. The Medical Faculty and University already knew what was required. The problem was money.

In 1930, thanks in large part to the organisational efforts of Dr Doris Gordon, the New Zealand Obstetrical Society raised enough to establish a Chair. Joseph Bernard Dawson, trained in England was practising in Adelaide when appointed. He was forty-five, had a keen interest in teaching and had wide experience in his field, including research in embryology and the development of ante- and post-natal clinics. He wrote later that, when he took up his duties in 1932 after a six-month tour of obstetric and gynaecology units in Britain, Europe and North America, his department was 'non-existent save for a set of old and faded wall diagrams, a dilapidated obstetric phantom and one female pelvis.' He supplemented his lectures with lantern slides and film, and began small-group teaching, in tutorials and in the labour room. He sent a terse report to the University Council outlining the conditions in which he was expected to teach. Clinical facilities, he said, were inadequate and staff quite insufficient. He had forty students, but access to only fourteen maternity beds, which were located in three separate hospitals. He described an occasion on which he had three patients in labour at the same time, one in the labour room, one in the bathroom and the third in the bed of a convalescent patient, who had had to be turned out to make room

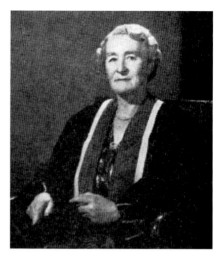

Dr Doris Gordon.
Back-Blocks Baby-Doctor, An Autobiography.

Doris Gordon, Secretary of the Obstetrical Society, 'If we cannot have an endowment from one benefactor, what is to stop us obtaining it from a dozen or twenty benefactors?
Back-Blocks Baby-Doctor, p. 179

for her. Such conditions, he asserted, were 'unsatisfactory, subversive of the interests of patients, damaging to the reputation of the institution and impossible from the point of view of instruction.' The teaching of obstetrics was well below the standard required by the General Medical Council. Much later, Dawson looked back on his first six years at Otago as having been fully occupied with 'the enhancement of the teaching programme and the struggle for the new hospital', itself a requirement for optimum teaching. The Government had promised a new maternity hospital when Dawson took up his chair, at a probable cost of £30,000, but reneged when the Depression deepened. It took much bitter negotiation and a personal appeal to the Prime Minister to get approval for a facility of reduced size, with twenty-six beds rather than the forty-four recommended. The new Queen Mary Hospital finally opened in 1937.[37]

Deans of the Otago Medical School & Deans of Faculty, 1891–2000

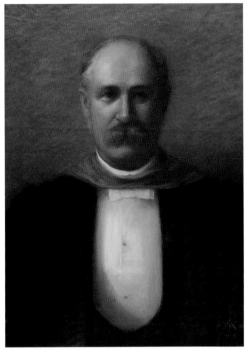

J.H. Scott, Sole Professor of Otago Medical School,
1877–1905; First Dean of Faculty, 1891–1914.
Frances Mary Wimperis, 1910.

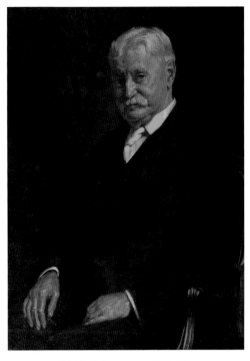

Sir Lindo Ferguson, 1914–36.
Archibald Nicoll, 1937.

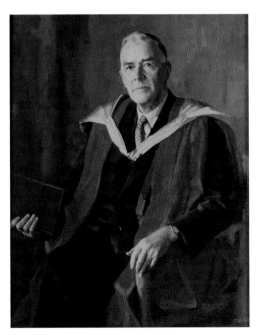

Sir Charles Hercus, 1937–58.
Sir William Dargie, 1958.

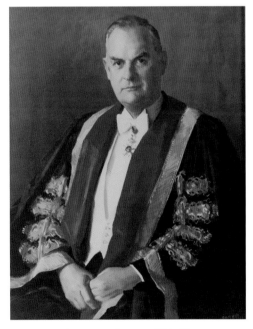

Sir Edward Sayers, 1958–67.
William Alexander Sutton, 1967.

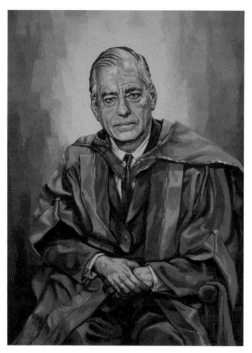

Professor William Adams, 1968–73.
John Gillies. A posthumous portrait, 1973.

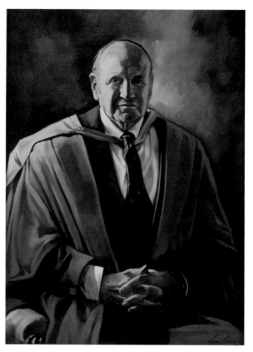

Professor John Hunter, 1974–77, 1986–90.
Dean, Christchurch School, 1982–85; inaugural AVC,
Health Sciences, University of Otago, 1989–90.
John Gillies.

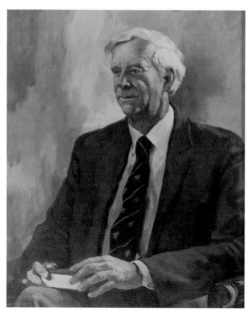

Professor Geoffrey Brinkman, 1978–83.
W.A. Sutton, 1985.

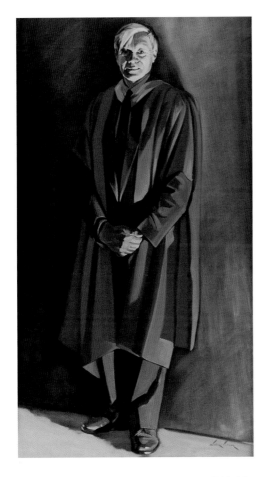

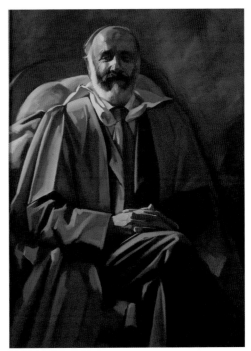

Professor John Campbell, Dean of Faculty,
1995–2004.
John Gillies.

Professor David Stewart, Dean of Faculty, 1991–95;
Dean, Otago Medical School, 1986–90; AVC,
Health Sciences, 1991–98.
John Gillies.

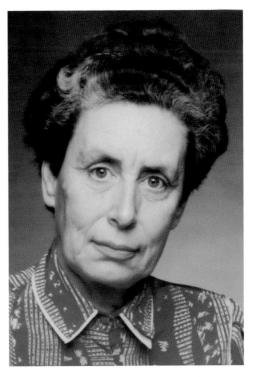

Professor Linda Holloway, Dean, Wellington School,
1996–98; Dean of Faculty 2005; AVC, then PVC,
Health Sciences, 1999–2005.

Dean, Otago School of Medical Sciences

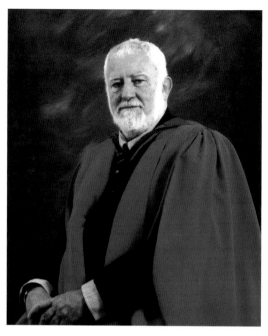

Professor David Jones, Otago School of
Medical Sciences, 1996–2006

Deans, Dunedin School of Medicine

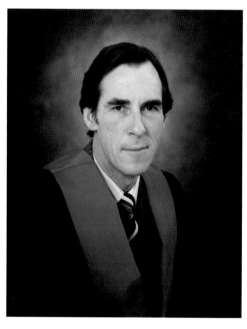

Professor Graham Mortimer, Otago Medical School,
1991–96; Dunedin School of Medicine,1996–97.

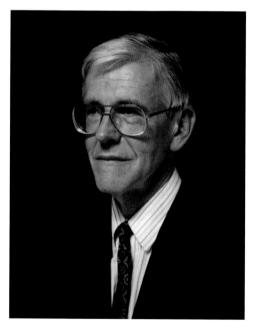

Professor William Gillespie, Dunedin School of
Medicine, 1998–2002.

Deans, Christchurch School of Medicine

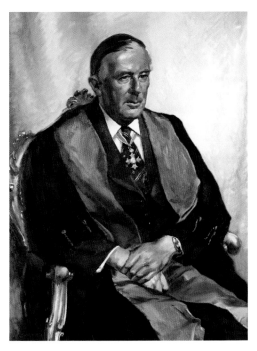

Professor George Rolleston, 1970–80.
W.A. Sutton.

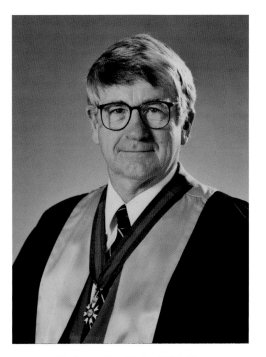

Professor Alan Clarke, 1986–93.

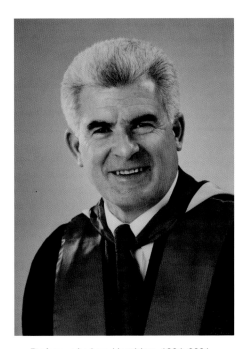

Professor Andrew Hornblow, 1994–2001.

Deans, Wellington School of Medicine

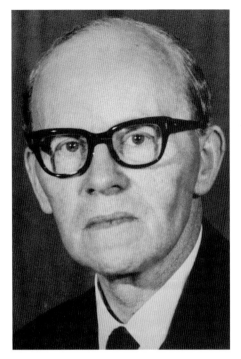

Professor Fr ancis Hall, 1972–75.

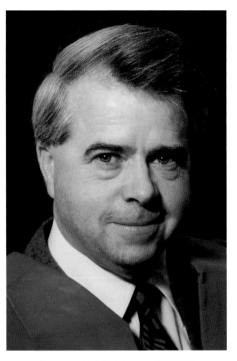

Professor Ralph Johnson, 1977–85.

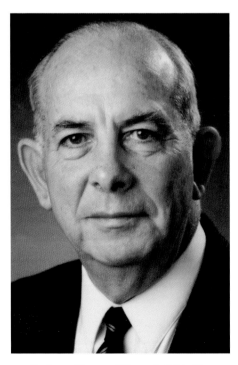

Professor Thomas O'Donnell, 1986–91.

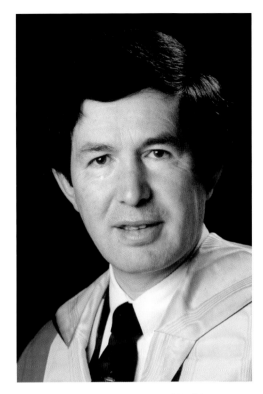

Professor Eru Pomare, 1992–94.

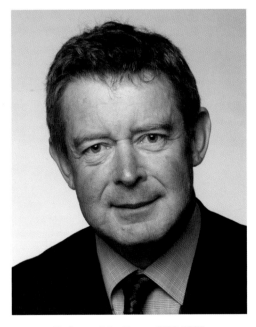

Professor John Nacey, 1998–2007.

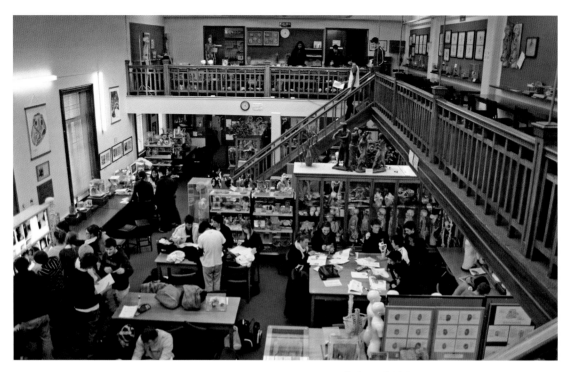

A class of third-year medical students
at work in the Anatomy Museum.
Photo: Chris Smith.

Cadaver Spoken Here

In the beginning were the words
(*artery, arcuate, acetabulum*)
and the words were pared from flesh
which had dwelt among us

Adolescent and absurd
in greasy short white coats
we sliced and sawed
from axilla (*a truncated space
bounded anteriorly by ...*)
down ligament, nerve and tendon
through anatomical space
into language

He was old and frowning
(*orbicularis oculis, levator palpebrae*)

His clenched hands
resisted dissection

In his dying what did they grasp?

Were terror, hope, yearning
audible over
arrest, arrhythmia, asystole?

Aged man, flayed man
generous man
why did we never think to thank you?

                    Rae Varcoe

The Changing Face of Anatomy

Rae Varcoe's poem, reprinted here with permission from her collection *Tributary* (Victoria University Press, 2007), reflects the unease generations of medical students have felt when faced with human dissection. Dr Varcoe, a graduate of 1968, is now a blood diseases physician at Auckland City Hospital.

The study of anatomy at the Otago Medical School still involves human dissection, but it also includes the use of X-ray images and dissected parts preserved by plastination, when the water in them is replaced with silicone. The Anatomy Museum is the centre for this study.

Since 2004 an annual thanksgiving service has been held for those who have given their bodies to the Medical School. Alternating between Dunedin and Christchurch, the service typically involves two to three hundred people: medical students and the families of the donors.

CHAPTER 10

The Clinical Club and the Monro Collection

I N 1915, Sydney Champtaloup invited a select group of his academic and clinical colleagues to form a Clinical Club. The group of eight to ten members met every few months, hosting the evening meeting in turn in their own homes, with supper provided. There were some 148 meetings in all, over the twenty-four year period before the club lapsed in 1939. The Clinical Club represented the younger and livelier leaders on the Medical School and Hospital staff. At first, it had seven members: the three recently appointed professors, Champtaloup, Drennan and Gowland, and a group whose appointments dated from 1905 or soon after, Malcolm from the Medical School and Fitchett, Stanley Batchelor and Russell Ritchie from the Hospital. When Champtaloup died in 1921, Hercus was invited to become a member. Physician and paediatrician Ernest Williams joined the group some time in the 1920s and Gordon Bell in 1932. The membership never rose above ten. After Champtaloup's death, Drennan provided the impetus behind the group and, when he left, Hercus took on the role. Although Gowland resigned in 1934, after eighteen years in the Club and to the general regret, most members stayed on, to form a stable core.[1]

It is not clear precisely why this particular group came together, but perhaps we need look no further than personal compatibility and a fascination with medicine, its various disciplines, its teaching and research. Although it was later claimed that Champtaloup wanted to bring together the academic and clinical sides of the School, this does not fully explain who was included and who was not. The absence of Professors Ferguson, Barnett and Riley, for example, can probably be accounted for by the fact they were from an older age group. However, we must assume that Professors Carmalt Jones, D'Ath and Dawson, either were not invited or declined to join.[2]

In spite of the acknowledged distinction of its members, the Clinical Club has been regarded as being outside the mainstream narrative of the Medical School, merely a social gathering of like-minded staff who enjoyed each others' company and whisky. The impression that the Club met simply for entertainment might also be inferred from the witty and light-hearted tone of some of its minutes. Hercus and Bell, both members, consign the club to an appendix of their history. It could be argued that it deserves more. As well as a social gathering, the Club was a high-powered seminar, at which members presented papers for the informed criticism of colleagues, reported on the latest developments in their various disciplines, and discussed the politics of advancing the Medical School. The topics for the meetings were circulated in advance to give members time to read up the relevant literature, the order of business was strictly adhered to and full minutes were kept.

John Hunter has analysed the volume of minutes from the last decade of the Clinical Club, 1928–39, and lists some of the topics

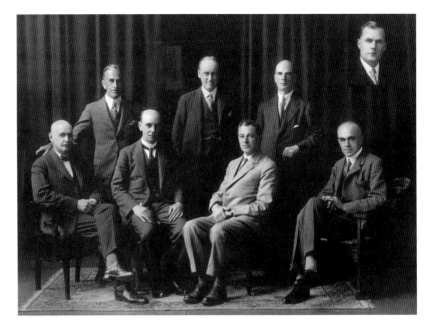

Members of the Clinical Club in the 1920s.
Standing, left to right: Ernest Williams, Russell Ritchie, Percy Gowland. Inset: Charles Hercus. Seated left to right: Frank Fitchett, John Malcolm, Murray Drennan, Stanley Batchelor.
Otago Medical School.

dealt with. In 1933, Williams compared and commented on the numbers of stillbirths and neonatal deaths in 1922 and 1933, and Bell discussed thyroidectomies for goitre in 368 cases over six years in the Dunedin Goitre Clinic. In 1934, Malcolm talked about dietary problems affecting the Byrd Antarctic Expedition. The same year Gowland introduced a wide-ranging discussion on arteriosclerosis and cholesterol, and Fitchett led a session on thyrogenic agents. The minutes also include various reports of overseas conferences. After the main topic of the evening, each member would draw attention to any recent developments in his own area of expertise, and hospital and private cases were brought up for diagnosis or discussion. Members discussed a variety of medical and non-medical publications and brought exhibits, ranging from the new electrocardiogram in 1938 to shaving devices and soaps. At the end of the evening there was supper and general discussion on the Medical School, its curriculum and progress.

The minutes, which were recorded by the host of the evening, are as varied in style, legibility and length as they are in content. They also offer a guide to the members' personalities: Gowland and Malcolm appear steady and reliable, unless provoked, Fitchett comes across

as an efficient practical physician who enjoyed mischief and inspired affection, while Hercus is more ponderous in tone. There are at least two outstanding set pieces, Fitchett's moving tribute to Champtaloup in 1921 and Drennan's whimsical account of the special dinner-meeting he hosted before his departure in 1928.

The Medical Library and the Monro Collection

During Ferguson's deanship the Medical Library took shape and gained what is still its most valuable asset, the Monro Collection. Under Scott the medical section, haphazardly built up from gifts or bequests from local doctors, was part of the main University Library. Both Scott and Malcolm also purchased journals in their own disciplines and Colquhoun was a steady advocate of the Library. It was 1909 before a regular annual sum – a princely £50 – was allocated for purchases for the medical section. Also in that year, the Otago Branch of the British Medical Association offered to donate their small working library and a modest sum of money annually, in return for access by their members.[3]

In 1917, the medical section of the University Library gained its own space in the new Medical

The 85th Meeting of the Clinical Club was held at Dr Drennan's residence, 26 Balmacewen Road, on 26th October, 1928, at 7.30 p.m.

All members were present.

The occasion was memorable, the meeting remarkable.

The occasion was the last on which the Club will meet under Dr Drennan's auspices before his translation to Belfast. The meeting differed from all its recorded predecessors in that it was inaugurated by an excellent dinner of which members partook as Dr Drennan's guests.

The table was tastefully decorated and the menu listed an appetising and delicious repast. Soup, whitebait, forequarter of lamb, kidney, potatoes, green peas, meringues, Norwegian trifle, fruit salad, savoury, dessert, coffee, sherry, whisky, claret, port, 48 liqueur brandy, freely ingested and rapidly assimilated put members in excellent humour.

The narcotising effect of the alcoholic liquors upon the highest cerebral centres was happily demonstrated by members generally in a sustained and merry loquacity.

The individual effect was best demonstrated by Dr Williams, probably by reason of heavier dosage. Freed from the natural restraining influence of his highest centres, he displayed an exuberance of scintillating wit that delighted the meeting. Dr Malcolm's natural expression was transfigured. A happy, beaming, guileless countenance needed only another layer of subcutaneous fat to make him another Pickwick.

The depressing weight of heavy financial responsibilities contracted as a direct result of his reproductive fertility was lifted from Dr Batchelor's shoulders and made him again the happy, genial, conversationally inconsequent Batchelor of the earlier years of the century.

The hypnotic influence of alcohol was demonstrated by Dr Hercus only. The heaviest man in the room, reclining weightily in the smallest chair, he slumbered peacefully, but in the watchful manner of the serpent, for a mis-statement of some microgrammic or grammatic measurement at once uncovered his heavily lidded eyes and stimulated to sonorous utterance his belly-rooted voice.

A subduing effect was demonstrated by Dr Gowland. Lengthily silent, he sat supporting chin in hand, a countenance sombre and intense. His relatively infrequent utterances were less reminiscent, less positive, more negative than usual. As the evening wore, the depression lifted and at the close, our Gowland was himself again.

Dr Ritchie's ready, dominating laugh was even readier and his keen scent for humorous situations even keener. To laugh loud at Dr William's sallies, to cap them and laugh again, louder still, was to stimulate the receptive centres of pleasurable sensations of all the members.

Dr Drennan, perhaps in the solicitous desire to serve his guests, had neglected to imbibe his share of the Divine fluid, and was his own dear self. As is his wont, he offended the nostrils of his fellow-members by introducing for their inspection, a portion of some dismembered human being, probably defunct.

The effect upon Dr Fitchett was not observed.

This thoroughly enjoyed, instructive, illuminating and revealing meeting was continued with unabated pleasure until one o'clock when, moved more by consideration for their host than because they felt they had exhausted the fund of entertainment, the guests departed.[4]

Minutes of meeting of 26 October 1928.
Otago Medical School.

School building and the Medical Library was born. Faculty set up a library committee and, from 1918 to 1922, the indefatigable Drennan added the post of part-time honorary librarian to his other responsibilities, during which time he introduced the Dewey system of cataloguing and organised a borrowing system. Carmalt Jones and Dr Crawshaw in turn succeeded him as librarian in 1922–23. In 1923, the Dean reported that whereas ten years ago the library had consisted of only seven hundred volumes (with only thirty-five published since 1900), it now contained three thousand volumes, thanks in part to appeals to the profession. The total amount spent on books for the year had been £291. Anatomy and Physiology had their own departmental collections and journals were maintained by the personal contribution of staff. In 1924, there were substantial additions. Dr James Young, the leading New Zealand authority of the day on medical history, gave the first of two important gifts of his own books and Ferguson, during a visit to the United States, purchased a huge collection of eleven to twelve thousand books, at ten cents each, from the College of Physicians' Library in Philadelphia. The College was disposing of duplicates, which proved on closer inspection to be of variable quality, but a later medical librarian pointed out that the purchase had enabled the library to secure a number of items it would not otherwise have been able to obtain. The new books required two thousand feet of additional shelving.[5]

This was the situation of the Medical Library when, in 1929, the most remarkable windfall arrived, a dazzling collection of some four hundred rare books and manuscripts. They had originally belonged to one or other of three generations of the Monro family, each called Alexander, who in turn had held the Chair of Anatomy in the Medical Faculty of the University of Edinburgh, over the 120 years from 1726 to 1846. The father of the first Alexander (later known as Alexander primus), John Monro (1670–1740), had studied medicine at Leiden, at the time the foremost European centre, and later became a surgeon-apothecary in Edinburgh. He conceived the idea of setting up an active medical school in Edinburgh, backed

by an appropriate hospital, and his son made the dream a reality. Appointed Professor of Anatomy, Alexander primus (1697–1767) gathered able colleagues round himself and took a leading part in setting up the Royal Infirmary. He engaged his own son in teaching from the time he was twenty, and Alexander secundus (1733–1817) duly succeeded to the Chair of Anatomy, taking the Edinburgh Medical School to the height of its influence. His son, Alexander tertius (1773–1859), who in turn succeeded his father, was less able and less dedicated however and, when he resigned in 1846, the family's extraordinary academic tenure came to an end.[6]

How the books and papers of this influential family came to find a home in Dunedin is one of the quirks of history, in particular of nineteenth-century British colonial family history. The fourth of Monro tertius' twelve children, Dr (later Sir) David Monro (1813–77) emigrated to Nelson in 1841, became a successful sheep farmer, a member of the first Colonial Parliament in 1854 and a respected Speaker of the House of Representatives. He received word of his father's death and his legacy of the family collection of books and papers in 1859, but it was some years before he arranged for their transport to New Zealand. 'There are some fine old books but they have been miserably badly treated', he wrote in his diary in February 1872, when he was unpacking some of the many boxes. After Sir David's death, the collection passed to his daughter and her husband, Sir James Hector, MD (Edin) and in 1907 to their son, Dr Charles Hector, who sent it to the General Assembly Library in Wellington for safe-keeping. His intention, and it seems that of his father, was to gift the collection to the Otago Medical School. This eventually happened in 1929, after some acrimonious correspondence between Dr Charles Hector and the General Assembly Library.[7]

Professor Douglass Taylor has made the Monro Collection a special study. He produced a booklet on the collection to accompany a display at the Medical School's centenary in 1975, was invited to give a paper on it at the 1976 Edinburgh University celebrations and published *The Monro Collection in the Medical Library of the University of Otago* three years later. In 2006, he co-curated an exhibition, 'In the Flesh: the Monro Dynasty, 1720–1846', at the University of Otago Library. In his book, Taylor describes the elements that make up the collection: books presented to one or other of the Professors Monro by their authors, commonly old Edinburgh students, and items which the professors regarded as necessary references; standard editions, of Hippocrates and Galen for example; a number of medical classics of the seventeenth and, especially, the eighteenth century, such as nine major works by Albinus of Leiden, and a number of works by Haller, whose eight-volume set of *Elementa physiologicae* (1757–66*)* was considered indispensable by William Sharpey, the pre-eminent British physiologist of his day, even a century later. As well there are volumes of splendid anatomical illustrations and books by Monros primus and secundus, notable among the latter being *Observations on the Structure and Functions of the Nervous System* (1783). The manuscripts in the collection, which are equally remarkable, include the index to casebooks of Monro secundus for forty-two years (1767–1808), during which period he saw 9384 patients. Unfortunately, the casebooks themselves are missing. Monro secundus lectured without notes, but at one point he actually bought back lecture notes that had been taken in shorthand and later transcribed by one of his students: there are two sets of lectures, both incomplete, one in ten volumes (1773–74), the other in twenty-five volumes (1774–75).[8] With the advent of the Monro Collection, the Otago Medical School Library became an archive of international significance.

In a footnote to the story, Dr W.J. Mullin, a graduate of 1890 and, in his retirement, medical librarian, recalled in 1954 how, on one occasion during his student days, Professor Scott had

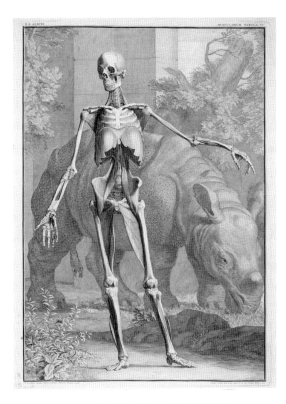

Bernhardus Siegfried Albinus (1697–1770) from
Tabulae Sceleti et Musculorum corporis humani,
one of nine works by Albinus in the Monro Collection,
Medical Library, University of Otago.

asked him which of the Professors Monro the foramen was named after. He had never heard of the Monros, so Scott told him about the three professors, primus, secundus and tertius, and that the foramen was named by secundus. 'Neither Scott nor I had any prophetic knowledge', he wrote, 'that more than 45 years later I would be called on to care for the books which had belonged to the three Professors of the Monro dynasty.' When the collection was handed over to the Medical School, Mullin presented a showcase for it, and in 1936 wrote the first account of the collection for the *New Zealand Medical Journal*.[9]

CHAPTER 11

Medical Students Between the Wars

'As Others See Us'

During the interwar period, medical students dominated extra-curricular student life at the University: in the Students' Association, the residential colleges, team sports, the Capping concert and student publications. Members of the largest faculty in the University, they stayed longer than most other students and often demonstrated real qualities of leadership. However, this did not always make them popular with students of other faculties.

The stereotype of the medical student at the University of Otago was established early and proved to be enduring. A strong element of envy runs through the humorous sketches of medical students that appeared, surprisingly frequently, in student publications over the decades. As early as 1893, in the *Otago University Review*, 'Semicolon Bijjj' refers to the nonchalance and exclusivity of the medical student. 'He plays tennis and fives, and for relaxation takes a class or two ... the Class is perfectly select; outsiders are not permitted.' A cartoon by Peter McIntyre in a 1930 number of the *Critic* captures the chief elements of the stereotype: his medical student is privileged, arrogant and God's gift to women.[1] Over time, additions were made, fairly or otherwise, to the picture, which was firmly delineated by the interwar years. The medical student was a hard drinker and a dedicated participant in Capping or other stunts. From his base in Knox or Selwyn College, he ruled student politics and sport. He favoured conservatism in politics and sexual innuendo in humour.

Open resentment informed 'Ray's' attack on the 'Number 1 Public Enemy: the Superior Medical', in a 1936 *Critic*:

> Why is he superior? Superior socially? Superior intellectually? Superior in his Samsonian attack upon the fundamentals of conventional religion? Superior in his two-gallon capacity? Or does his superiority lie in his bawdy humour and in having acquired intimate knowledge of a few facts of life and a bedside manner?[2]

Unfair as it was in most cases, the stereotype was nonetheless an acknowledgement of the special position medical students held in the Otago University student population.

Knox and Selwyn Colleges were at the heart of medical student culture. Both provided a home base for a high proportion of medical students and contributed hugely, in support, friendship and fun, to their experience at Otago. In its 'A' rooms, Knox provided the luxury of two bedrooms with a shared sitting room between but it also offered more than just physical comfort. Bill Anderson, for example, who had no family in New Zealand, came to Medical School in 1914 after four years in Gisborne Hospital with spinal injuries from a riding accident. When he became ill again in 1916 and was ordered to be immobilised in bed for three months, his friends brought him class notes and the Master, the Reverend Hewitson, arranged for another medical student, Robert

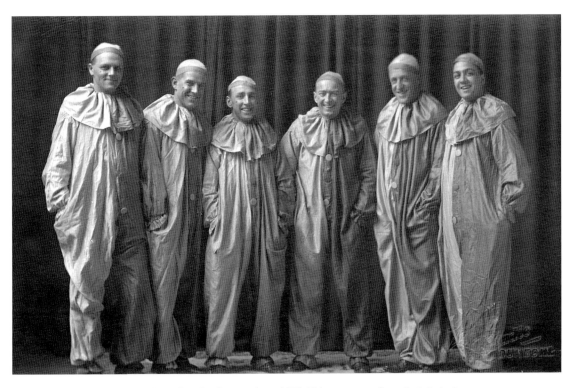

The traditional Capping Sextet, about 1922. This group are all medical students.
From left: Eddie Butler, Archibald McIndoe, Peter Quilliam, James Maunsell, Robert (Robinson?) Hall, Moe Kronfeldt.
Most went on to practise in New Zealand but McIndoe, later Sir Archibald, settled in Britain,
where he took plastic surgery on burn victims to a new level in World War II.

Hocken Collections, Uare Taoka o Hakena, University of Otago, Maunsell Collection, Acc. No. P 92-001b.

Burns Watson, to stay over the vacation to look after him. Both describe the episode, which cemented a long friendship, in their published memoirs.[3] Francis Bennett was a poor examinee whose medical studies began badly, twice: once before he went overseas on military service and the second time after he returned. On this second occasion, the Master and a group of friends at Knox persuaded him not to give up. The Master paid his fees for two terms and arranged coaching for him.[4] Patrick Eisdell Moore, who spent four years at Selwyn in the late 1930s, begins the Otago University chapter of his autobiography, 'One of the best things about going to Dunedin was Selwyn College.' He remembered fondly the benign influence of Warden Archdeacon 'Algy' Whitehead, whose 'authority was intangible, all-encompassing and wholly effective.' Selwyn provided him with a base for his many activities: rugby, playing the piano for dances, editing the

Medical Digest (for which he produced some excellent cartoons) and serving a term as college president. He found it necessary to move into private digs in his final year to be free from distractions.[5]

Private board was still common and the traditional baiting of long-suffering landladies might have reached its peak with the antics of Terry Maunsell in the 1930s. One landlady of generous proportions was enjoying a bath when he dislodged the plug by pushing a wire up the drain pipe, emptying the bath and leaving her, as he imagined, 'like a stranded whale'. Maunsell claimed to have been evicted from every boarding establishment in town and spent some months sleeping in the Student Union and, when evicted from there, in a tent on Opoho hill.[6]

The proportion of medical students at St Margaret's College remained high as the College grew, twenty-two out of sixty residents in 1917 and twenty-five out of 102 in 1924. Typically they stayed throughout their course: six of the seven women to graduate in medicine in 1922 were St Margaret's residents, seven of the eleven in 1923 and five of the eight in 1924. In 1920, OUSA adopted a new constitution that included a Lady Vice President – the first was the outstanding medical student, Alice Rose, who would be the first woman to take up a Travelling Scholarship, in 1925. However, women were still excluded from performing in the Capping concert and, in the case of medical students, from attending the fifth-year medical dinner. In 1920, after heated debate, the Medical Students' Association voted by a large majority to continue to exclude women. The *Review* sometimes ran articles hostile to women medical students. At Knox, the Misogynists' Society flourished between the wars and the developing college culture of initiations, drinking and sport was strongly masculine.[7]

The medical student population remained overwhelmingly European. The first non-European woman to study medicine at Otago was also the first Chinese person to do so. Kathleen Pih came to New Zealand as a small child with a returning missionary and was granted permission to remain, despite restrictions at the time on Chinese immigration. After graduating in 1929 she went to work at the Canton Villages Mission. She took leave to gain her Diploma

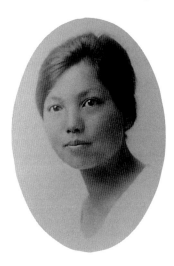

Kathleen Chang, the first Chinese graduate of the School. Otago Medical School.

in Ophthalmological Medicine and Surgery in London in 1935, returning to work on through the Sino-Japanese war before her marriage to Kwong So Francis Chang, Professor of Anatomy at St John's University, Shanghai. The couple taught there through World War II, the civil war and the communist takeover until 1950, when they moved to the universities of Malaya and Hong Kong. They retired to New Zealand in 1969 and Kathleen Pih-Chang died in 1991.[8]

The example of Peter Buck and Wi Repa at the turn of the century did not lead to an increasing Maori presence in the Medical School. It was 1919 before the next Maori medical student, Edward Ellison, graduated and a further decade until the next, Louis Potaka. Like their predecessors, both excelled at rugby, but their careers proved very different. Born in 1884, Ellison was only a few years younger than Buck and Wi Repa and, like them, had attended Te Aute College, but he could not raise the money to attend Medical School until 1914, when he was a married man of thirty. Some years after graduation he returned to Otago to specialise in tropical medicine and, apart from four years as Director of the Department of Maori Hygiene, he made his career in the Pacific. He served in Niue, Samoa and Fiji and finally as Chief Medical Officer to the Cook Islands from 1933 to 1945, making his mark as an administrator with a cool head in a crisis. His contribution to the health of the Polynesian people was outstanding. Potaka's life was shorter, sadder and more stormy. Born in 1901, he entered Medical School in 1920, remaining nine years to complete the course. After a time on the West Coast, which ended in dispute, he joined Admiral Byrd's 1934–35 expedition to Antarctica. It was the high point of his career, but left him with snow blindness. A locum position in Nelson then led to a falling out with a local doctor, a breach with the local branch of the BMA and serious financial troubles. In 1936 he took his own life.[9]

In the 1930s the first medical students from Fiji entered the School. The first, in 1930, was Ratu Dovi Madraiwiwi and he became the first fully qualified Fijian doctor. On graduation, Dovi proved reluctant to return to Fiji, taking up house surgeon positions in Gisborne and Hamilton until some pressure was applied. Resentful of being appointed to a position of lesser dignity and pay than his Western counterparts, he was glad to leave Fiji during World War II to serve with the NZEF in the Solomon Islands. He did not return permanently until 1956. In 1934, the first Indo-Fijian student, Mutyala Satyanand, entered the School. He too preferred to settle in New Zealand on completion of his course, heading the Accident and Emergency Department at the Auckland Hospital. He was subject to manpower regulations during the war and he and his wife were later naturalised.[10]

Student Affairs

Medical students maintained a tight grip on the presidency of the University Students' Association from 1914 to 1924, a decade which marked the beginning of much greater responsibility for the Association. In 1914, when a new student complex opened, which included Allen Hall, a meeting room for the executive, men's and women's common rooms, dressing rooms and a buffet, OUSA had almost complete financial and administrative control. The 1920s saw a further increase in responsibility. As the student roll rose, OUSA imposed compulsory fees, controlled its large profits from Capping and in 1923 purchased the student canteen. From 1933 it employed a full-time secretary. Medical students were in the vanguard of student activities. The 1922–23 OUSA Executive, for example, included the remarkable group, J.A.D. Iverach, as President, Arthur Porritt as Vice-President, and Derek Denny-Brown as Social Representative. 'I believe that my year was generally regarded as a good one', Iverach wrote years later.[11] Francis Bennett, in spite of anxieties about coping with his course, became Junior, then Senior Secretary of the Medical Students' Association and a member of Student Council. He joined the Debating Society and served as President of the Student Christian Movement. He wrote for all the student publications of his day, except *Critic* and the Capping magazine, and edited most of them. As Intellectual Affairs representative on OUSA in 1925, he founded *Critic*.[12]

A great opportunity arose for OUSA when land near the University, reclaimed to accommodate the New Zealand and South Seas exhibition of 1925–26, became available as sports grounds. The University leased 3.8 hectares for 99 years and OUSA provided more than £10,000 for a grandstand and for ground preparation, fencing and so on. Sir Louis Barnett, who donated £2000 to the project, opened the grandstand and sports area on 5 April 1930. He was accompanied by the OUSA President, medical student Jack Stallworthy. On that first day, medical student and later Rhodes Scholar and Olympic gold medallist Jack Lovelock took nine seconds off the club's mile record. Access to a home ground at Logan Park enabled the University Cricket Club to be re-formed. It was an exciting beginning, although ongoing maintenance of the asset proved a heavy burden for OUSA.[13]

The OUSA executive alienated a number of students at this time, either because it was controlled by 'allegedly superior and obviously brainless meds of long standing', as an arts student put it in 1930, or because its perceived stuffiness offended the flourishing boozy, bohemian elements in the student body. There were, of course, medical students on both sides of the conservative/disorderly divide. Some 'chronics' enjoyed the pleasures of the student life so much that they wanted to prolong them and they were permitted to complete, no matter how long it took. 'Hatch' Fookes famously spent ten years qualifying in medicine because he played so much football. In three quite dramatic episodes medical students fell foul of university authorities. A third-year medical student was sent down for a year in 1931 for drunkenly insulting a lecturer at an Allen Hall hop. When *Critic* took the view that the penalty was too harsh, the Professorial Board forced its editors to back down. The next year talented medical student Joe Small took over *Critic*, changing its tone to the racy and provocative. 'Concerning drink', he wrote, 'there are two choices – the gin and squash and the gin and two. Both are good.' He used *Critic* to object in the strongest terms when the University Council banned the Capping procession and ball because of drunkenness

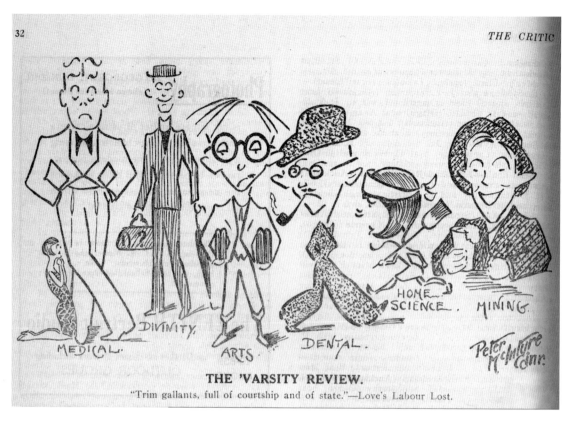

THE 'VARSITY REVIEW.

"Trim gallants, full of courtship and of state."—Love's Labour Lost.

Peter McIntyre's impression of students of the various Faculties. *Critic*, 1 May 1930, p. 32.
McIntyre (1910–1995) spent one year at Otago University in 1930 before moving to London to study at the Slade School.
He was New Zealand's official war artist from 1941 to 1945, and later achieved eminence as a painter of landscapes.

Hocken Collections, Uare Taoka o Hakena, University of Otago, j.

the previous year. He too was sent down for a year and the Council tightened its regulations by creating a new Board of Discipline. In the third case, OUSA President Douglas Kennedy, a medical student famed for stunts at Knox and in Capping who would one day become Director General of Health, came up against more sedate elements in the student administration itself. In 1937, when the Intellectual Affairs representative banned an issue of *Critic* because of a cartoon the Senate found insulting, Kennedy himself distributed the paper at dead of night throughout North Dunedin, to the fury of the Executive and Student Council. During the war a contemporary remembers him being lowered from the main Dunedin Post Office with an open umbrella, in imitation of Hess parachuting into Scotland.[14]

Conman Murray Beresford Roberts was in quite a different league as a prankster. In 1937, his first year as a medical student, he and a companion enjoyed the hospitality of a number of Dunedin homes by masquerading as house surgeons. He cheated in his second year written anatomy exam, was exposed by Professor Gowland in the oral, and had to relinquish his place. This did not prevent him taking a position as a locum for a doctor in Canterbury in 1944 and fraudulently signing a death certificate, an escapade which earned him a two-and-a-half year prison term. Among other medical impersonations (and there were many non-medical ones) he posed as Assistant Medical Director of the 3rd New Zealand Division, a Professor of Neuropsychiatry, a Naval Surgeon Commander and Lord Horder, Physician to the Queen.[15]

The *Medical Digest*

In October 1934 the Medical School reached a new stage in developing a community of its graduates and students, with the appearance of the *Medical Digest*. For the next four decades, the *Digest* would provide a unique record of the School's activities and an idiosyncratic and highly readable blend of serious medical opinion and dubious medical student humour. The first number announced itself as 'an annual publication from the Medical School, University of Otago, Dunedin, New Zealand' and 'a journal for Otago graduates and students'. The second number, in November 1935, stated that it was published under the auspices of the Medical Students' Association. The earliest *Digests* were about forty pages in length, with additional pages of advertisements at the end, and sold for 2/- a copy. Contributors were people of standing. Sir Lindo Ferguson had pride of place on the first pages of the first issue with a memoir of the old hospital block, 'A Landmark Passes'. Dr Arthur Porritt, who had left Otago on a Rhodes Scholarship in 1923 and at the time was Assistant Professor of Surgery in the University of London, contributed 'Recollections of Russia', a country he had recently visited with a rheumatism commission; Professor Carmalt Jones contributed a solicited article and there was a tribute to the late Dr F.R. Riley, 'a beloved physician'. Dr Benno Monheimer, recently arrived as the first of the German medical refugees from Nazism to settle in Dunedin, described medical studies in Germany, and Dr Charles Burns wrote on 'Postgraduate Study'.[16]

This first number appeared with a plain cover, but it contained some cartoons by the young Russell Clark. Described as 'a leader of the modern School of Art in New Zealand', Clark was thanked for the stimulating interest he had taken and the help he had given towards the founding of *Digest*. For the 1935 *Digest*, Clark provided a cover illustration, as well as cartoons of the Dean and Professor Gowland and, for the 1936 issue, some four pages of illustrations, including the striking study, 'The Operating Theatre'. The editors believed that his cartoon portraits of the professors were largely

Readers of the first issue of *Digest* were treated to a purportedly more accurate version of 'John Brown's Body', such as a 'modern poet of the *vers libre* school, with a Sydney Smith in one hand' might have written:

'John Brown
is undergoing
putrefaction
rigor mortis has
passed off and there is a green
colouration in the region of the
caecum
his tissues are all
emphysematous with
gas
poor old John'

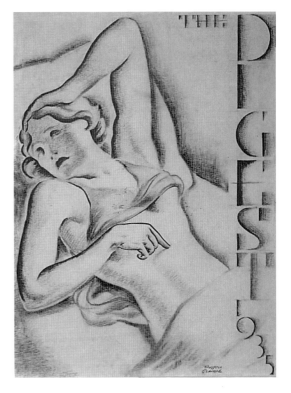

Russell Clark's cover for *Digest* 1935.
Otago Medical School.

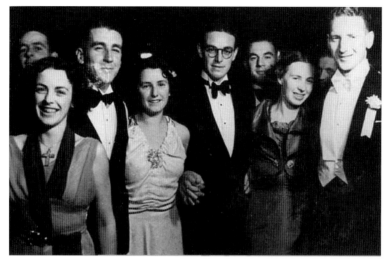

The Medical Ball, 1938.
The ball, organised by OUMSA, became firmly established as the highlight of the social year.
Hocken Collections, Uare Taoka o Hakena, University of Otago, Alumnus Association Collection. MS 1537/338.

responsible for the immediate success of the *Digest*. The collaboration ended when Clark left Dunedin in 1937 to become, in turn, an illustrator for the *Listener*, official New Zealand war artist in the Pacific and lecturer at the Canterbury School of Art.[17]

The *Digest* continued to feature articles by senior School staff and other prominent persons connected with medicine. In 1935, for example, Col F.T. Bowerbank, Director of Medical Services, wrote on 'The Medical Arm in Warfare', Professor Dawson on 'The Man Midwife' and Professor Bell on 'Postgraduate Education in Surgery'. Dr D.G. McMillan, chief architect of the health scheme of the new Labour Government, contributed a piece on the future of medical practice, and Professor Hercus provided a solicited memoir on his wartime experiences.[18]

By the end of the decade the *Digest* was including more OUMSA news, and it became customary to include lists of its office holders and patrons and the President's annual report, as well as reports of meetings of clubs such as the Otago Medical Society, the Clinical Society, the Medical History Society and the Medical Debating Society, and the Otago University Medical Corps. Other regular features were obituaries of former staff (usually written by other staff), welcomes to new staff, and articles on early days in the School. When the *Digest* celebrated its 'coming of age' in 1954 the Dean, Professor Hercus, wrote that its policy 'was not to publish scientific articles but rather to serve as a medium to record the social life of the School and maintain the community of interest between staff, students and graduates'. To a large extent it had succeeded.[19]

≈ Anatomy of a Medical School ≈

CHAPTER 12

The Dean's Assessment

IN FERGUSON'S clear, measured annual reports to the Chancellor we can follow the progress of the Medical School under his guidance, its immediate requirements and his aspirations for its future. The main themes addressed in the reports recur throughout: staff changes and shortages, fluctuations in student numbers, the need for more money, the need for more space, a separate library building and a new maternity hospital. In his last report, in 1936, Ferguson took the opportunity to review the fifty years since the inauguration of the complete course, which was also the period during which he himself had been associated with the School.

Ferguson's final report to the Chancellor tells a story of growth, beginning with student numbers. Over the twenty years from 1887 to 1907, 107 students graduated, an average of only five or six a year. Of the about fifty-five doctors who added their names to the medical register each year, only one in ten was locally trained. The School was handicapped by a lack of funds and was dependent on the 'self-sacrificing services of a small group of teachers who were receiving merely nominal sums in recognition of their work.' When student numbers began to build up after 1907, the School's limited accommodation and equipment were severely taxed. The sole lecture room was occupied practically every hour of the day, with no time between lectures to change diagrams or set up apparatus and exhibits. Ferguson considered it 'almost unbelievable' that any attempt at systematic work should have been

carried out under such conditions. Even after the extensions to Physiology added a second lecture theatre, only the cooperation of Professors Scott and Malcolm made lectures in other subjects possible. After about 1910 the School grew rapidly, with almost two hundred students graduating by 1914. At last, new buildings opposite the Hospital, for Bacteriology and Pathology in 1916 and Anatomy and Physiology in 1926, provided adequate space.

Between 1916 and 1936, the School produced more than eight hundred graduates. In 1907, there had been about six hundred medical practitioners on the New Zealand medical register, of whom only 16 per cent were locally trained. By 1936 there were more than fourteen hundred, 53 per cent of them New Zealand-trained. About one third of the graduates, 334 of roughly one thousand, completed higher qualifications in Britain. It was evident that the School would supply an increasing proportion of the doctors practising in New Zealand and would thus have an enormous influence on the health and welfare of the community. To fulfil this responsibility, by maintaining training at the highest possible level, the School urgently needed a Library Block, a Public Health Block, extensions to the Pathology Department, animal houses, a class room for the fifth-year subjects and accommodation for research workers.

Many of the issues Ferguson chose to address have a modern ring. Was the School, he asked, equal to the task of supplying the demand for practitioners in the Dominion? He argued that the problem was not so much a shortage of doctors as their uneven distribution, with isolated practices proving hard to fill. Would graduates who went overseas for further qualifications and experience return? Of the thirty-three graduates of 1933, twenty-seven were in London at the time of his report and some would certainly find openings in Britain, where the opportunities were greater than in a small community such as New Zealand. Ferguson warned of the effect recent legislation passed by the Labour Government, concerning rates of pay and hours of work, was likely to have on their decision. He suggested that graduates working overseas would not unnaturally think that if a clerk at age twenty-six must receive £6.10 for a forty-hour week, with a holiday on full pay, then their nine or ten years' work at an outlay of

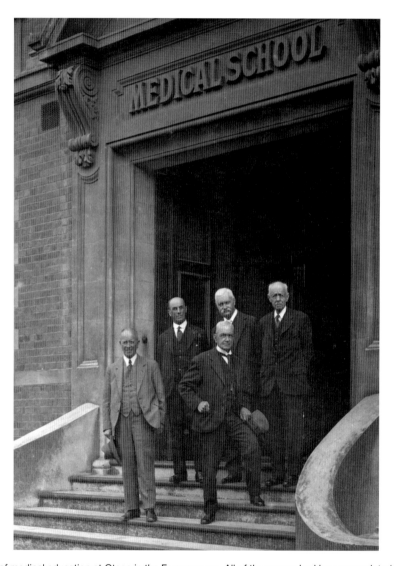

Veterans of medical education at Otago in the Ferguson era. All of these men had been associated with the Medical School for more than half a century when the photograph was taken in the early 1930s.
At the back, from left: Sir Louis Barnett, Sir Lindo Ferguson, Dr D. Colquhoun.
In front: Dr W.J. Mullin and Dr W.S. Roberts.

From L.E. Barnett, 'The Evolution of the Dunedin Hospital and Medical School: a Brief History', *Australian and New Zealand Journal of Surgery*, April 1934. Hocken Collections, Uare Taoka o Hakena, P97-104 a.

some £1500, in a profession where they could be called on day or night and in which there was no holiday pay or refresher leave, should command a better reward.

High student numbers were a serious concern in 1936. The economic depression of the previous four or five years had led large numbers of young men, who would normally have found careers in business, to seek admission to the professions. At the Medical School this resulted in large classes and consequent problems in clinical training. The Hospital Board had agreed to increase teaching facilities within Dunedin Hospital, but building had been delayed. The School would have to continue calling on hospital staff in the other three main centres to provide clinical training for sixth-year students. Ferguson recommended that the position of the teaching staff at these hospitals should be standardised and went into some detail describing how teaching should be correlated and uniform standards established in the scattered centres. The School should have a salaried representative on the staff of each hospital – a 'local sub-dean' – with the status of a member of Faculty. The clinical teachers should be recognised as members of the Otago Medical School staff, receive some payment and be visited periodically by the Dean.

In his final report, Ferguson also looked back on the busy year just past. The thirty-nine graduates had all found hospital positions as resident officers. He expected there would be fifty-six graduates in 1937, a number that should fully meet all requirements. Staffing was always to the forefront of his concerns and he paid tribute to those long-serving staff members for whom, like himself, the year marked the end of their career: Dr Benham, who had given foundation training in biology for thirty-nine years; Dr Newlands,

who had been on the staff of the Hospital for thirty years and an assistant lecturer in surgery under Sir Louis Barnett, was still a valued member of the Hospital Board and the Senate of the University of New Zealand; Dr North, tutor and assistant lecturer in gynaecology, who was currently in Britain and who would, on his return, also have reached the age limit which would terminate his active connection with the School. Ferguson himself had already retired from the staff of the Hospital, being replaced by Dr Carswell as head of the Department of Ear, Nose and Throat and lecturer in Ophthalmology. He took one last opportunity to protest staff shortages caused by poor remuneration. Professor Hercus urgently needed lecturers in Bacteriology and Public Health. However, no suitably qualified person would be likely to accept a position teaching in Public Health at £350, when he could get a permanent position in the Public Health Department at twice that salary, or in Bacteriology, when he could obtain a Hospital Board post at £700–£900. Finally, Ferguson thanked his staff for their loyalty and devotion to their duties and Dr Hercus for his whole-hearted cooperation during his thirteen years as Sub-Dean.[1]

The Dean's report summed up well the achievements of the School under his guidance, acknowledged its problems and provided some guidelines for its future. Its smooth narrative of progress describes an inward-looking School, focused on its own interests, apparently sheltered from what was going on outside its walls: the distress and anger caused by the economic depression of the early 1930s or the turmoil that arose among medical practitioners in response to the first Labour Government's plans to change the landscape of health care in New Zealand.

PART III

Research and Expansion:
The Hercus Era
1937–1958

World War II

LIKE his predecessor in 1914, Professor Charles Hercus took office in a brief phase of optimism before the onset of a world war. World War II dominated his early years as Dean and, like Sir Lindo Ferguson, Hercus not only met head-on the challenges wartime conditions posed in the management of the School, but also took full advantage of the opportunities they offered. In each case, although the war meant crises of staff shortages and overcrowding of classes, the need for more doctors to serve with the fighting forces, or to replace doctors who were doing so, gave the Dean powerful leverage with the Government of the day. If World War I had established the Medical School as the dominant faculty in the University, World War II strongly confirmed this predominance.

The mood in 1937 was buoyant. The worst of the economic depression of the early 1930s was over and the University was looking to expansion. A planning committee set up in 1937 felt confident enough to propose an ambitious development of new buildings to the north of the University complex.[1] The Medical School could boast a growing staff, more specialisation, a developing research culture, very good accommodation and facilities and, more recently, new clinical lecture theatres at the Hospital and access to the new Queen Mary Maternity Hospital. The change of Dean could not have been smoother. Professor Hercus, who had been Sub-Dean for thirteen years and Acting Dean throughout 1927, had gradually been assuming more and more

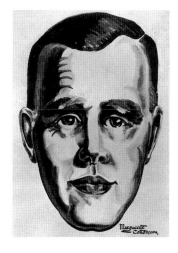

The New Dean. Marguerite Cotton's admiration for Charles Hercus is evident in her frontispiece for the 1937 *Digest.*

Medical Library, University of Otago.

responsibility over the previous decade. His initial survey of the needs of the School, which covered familiar territory – more money, more staff, more accommodation, the development of research and the development of the teaching hospitals in the other centres into well-organised Branch Faculties – was promptly endorsed by the Medical Faculty, the Professorial Board and the University Council. In June, the School tapped in to the upbeat mood of the times by holding a successful open night which, as *Critic* noted, was the 'first conversazione since the dim ages'. At least five hundred 'bewitched and gazing sightseers' were moved briskly from one demonstration to another, their passage up and down stairs expertly directed by the Professor of Anatomy who appeared, in the admiring opinion of the paper, 'to have a flair for traffic direction'.[2]

In 1939, there were a record 391 students on the School register and sixty-five students graduated during the year.[3] The outbreak of war in September shattered the optimistic mood, disrupted any prospect of orderly progression and forced the School to substitute day-to-day crisis management for long-term planning.

The Initial Impact: 'Foreign Medical Practitioners'

In the Medical School's report for 1939 we sense, for the first time, reverberations of the trouble in Europe, in an issue that roused public feeling to a degree apparently disproportionate to the numbers involved. Under the heading 'Foreign Medical Practitioners', the report notes that thirteen refugee doctors had been admitted to the Medical School to re-qualify, by taking the last three years of the medical course and the corresponding examinations. They included men and women, Christians and Jews, and they came from Germany, Austria, Hungary and Poland. Because the Customs Department had granted them residence in New Zealand and the Medical Board had accepted them, the University Council felt obliged to allow them to enter the Medical School. However, the Council thought their numbers were unduly large and protested to the Customs Department. In view of the overcrowding of the School, the Council decided to admit no more than three refugee doctors a year, unless the circumstances were very exceptional.[4] As reported in the local press, it was clear that 'whatever might have been the policy in the past there [was] not much likelihood of any further applications from refugee medical men and women for admission to the School being accepted.'[5] The item caused sharp dissension in the New Zealand University Senate when the report came up for discussion. A Hamilton member thought it extraordinary that 'an academic body connected with a humanitarian profession should go out of its way to close the doors to those who had to flee the worst tyranny the world had seen' and urged Senate to dissociate itself from the Medical School's actions. The Otago Chancellor felt obliged to explain that the Dean's report had been written in haste on his return from overseas (like his predecessor in 1914, Professor Hercus was out of the country when war began) and gave the wrong impression. The real issues, the Chancellor explained, were the overcrowding of the School, which was trying to cope with an intake of 122 in accommodation designed for a hundred, the fact that the Medical Council had no authority to accept the refugee doctors, and that the doctors themselves seemed to have been misled into believing that entry to New Zealand automatically meant entry to Medical School.[6] In the event, the language of the relevant section of the report was softened, with 'protest' to the Customs Department being replaced by 'communication'. The School's difficulties in accommodation were also spelled out and it was made clear that in future years only a small number of re-qualifying doctors from overseas could be accepted, not more than three in any one year.[7]

It is surprising that, in an annual report dated December 1939, Hercus did not mention the outbreak of war. His earlier work with the OUMC is practical evidence that he was aware of the likelihood of war and of the role medical graduates would be called on to play if it eventuated. The sense of foreboding felt in 1939 was perhaps most poignantly expressed by Carmalt Jones, who turned sixty-five that year and had planned to retire to England. As speaker at the May graduation ceremony, he concluded his address in sombre tone: 'It is no hyperbole to say that our civilization is trembling in the balance.'[8] Carmalt Jones was Acting Dean when war was declared on 3 September. He called all the medical students together to explain what war would mean to them. Then, as Neil Begg recollects, ashen-faced and to general embarrassment, he broke into a wavering rendition of the national anthem. Sympathetic students stood and some joined in and then, too choked with emotion to speak further, Carmalt Jones left the room.[9]

Over the war years, at least until 1944, there were few new developments at the Medical School, as priority was given to finding solutions to immediate problems of staffing and accommodation. Provision of a new building for

Pathology, Bacteriology and Preventive Medicine, which had been considered 'imperative' in 1939, had to be deferred until the end of the war.[10] The last professorial appointment until 1944 was the Chair of Medicine in 1940, to replace Carmalt Jones and Fitchett.[11] Although some appointments were made at a more junior level, staff losses were the norm. In 1940, Dr Muriel Bell resigned as Lecturer in Experimental Physiology to join the Department of Health. Other staff collaborated with the Defence and Health Departments on medical problems arising from the war. In 1940, eleven teaching staff were listed as being on active service. In 1942, Hercus reported that more than three hundred graduates of the School were serving in the armed forces. Twenty-seven were prisoners of war.[12]

Medical Students and Military Service

As had happened in World War I, there was intense debate over the medical students' military obligations, a sharp increase in student numbers and pressure from the Government to shorten the medical course. In September 1939 *Critic* ran a long, sombre editorial, expressing fears that the war just begun 'looks as if it may be World War II ... [and] may be more fearful than the last.'[13] In June 1940, in the wake of the collapse of France and the withdrawal of British troops from Dunkirk, the Medical Students' Association called a special meeting to discuss the place of medical students in the war effort. The Medical Faculty had been told at the outbreak of the war that medical students were to carry on with their course, but there had been 'peculiarly acrimonious comment' in the community about their apparent unwillingness to enlist. The meeting was intended to show that rather than evading action, the students were steadily preparing for service in the military, so as to give their best for the country instead of taking the easier and poorer way of enlisting as half-trained, inexperienced men.[14] At a subsequent gathering, the Dean responded to questions raised at the meeting. The issue of enlistment, he said, would be settled when the National Service Emergency Regulations, instituting call-

up by ballot, came into force on 22 July. Those in essential occupations could seek exemption by appealing to the National Board of Appeal if they were conscripted. It was 'fairly evident' that medical students would be exempted. As yet there was no urgent need for medical officers, and a year's postgraduate work as a house surgeon was required by the army authorities before new graduates were accepted. Medical students had offered themselves at the outbreak of war, but the Government considered they were doing a better job by continuing with their studies.[15] By early 1941 the regulations had been clarified. Third and fourth-year students called up in the ballot had their obligation to serve postponed indefinitely. First and second years were entitled to seek postponement. Thirty medical students who had completed two years' study had already appealed and Professor Hercus had appeared on behalf of each.[16] A letter to the *ODT* on 13 July 1941 drew attention to the 'senseless attitude of Government to second years'. If called in an overseas ballot they had to go. Of the current class of a hundred students, thirty-eight could expect to be called by the end of the year, but would be allowed to complete their second year. If they were allowed to complete their whole course, which would take until 1944, they would be able to serve as fully trained medical officers.[17]

Medical students may not have been expected to serve in the armed forces, but they were expected to undergo military training in the Otago University Medical Corps. Geoffrey Brinkman, who did his Intermediate year in Dunedin in 1939, recalls that within a month of war being declared, all those registered as medical students, including first years, received a letter from the army offering them the choice of volunteering to serve in the OUMC or being liable for the draft. They chose the OUMC. In December, as soon as exams were over, hundreds of medical students assembled at Burnham Military Camp, where they spent the summer as cadet officers. They had all the privileges of the officers' mess, but were not saluted by the other troops. Not surprisingly, their special status was resented by some of the recruits. The night the First Echelon left for overseas, they boasted that they were coming over to beat up the medical students and, as a precaution, the students were taken out on manoeuvres on the Canterbury Plains for the night and slept under the stars. At the end of the camp, they were granted leave without pay to resume their medical studies. Theoretically, they were under army control for the duration of the war. All vacations, including long weekends, were spent in camp or in barracks in Dunedin. Initially they were trained as infantry, but once they had reached the clinical years, they were given clinical assignments in one of the armed forces. Brinkman served at Taieri, Wigram and Rongotai.[18]

The outbreak of World War II upset the established routine of the OUMC in an unexpected way. At the beginning of 1941, what Hercus describes as an 'amazing metamorphosis' occurred. The unit abandoned its training of medical students in the principles and methods of medical field service in favour of general infantry training with other student recruits. It took many conferences in Wellington, Christchurch and Dunedin to reverse the decision, but later in the year the unit resumed its original function under Hercus's command.[19] With fears of an imminent Japanese invasion, it provided medical and dental care for the troops and the Home Guard mobilised for the defence of the South Island. Early in 1942 full mobilisation of the New Zealand forces was ordered, and the University released all medical and dental students serving with the OUMC for military duties. During this period, the OUMC trained and mobilised fifty Resident Medical Officers and posted them to South Island Formations in the field from Blenheim to Dunedin. It also supplied a full Field Ambulance to Rakaia, a Fortress Field Ambulance and a Field Ambulance Company at Blenheim. The OUMC thus fully justified its role in a country under military stress, with a third of its medical profession serving with the Expeditionary Force overseas.[20]

To make more trained medical officers available for the armed forces, or to replace those serving overseas, the Government urged the Medical School to shorten its course, as had been done in World War I. The request to cut six months

off the course presented problems. The General Medical Council of Great Britain insisted on a minimum of fifty-seven months' undergraduate training, excluding the Intermediate year, if a medical degree was to be recognised throughout the Commonwealth. This meant a full five-year course, so Otago could not shorten its course unless the GMC changed its regulations.[21] As a compromise solution, sixth-year students, in the last six months of their course, were made available to replace house surgeons at eleven New Zealand hospitals which had a staff of three or more house surgeons.[22]

Pressure of Numbers and Refugee Doctors

The Defence Department's demand for more doctors exacerbated the problems the Medical School already faced from a sharp increase in student numbers. In 1939 the Dean had signalled the problem of overcrowding when, in addition to the record 391 students in the medical course, there were another 166 in the Intermediate year. The following year, when the numbers rose to 452 medical students and 174 intermediates, the University Council limited the number entering second year in 1941 to one hundred. Careful consideration was given to the selection process. Preference was given to students who had failed second year but were allowed to repeat because they were favourably reported on by staff, and to graduate entrants. The other places were allocated on the basis of Intermediate examination marks, in proportion to the number of candidates in the various centres. Of the 185 applicants the eighty-three who had passed the Intermediate examination were all admitted. Medical School staff regarded the process as satisfactory and recommended that it should be repeated for the 1942 intake.[23]

Despite the care taken in selection, limiting the number of entrants was unpopular in the wider community. It fuelled the controversy over refugee doctors being admitted to the School and led to demands from Auckland for a medical school of its own. The issue of refugee doctors appears only briefly in Otago Medical School records, but it exercised the University Council from time to time after 1939, as individual cases were considered, and it smouldered on in the press. In February 1940, just after the Senate debate on the Medical School's 1939 Annual Report, the *Otago Daily Times* ran a four-column report on the Council's reconsideration of the cases of five applicants previously refused entry to the School. It seemed that the doctors had been told at New Zealand House in London that they could enter Medical School to requalify, if the Customs Department accepted them. As a consequence, the Medical School felt morally bound to admit them. The decision was not uncontroversial: indeed, a call for a total ban on refugee doctors was lost by only one vote. By this time, as Professor Hercus reported to the Council, applications from sixty-seven refugee doctors had been dealt with by Customs. Of the fifty permitted to enter New Zealand, thirty-nine had done so. Of these, seventeen had entered Medical School and another nine expected to do so. Eight were in private practice and five in other occupations. He complained that the question of who should decide whether to admit the doctors to the Medical School was like the old army game of 'passing the buck': the Customs Department handed it on to the Medical Council, the Medical Council to the University Council and the University Council to the Medical Faculty – the function of which, he asserted, was to teach and examine, not to make far-reaching decisions of policy.[24] In an editorial two days later, the *ODT* was quite clear that the decision should rest with the University Council.[25]

The number of refugee doctors may not have been large, but the question of whether they should be allowed to take places at the Medical School ahead of New Zealand students and whether, once qualified, they should be allowed to compete in private practice with New Zealand doctors, aroused intense public feeling. In May, the President of the Auckland Branch of the British Medical Association warned that at the same time over a hundred patriotic medical practitioners were serving in the war, fifty German doctors were practising in New Zealand.[26] 'Diversity of opinion' on the question was reported from the University Council meeting in June and the press report was followed by a spate of correspondence in the *ODT*, some of it strongly anti-German and most of it pseudonymous. 'J'accuse' was particularly outspoken. Other correspondents, including a fifth-year medical student, strenuously defended the foreign doctors.[27] The Returned Servicemen's Association (RSA) entered the fray, alleging subversive activities among University staff, and the *Truth* newspaper jumped on the bandwagon with an inflammatory piece headed 'Aliens Come First', in which it claimed that New Zealand medical students were losing places to foreigners. It was 'a pitiful reflection on the administration at the University of Otago that a year after admitting more than a dozen aliens to the Medical Faculty … the announcement is made that native-born second-year students in 1941 will be drastically limited'. The University Council responded by publishing its selection policies for medical students.[28]

Early in 1942, as married men were being called up to serve in the armed forces and places in the Medical School were restricted, the issue flared up again. This time the RSA claimed that refugee doctors were building up lucrative practices while New Zealand doctors were serving overseas. There was an 'overdose' of medically trained refugees, which would create problems when New Zealand doctors returned from the war. Foreign doctors should be used to staff hospitals, not permitted private practice.[29] The Senate of the University of New Zealand debated the question in committee, again with a reported divergence of opinion. Medical School staff member Dr Newlands, who was Chairman of the Medical Council, and a member of Senate, gave a press release explaining the background to the New Zealand Medical Council's policy of accepting no refugee doctors during the war. Two days later he had to defend the Medical Council against accusations that New Zealand was 'the most exclusive country in the world'.[30] When two further cases came before Senate in January 1943, the same arguments resurfaced. The Medical Council was against admitting them to the Medical School, but Senate questioned the Council's right to refuse entry to the School to any refugee doctor who had been accepted into New Zealand and voted to admit them. When the Otago University Council heard of the decision, one member expressed his disgust that Senate had 'foisted' two more refugees on the Medical School.[31] The Minister of Health made a statement on government policy: no more refugee doctors would be admitted during the war. He noted that those already in place were proving very useful, generally accepting the Government's direction as to where they should practise.[32]

The Clamour for More Doctors

The limitation on places at the Otago Medical School added impetus to Auckland's demand for its own School. As early as mid-1940, the Member for Onehunga used a parliamentary question to the Minister of Health to advocate establishing a medical school in Auckland.[33] The following July an *ODT* editorial commented on 'a variety of complaints and a good deal of loose talk, generally in Auckland, about the Medical School.' The Chairman of the Auckland Hospital Board, Mr Moody, threatened to withhold doctors from military service unless the Otago University Council modified its admission policies. Moody acknowledged that his intention was to '[drop] a bomb among the University people in Dunedin', adding that until Auckland had a medical school there would be a shortage of doctors, even if there was no war.[34] The Health reforms of the Labour Government necessitated more doctors and the restriction on medical student numbers was sharply criticised in Parliament.[35] Dr McMillan, principal architect of the reforms, urged that preparations should be made so that a medical school could be opened in Auckland as soon as possible after the war. Opinion on the issue divided on geographical lines. The *ODT*, predictably enough, took the view that it would be economically unsound to establish a second medical school in a country the size of New Zealand.[36] When the Auckland branch of the National Council of Women came out strongly in favour of an Auckland school, members of the Dunedin branch consulted Hercus, who told them that a new school would cost an initial £400,000

to £500,000 and, thereafter, £400,000 a year, a huge drain on resources when the existing School was not yet fully equipped and staffed.[37] Hercus repeated the same arguments, more forcefully, in 1943. In February, as the Medical School succumbed to pressure from the Government to increase its intake to 120, Hercus made it clear that this was the absolute maximum possible with current facilities. Precious resources must not be stretched over two institutions while the existing Faculty of Medicine was not yet a 'real' School. There was still insufficient specialisation, the Medical Library was inadequate, and levels of staffing and equipment were unsatisfactory. Until the Otago School was fully staffed, he said, any attempt to establish one in Auckland was inopportune. His arguments did not convince the Auckland lobby. Dr McMillan claimed that New Zealand needed a full two hundred medical graduates a year, prompting the Chairman of the Auckland Hospital Board and the Labour Member of Parliament for Otahuhu jointly to issue a statement that an Auckland medical school would be set up as soon as the necessary equipment was available. The *ODT* labelled this 'impudent propaganda'. Fuel was added to the flames when some of Auckland's 1943 Intermediates failed to gain places in medicine at Otago.[38]

The increase in the second-year intake to 120 might not have been enough to satisfy northern critics, but it was certainly enough to create tension and even distress within the Otago Medical School. The preclinical departments were already under heavy strain and the clinical teachers agreed that even a hundred students was well above the optimum of sixty or seventy for teaching with the hospital resources available in Dunedin. The Medical Faculty and the University Council had agreed to the increase only after emergency meetings and with the greatest reluctance.[39] Two of the most senior professors, with sixty-eight years' service to the School between them, could not accept the decision. John Malcolm approved the increase, but at the age of seventy and after almost forty years heading the Physiology Department, felt that he could not cope with its implementation. Percy Gowland also resigned, a few months

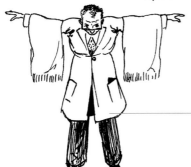

This item from *Digest* **1942 suggests that even at the end of his teaching career, Gowland's vividly illustrative teaching style could still make an impact:**

'We feel we cannot but admire
That earnest anatomic sire
Who, in attempts to tutor us
So oft becomes a uterus.'

Digest 1942, p. 52.

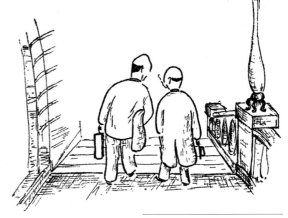

'The Old Order Changeth':
The departing figures of Gowland and Malcolm illustrate an
affectionate tribute from J.A. Begg to the professors
whose departments were 'the focal point and
essential foundation of the medical course.'
Digest 1943, p. 13.

before retirement age, in protest at the extra pressure on the already over-worked Anatomy Department. At the end of 1943, Hercus reported that the School was having to deal with twice the normal number of students and was 'absolutely at bedrock' in staffing.[40] Nevertheless, the outcome of this crisis was more advantageous than might have been predicted. The University agreed, for the first time in its history, to fill a chair by invitation. Dr W.E (Bill) Adams, an Otago graduate who was at the time Senior Lecturer in Anatomy at the University of Leeds, accepted the invitation to become Professor of Anatomy and arrived in Dunedin at the beginning of 1944. The Chair of Physiology was advertised and Dr J.C. (Jack) Eccles, then Director of the Kanematsu Institute in Sydney Hospital, applied and was appointed. They were new men for a new era.[41]

By 1944 there were other signs of new times ahead. The Dean had driven a hard bargain with the Ministers of Education and Health: in return for the increased student numbers the Government agreed to make an immediate start on a third medical building on Great King Street. At first known as the South Block, it was intended to house Pathology, Bacteriology, Public Health and Medical Jurisprudence and to provide space for research and animals, together with some space for clinical departments. Substantial alterations were also approved for the Scott Building. The Government immediately increased its annual grant to the School, which had been £8000 before the war, to £13,000. It also promised to increase the funding needed to bring the various departments up to strength, on the basis of a detailed statement drawn up by Hercus of the needs of each department.[42]

Meantime student numbers continued to rise. The 1944 session opened with another record 605 students in the Medical School, as well as 333 students enrolled in the Intermediate course in the four centres. Part of the increase was probably due to the fact the Government had made available a hundred medical bursaries. No wonder the Dean referred in his annual report to 'another extremely difficult year'.[43] As the end of the war came in sight, the prospect also arose of an influx of demobilised servicemen wanting to study medicine.

Otago Medical Graduates at War

From one point of view then, the Medical School during World War II was an institution struggling with almost unmanageable numbers in over-crowded accommodation and an atmosphere of acute stress. For graduates of the School who served with the fighting forces, the war had a very different aspect. Their experiences were varied, sometimes heroic, sometimes amusing, often horrific. In 1946, the *Digest* published a list of their names, carefully drawn up by the Dean's secretary, and prefaced by a list of those who had lost their lives in the war. Hercus wrote that the OUMC had provided 682 officers, of whom twenty had lost their lives. The *Digest* lists twenty-two fatalities: the two who had not been trained in the OUMC were the only women on the list, sisters Florence and Tessa Craig (later Thompson), both graduates of 1932, who died in the fall of Singapore, fulfilling their medical duty of care to the end.[44] Some of the graduates have published their stories. Lindsay Rogers, for example, wrote of his time with Marshall Tito in Yugoslavia as a 'guerrilla surgeon'. *Time* magazine, referring to him as 'Doctor X', said he had asked to be transferred to Yugoslavia after performing 9000 operations in Africa. Instructed by Tito to set up a hospital in a farmhouse, he drove out the pigs and chickens and went to work, using a carpenter's hammer, hacksaw and chisels as his instruments and salt water for antiseptic.[45] John Borrie, in *Despite Captivity*, an account notable for its broad humanity, described his four long years as a prisoner of war, from his capture in Greece in April 1941 to his release in Germany in April 1945. He was later awarded an MBE for his services to fellow POWs.[46] Neil Begg described his service in Egypt and Italy in his autobiography, *The Intervening Years.* He completed his medical course in the early months of the war which, when he wrote fifty years later, seemed to be 'quite separate and unconnected' with his life before and after. He began as the Officer Commanding 102 Mobile Venereal Disease Treatment Centre in Egypt and from 1943 served in Italy with the 2nd Division.[47] For some medical officers trained in the OUMC, it was the second time around. Montie Spencer, for example, who had gone via Egypt to Gallipoli as a medical student, returned as Officer Commanding the 2nd New Zealand Hospital at Helwan and later in the desert near the Suez Canal. His letters home, published by his daughter, give a vivid picture of day-to-day life in the Hospital and its surroundings, suddenly ended by his death from typhus fever in 1943.[48]

Medical units began training in Burnham and Trentham in September 1939 and left New Zealand with each of the three echelons. They served in Greece and dealt with the wounded from Crete, sweltered in the heat and sand of North Africa, slogged from Sicily up the length of Italy, were engaged in the Middle East and the islands of the Pacific. They provided mobile units near the front line, well-equipped general hospitals in safer areas and hospital ships. They could close down, pack up and move at short notice and open at a new location with the maximum of efficiency and the minimum of fuss. The aim was to have a short and rapid line of evacuation so that the wounded could have the benefit of prompt early dressing and surgery. The evacuation of wounded soldiers by ambulance or air was far more speedy than it had been in 1914–18 and surgical theatres were closer to the front line, so that the wounded had a better chance of surviving. It has been estimated that one in twenty of the wounded died, compared with one in ten in World War I. As the war drew to an end, General Freyberg paid high tribute to the New Zealand Medical Services:

> In the opinion of 2NZEF, and this opinion is borne out by comments from outside sources, the New Zealand Medical Services are without equal. The standard of surgical and medical treatment and administration of hospitals, casualty clearing stations, field ambulances and convalescent depots has been most important in keeping up the morale of the force overseas. The personal interest shown by the medical staff has established a sense of confidence in all who have come under their care.[49]

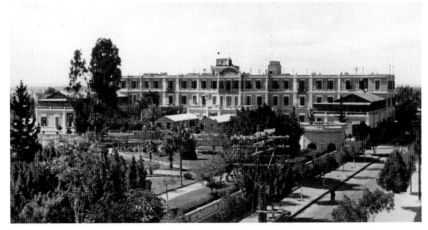

Second New Zealand General Hospital Cairo, formerly the Grand Hotel.

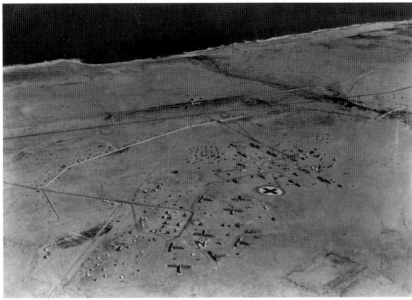

Very different accommodation: Second New Zealand General Hospital Gerawla, from the air.

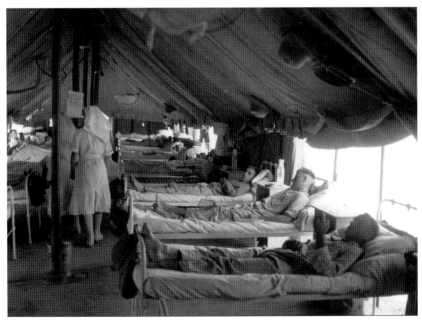

Inside a tent ward at Gerawla.

Photographs, Christine Daniell, Montgomery Spencer collection.

As in World War I, the need to treat war injuries stimulated the development of new medical techniques. New discoveries, sulphonamide antibiotics, developed in the 1930s, and the widespread availability of penicillin from 1943 dramatically reduced the chances of infection. Begg wrote excitedly of the advent of penicillin that he had 'taken part in a medical revolution'. Dramatic advances were also made in plastic surgery by Otago's Archibald McIndoe and his team. Although burn injuries, a particular hazard for fighter pilots, could be treated with saline baths, the disfigurement to facial features remained. Plastic surgery could partially repair the damage. Sir Harold Gillies, who had developed the specialty of plastic surgery at Sidcup in 1914–18, had persuaded his Dunedin cousin, Archie McIndoe, to specialise in this field and McIndoe was already Consultant in Plastic Surgery to the Royal Air Force when war began. At East Grinstead in Sussex he developed a centre specialising in the treatment of air force casualties with facial burns and injuries. His work included not only operating on the men, but rehabilitating them as well. It was commonly said that it was his personality that pulled his patients through. After the war former patients continued to meet regularly in the famous and exclusive Guinea Pig club.[50]

Many of the Medical School staff of the post-war decades shared the experience of military service. Lawrence Wright, who served in North Africa and Italy, was demobilised in Britain and completed his pre-war scholarship before his appointment to the Chair of Obstetrics and Gynaecology in 1952. John Borrie also spent the immediate postwar years gaining further qualifications and winning some prestigious awards in England, before returning to Dunedin in 1952 to serve as senior thoracic surgeon for the southern region and lecturer at the Medical School. The Australian Michael Woodruff, Professor of Surgery in the mid-1950s, studied vitamin deficiency diseases at first hand during his four years as a POW in the notorious Japanese Changi prison camp. With the help of engineers, who constructed a chopping machine for him, he turned the grasses round the camp into a foul-tasting liquid containing the B-group vitamins. In one year they made 20,000 gallons of the extract, with strikingly beneficial results for those who took the mixture. Stanley Wilson, who was on the visiting staff of Dunedin Hospital for many years before and after the war and was senior lecturer in surgery in the Medical School from 1952 to 1965, served with the NZMC in the Middle East and the Pacific from 1940 to 1944. In the Western Desert he won a reputation for pre-eminence in battle surgery. He was largely responsible for developing the use of nasogastric suction and intravenous fluid replacement in battlefield abdominal injuries.[51] Wilson and Norman Speight, who was in charge of 6 Field Ambulance, were captured when it was overrun at Sidi Rezegh. Wilson was able to escape and Speight was released in an exchange of prisoners a few months later. Both men, together with Walden Fitzgerald and Victor Pearse, returned from active service to teach in

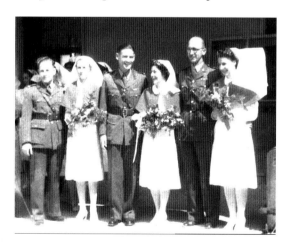

A wedding of army medical staff at Caserta, Italy, in April 1945. The wedding party, from left, are Major Albert Adams, Sister Audrey Hobson, the groom, Major Lawrence Wright and bride, Sister Isobel Henderson, Major Alex Borrie and Sister Mary Howden. The Colonel and the Hospital Matron acted in loco parentis and the groom said the wedding was viewed as a 'sideshow' to the party afterwards. All the men were Otago medical graduates.
Photograph, Lawrence Wright.

the Medical School.[52] The postwar School had more students and more staff, more academic visitors, a new building, a revised curriculum, a stronger emphasis on research and increased financial support from government through the new University Grants Committee, which for the first time placed the finances of the School on a stable basis. For all the problems and distress the war had brought, it provided an important stimulus for increased government support for the Medical School and marked a new stage in its development.[53]

Sir Charles Hercus, 1888–1971
Dean of the Otago Medical School, 1937–58.

WHEREVER you look in the records of the Otago Medical School for the first half of the twentieth century, you are likely to find Charles Hercus. Born in Dunedin in 1888, he was brought up in Christchurch and returned south as a dental student in 1908, the year the Dental School opened. He was one of the first group, of three, to graduate in 1911. He appears in a photograph on the wall at Knox College, taken in 1909, as one of the first intake of students to the College. He was a foundation member of the Otago University Officers' Training Corps, the forerunner of the Otago University Medical Company. Graduating from Medical School in 1914, he took part in the Gallipoli campaign and served with distinction throughout the war, being mentioned in dispatches four times, and awarded the DSO in 1917 and OBE in 1919. Hercus married Isabella Rea Jones in 1923. They had two sons and two daughters.

Ahead of his time in his commitment to public health, Hercus took an MD and Diploma in Public Health after the war, joined the Department of Health and resumed his association with the Medical School in 1921 as Professor of Bacteriology and Public Health. This was the beginning of an unbroken service to the school that lasted thirty-seven years, until 1958 – and even beyond, if one accepts the story that for some time after his retirement he regularly came in to look at the mail. To outsiders, and others in the University, he seemed to personify the School itself.

Hercus's determination to foster research was backed by his own record in seeking a preventive for the goitre that affected a fifth of the New Zealand population in the 1930s. As a teacher he was respected – the great armful of books be brought to lectures impressed students – rather than exciting, but the public health thesis he introduced for senior students has created a remarkable archival resource.

After his retirement, Hercus was active in the Taieri hydatid station, and collaborated with Sir Gordon Bell in writing a history of the Medical School, notable for its detailed knowledge of events and persons. He died in 1971 after some years of failing health.

Hercus is honoured by two prestigious awards in his name. The Sir Charles Hercus Health Research Fellowship, established by the Health Research Council of New Zealand in recognition of his contribution to biomedical, clinical and public health research, is a four-year postdoctoral fellowship for a researcher whose scientific field has the potential to contribute to the health and economic goals of the Government's investment in research, science and technology. The Sir Charles Hercus Medal of the Royal Society of New Zealand, established in 1996, recognises outstanding research in the biomedical and health sciences.[54]

CHAPTER 14

Research and Expansion Under Hercus

The First Decade: Focus on Research, 1937–1947

When Sir Gordon Bell came to write a tribute to his co-author of *The Otago Medical School Under the First Three Deans*, he chose the words 'He fostered research' to sum up the core aspect of Sir Charles Hercus's multi-faceted achievement as Dean of the School from 1937 to 1958. Hercus was an innovative teacher, a superb administrator with particular skill in financial matters, and a far-sighted academic diplomat – the apt pupil in this of Sir Lindo Ferguson. However, research was the foundation on which all else rested, both cause and effect of the remarkable expansion of the Medical School in the Hercus era.

Until the mid-1920s, Bell elaborated, the Medical School had been largely a vocational institution, its early professors too burdened by routine duties and lacking time and funding for regular research.[1] Emeritus Professor Fred Fastier, who held a research post from 1940 in the Department of Medicine, put it more strongly, referring to a 'dismal attitude to research' as one of the 'glaring faults' of the interwar School. 'Most of the medical faculty', he wrote, 'were content to accept the view that worth-while research could not be carried out in New Zealand.'[2] Hercus changed this attitude. Under his deanship, the research culture that made the Faculty of Medicine a true University School, qualified to add to knowledge as well as impart it and underpinned by funding generous enough to permit a massive increase in

staff at all levels and in a variety of areas, began to flourish in the years after World War II.

In 1950, five years after the end of the war and when he was well into the second decade of his deanship, Hercus used a lecture to the Wellington branch of the Royal Society of New Zealand to affirm his credo on research. Under the title 'New Zealand and Medical Research', he gave a detailed and lucid exposition of the role of research in the Otago Medical School. Hercus's definition of medical research was all-encompassing. Far from being limited to the field of disease, it was concerned with the study of health and normal development and with the study of man's environment in so far as it affected his physical and mental well-being or, as he put it, the 'right use of the human body'. For what Hercus had in mind, the term 'human research' was more appropriate than 'medical research'.[3] Such research found its natural home in the University and its development was the responsibility of every professorial head of a University department. 'Unless the professor undertakes some research of his own, at the same time encouraging and stimulating his staff continually to do likewise, there will be no vitality in his department.'[4] More than a credo, this was a statement of policy.

The foundations for such an all-pervasive research culture in the Medical School had been laid in the late 1930s. When funding, both public and private, became available, enabling teams of researchers to combine on broad projects, the Medical School was ready to take advantage of the new opportunities. The breakthrough came in 1937 when the Government set up a Medical Research Council (MRC) in the Department of Health. Modelled on the British Council of 1911 and under the chairmanship of the Director-General of Health, its purpose was to advise the Minister on research funding. Hercus had supported the Director of Health, Dr Michael Watt, in setting up the Council and he and Muriel Bell were appointed to it. The Council received an annual grant of £35,000. At its first meeting Peter Fraser, the Minister of Health, emphasised the active interest his Government took in medical research and indicated that, in the meantime at least, this should be concentrated on subjects of vital concern to New Zealand. In a decision of great import to the Medical School, the Council chose to support research in the University, either through departments or in separate research units, rather than create a new research institute. Specialised committees under the Council were set up to propose research programmes, estimate the cost involved, and supervise the work. By 1938, committees had been appointed for research into nutrition, chaired by Malcolm, hydatid disease, chaired by Barnett, goitre, chaired by Hercus, and obstetrics, chaired by Dawson.[5] It was a splendid opportunity for the Otago Medical School and, in his annual report in 1938, Hercus urged the Government to go further and establish a Department of Medical Research within the School. He repeated the recommendation the next year, when he reported on the difficulties of carrying out research into nutrition, thyroid disorders and hydatid disease with workers dispersed in different departments of the School. A new building, given over to medical research, was needed to house these workers.[6] It did not happen at this stage.

The need to provide additional space for research was given urgency by a major bequest. The trustees of the W.H. Travis Trust, of Christchurch, allocated £12,000, over seven years, towards tuberculosis research in the Medical School. Dr Norman Edson began work as a Travis Fellow in 1940. A brilliant Otago student, the first to take the degree of Bachelor of Medical Science, winner of the Travelling Scholarship in 1930 and

a Beit Memorial Fellowship which enabled him to complete a PhD at Cambridge, Edson had been a lecturer in biochemistry since 1937 and would later become foundation professor in the discipline. After some thirty years' association with the department, he summed up: 'It would be difficult to exaggerate the importance of the Travis Laboratory as a factor contributing to the creation and strength of the Biochemistry department.' The trustees had been generous in providing expensive equipment for the laboratory, which enabled modern techniques to be employed, such as electrophoresis, ultracentrifugation and the use of the radioactive isotope of carbon. They founded scholarships for research students and brought stimulating visitors to the department for six-month periods. They thus facilitated the unification of teaching and research and the amount of money they made available for both 'would have been regarded as an unbelievable sum 25 years ago'.[7]

In April 1939, the threat of war in Europe brought a medical researcher of the first rank to Dunedin, Dr Walter Griesbach. A dignified and cultured man, already over fifty, experienced as a clinician, university lecturer and researcher and the author or co-author of twenty-eight scientific publications, he had left Germany to escape Nazi persecution and come to Dunedin because of his wife's connections. He was appointed as a research fellow and began the research on the pituitary gland that would occupy him for the next twenty-seven years, most of it in the Thyroid Research Department of the Medical Research Council. During this time he was author or co-author of another forty-four papers, which greatly enhanced the reputation of the Medical School. Muriel Bell, at this stage a lecturer in physiology and experimental pharmacology, wrote that he must have 'pined for the contacts he had been accustomed to, among the élite brains of Europe'. Together with Bell, he taught physiology in a more down-to-earth style. 'When the study of the pituitary-thyroid relationship was proposed', she continued, 'we collected pituitaries from the skulls of sheep slaughtered at Burnside and Balclutha before morning classes began, in order to obtain material for histology and for making thyrotropic hormone.' By this time, there was a small but impressive medical research community at Otago, into which Griesbach readily fitted. The most significant contact was H.D. (Dick) Purves. Duncan Adams, himself part of the group of thyroid researchers, affirmed that 'the great good fortune of Dr Griesbach's exile from Europe [was] that it resulted in his collaboration with Dr H.D. Purves.' A chemistry graduate, Purves had started as Hercus's research assistant in 1932, completed a medical degree in 1941 and become director of the Medical Research Council's Thyroid Research Department. The collaboration, as Adams described it, was 'a marriage of the systematic morphological type of study of the old Austro-German school with the functional, physiological approach characteristic of Anglo-Saxon investigators.' Together they identified the six pituitary cells which produce the six different pituitary hormones and wrote a number of joint papers.[8]

The appointment of Professor Horace Smirk, on the eve of World War II, underlined the thrust towards research during the late 1930s and foreshadowed its expansion in the post-war period. It had long been decided that when the two part-time Professors of Medicine, Carmalt Jones and Fitchett, retired they should be replaced by a full-time professor. Both had made contributions to clinical research, but had been too heavily engaged in teaching and administration and the demands of private practice to undertake long-term research projects. The new professor was to be free of the demands of private practice and able to devote himself entirely to clinical and theoretical teaching and the development of research. When the post was advertised in Britain, Australia and New Zealand, it attracted twenty applicants. Hercus went to Britain to join the selection panel in interviewing candidates. Dr Horace Smirk, Manchester-trained, with experience at University College, London and in Vienna and, since 1935, Professor of Pharmacology in the Medical School of Cairo, was already widely known for his research in hypertensive disease. It is indicative of the new focus of the chair that the University Council did not think it necessary

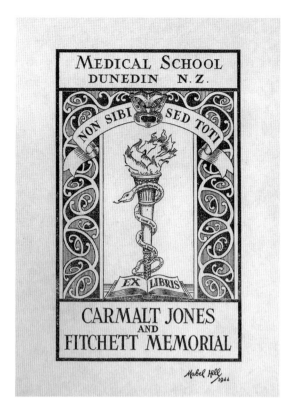

Bookplate by Mabel Hill, designed for books purchased for the Medical School Library from the fund collected at the retirement of Professors Fitchett and Carmalt Jones in 1939. Selected by the professors, the plate incorporates design motifs embodying Medicine, a School of Learning, a Library and New Zealand.
Digest 1944.

to consult with the Hospital Board before appointing him. The Department of Medicine had broad responsibilities, overseeing the teaching of paediatrics, psychiatry, therapeutics and pharmacology, and it had been agreed that Professor Smirk should head an enlarged department, built up by the appointment of a senior lecturer, two full-time assistant lecturers and two part-time lecturers. On his arrival, Smirk argued convincingly for more staff, and was also sharply critical of the accommodation provided for him and the inadequacy of laboratory services. By early 1941, he had obtained three full-time senior lecturers, four full-time juniors, a senior visiting physician, two junior visiting physicians and three acting assistant physicians. The School was equally prompt in providing

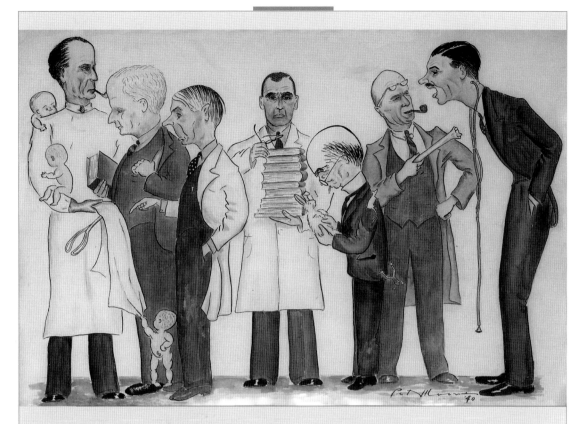

The best-known, and best-loved, caricature of Medical School staff was done by Pat Moore (now Sir Patrick Eisdell Moore) for *Digest* 1940. From left to right are: Professors Dawson, D'Ath, Bell, Hercus, Malcolm, Gowland and Smirk. In his autobiography sixty-four years later, Moore commented on the cartoon and the professors' first reactions to it:

'The central figure was Hercus. To me his bland and correct features defied the caricaturist. All I could do was load him with the piles of books he invariably brought to each lecture … I failed, I think, with Bernard Dawson, the obstetrician. I watched as he opened his copy of the *Digest* and stared long and silently at the page. His barely controlled expression of dismay revealed that I had not quite captured the air of handsome arrogance of which he was so proud. Johnnie Malcolm was amused. Percy Gowland was delighted, but it was Horace Smirk, to whom I had been the most fiendish, who appreciated it the most. I had kept his yellow complexion and portrayed him in the act of leaning forward and barking. He had an immensely long stethoscope, which held some special magic for him and this occupied a prominent position in the group.

'I was in the vestibule when he came up to me, waving his copy.

'"Is this how you spend your days, Moore?" he queried, "You're wasting your time doing medicine." And he went off to the sales table and bought another dozen copies.'

P. Moore, 'The Professors', Otago Medical School.
So Old So Quick, pp. 87–8. Cited with the author's permission.

Sir Horace Smirk, 1902–1991

Professor of Medicine, 1940–61, Research Professor and Director of the Wellcome Institute, 1962–68

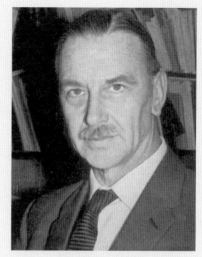

Sir Horace Smirk.
Hocken Collections, Uare Taoka o Hakena,
University of Otago, Acc. No. c/n E 3605/23 c.

THE arrival of Horace Smirk in 1940, as Professor of Medicine, made an instant impression. One of his students, Patrick Moore, viewed him with the sharp eye of a talented cartoonist: 'direct from Cairo, a Lancashire man, immensely tall, with a bristling moustache and an astonishingly yellow complexion (due to anti-malarial drugs which had not yet worn off) .... He had a habit of leaning forward, as if his long legs were stilts, and barking his words out in a staccato North Country accent'. The 1940 *Digest* described his lean, energetic figure 'striding about the school at a furious pace and with incredible purpose'. He is remembered arriving at Allen Hall to inaugurate the 1941 session, 'two yards of pump water on a bicycle, with his gown a-flutter and his MD bonnet jammed down against the slipstream'. But the students found him very kind and appreciated – nervously – rostered Sunday afternoon visits to his home. Smirk had married Aileen Bamforth in 1931 and the couple had four children.[9]

Smirk built up the Department of Medicine, engaged wholeheartedly in research and fostered future researchers among his students through the BMedSc and PhD degrees. A number entered the Department of Medicine through the Science Faculty. He encouraged junior staff to take the Membership of the Australasian College of Physicians, which could be obtained locally. Generous funding from the Medical Research Council, insurance organisations and pharmaceutical companies enabled him to set up units specialising in psychopharmacology and rheumatology and bring other research interests into the department.[10] The expansion of the department, and its increasingly scattered accommodation, made administration unwieldy. At one stage Smirk oversaw ninety staff and, with the Dean at the time Sir Edward Sayers, he explored the idea of separating the components of his chair into research and clinical teaching. A generous grant from the Wellcome Trust in London provided a new building in 1962 to house him as a research professor, together with his research team, regular overseas visitors and a colony of specially bred hypertensive rats. An experiment to further raise the rats' blood pressure was to expose them to a motor horn, turned on daily at exactly 5 p.m. – which came near to inducing hypertension in members of the nearby Pathology Department as well.[11]

Smirk received numerous honours. He was knighted in 1958. At his retirement, in 1968, a special issue of the *New Zealand Medical Journal* was produced in tribute to him. In a guest editorial, the director emeritus of the Cleveland Clinic Foundation in Ohio praised his success in undertaking 'the building in New Zealand of what has become one of the great research centres of the world'. At the centenary of the Medical School in 1975, he was one of a distinguished group to receive honorary degrees. In 1987, he was awarded the Medical Research Council's silver medal, but by that time was not well enough to receive it in person. Horace Smirk died after a long illness in 1991.[12]

the requirements for Smirk's research. When he arrived, there were no technicians and a lack of equipment necessitated some ingenious recycling – references to Frankenstein's monster were common. The department had no fume cupboards and the only electrocardiograph was a reject from the Hospital. Soon after he arrived, however, Medical Research Council funding enabled Smirk to engage in the long-term study of hypertension and cardiovascular disorders which would make his name internationally and around which a whole school of research would grow. Hercus lauded the developments as the beginning of a new age of research in clinical medicine.[13]

It was fortunate that the building blocks for a research culture in the Otago Medical School were in place by 1939, before the demands of war took precedence over all other concerns. Research continued, however, under the auspices of the MRC and the Travis Trustees. In 1942, the MRC gave an additional £1000 per annum for research into clinical medicine. From 1943, after the appointment of Mr Murray Falconer as neurosurgeon, it provided money for his research into prolapsed intervertebral discs and leaking intracranial aneurysms.[14] For some, the war offered new research opportunities and responsibilities. The medically qualified nutritionist Muriel Bell, who had gained an MD in 1926 for a thesis on basal metabolism in goitre in New Zealand and spent five years in London developing her lifelong research in nutritional science, was a prime example. As State Nutritionist in the Department of Health from 1940, she made recommendations on food rationing and sought answers to dietary problems caused by shortages of imported foodstuffs, such as oranges and cod liver oil. In this case, her answer was rose hip syrup, rich in vitamin C and made up from a recipe she had created in her own kitchen.[15]

The two dynamic professors who joined the staff at the beginning of 1944 were met by a massive teaching workload. Dr Bill Adams found his staff in Anatomy – a senior lecturer, a junior lecturer and two demonstrators – totally inadequate to cope with the number of students and the work of his department. Most of the teaching fell to him,

as it had done to his predecessor. Until he could build up his staff, which was a gradual process, research had to take second place.[16] Adams had been a lecturer at Otago in the past and already had a reputation as a 'fine teacher but a hard man'. He asserted his authority at his first lecture as Professor, by throwing out one of a restless group in the back row, the embarrassment of the student concerned compounded by the fact that his friends had confiscated one of his shoes. It was not an isolated incident. 'Who will forget', asked Professor David Cole rhetorically in a formal speech at the Medical School centenary in 1975, 'his first few lectures each year, the memorised roll call, or the almost inevitable ejection of the talkative or clowning student?' Adams lectured 'very well indeed', one of his students recalled, 'in a firm, even dogmatic style.'[17]

The new Professor of Physiology, Jack Eccles, just thirty-nine and tirelessly energetic, came to the Medical School 'with a rush and a roar' and made an even greater impact. Eccles' whole background had been in research and his work in neurophysiology had already gained him his FRS. He had travelled from his native Melbourne to Magdalen College on a Rhodes Scholarship in 1925, joined the team working with Sir Charles Sherrington and gained first-class honours in physiology and biochemistry. Although well established in Oxford, he decided to return to Australia in 1937. He established a research team in Sydney which studied neuromuscular transmission in cats and frogs. By 1943, however, he was looking for another base and moved to Dunedin in January 1944. He remained only six years, but it was long enough to give a strong boost to the research culture of the Medical School and to inspire a number of the best students.[18] His own teaching attracted both praise and criticism. A student of his first class remembers one lecture as 'a revelation of clarity and biological beauty', realising much later that the material was fresh in Eccles's mind from keeping a few pages ahead of the class in the textbook of the day.[19] His practical classes had real experiments, but he tended to concentrate heavily on his own interests. His successor, Dr Archibald McIntyre, believed that his teaching was unbalanced, with too much time

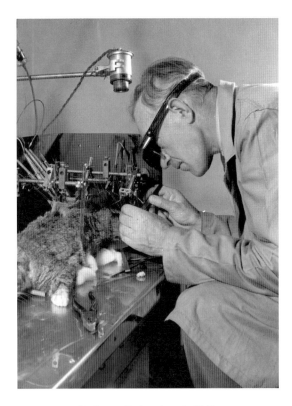

Professor Eccles at work, 1949.
Hocken Collections, Uare Taoka o Hakena, University of Otago,
Acc. No. 82.189 g.

the development of knowledge as a growing and living thing. In addition to being evidence based, the presentation of medical knowledge must include demonstrating the lines along which it is going and the patterns and underlying concepts that appear in it. For Eccles, research was the key. The status of a medical school, he maintained, was judged abroad 'by its contribution, and the contribution of its graduates, to medical science and virtually not at all by the standards of its examinations.' What had been achieved to date at Otago had been due to the 'heroic efforts of a few in the face of great difficulties' and on 'a very few thousand pounds a year.' There was a dire need for a much more generous policy in the endowment of research.[21]

Despite an enormous teaching load, Eccles lost no time in re-establishing his own research laboratory, assisted by Jack Coombs, a talented electronic engineer, and recent graduate Dr Lawrence Brock. Eccles' presence at Otago attracted a stream of prestigious overseas visitors. He invited the philosopher Karl Popper, then at Canterbury College, to give a series of lectures. His contribution to what has been called a golden age of the Otago Medical School was immeasurable. When the Auckland Medical School opened in 1968, Eccles was proud to claim that most of the senior faculty had been his students.[22]

Eccles' demand for more staff led to two appointments of importance for the future. Norman Edson returned to Biochemistry as an Associate Professor and when Physiology and Biochemistry were separated in 1949, he was promoted to the Chair.[23] Also in 1949, Eccles persuaded Dr McIntyre, who had been a former close colleague in neurophysiological research in Australia, to come to Otago as a senior lecturer. When Eccles left the following year to become Professor of Physiology at the Australian National University and his position was advertised, McIntyre was appointed.[24] Like Eccles, he placed the utmost importance on research.

In Canberra from 1953, Eccles' career soared. The new research university was well funded and he was able to draw together a distinguished team.

spent on controversial neurophysiological topics and not enough on the more clinically applicable aspects of physiology, but that it also had 'the great merit of keeping the students in touch with at least part of the growing frontier of knowledge'. McIntyre believed that while many of Eccles' lectures may have bewildered students of average and less-than-average ability, they stimulated the most able and to some 'opened up new worlds of intellectual excitement and endeavour'. In a significant addition to the curriculum, Eccles introduced a BSc course in physiology.[20]

Eccles lost no time in nailing his colours to the mast with an article in the *Digest* (the same issue that welcomed him to the School), on 'Research and the Medical School'. A doctor graduating from Medical School, he argued, was only partially trained. He must continue his self-education throughout life by practising as an applied scientist. He argued passionately for the influence of research on teaching and

His work focused on processing information in the cerebral cortex, cerebellum and hippocampus. He was made Knight Bachelor in 1958 and, in 1963 he shared the Nobel Prize in physiology and medicine for his contribution to the ionic nature of synaptic transmission in the central nervous system. He was made a Companion in the Order of Australia and in 1963 Australian of the Year. His last years were less rosy. Faced with compulsory retirement at sixty-five, he chose to leave Australia for the United States, eventually settling at the State University of New York. When his laboratory career finally ended in 1975 he moved to Switzerland. Eccles died in 1993.[25]

A further stimulus to the research culture, and its integration into the teaching of the Medical School, was the revival, after some years in abeyance, of the degree of Bachelor of Medical Science and the institution of a Master of Medical Science in 1945. The BMedSc had been introduced in 1926 to enable a few selected students to take a year out from the medical course to concentrate on one of the preclinical sciences and serve an apprenticeship in research. Gowland had been instrumental in its introduction and Eccles and Adams revived its popularity, which this time proved durable. Hercus and Bell describe it as an outstanding success, producing a 'more or less steady stream of medical graduates who entered into clinical careers and also into medical teaching and research careers.' David Cole and Gavin Glasgow were among the five who took this 'sideways move' in 1945 and both acknowledged that it had led to more academic and interesting careers than might have eventuated otherwise. In an unpublished memoir, Cole describes their two-part joint project and the excitement and sheer entertainment of working with Eccles (to reproduce experimentally in cats the effect of the protruded intervertebral disc on the nerve roots to the legs) and the young neurosurgeon Murray Falconer, fresh from the wartime head injury unit at Oxford (to investigate numb patches on the legs occurring in sciatica). The tight little group of five students experienced the heady pleasure of Oxford-style seminars on various neurophysiological topics and the sense of working close to the edge of scientific knowledge.

The sight of Eccles in his own laboratory, a huge cage of chicken wire, was, as Cole described it, 'almost a caricature of the mad scientist amongst his oscilloscopes, wires and animals.' The MMedSc was more restricted in scope. It was designed for holders of the BMedSc who could continue for a further year on an approved course of study and supervised research. They would then be ready to proceed to PhD study. Candidates for the MMedSc were examined by two written examination papers and oral examination and a research thesis.[26]

The postwar focus on medical research at Otago fitted into a much broader international context. Spectacular advances in the application of science, particularly in the medical field, had been stimulated by the war. In 1946, Hercus attended a British Empire Science Conference in London, which led to new research for the Medical School: its extension to those Pacific Island territories for which New Zealand had administrative responsibilities. Working with the South Pacific Commission, the Medical School would provide research facilities for members of the health services working in the region and would initiate research into problems specific to it.[27] The Medical Research Council supported the work through a special committee and offered two fellowships to researchers. In 1950, Hercus could report that an Island Territories research team was working in collaboration with the medical department of Samoa and the Cook Islands on the health problems of their people. Expeditions had worked over the summer vacations of 1948–49 and 1949–50 on the endemic problems of yaws, filariasis, hookworm and tuberculosis, as well as the general nutritional status of the people.[28]

Research expansion into the South Pacific area was only one aspect of the increased contact of the Otago Medical School with the outside world made possible by the end of the war. Staff also participated in overseas conferences and took research leave, and distinguished visitors travelled to the School. The visitors began arriving even before the war ended. In 1944, Sir Howard Florey gave lectures to staff and students over a three-day period and discussed possible modifications to the conditions of the Nuffield Trust for the endowment of demonstratorships and clinical assistantships for Dominion university graduates at the Oxford Medical School.[29] The same year, the formidable Dr Edith Summerskill, British doctor and Labour MP, who had studied welfare and maternal services in Europe, the USA and the USSR, as well as in her own country, inspected and, was impressed by, the work of Professor Dawson. She was also impressed by Hercus, commenting to the *Evening Star,* 'I have met today with the most progressive dean of any medical school I have visited during my travels.'[30] In 1948, the centenary of Otago province brought a large number of overseas visitors to the School. Some attended gatherings, such as the annual meetings of the Royal Australasian College of Surgeons and the British Medical Association. Others visited as individuals, among them Professor Hugh Cairns, the first Sims Commonwealth Travelling Professor, who spent ten days at the School, Professor J.C. Spence of the Medical Research Council of Great Britain and Dr Leech of the American Rockefeller Foundation.[31]

The Second Decade: Medical Education, Research and Expansion, 1948–1958

In the immediate post-war years, the University of Otago struggled to cope with a bulging student population in limited accommodation. The Medical School was spared the worst of this problem, as its numbers were restricted by government, albeit at an uncomfortably high level, and it had a major new building under construction. The completion of the South Block, promised to the School in 1943, was fraught with difficulties. The land had to be purchased from private home owners, there were complications over the foundations because of water-logged subsoil, and serious shortages of labour and building materials. Hercus had warned of the difficulties of teaching the enlarged class of fourth-year students in 1945 if the building was not ready for use. It was not. In 1946, he had to acknowledge that 'exasperating but inevitable delays' meant it was unlikely it would be ready for occupation before March 1948. Not surprisingly,

an attempt to use the ground floor of the new block while construction proceeded overhead had to be abandoned because of the noise. Throughout 1947, work in the Departments of Pathology, Bacteriology and Preventive Medicine and in the library was seriously handicapped. It was September 1948 by the time the Minister of Education could open the new building. Five storeys high and with a total floor space of one and a quarter acres, it contained more than two hundred rooms. The ground floor housed the Preventive Medicine Department and various laboratories and consulting rooms, the first floor, Pathology, and the second, Bacteriology. The third floor was given over to research, with seventeen laboratories and various support services, such as glass blowing, workshop and photographic rooms. Above this was the animal floor. The new building would provide excellent accommodation for the period of research expansion to come. Appropriately, it would be named for Hercus in 1969.[32]

As the war drew to a close, the whole question of medical education opened up. In 1944 a British Interdepartmental Committee (the Goodenough Committee) investigated and sharply criticised the British medical curriculum, as established by the General Medical Council and followed by the Otago Medical School. The Committee called for an overhaul of the entire curriculum, to

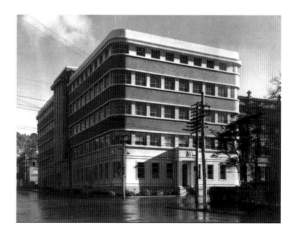

The new South Block (later the Hercus Building) in 1949.
Hocken Collections, Uare Taoka o Hakena,
University of Otago. c/n/E 5824/2A.

Around the Medical School, 1949

All photographs Hocken Collections, Uare Taoka o Hakena, University of Otago.

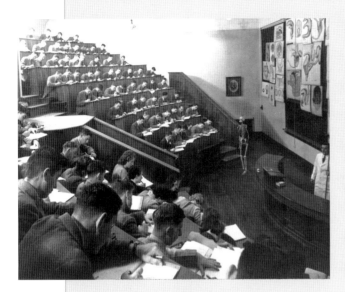

An Anatomy lecture in progress.
c/n E5994/22. S07055a.

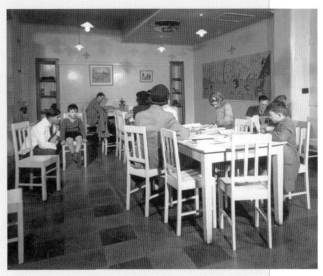

Waiting room, Department of Preventive Medicine.
c/n E 5995/36A d.

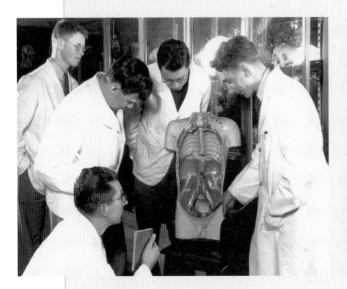

Group of students with Dr Trotter, Anatomy, (right).
c/n E 5994 25 c.

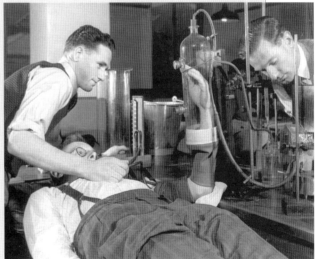

Medical students conducting experiments
in the Physiology Department.
c/n E 975/36A SO4-180 e.

increase its educational, rather than vocational, aspects. It recommended shortening the course, reducing its factual content and requiring that all students hold a house appointment for a year before registration. These recommendations were eventually incorporated in a Medical Act, which came into force at the beginning of 1957. In May of that year, the General Medical Council issued an entirely new set of recommendations for medical education. Hercus and Bell, writing at a time when these had yet to be implemented, were enthusiastic at the prospect, praising the new 'spirit of freedom' in what they called the 'Magna Carta for medical education'. In line with the report of the Goodenough Committee, the recommendations called for lighter and more flexible curricula that allowed for more experimentation in its order. They affirmed that the memorising of factual data should not interfere with the primary need to foster the critical study of principles and the development of independent thought. They endorsed a compulsory sixth year of hospital experience before registration. The Otago Medical School welcomed the tone of the Goodenough report and the consequent changes, which began well before the Committee's recommendations were given legislative form.[33]

The Senate of the University of New Zealand also undertook a review of medical education at the end of the war. Its aims were practical: to determine the number of doctors the country would need in future years and assess whether Dunedin could provide enough clinical experience to train them adequately. In 1946–7 a committee, convened by the Vice-Chancellor of the University of New Zealand and including the Dean of the Otago Medical School, reviewed medical education in Dunedin, Wellington and Auckland. It concluded that the training provided by the Otago Medical School was generally sound, although more staff and buildings were required. It considered the current output of eighty new doctors a year to be adequate for some time. In relation to the curriculum, the committee recommended that the workload in fifth year be reduced by transferring some subjects to sixth year, that a medical and a surgical tutor be

appointed in each of the Branch Faculties and that graduates spend a compulsory hospital year before registration.[34] The report was adopted by Senate and its principal recommendations were gradually implemented. Improvements were made in the staffing and facilities of the Medical School, although they remained below what Hercus thought desirable. Congestion in the heavy fifth-year programme had already been addressed in 1945 by removing Applied Anatomy and Physiology from the Third Professional examination, and the programme was further lightened by transferring the teaching in Practical Obstetrics and Gynaecology, and in Eye, Ear, Nose and Throat from fifth to sixth year. There was a major change in 1950 when, in accordance with a 1947 recommendation of the General Medical Council, the course of Anatomy, Physiology and Biochemistry was reduced by a term, leaving the last term of the third year available for an introductory clinical course. The change was made reluctantly, because staff believed they needed a full six terms to teach the basic medical sciences. There was a lack of staff and facilities for clinical and para-clinical instruction in the new course and the change also meant transferring the First Professional examination from the end of the year to August.[35]

The burden of high student numbers, partially eased by the Branch Faculties, hung heavy over the Medical School in these years. In 1948, the hospitals in Christchurch, Wellington and Auckland were each given part funding for a medical and a surgical tutor with senior qualifications and, in 1955, additional government funding enabled the setting up of full-time medical units with a senior specialist, a registrar and thirty beds. A compulsory hospital year before full registration was instituted in 1952. In spite of this assistance at the clinical level of training, staff generally favoured a reduction in student numbers. Hercus himself thought an annual intake of sixty would be the optimum. In 1952, another Senate committee was set up to consider whether, where and when a second medical school should be set up. It recommended that planning begin for a medical school in Auckland to open in fifteen or twenty years' time.[36]

The *Digest* and Medical Education

After the war, renewed international contacts and, perhaps, the presence of older, more critical returned servicemen in the Otago classes, provided a stimulus to student debate on medical education. The theme runs as an increasingly strong thread through the *Digest*, from its first appearance in 1934 to its eventual demise in 1978. Taken as a whole, the *Digest* articles give the lie to any claim that there was little interest in the topic, or that students accepted the Otago course unquestioningly. The articles fall into three main categories: specific teaching recommendations, reports on innovations in overseas schools and (often trenchant) criticism of the Otago course, which peaked about 1967. Only a few articles on medical education appeared during the first decade of the *Digest* and these usually came from staff. In the 1936 issue, for example, there was a plea for a diploma in psychological medicine, and articles on proprietary medicine and Maori medicine. In 1937, Professor Edson contributed a quite lengthy piece arguing for fewer examinations and an extension of the tutorial system, to combat student inertia. Another dominant theme of the *Digest*, student inertia, was often blamed on the curriculum and how it was taught.[37]

Within a few years of the end of the war, the tone became more critical. The 1947 *Digest* included a fairly traditional plea from staff member J.L. Malcolm that the Medical School should make more use of visual aids, especially film, but by 1948 more fundamental issues had begun to emerge. That year, the editors broached the question of whether the Otago course fitted the student for medical practice, concluding bravely that 'complete reform of the course may perhaps be the goal at which to aim …' The following year, in a 'Letter from Brooklyn', Chandler M.C. Brookes, who had been associated with the Physiology Department between 1941 and 1947, brought up the crucial question of the crowded timetable. He 'never could see where and when the medical student at Otago had opportunity to study'. Brookes argued that a bigger library and fewer lectures would free up the overworked faculty and 'place a greater responsibility on the students' shoulders, where it rightly belongs.' He sensed a 'subtle antagonism between students and professors'.[38] In 1950, the University's recently appointed Vice-Chancellor, Dr R.S. Aitken, himself a graduate of the Otago Medical School, challenged it to deliver a 'vocational' course in a 'liberal' way. Medicine, he said, was 'as much an art as a science'.[39]

Rumblings of discontent continued intermittently through the 1950s. In 1955, for example, one writer complained that the medical course was producing too many specialists, who knew next to nothing about general practice and cared even less. The same issue contained a quite detailed report on the innovative medical course at the University of Western Reserve, Cleveland, Ohio. This course had been introduced because students had been dissatisfied with the burden of factual learning, the splitting of medicine into numerous departments and the schism between preclinical and clinical sciences – all issues relevant to Otago. Two years later, an editorial referred approvingly to the recommendations of the General Medical Council of Great Britain for more interdepartmental teaching and a less abrupt divide between the preclinical and clinical years. In the last year of the decade the editors claimed that all over the world it was being acknowledged that passive instruction could never satisfactorily replace active discussion and criticism.[40] Both the specific causes of discontent with the Otago course and possible ways to remedy them had been identified by the end of the 1950s.

Expansion of Staff

The first two or three years after the war were characterised by staffing difficulties in a medical school whose student population was swollen by returned servicemen. The 1946 roll of 676, including Intermediates, would not be reached again until 1953, and would not be maintained after that. By 1948, the situation had stabilised and the second decade of Hercus's deanship was an outstanding period for the Medical School, despite his contention that staffing was difficult because the salaries Otago could offer did not meet the international market and prospects in Britain were particularly good at this point.[41]

In the 1950s there were some significant professorial appointments. In the Department of Surgery, Sir Gordon Bell was succeeded in 1953 by the first full-time professor, Michael Woodruff, FRCS (Eng). Born in London in 1911, but brought up and educated in Australia, where his first degree was in engineering, with honours work in mathematics, Woodruff had passed the primary examination of the Royal College of Surgeons while still a medical student. Although he was commissioned in the Australian Army Medical Corps in 1940, he was not called up until he had completed his Master of Surgery the next year. Posted to Malacca, he then spent most of the war as a prisoner of the Japanese. After the war, he completed his FRCS in Britain and began his lifelong research on immunology and transplantation. He was Assistant Surgeon in the Children's Hospital in Aberdeen when he accepted the Chair at Otago. Woodruff stayed only four years at Otago before he was appointed, without even the formality of an interview, to the University Chair of Surgery at the Edinburgh Royal Infirmary. Nevertheless, these years were very productive for him scientifically and were a stimulus to the Medical School's research programme, as he published major papers describing 'an immunological phenomenon known as runt's disease, the anterior chamber of the eye as a privileged site for foreign grafts and the use of banks of frozen skin in the management of burns.' At Edinburgh, where he remained until his retirement in 1976, Woodruff's career was stellar. He built up an outstanding department of surgical science focusing on transplantation biology and tumour biology, with a special interest in immune response to tumours. He established the first transplant unit in the United Kingdom and in 1960 performed the first successful kidney transplant in the United Kingdom between identical twins. He published *The Transplantation of Tissues and Organs* in the same year. The Medical Research Council funded an MRC Research Group under his direction and the Nuffield Foundation built a specially designed building for transplantation at the Western Infirmary, with him as Honorary

Director. He was knighted in 1969 and received numerous other honours and awards. In 1958, Gustav Fraenkel MA MCh (Oxon), who had been engaged in research at Oxford into wound healing, replaced him as Professor of Surgery in the Otago School.[42]

In Obstetrics and Gynaecology, Sir Bernard Dawson retired after thirty years, to be replaced in 1951 by an Otago graduate, Lawrence Wright FRCS (Eng) FRCOG, who was working as First Assistant in the Obstetrical and Gynaecological Department of St George's Hospital and Medical School in London. Wright had been studying and working in London since the end of the war and was persuaded by Hercus to return to his alma mater. He would serve the Medical School with distinction until 1981.[43]

In 1955 the long-planned division of Professor Hercus's Chair came to pass. He retained Preventive and Social Medicine and John Miles MD (Cantab), Research Fellow at the Adelaide Institute of Medical and Veterinary Science, was appointed to the newly created Chair of Microbiology, as Bacteriology was renamed. He would hold this post for twenty-three years, constantly fostering the links between science and medicine. A medical scientist of distinction, with a long list of publications, Miles is regarded as the father of microbiology as a tertiary discipline in New Zealand and was the driving force behind the development of the Department of Microbiology and Immunology into an outstanding centre for teaching and research.[44]

There were other appointments of importance for the future during this time. Dr Wallace Ironside MD (Aberdeen), arrived from a lectureship at Leeds to a post as special clinical lecturer in psychiatry and would later head a separate department as Professor. Mr John Borrie MBE ChM FRCS, was appointed lecturer in thoracic surgery. He later advanced to Associate-Professor in his specialty and he also served the Medical School in other ways. In 1957 he founded the postgraduate course for specialists in basic medical science, which gained an international reputation and for which he was awarded the Royal Australasian College of Surgeons' medal for services to postgraduate education. Fifty years on, the course was attracting ninety Australian and New Zealand surgical trainees. After his retirement in 1980, he became a dedicated honorary curator of historic medical artefacts, a role recognised in the naming of the John Borrie History Hall after him. Frederick Fastier MSc (NZ) DPhil (Oxon), became senior lecturer in pharmacology. He was promoted to a personal Chair in 1969 and, in 1976, became head of the new Department of Pharmacology.[45]

Research

Research in the Medical School flourished during this period and the Medical Research Council was central to its development. In 1951 the Council ceased to be a committee of the Department of Health and achieved independent status, with an increased budget and a proliferation of sub-committees. In 1956 it produced a glossy, well-illustrated booklet describing its work. Prominently displayed on the first page was a large photograph of the Hercus building with the proud statement. 'Headquarters of medical research in New Zealand is the new block of the University of Otago Medical School, where most of the work supported by the Medical Research Council is undertaken.'

In the pages that follow, the work of each of the MRC's eleven committees is concisely described and generously illustrated. The Otago Medical School had a virtual monopoly. A Dental Committee (from 1947), located along the road at the Dental School, was the only research committee not housed in the Medical School. The booklet reports that the research of the Clinical Medicine Committee (established 1942) on heart disorders and drugs affecting the heart, resulted in a method of treatment that gave relief from high blood pressure. The Nutrition Committee, one of the original committees, established in 1938, was engaged in a survey of the foods eaten in New Zealand households on the basic wage, and by Maori families, and was investigating the vitamin and other nutrient value of New Zealand foods. The Microbiology Committee, established in 1947 by the amalgamation of the former Hydatid and Virus Research Committees, was

investigating infectious diseases caused by three groups of agents, bacteria, fungi and viruses. The Endocrinology Committee was carrying out work begun in 1924 on goitre and its prevention, and the treatment of thyroid disease. The principal aim of the Neurophysiology and Neuropathology Committee (1944) was to further elucidate the nature of the process underlying brain and spinal cord activity, with the aim of diagnosing and treating nervous diseases. Research was undertaken by the Cancer Committee in two sections, the study of the development of tumours and the effect of radiation on living tissue. The Obstetrical Research Committee (1951) was interested in the practical problems of childbirth in all its aspects, as well as the wider field of gynaecology. The Surgical Research Committee, dating from 1953, was engaged in four fields: tissue transplantation, experimental cardiac surgery, the metabolic response to surgery and the genetic study of a family with multiple polyposis of the colon. The Island Territories Committee (1946) was collecting information on health and disease in the Pacific area with a view to solving health problems specific to the region. The Toxicology Committee (1953) was investigating possible dangers arising from the use of food additives. The Chest Diseases Committee (1951) had been set up to consider the development of a policy on thoracic surgery.

The last section in the booklet informs readers that the £55,000 per annum allocated to the MRC for 1956 and 1957 was quite inadequate to carry out all these activities and that the Council was seeking donations or bequests.[46] Although individual researchers are not identified in the publication, except in captions to some of the illustrations, the MRC's overview of its activities demonstrates the vigour of the research culture at the Medical School in these years, thanks to the group of professors and senior academic staff appointed after the war and to some new arrivals taking up research positions. In the 1950s, a number of MRC researchers working in the School were given honorary lecturer status.

Outstanding researchers among the new arrivals were Drs Franz and Marianne Bielschowsky, who arrived in 1948. Born and educated in Berlin,

Franz Bielschowsky had held a research post at Dusseldorf before he was dismissed by the Nazis, on racial grounds, in 1933. He was living in Madrid when the Spanish Civil War broke out and he served in a hospital for the Republican army. Then in Britain, from 1939, he began work for the British Empire Cancer Campaign. The Cancer Society of New Zealand brought him to Dunedin as Director of Cancer Research in the Hugh Adam Department of Cancer Research, where he remained, despite attractive overseas offers. He began work on the relationship of the endocrine glands and cancer. He needed pure-bred strains of mice for this research and Dr Marianne Bielschowsky undertook the breeding programme, developing several unique strains. The obese hyperglycaemic mice, a strain with autoimmune haemolytic anaemia and mice with megacolon, created world-wide interest and requests for colonies. Franz Bielschowsky became a leading authority on the influence of hormones on carcinogenesis.[47]

Dick Purves, who headed the Endocrinology Committee, played a central role in many of the School's most significant research activities. He carried Hercus's work on the prevention of goitre to a successful conclusion, by establishing the proportion of iodine that needed to be added to salt in the New Zealand diet to be effective. The standard (one part potassium iodide per 20,000 parts of salt) was adopted by the Department of Health in 1941–43. John Hubbard, a later Professor of Physiology, wrote that Purves deserved 'the eternal gratitude of his fellow citizens for his leading role in the abolition of the thyroid enlargement (goitre) which had once disfigured nearly 20 per cent of the population'. In addition to his work with Griesbach, on the physiology of the anterior pituitary and the thyroid glands, Purves collaborated with T.H. Kennedy in the identification of anti-thyroid drugs to treat Graves' disease. Working with Duncan Adams, he proved that Graves' disease was caused by autoantibodies. The scientific papers resulting from these and other collaborations run from 1933 to 1977, with several typically published each year. Purves demonstrated that the highest international esteem could be achieved from Dunedin, with local training. National and international honours included an honorary DSc from Otago in 1972. Purves retired in 1973 and died in 1993.[48]

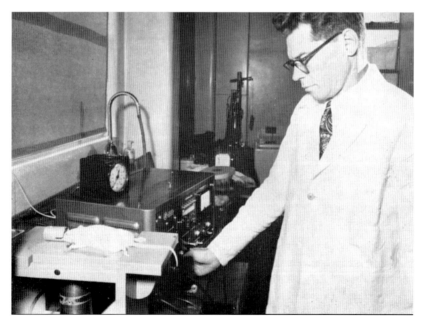

Dr H.D. (Dick) Purves.
Medical Research Council booklet, Medical Library, University of Otago.

Horace Smirk's research into hypertension also won international plaudits during this period. His quest for a drug that would lower high blood pressure had begun in Cairo between 1935 and 1940, when he tested nearly 1500 chemical compounds on the stray dogs that roamed the city. In Dunedin, using wild rabbits and later specially bred rats, he tested a similar number until, in London in 1949, he learned of hexamethonium. He wrote a series of ground-breaking papers demonstrating the effectiveness of the drug and established a clinic where it was successfully used to treat hypertension. Fastier noted, 'From the patient's standpoint, hexamethonium was a vile drug ... but it pointed the way to effective therapy.' In 1958, Smirk summed up his research in a major monograph, *High Arterial Pressure*.[49]

For almost twenty years after the war, Muriel Bell continued to make her energetic and forward-looking contributions to public health. She worked with an influential network of professional women, notably Dr Elizabeth Gregory of the Home Science School and Dr Helen Deem of Plunket. Nevertheless, her work was sometimes underestimated by the academic community, perhaps because of its practical nature and her effectiveness in popularising it. She had advocated free milk ('our best food') in schools since 1937 and she served on the Milk Board from 1945 to 1974, the year of her death. She planned diets for people living on remote islands and, in her weekly columns in the *Listener*, she explained nutritional research in everyday terms. She wrote *Lecture Notes on Normal Nutrition* for nurses. She campaigned against some powerful opposition for the introduction of fluoride into public water supplies, dubbing herself 'battle-axe Bell' as a mark of her determination. In the 1950s, she conducted research into cholesterol and heart disease and vainly tried to persuade insurance companies to collect statistics on obesity. In 1956, she devised highly successful rations for both men and dogs for the New Zealand Trans-Antarctic expedition. Bell retired in 1964 and was awarded an honorary DSc by Otago University in 1968.[50]

'All who have been brought up in this country or have brought up their children here ... are indebted to Dr Bell's persistent and inquiring interest in the welfare of women and children during her long career ... [she] campaigned with unexampled energy to make the findings of research available for the common benefit – from rose hip syrup to fish liver oil, from the extraction rate of flour from wheat, from milk in schools, to fluoride in the water supplies.'

Citation for the award to Muriel Bell of the degree of Doctor of Science, honoris causa, University of Otago, 1968. Registry, University of Otago.

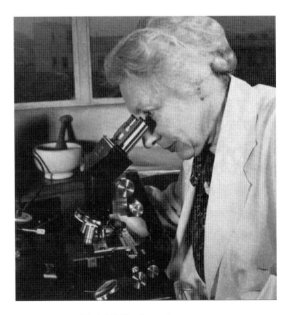

Muriel Bell at her microscope.
Medical Research Council booklet, Medical Library, University of Otago.

CHAPTER 15

Medical Students in
the Mid-Twentieth Century

In the Shadow of War

War dampened the ebullient student mood, typical of the 1930s at Otago, to one of greater seriousness. With the high proportion of male students on active service, it also intensified the medical students' domination of student affairs. In 1941, the editor of *Critic* warned of the need to guard against 'the complete control of OUSA by the Medical School'. He reminded readers of the bitterness their ascendancy had aroused after the previous war, when the last general student meeting had ended in a 'free-for-all fight, Medical and Dental v. the rest of the Varsity'.[1] Medical students made up 90 per cent of the male student population for much of the war and filled the presidency of OUSA continuously over the years 1942 to 1945. The residential colleges continued to be at the heart of student activities, and medical students continued to predominate in them. At Knox College in 1944, they numbered eighty, out of one hundred and eight residents, and they commonly stayed for the entire length of their course. Ian Prior, who began University in 1940, when he was just sixteen, thought that the most satisfying thing about being there was getting into Knox. He roomed with several 'great people', who remained his friends, and he appreciated the tutorials in the compulsory subjects for Intermediate that were held at the College. David Cole, who entered Knox in 1942, also shared rooms with a succession of four friends ('wives') over the years. He thoroughly

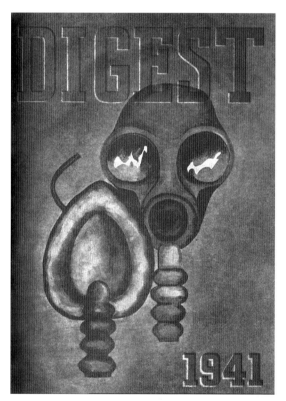

The cover of *Digest* 1941 reflects the sombre mood.
Medical Library, University of Otago.

enjoyed the 'happy communal life', with all main meals provided and facilities laid on to make scrambled egg suppers. He relished the initiation ceremonies and sports, including bombing hapless passers-by from the central tower block with water-filled paper bags.[2] Student activities were restricted during the war, however.

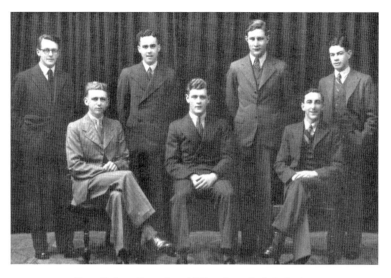

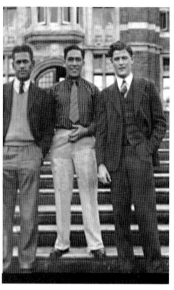

Knox College Executive, 1945 – all medical students.
Back row, left to right: Norrie Roger, Hugh Fleming, Bruce Harvey and John Phillips. Front row: Geoff Walton, Ian Prior and Jim Baird.

Rugby friends on the steps of Knox College. Voselegi, a dental student from Fiji, and medical students Nitama Paewai and Ian Prior.

Capping celebrations were suspended and, from 1942, there was no procession, concert or ball, and no Easter Tournament. Medical students did not have the time to organise these events, even if they had been thought appropriate to the times, because they were technically on leave from the army and spent their vacations and some weekends in camp.[3] The *Digest* continued publication, but focused on war-related items.

University sport slumped during the war, although rugby was less affected than cricket. Ian Prior remembers playing a lot of rugby and captaining the University A team for a time. He and a fellow medical student, the brilliant half-back Nitama Paewai, played together for Otago, for the New Zealand Army (as members of the OUMC) and for the South Island versus the North. That was as far as it was possible to go during the war, because there were no All Blacks.[4] In the case of cricket, Griffiths claims, the war turned decline into almost total collapse and cut off the careers of many promising individual players. One cricketing fixture that was maintained was the annual match between Knox and Selwyn Colleges. In 1944, it provided one of the great University sporting stories. Playing for Knox, a six foot three medical student from the Fijian

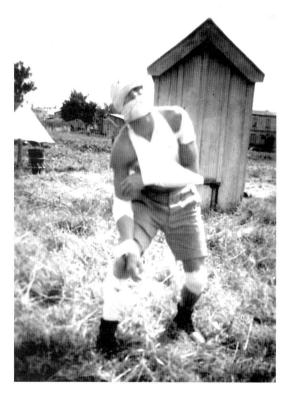

Bandaging was part of the army training for medical students in camp at Blenheim. Tangi (Richmond) Martin was said to be a willing subject.

All photos, Ian Prior collection.

royal family, Ratu Kamisese Mara, demolished Selwyn with an exhilarating innings of 147 runs, which included twelve sixes and twelve fours, as well as taking five wickets for twenty-six. The next year he was equally deadly in his shattering of an Albany Street window.[5] Mara, as he was then known, also excelled as a line-out forward in rugby and won the high jump, discus, shot and javelin at the inter-faculty sports. He earned a triple blue in rugby, cricket and athletics, won the Drinking Horn at Tournament with a new record, played the triangle in the Capping band and was a huge, and hugely successful, female impersonator in the post-war Capping concert. At the beginning of his fourth year, Mara was recalled by the Council of Fijian Chiefs to train as an administrator at Oxford. As Ratu Sir Kamisese Mara, he later served as the Prime Minister of Fiji for many years.[6]

The war might have been expected to open opportunities for women medical students to take a fuller part in university life. However, although the proportion of women among the student population rose, to an impressive 75 per cent in arts, there was little change in the balance of the sexes at the Medical School. One medical student, the multi-talented Diana Shaw, became the first woman to edit *Critic*, in 1942.[7] *Critic* had no patience with conservative male attitudes at this time. On one occasion, a correspondent suggested that the acute shortage of space in the Medical School, that arose after the intake was raised to 120, might be resolved by excluding women. 'There are 21 women in second year', he wrote, in April 1943, 'of whom about two will qualify' and they would be better off studying Home Science. 'Med' responded sharply that forty of the forty-one women who had recently completed the course were already in employment.[8]

Entering Medical School when the war was at its height, Barbara Heslop was struck by the subdued atmosphere. Professor Adams reminded the second-year class, on their first day, that New Zealanders were dying overseas while they enjoyed the privilege of being students. 'In the circumstances', she commented drily, 'it would have been almost subversive to have complained

Fee for Parts

And when you died
There was no one,
No one who could say
To red-eyed daughters, tight-lipped sons
That you had tried
Had done your best
Had been a friend, a grand old man;
No one, when they tiptoe in and lift the shroud
To say, how beautiful
You are, with face unfevered, brow unlined,
At rest.

Yet the mystery just lately
From your cells departed
Is the same that leaves all others' cells
Masterless, and inco-ordinate.
And we with knives and weighty tomes
Would probe, examine and dissect
This lump of clay.
Vainglorious we try to understand
Your mystery
Unpenetrated and
Impenetrable

There were
No flowers for you, nor psalms,
Nor cool green earth;
But integers metallic; ribaldry
And young irreverence.
Injustice? Still they say:
'No sparrow for a farthing sells
But God the Father ...
And of your head each hair the Angels number.'
But even then
I wonder.

W.D.T., better known to later students as Professor Trotter of Anatomy. *Digest* 1943, p. 34. Medical Library, University of Otago.

of our lot.' She was one of fifteen women who graduated in 1948. On the roll of women graduates, they numbered 186 to 200 out of a total which, when she wrote in 1993, had almost reached 1500.[9] One of the fifteen was the first Maori woman medical student, Rina Ropiha. From a privileged European-style background and with supportive parents, she began her course in 1943, married a law student in her second year, had a child the following year, and graduated in 1948. She completed her clinical training by commuting from Nelson to Wellington each week, leaving her baby with her husband and in-laws. Later, as a practising psychiatrist in Nelson, with four children, she became frustrated at the impossibility of undertaking postgraduate training to progress in her specialty.[10]

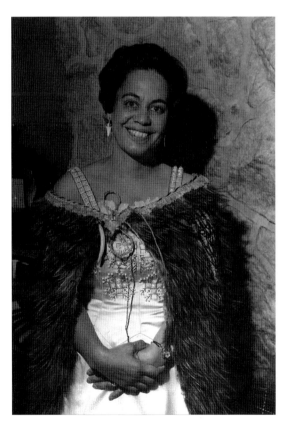

Rina (Moore) née Ropiha.
Private collection.

The Post-War Era: Traditions Re-asserted

After the war, male medical students resumed their role centre stage in the University. Elworthy calls the section of his book on the late 1940s and the 1950s, 'the post-war consensus'. He describes the period as prosperous, conservative and hard-drinking, with signs of a 're-domestication of women within the university'. The confident mid-twentieth century medical student enjoyed his place in the established hierarchy, a paragon of conformity in a notably conformist period of student culture. In a 'Then and Now' piece for the 1975 *Medical Digest*, Associate Professor James Gwynne wrote nostalgically of the late 1940s, when he had been a student at Otago. 'Our acceptance of the Establishment was complete … most of us were so proud to be medical students that it never occurred to us to be anything but satisfied with our environment.' The outward appearance of medical students reflected this conformity: brown or green sports coats and brown or grey trousers and 'it never occurred to us to attend the medical school without a tie'. Medical students were clean-shaven, their hair cut short back and sides.[11] In a 1954 *Critic*, 'Pamela' made fun of the carefully tasteful attire of the medical students of the day. Their accoutrements, she wrote, consisted of 'a sports coat of quiet design and exemplary cut and a quiet Donegal tie – grey bags, well pressed and touched only with a subtle scent of the dissection room', brown or black shoes, never tan, a gaberdine raincoat and an umbrella which 'must never be unfurled, even in the unlikely event of rain.'

Of their confident pre-eminence in the University, 'Pamela' wrote:

> It is generally recognised that the aristocracy of the university have their headquarters at the Medical School, and indeed no-one apart from the less educated of the other faculties would dream of questioning this …. The serene supremacy of the medical student is achieved through that ancient philosophy … that although the medical student may hold offices, make up Students' Exec., take every place in the Tournament teams, win the

drinking horn, act Don Juan successfully twenty-four hours a day – yet he must do this, as it were, without effort and without seeming to notice his own prowess.[12]

Medical students joined in this characterisation of themselves. In the 1950 *Digest*, for example, 'The Microscope' describes their characteristics year-by-year. At no point did any of the sketches of the stereotypical medical student include women.[13]

In 1949, senior medical students resumed the grip on the OUSA presidency that they had established during the war. They held the office from 1949 through to 1957, with the exception of one year, and for five of the subsequent eight years. Under their steady guidance, during a period when university education was government-funded and holiday jobs were plentiful, student life became more cohesive. During this time, OUSA tended to avoid politics and consolidated its position within the University. The Association gained representation on the University Council, worked for a new Student Union building (opened in 1960) and became an incorporated society, which enabled it to own land in its own right and removed liability for debt from individual executive members.[14] It won respect from other New Zealand student bodies. Otago's senior status in NZUSA, as well as his own ability, enabled medical student Bill Smith, president of OUSA in 1955 and 1956, to represent New Zealand students at an International Student Conference in Birmingham. He was the first person from outside the NZUSA Executive to do so.[15] In 1960, the incoming OUSA president, fifth-year medical John Cullen, spoke to *Critic* about his perception of his role. He intended to confine the interests of the Students' Association to internal student matters and hoped it would not have to concern itself with what students did outside the university precincts. The new Union building, with its attendant organisational problems, would present novel and exacting tasks and there was planning to be done for a new gymnasium.[16]

At the end of the war, after a lapse of three years, Capping resumed its place as the highlight

'As Others See Us'

Second Years:- These are easily recognised. They wear white coats with name upon the lapel. A heterogeneous crowd, some shy, some bold, but with a touch of the schoolboy still about them. They hunt in packs, usually avoiding the female. They attend lectures.

Third Years:- These wear off-white coats, usually labelled with someone else's name. They are men of the world; wine women and song their theme. Often suffer from an obscure disease called 'morning after'. Can always be heard, even if not seen, only an 'oral' reducing them to comparative silence. They attend lectures – usually.

Fourth Years:- These are serious souls; the ills of the world already weighing heavily upon their shoulders. They dash madly from classroom to clinic, usually clutching some weighty tome. They talk shop, in season and out; their relaxation a p.m. on the last exam paper. They attend all lectures – late.

Fifth Years:- These wear anything, mostly a hectic colour scheme. They are so blasé, to them all things are known. For a short space they go into retreat from whence they emerge Q.M.-plus. They attend lectures, occasionally, – for a quiet nap.

Sixth Years:- These are gorgeous creatures, garbed in spotless white of the neck to knee variety. Worn nonchalantly open, the implement of the profession peeps coyly from a pocket. Gone are the days of shapeless bags, a knife-edged crease dissects their strides. They have acquired the medical murmur and can only be heard with a hearing aid. They practise – a bed-side manner.

'The Microscope', *Digest*, 1950, p. 30.

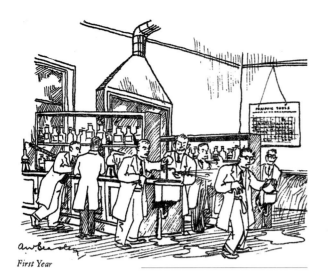

First Year

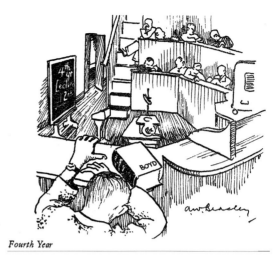

Fourth Year

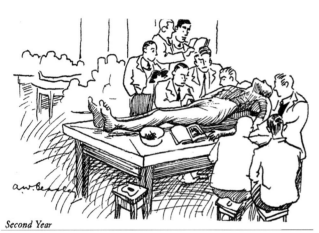

Second Year

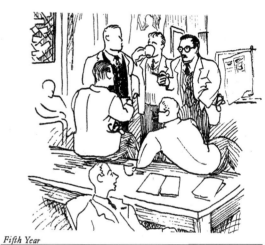

Fifth Year

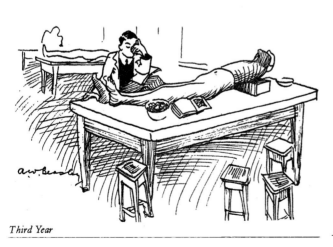

Third Year

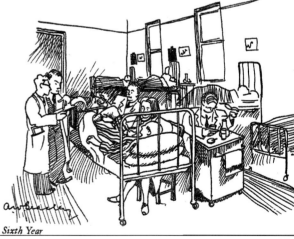

Sixth Year

A.W. Beasley casts a cynical eye over his fellow medical students as they progress through their course.
He became an orthopaedic surgeon, Clinical Reader in the Department of Surgery of the
Wellington School of Medicine and, in retirement, an historian.
Digest 1949.

of the student year. David Cole was Director of the Capping concert for three consecutive years, 1945–7. The traditional elements of the all-male show were revived. The sextet (a quartet was all they could manage the first year) again sang ribald or satirical songs, beautifully. The Selwyn ballet and the Knox farce reappeared. As in the past, excessive drinking made the chorus the most 'risk-prone' section of the concert. The opening night of the 1945 concert and the Capping procession were held on 5 May, a day made memorable by the end of the war in Europe. In 1947, women were included in some items in the Capping concert, thanks largely to the determination of medical students Jean Lyness and Diana Montgomery. David Cole wrote nostalgically of his three Capping concerts, which summed up for him 'a lot of what was special about Dunedin in the 1940s'.[17]

More than a decade later, senior medical students were still running Capping. In 1959, under the heading 'Medical Stranglehold on Capping', *Critic* complained:

> The Capping Controller's job is held by a fifth year med and has been as long as anyone can remember. The Procession Director, the Amenities Controller, both Book editors, the Book Sales manager, the Front-of-House manager and Grads' Convener and the Concert Director and his numerous underlings are all senior medical students. The situation recurs year after year.

Critic objected especially to the perks that went with the positions.[18]

Student interests within the Medical School continued to be served by their own Association. The minutes and annual reports of OUMSA show a stable pattern of day-to-day activities, of which social occasions were an important element. Departing or retiring staff were farewelled and newcomers welcomed, meetings of the Medical History Society and the Clinical Society were held, with variable attendance, and the medical ball was invariably described as a 'great success'. In 1946, the third-year representative on OUMSA was Norm Wimsett, one of the memorable characters among the medical students of his day.

Deciding to use his position to learn something about the external examiner for the approaching First Professional exam, he wrote to the president of the Melbourne Medical Students' Association asking for information about the foibles of their Professor of Anatomy, Sydney Sunderland. Did he have any peculiarities Dunedin students should know about? An answer duly arrived, with a quite detailed account of the professor, ending with the comment that he was not such a bad fellow. It was signed, Sydney Sunderland. A postscript explained that in Melbourne the president of the Medical Students' Association was always a staff member.[19]

After the war, medical students resumed their pre-eminence in sport. Cricket was included in Tournament from 1949 and Otago did well in inter-university matches in the 1950s, though less so in club games. The hero of post-war Otago rugby was medical student Ron Elvidge. He represented Otago on thirty occasions between 1942 and 1950, captaining the teams that won the Ranfurly Shield in 1947 and beat the touring British Lions in 1950. He played nineteen matches for the All Blacks from 1946, touring South Africa in 1949, and leading the side twice. As captain of the All Blacks in 1950, he was seriously injured in a test match against the Lions. Nevertheless, he insisted on returning to the field, to score the only try of the match. He did not play again.[20]

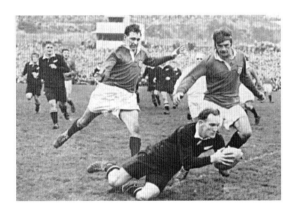

Ron Elvidge scoring a try.
Photograph, Dr Elvidge.

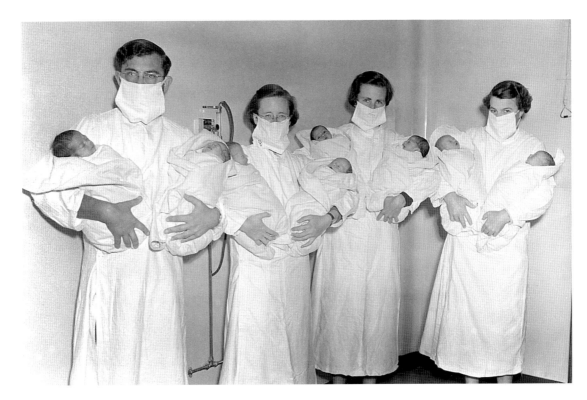

Gaining obstetric experience at the Queen Mary Maternity Hospital was a memorable and satisfying part of the medical student's training. Here, a group of them hold four sets of new twins at Queen Mary.
Otago Daily Times, 19 February 1954.

Women medical students did not share the easy assumption of leadership roles enjoyed by their male colleagues. James Gwynne recalls the dismissive attitude to them in the postwar Medical School:

> There were very few females ... and their inferiority and general unsuitability for a career in medicine was generally accepted at the beginning, although as the course progressed it became apparent to us that the opposite sex was making notable contributions in several directions. We were most impressed when two of their number married returned soldiers before we reached fourth year.[21]

That academic aspirations, especially in the sciences, were regarded as a danger to womanliness is a reflection of postwar attitudes.

Women medical students simply accepted their continued exclusion from the main common room and the fifth-year dinner. Barbara Heslop did not think that any of the women in her class would claim to have been persecuted because of her sex, 'but' she commented, 'I'd hate to imply that overt sexism wasn't alive and well. As students we simply lived with it, ignored much of it and probably became immune to it.' Some aspects of medical education were 'so far removed from today's classes that it might have been another incarnation.' 'Eefie' White, for example, would often ask one member of the class to come out to the front with him during a lecture or clinic. If he chose a girl, he would 'conduct most of the class with his arm around her waist .... Medicine was still very much a "gentlemen's club" whose members tolerated us.'[22]

In 1954, the perception of appropriate masculine and feminine behaviour formed the backdrop to a sensational and tragic event which cast the Medical School and its recent graduates into the full glare of the public spotlight. On 11 December, Dr Senga Whittingham fatally shot her former fiancé, Dr Bill Saunders, in a toilet at the house surgeons' quarters of the Dunedin Hospital. The event had all the elements to engage the avid attention of the press and the public. The newspapers highlighted Saunders' sexual exploits and the devastating effect on Whittingham of his abrupt termination of their relationship when, at his insistence, she had aborted his child. The contrast was drawn again and again, by her lawyers and the press, between the brilliant, arrogant 'Sexy Saunders' and the gentle, reserved Whittingham, driven to desperation by the defection of her lover and with her health undermined by months of intense pain. From 13 December 1954, when the first account of the shooting made headlines and, especially during the court case from 8 to 15 February 1955, the affair dominated the news. The jury found Whittingham guilty of manslaughter, recommending the 'utmost leniency' and she was given a sentence of three years. Throughout, she was portrayed as a victim, driven beyond endurance. The media depiction of the house surgeons' lifestyle of womanising and wild parties, which it was claimed Saunders exemplified, cast a lurid light on the Otago Medical School. A year after

the event, the 1955 *Digest* was notably circumspect in its reference to the whole episode, confining itself to an obituary for Saunders which referred to his 'tragic death', listed his many academic and sporting achievements and mourned a brilliant career cut short.[23]

Throughout the 1950s and into the 1960s, many women medical students continued to feel they were there on sufferance. Some of them told their stories in a collection published in 1994. Susi Williams called her contribution, 'Sober Suits and Low Heels – And Don't Dare be Pregnant', and Glenys Arthur entitled hers, 'Swimming Against the Tide'. Both resented sexist comments and jokes from staff. Robyn Hewland, who commenced second year in 1958, said women were often reminded they were 'taking a man's place'. The comment of one professor, that girls were useful only for routine duties such as dishes and anaesthetics, and of another, who taught that premenstrual tension was more common in women who had not adapted fully to woman's role in society, still rankled almost forty years on.[24] Nevertheless, the stories of their careers are a record of achievement in their chosen profession.

CHAPTER 16

A Formidable Dean: Charles Hercus in the School and the University

THE ROLE of the Medical School within the changing University environment of the post-war years was of the utmost importance, although university historian Morrell claims that the explosive growth of other faculties made its dominance less striking than it had been before the war. In the immediate postwar period, he argues, the University was 'preparing to advance on a broad front'. A great influx of students, many of them returned servicemen assisted by a generous government rehabilitation policy, strained staff and facilities almost to breaking point. When enrolments levelled off, it was at a figure around a thousand higher than the pre-war average.[1] It is debatable whether the relative influence of the Medical School in this enlarged University was lessened. Certainly the ability of Sir Charles Hercus, both in his position as Dean and in his capacity, as an individual, to envisage new developments beyond his area of immediate responsibility and provide the impetus to bring them to pass, was an outstanding feature of the University in postwar years.

The environment in which Hercus worked had several potentially limiting features. One of these was the appointment of an executive Vice-Chancellor. The strains of the war and its aftermath on the University's administrative structure had demonstrated the need for a full-time administrative head.[2] Although the position was approved by Council in 1944, nothing more could be done until the war had ended and until the Government agreed to pay a salary at least equal to that of the highest paid professor. It was 1948 before Dr Robert Aitken was appointed. A graduate of the Otago Medical School, winner of the Travelling Scholarship in 1923 and a Rhodes Scholarship in 1924 and, at the time of his appointment, Regius Professor of Medicine in the University of Aberdeen, Dr Aitken was warmly welcomed by the Medical School as one of their own.[3] By 1964, when Hercus and Bell published their chapter of tributes to the University's successive Chancellors, their tone was less wholehearted. They noted with concern that the appointment of Dr Aitken (by then Sir Robert Aitken, Vice-Chancellor of the University of Birmingham) as full-time Vice-Chancellor had materially reduced the responsibility of the Chancellor. They deplored the fact he had abolished the Council's Sub-committee of Medicine and Dentistry and replaced it with a lay Council member as Visitor to the Medical School. They believed the new system was 'too informal' to meet the needs of a growing school.[4] It was an indication of things to come.

The new Vice-Chancellor had his own views on medical education and did not hesitate to make these known. In an address to the Otago Branch of the Royal Society in July 1950, he addressed the question of the role of medicine within the University. The physician of today was well grounded in the rudiments of science, he told his audience, but halfway through his training the student had to make 'that violent crossing from the world of scientific order to the world of clinical disorder … to a world of miscellaneous sick human beings, a good half of which makes no chemical or physical sense at all.' The 'human urgency' of medicine was a profound disturbance to a mind trained in the delicate precision of physical science. Some met it by studying not only the physical ailments but the whole lives of their patients. He spoke of the developing interest in social medicine. Medicine, he explained, was passing out of its preoccupation with physical science, to explore 'those wide fields of human experience and human behaviour which have hitherto belonged to the humanists.' It was as much an art as a science, capable of reconciling the conflicting views of the humanities and the sciences.[5] Not all of this sat comfortably with the research focus or style of teaching of the postwar Medical School.

Dr Aitken served nearly five years as Vice-Chancellor before moving to Birmingham and, in this time, he impressed with his wisdom and breadth of vision. For a few months in late 1953,

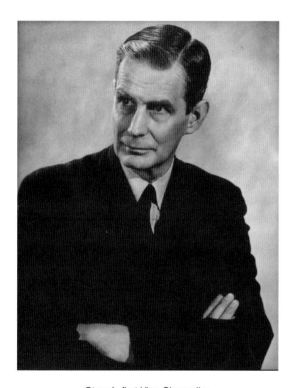

Otago's first Vice-Chancellor, Otago medical graduate Dr Robert Aitken.

Registry, University of Otago.

Sir Charles Hercus took on the responsibilities of acting Vice-Chancellor until Dr Frederick Soper, Professor of Chemistry at Otago for the previous eighteen years, was appointed. Soper filled the position until 1963 but Registry insiders believed that he was not strong enough to stand up to the dominant and experienced Medical School Dean.[6]

Another postwar administrative change, with far-reaching implications for the Medical School, affected the University of New Zealand as a whole. In January 1948 it set up a University Grants Committee (UGC) composed of the Chancellor, Vice-Chancellor and five members appointed by Senate. Early in 1949 the UGC visited the Colleges and presented its budget to the Minister of Education. A formula to provide a block grant to each institution for the next five years was then worked out between the University of New Zealand and the Education Department.[7] The special schools were visited by the Committee but were not bound by the (controversial) formula. This separate status of the Medical and Dental Schools proved very favourable, because the University of Otago was authorised to make separate representations on the salaries of their staff.[8] Hercus was understandably an advocate of the new system, believing it 'brought a new spirit of realism into the financial scene' and for the first time placed the finances of the Medical School on a reasonable and stable basis. The 1949 grant was £37,780, itself a great increase on the £8000 government grant at the end of Ferguson's deanship. On the recommendation of the UGC, it rose to £67,667 in 1950 and continued to climb steadily until, in the last year of Hercus's deanship in 1958, it reached £182,532. Although the increased government support was welcome, the restrictions that were placed on its spending were not. The money had to be used for the precise purpose for which it was granted. Especially irksome was the requirement that salaries had to conform to government regulation, which meant that they could not be raised to the level of overseas medical schools – and even a 15 per cent rise in 1951 did not close this gap. The difference in salaries between clinical and non-clinical teachers made filling the latter posts difficult and, in 1952, no fewer than fifteen senior positions were unfilled.[9]

Buildings were not, at first, part of the brief of the UGC and the general rule of one major building at a time was an ongoing frustration to the University of Otago. In 1949 a Dental School building was top of its list of priorities, but the new National Government of that year deferred the project. The Dental School did not eventuate until 1954, nor did any other government-funded buildings at Otago during this time. The Medical School had been fortunate to have completed its imposing and expensive South Block in 1948, in an otherwise bleak period.[10] But more was needed and a major crisis erupted in 1954 when Professor Woodruff, newly arrived and eager to begin research, insisted on better accommodation and facilities. Hercus persuaded the University Council to use £35,000 that had accumulated in salary savings from unfilled posts over the previous four years to erect a single-storey building of about 5000 square feet, as temporary accommodation for Surgery and also Obstetrics and Gynaecology. The UGC objected, arguing that because the Medical School had accumulated reserves, it should not get the large increase in its grant that it had requested. The Minister of Education confirmed that the reserve account could not be used for the proposed clinical building, but had to be used to finance the developments in the School the UGC had recommended for the quinquennium beginning in 1955. 'No doubt', Morrell comments, with a rare expression of personal opinion, 'the real obstacle was the well-known Treasury view that the proper thing to do with savings was to return them to the Consolidated Fund.' Eventually the Government backed down and the building, financed half from savings and half from an opportune bequest, was opened in June 1956.[11] Located, as it was, to the north of the Scott Building, Hercus could refer to it as the last phase of the Lindo Ferguson plan for a Medical School extending along the full block on Cumberland Street opposite the Hospital. 'At last the Department of Surgery had a laboratory with adequate facilities and admirable provision for experimental surgery', he wrote later, with evident satisfaction. On the other hand, the University Registrar of the day believed that Hercus's reputation with the UGC never recovered from what they viewed as indefensible practice: he had been given money for one purpose and used it for another.[12]

Any developments in the Dunedin Hospital's building programme also directly affected the Medical School. In 1956, the School benefited from the opening of a new hospital on the edge of the city, in the hill suburb of Wakari. The hospital

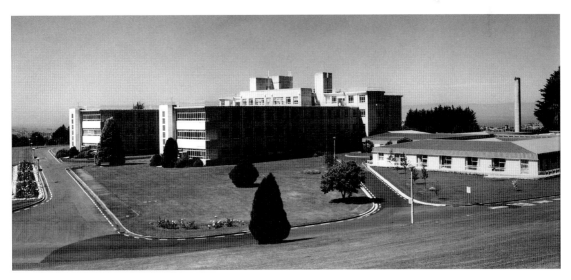

Wakari Hospital, in the 1960s.
Archives New Zealand, Te Rua Mahara o te Kāwanatanga, Dunedin Regional Office – DAHI/D274/193.

had been long under consideration. As early as 1944, the Joint Relations Committee of the Otago Hospital Board and the University of Otago had submitted a set of building priorities to the Hospital Board. The list was depressingly long, and included a new physiotherapy block, a nurses' home, kitchen, lecture block and new residential wing, an outpatients' block, additions to the Queen Mary Maternity Hospital, house surgeons' quarters, a new two-storey children's block to replace the old Victoria and Jubilee Pavilion and a four- or five-storey surgical and theatre block. The last of these was regarded as the first priority, but in the meantime some temporary improvements were made at the Dunedin Hospital. In 1945, a new Otago Hospital Board, chaired by Dr McMillan, opted for something quite different, the development, on the Wakari site, of a large hospital, with nurses' home, kitchen, theatre block, and provision for students and resident staff. It would be complementary to the Dunedin Hospital, but would have full surgical and medical facilities. The project had its disadvantages. It was too big to be carried out at the same time as a thorough upgrade of Dunedin Hospital, so this much-needed work had to be deferred. The proposed site was a long way away from the School, which would be inconvenient for students. Nevertheless, work began in 1948. The historian of the Otago Hospital Board called the decision to commit to a major hospital on the Wakari site 'one of the most important the post-war Boards had to make'.[13] He described the long process of building as plagued by indecision, changes of direction and inadequate planning. There were also practical problems, which required calling in a consultant architect, and doubts simmered on about the wisdom of the whole enterprise. Finally, in December 1956, the OHB took over the £1.5 million hospital. It consisted of six wards – for paediatrics, children's surgery, burns, thoracic surgery, general medicine and general surgery – and a nurses' home for 130 nurses and thirty domestic staff. Although students did indeed find travelling to the new hospital time-consuming and inconvenient, the Medical School benefited from it in several ways. There were modern operating theatres,

described as 'luxurious', for thoracic surgery, facilities for the treatment of burns and generous accommodation for radiotherapy, which allowed radiodiagnosis to take over space in the Dunedin Hospital and both departments to expand. The Dunedin Hospital, on the other hand, was left in an unsatisfactory state.[14]

The government grant through the UGC was not, of course, the only income of the Medical School and, like his predecessor, Hercus nurtured any additional monies and used them carefully. In addition to research funds from the Medical Research Council, the Travis Fund and the British Empire Cancer Campaign, there were a number of special funds, such as that for the library. In 1949 Hercus set up a Special Purposes Fund, which was available for purposes agreed to by Council, without requiring the approval of the UGC. Salaries for the endowed chairs – the Mary Glendining Chair of Medicine, the Ralph Barnett Chair of Surgery, the Obstetrical Chair and the Wolff Harris Chair in Physiology – were henceforward paid through this fund. It was also used for extra-to-establishment positions. A gift of £5000 in 1946, in honour of Dr Harold Chaffer, was for encouraging distinguished visitors to come to the School. In 1953, the Russell bequest enabled the Medical School to purchase a small farm on the Taieri for breeding animals used in medical research.[15]

Innovative and far-sighted as a leader of the Medical School, Sir Charles Hercus also used his immense energy in the service of the wider University, especially in health-related areas. He had great influence on the Schools of Dentistry and Physical Education. It was natural, in view of the fact that his own first degree was in dentistry, that the Dental School should have found in him a staunch ally. He was a good friend of Dr (later Sir) John Walsh, who arrived from Melbourne as the new Director of the Dental School in 1946. Both held qualifications in medicine and dentistry, both were dynamic and determined, both were researchers and writers. Each was behind a major public health initiative – the iodisation of salt in the case of Hercus and the fluoridation of water in the case of Walsh. They made a powerful duo.[16] Sir Charles also exerted sustained pressure to secure a School of Physical Education for Otago. In 1937, a scheme to provide a three-year physical education course within the Medical School was mooted, but it fell through. Hercus studied the question when he was on leave in 1939 and presented a comprehensive report on physical education in Britain and North America to the University Council. The war put a stop to further developments at this point but the matter was taken up again in 1944. In 1947, Philip Smithells, Superintendent of Physical Education in the Education Department, accepted the directorship and a School of Physical Education opened in 1948 with thirty students, in the former Teachers' Training College building. It was not part of the Medical School, as had been suggested earlier, but Hercus was instrumental in bringing this new special school to Otago.[17]

A development of importance to the health of Otago University students in general arose from the activities of the Department of Preventive Medicine. From the time he was appointed in 1922, Hercus had expanded the time in the curriculum given to public health and emphasised its practical aspects. He increased the staff and made connections, through lectures and seminars, with government, local authority and voluntary services in areas of maternity, infant and child welfare, and adolescent and industrial health. In 1946 a health clinic he had set up to introduce fifth-year medical students to social, economic and community influences in medical care was made available (at the request of the University Council) to all students, especially those from outside Dunedin. Students were given an annual physical examination, including a chest X-ray. The service, which was funded by a grant from the Social Security Fund, evolved into the Student Health Service. All fifth-year students were attached to the clinic for a week, giving them the chance to see for themselves 'some of the less tangible social, economic and community factors important in the aetiology, control and prevention of disease and in the promotion of mental and physical health.'[18] Students in Hercus's course also carried out practical research, sometimes working in pairs, on some aspect of public health, presenting their findings orally to their class and then in written form. A number of the best of the theses were published in the *New Zealand Medical Journal*.[19]

The personal prominence of the Dean reflected the dominance of the Medical School in the University. It seemed he was called on to act as chairman whenever a major project needed to be pushed along. For example, in July 1948 when the Council set up a Union Building Committee to appeal for funds to replace the old student union, which dated from 1914 and was long outgrown, Hercus was its first convener. He also had a large share in formulating the University's long-term plan.[20]

The Dean's summing up

In 1958 Hercus reached the mandatory retirement age of seventy. As Ferguson had done before him, he used his final annual report to review the principal developments during his deanship and to signal the immediate problems he believed were confronting the School. His overall theme was growth, 'reflecting the phenomenal expansion and widening of scope of medicine in the last 21 years'. He listed new departments: the Department of Physiology had been split into Physiology and Biochemistry, and Bacteriology and Public Health had become the Departments of Microbiology and Preventive and Social Medicine. Sub-departments under full-time staff had been developed in Medicine and Surgery and some would soon reach independent status: in the Department of Medicine, Paediatrics, Psychiatry and Neurology and, in the Department of Surgery, Thoracic Surgery, Ophthalmology and Anaesthesia. The growth of administration and special services had led to the establishment of the Dean's Department, which included the Branch Faculties in Christchurch, Wellington and Auckland and the administrative offices, library, photography and artist, glass-blower, caretakers and animal department in Dunedin.

A striking increase in the number of academic staff and students had accompanied this expansion of departments and sections. The eight professors, fifteen lecturers and twenty assistant lecturers of 1937, had risen to nine professors, four associate-professors, thirty senior lecturers, and fifty-nine lecturers and assistant lecturers by 1958. Support staff also rose proportionately during this time. The Branch Faculties had developed strongly, with full-time senior lecturers being appointed in Auckland and Christchurch and a similar appointment planned for Wellington. The number of students had risen from 378 in 1937, to 515 in 1958. There had been 1913 graduates over the period. Almost three-quarters of the doctors on the New Zealand medical register were graduates of the School. The School's undergraduate teaching had moved beyond medical students, to take in dental, physical education, home science and nursing students, in considerable and increasing numbers.

In his complaints about space and money Hercus covered familiar territory. Accommodation, he said, had been a major problem throughout his deanship and it was only partially solved by the completion of the new South Block in 1948 and the building to house Surgery and Obstetrics and Gynaecology (intended long-term for a staff and student cafeteria) in 1956. The Department of Medicine was still stretched over several locations and the Medical Library was desperate for space, with some of its books having to be stored in the basement at Wakari Hospital. By 1956 the animal department had become so congested that the University used money from a bequest to buy land on the Taieri for it. Part of a hangar at the Taieri Air Force Station was also brought into use for the hydatids research unit.

The struggle for finance had been incessant. The system of quinquennial grants, negotiated through the University Grants Committee, marked an advance in financial policy, but the practice of strictly ear-marking allocations allowed the Medical School no freedom of manoeuvre. The School benefited from a slow but gratifying increase in private gifts and bequests, which had reached the sum of £201,000, despite heavy taxation and the Government's refusal to give a pound for pound subsidy on gifts.

Debate about the aims and content of the medical curriculum had continued with increasing tempo. Overseas, agreement was emerging in favour of a broader, educational approach, to develop 'an educated person equipped to learn and trained in habits of logical and critical thought and with a close appreciation of the humanistic as well as the technological aspects of medicine'. However, Hercus thought it would be many years before this would be fully reflected in the traditionally vocational medical curriculum at Otago.

Interest had been maintained in postgraduate training, both in the compulsory intern year and the subsequent training of graduates in the various branches of medicine. A short course held for candidates for higher qualifications attracted twenty-eight enrolments and a refresher course for general practitioners, thirty-one. Three postgraduate newsletters had been circulated throughout the hospitals of the Dominion.

Research had increased substantially, both within departments and in research organisations housed within the Medical School. International recognition had been achieved in several directions, as shown by invitations to international congresses, by scientific publications and by requests from overseas workers to come to the School for further experience. The policy of concentrating medical research around the School created an atmosphere of research, stimulating to staff and students alike. In 1958, three numbers of the *Proceedings of the Otago Medical Research Society* were published, containing twenty-eight papers.

The immediate problems the School faced, which needed to be resolved before the proposed second medical school in Auckland proceeded, centred on finance. Securing and retaining staff of first-rate calibre in teaching and research was the fundamental challenge. The Otago School was doubly handicapped, by the geographical isolation of New Zealand and by the reluctance of the New Zealand people to realise its unique significance and be prepared to support it adequately. The solution was to attract the school's own best students to train for academic medicine. The Bachelor of Medical Science had been fruitful in providing staff of the highest quality but over the past thirteen years only four or five per cent of students passing the First Professional examination had been able to afford it. Financial assistance of about £300 per year for each candidate, together with a scheme to employ them after registration, travel facilities for overseas study and a guarantee of employment for a time on their return would secure a steady stream of potential teaching and research staff. There was also an urgent need to secure equality of salary scales between the medically qualified staff of the Medical School and the hospitals of the Dominion. New Chairs were required, in psychiatry and child health, for example, as well as more associate professorships.

Hospital accommodation designed to include teaching and research was absolutely essential. While the opening of a 180 bed hospital at Wakari was a step forward, the Dunedin Hospital was 'entirely inadequate for modern teaching and research purposes'. Plans for its reconstruction had been drawn up, but the difficulty of securing finance was likely to delay the building. Hercus believed it should have the highest priority in the Dominion's hospital building programme.

Throughout his deanship Hercus served on the University Council as a Professorial Board representative. He recommended that the Dean of the Medical School should have this right ex officio and that the Council set up a special committee to consider all Medical School problems. There should also be University representation on the Hospital Board, to reciprocate the Board's representation on the University Council, and on the Advisory Council of the Department of Health. Such representation would advance policies, such as the regionalisation of hospital services and the ultimate provision of private paying wards in public hospitals, both of which would contribute substantially to clinical teaching in Otago.

'The School', Hercus concluded, 'is moving steadily, if slowly, towards the goal of a modern Medical School. While much remains to be done, the School has achieved an international reputation and its graduates are regarded with favour throughout the British Commonwealth.'[21] It was a fair assessment.

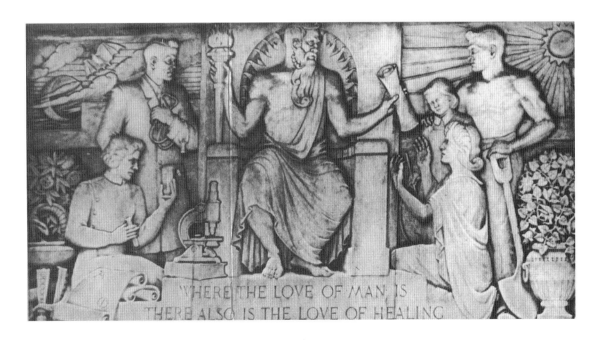

Marble plaque above the entrance to the Hercus Building, Hanover Street. The central figure is Hippocrates, who holds a torch and a scroll. To the left are two medical scientists and to the right a man, woman and child, to whom he is passing the scroll of medical knowleddge. The words come from Hippocrates' *Precepts*.

John Borrie, *Art and Observables in the Otago Medical School*, p. 13. Hocken Collections S08-508

PART IV

The Medical School
in a Changing Environment
1959–1981

CHAPTER 17

From Crisis to Christie
1959–1969

The Future of the Deanship: Professor Edward Sayers

For the first eighty-three years of its existence the Otago Medical School was guided by three Deans, each of whom served a term measured in decades rather than years. Dr John Halliday Scott was Dean for thirty-seven years, from 1877 until his death, while still in office, in 1914; Sir Lindo Ferguson served for the next twenty-three years, until he was edged into retirement at the beginning of 1937, when he was seventy-eight; and Sir Charles Hercus led the School from 1937 until he reached the maximum retirement age allowable, seventy years, in 1958. Each left his mark strongly on the School and each, it is generally acknowledged, was the man for his time. Over this long period the Medical School, and the individual Deans, held a dominant position in the University. However, by the end of the 1950s, the size and complexity of the School's operations and a rapidly changing environment in the New Zealand and Otago University systems, meant that the task had grown beyond the capacity of any one man. The age of the 'God-Professor' had passed and, in the new environment, there was no longer any room for the omnipotent medical Dean. Tellingly, Hercus's obituary in the *New Zealand Medical Journal* refers to him as 'the last of a generation that was expected to and was able to run single-handedly a faculty of medicine.'[1]

Later Deans were men of influence, but they would measure their service in years, not decades. There were four over the next twenty-one years, the length of Hercus's term of office: Sir Edward Sayers, from 1959 to 1967, Professor William Adams, from 1968 to 1973 (after eight months during which Professor J.R. Robinson was Acting Dean), Professor John Hunter, from 1974 to 1977 and again from 1986 to 1990 and Professor Geoffrey Brinkman, from 1978 to 1985. Not only did these men serve for much shorter terms than their predecessors, they also operated in a quite different academic environment, one in which it was necessary to adjust to, or circumvent, what the Deans saw as encroachments by Otago University and the University of New Zealand on their autonomy and that of the Medical School.

Hercus's impending retirement made the future role of the Dean an issue of intense and immediate concern. Hercus himself opened up the debate in a memorandum to Faculty at the end of May 1957. The Dean, he reminded members, was currently elected triennially by Faculty, with a tradition of automatic re-appointment. As the Medical School had grown, his responsibilities, in relation to administration, visitors to the School and research, had also grown hugely. He recommended that, in the future, Deans should sit ex officio on the University Council and that they should do less teaching, to enable them to spend time with the Branch Faculties.[2] Senior staff then contributed written opinions. Everyone acknowledged that the present Dean was carrying an excessive load and that it was essential to make the office more tolerable. At the same time, staff were concerned that the personal authority of the Dean needed to be balanced with his democratic responsibility to Faculty and his participation in the School's teaching programme. In September, a special Faculty meeting found enough common ground to endorse the existing system.[3]

The matter was then handed over to a sub-committee, chaired by Smirk, which reported at the end of the following February. It began by summarising the duties of the Dean. First, as Chair of Faculty and ex officio member of its committees, he had to communicate with the University of New Zealand, prepare Faculty business, conduct interviews with students and others, and work with the University's Professorial Board and Vice-Chancellor. Second, as Dean of the Medical School, he had responsibilities in relation to the Vice-Chancellor, the Hospital Board, the Branch Faculties, the Medical Council of New Zealand and the Medical Research Council. He also had to prepare the quinquennial budgets. Third, within the Medical School, the Dean's Department had to supervise the central office, caretakers, maintenance, animals, glass blower, photographic department and artist's department. In view of this multiplicity of duties, the committee recommended that an incoming Dean should spend only a small proportion of his time (say 25 per cent) teaching and that a qualified secretary should be appointed to assist him. It favoured an internal appointment and concurred with Hercus's opinion that the Dean should ex officio have a seat on the University Council. Faculty unanimously adopted the report.[4]

In the event, Faculty did recommend an external candidate, although the *Otago Daily Times* headline, 'Auckland Physician New Medical Dean', suggests less familiarity with the Otago Medical School on the part of the appointee, Dr Edward Sayers CMG, than was the case. An Otago graduate of 1924, Sayers was Sub-Dean of the Auckland Branch Faculty and an external examiner for the School in pharmacology and therapeutics. At fifty-five years of age, he was at the pinnacle of his career, one of Auckland's most senior physicians and a dominant figure in New Zealand medicine, with an enviable reputation for personal integrity. His

ward rounds at Auckland Hospital were a show place for open discussion and informed criticism. He was a specialist in tropical medicine, with a long list of publications to his name. A Chair of Therapeutics was created for him in the Medical School. The Otago University Vice-Chancellor, Dr Soper, spoke for the Faculty as a whole when he welcomed the incoming Dean as someone who 'at a time of rapid advances in medical education will both maintain and enhance the reputation of the School'.[5]

Bright Beginnings:
the Wellcome Research Institute

Sayers' deanship began with high hopes. Not only was the new Dean a man who commanded respect in the highest circles, it could also be expected that his brilliance as a clinical teacher would give a boost to the Medical School in an area of acknowledged weakness. That medical education was a top priority for Sayers was evident from his first annual report, which included accounts of his attendance at the 'unforgettable' Second World Conference on Medical Education at Chicago and his tour afterwards of most of the Canadian and a number of American and British medical schools. He had also attended the annual meeting of the Association of American Colleges. Sayers made a prompt start on remodelling the fourth- and fifth-year courses at Otago, to reduce the time given to lectures and increase that spent on clinical work in the wards. More time was allocated to psychiatry and preventive and social medicine and instruction commenced in radiology and clinical pathology. Further curriculum development was entrusted to a curriculum committee of 'Young Turks', without departmental heads.[6]

In Sayers' initial assessment of the needs of the School, the Department of Medicine came in for special attention. It was, he declared roundly, operating under 'sub-standard, cramped and unhygienic conditions', partly located in a local Sunday School building. Smirk's report, as Head of Department, filled in more detail: not only was the department overcrowded, its accommodation was spread over five separate locations and many of its laboratories were situated in a basement, with poor ventilation and light. Duties undertaken for the Dunedin Hospital were conducted in no fewer than six different buildings, as well as in different parts of the same building.[7] There was also a feeling in some quarters that the strong focus on Smirk's own research area of hypertension had thrown the department's clinical teaching out of balance.[8]

These problems were largely resolved by the greatest coup of Sayers' deanship, the separation of the clinical teaching and research components of Smirk's responsibilities through the establishment of the Wellcome Research Institute. In 1960 Sayers flew to London to negotiate a gift from the Wellcome Institute to the Medical School of £100,000, the largest sum it had ever been given, which was later increased to £120,000. The gift was in honour of Smirk's work on hypertension and was tied to his appointment as a research professor and director of a Wellcome Research Institute within the Medical School. During 1961, the Council duly appointed Smirk to a Chair and construction of the new Institute quickly got under way, with the building being opened early in 1963. At the end of that year, the Dean was able to report that, under Sir Horace's leadership, vigorous and active research in many fields was being conducted in excellent conditions. It was satisfying that, of the comparatively large staff, only the professor, a research assistant and two

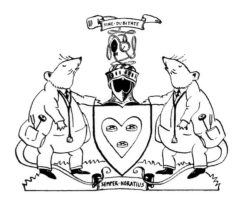

Medical students paid their own tribute to Smirk's research, and the rats that contributed to it, in this coat of arms, which first appeared in the 1958 *Digest*.
Otago Medical School.

technicians were a charge on the University, the rest being maintained by various research funds. Moreover, the new building freed up precious space elsewhere, previously occupied by the researchers.[9]

In 1962 Professor John Hunter took over the Department of Medicine, as Mary Glendining Professor. The top student of 1948, Hunter had joined the staff in 1956, fresh from postgraduate training in cardiology in London. At Otago he brought a New Zealand perspective to research that was gaining ground overseas, into the links between high blood cholesterol levels and coronary heart disease. He established the first coronary care unit in Dunedin for the intensive management of coronary patients in hospital. At Sayers' request, he had already reorganised the clinical attachments for fourth- and fifth-year students; now he set about the 'long and difficult task of building up medicine cross the board', creating an enlarged and more balanced depart-ment by setting up special units in areas such as endocrinology, neurology, gastroenterology and metabolic-endocrine diseases. He was given a free rein in appointments and, in some cases, was able to separate out whole new departments. He attracted back to Otago graduates who had gained overseas expertise in specialist areas, such as cardiologists Norma Restieaux and Pat Molloy. In 1962, Wallace Ironside, who had been at Otago since 1953, was promoted to Professor

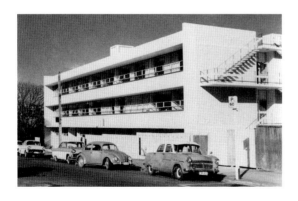

The Wellcome Building, soon after opening.
Photograph, Ted Nye.

of a new Department of Psychological Medicine, which he would head until he moved to become foundation Professor in the discipline at Monash in 1969. In 1963, Pharmacology and Pharmacy moved into renovated premises in the former Dental School, as an independent department under Dr Frederick Fastier. In 1966, James Watt became the first Professor of Paediatrics and Child Health.[10]

There were other changes in departmental leadership in these years. When Archie McIntyre left the Physiology department in 1961, James Robinson was invited to take over. A Cambridge graduate, Robinson had been recruited by Hercus in 1957, after he and his wife Marion, an Otago graduate, spent a sabbatical in Dunedin in 1954. He had been very impressed with the School and with McIntyre's Physiology Department. After Robinson arrived, the department shifted its focus from neurophysiology, to his own area of interest, cell physiology. Robinson was head of Physiology until he retired in 1980 and, under his efficient and benign leadership, the department expanded in student and staff numbers and in research. In 1963, Eric D'Ath's long reign in Pathology ended and Alun Wynn-Williams was appointed in his stead. When Hercus retired, the Chair of Preventive and Social Medicine went to Cyril Dixon, a Londoner with a broad range of medical qualifications and experience as a Medical Officer of Health in wartime England and postwar New Zealand. He came to Otago from a readership in epidemiology at the University of Leeds and as a recognised authority on smallpox. His eighteen years at Otago would be noted for research on the most effective provision of medical care and the training his department gave to many Directors of Health from the Pacific region. Dixon's first assessment of the department was heavy with criticism of the 'cumbersome deficiencies of a great many years.' In his view, the staff had been too much involved in work of a non-academic nature. He set about changing the emphasis by incorporating more tutorial teaching into the undergraduate course and altering its content and focus. Dixon reviewed the responsibilities the department had assumed in the Student Health Service, in inoculation work and in the public health field for the Health Department, with the aim of providing better services with maximum economies of staff. He warned that a considerable increase in staff and money would be required for his plans.[11]

When the University held its annual open day in 1960, the Medical School opened all its departments. The staff showed Council, University staff and friends around the School during the day and, in the evening, they welcomed some 2500 members of the public. Sayers acknowledged that such an event interfered with teaching but thought it was well worthwhile from the point of view of public relations. There were thirty-one academic visitors to the School in 1960 and forty-four the next year. Student numbers kept up, while the proportion of non-medical students increased in the basic sciences. Research was maintained during this time. The animal breeding station on the Taieri, a well-planned modern unit with room for expansion, was completed late in 1961. Although the deteriorating state of the Medical Library, traceable in the annual reports of these years, was a continuing frustration, there was a real sense that things were on the move.[12]

Gathering Clouds: the Medical School in an Autonomous University

The high staff morale evident in the Medical School at the beginning of the 1960s did not survive changes in the academic environment, both in the University of Otago and, more broadly, in the University of New Zealand, that threatened the School's privileged position as a national institution. In 1959, in the expectation that the number of students attending University would double within a few years, the Government appointed a committee to review tertiary education in New Zealand. Chaired by Sir David Hughes Parry, recently retired Professor of English Law in the University of London, the committee worked intensively from September to December 1959, reporting in that month. Its recommendations, which were far-reaching, were accepted both by the Labour Government to which it reported and the National Government

Sir Edward Sayers, 1902–1985
Dean, Otago Medical School, 1959–68

EDWARD SAYERS was born in Christchurch to a family in straitened circumstances, but he won a scholarship to Christs' College and, two years after leaving school, was helped by his Church to study medicine. On graduating in 1924, Sayers did further study at the London School of Hygiene and Tropical Medicine. He then spent seven years in charge of a Methodist mission hospital in the Solomon Islands, from where he sent malarial blood, film and other teaching materials to the School of Tropical Medicine in London, and snakes to the British Museum. In 1935, he gained membership of the Royal College of Physicians of London and returned to practise for a time in Auckland, before war broke out and he enlisted. Sayers' expertise in tropical medicine was highly valued by the military, and he was moved from Greece (where he was briefly captured but escaped) to Egypt, then to the Pacific, as the army's malaria expert. As consulting physician to the armed forces he was responsible for anti-malarial policy and could take much of the credit for the fact that New Zealand lost no one to the disease during the war. His handbook on malaria became a standard text. Sayers was also adviser on tropical diseases to the American forces in the Pacific, who recognised his work by awarding him the US Legion of Merit.

After the war, Sayers returned to Auckland, where he built up a fine reputation as a consulting physician and clinical teacher, chaired the Medical Council and served as Sub-Dean of the Auckland Branch Faculty of the Otago Medical School and on the Clinical Research Committee of the Medical Research Council. Sayers was the first New Zealander to become President of the Royal Australasian College of Physicians, serving from 1956 to 1958. He was made a CMG in 1956.

In 1959, the year between assuming the deanship of the Medical School, and negotiating in London the setting up of the Wellcome Research Institute, Sayers found time to complete his MD on malaria. It also reflects his priorities that he maintained a strong clinical commitment while performing the mainly administrative role of Dean, in a difficult period for the Medical School. As Professor of Therapeutics, Sayers continued to see patients and his Saturday morning ward rounds at Wakari Hospital were regarded by many as a highlight of the week. He always maintained that the graduates who mattered were 'the great number of unremembered but devoted general practitioners who, in the cities and the country towns of this land, have served their fellows with patience, with what skill they possess, and with honour and integrity.' Sayers was made Knight Bachelor in 1967.

Sayers married twice, first in 1928 to Jane Lumsden Grove, with whom he had six children, and after their divorce in 1971, to Patricia Dorothy Coleman, Dean of the School of Home Science at Otago. He died in 1985. [13]

---

that replaced it. The committee recommended disestablishing the single University of New Zealand in favour of four autonomous, degree-granting Universities. It argued that the powers of the University of New Zealand had already been so far eroded that the question of propping up the old federal structure simply did not apply. It also identified what it bluntly called a 'crisis of the first magnitude' in the areas of staffing, buildings,

conditions of study, university governance and finance. It did not intend, however, to have the newly autonomous universities compete with one another in badgering the Government for funding to cope with these problems. All the institutions would be resourced through an enhanced University Grants Committee, which would have the capacity to make academic as well as financial decisions. [14] All university requests to the Government were to be channelled through the UGC. Its terms of reference were accordingly very broad. The UGC would collect and publish information about university education, and then assess the country's need for those educational requirements and the financial needs of the institutions providing them. The Committee would also plan, in conjunction with the universities, a balanced development of the whole university system, allocating state grants and overseeing how they were spent. The Parry Committee was adamant that the UGC should be operative *before* the University of New Zealand disappeared, so that it could play its part in the transfer of power. Clearly the UGC was a major new player in the New Zealand university system. It is not surprising that it tried twice, in the early months of its existence, to change its name to something that reflected its wide powers, such as the New Zealand Universities' Commission or The University Commission, or that there was widespread resentment of its powers.[15] Staff at Otago certainly believed the universities' vaunted autonomy was more apparent than real. Writing at the end of the 1960s, Morrell summed up the generally held view that 'the principal beneficiary of "autonomy" was in fact the University Grants Committee' and that the universities, independent in name only, were really part of a federal structure with a strong central power.[16]

The University Grants Committee that emerged from the Parry committee's recommendations replaced the old UGC, which had provided advice to the Senate of the University of New Zealand on the needs of university education and considered applications for grants from the universities. Its system of quinquennial grants had worked well for staffing, less so for building projects. There was some continuity of personnel between this body and the new, more powerful UGC. The choice of its first chairman was of the utmost importance. Within a remarkably short time, and without formal advertisement, Dr F.J. Llewellyn, Vice-Chancellor of the University of Canterbury, was appointed. The Committee met in January 1961 and flung itself into the task of reform. The historian of the UGC, John Gould, believes that,

in the brief years of Llewellyn's chairmanship, the most thoroughgoing transformation ever brought about in the New Zealand university system was accomplished.[17]

From the point of view of the Medical School leadership, the transformation was almost wholly bad. The autonomy of the University of Otago (imperfect as this was perceived to be in Dunedin) seemed to pose a new threat to the autonomy of the Otago Medical School. In a letter to the Otago Vice-Chancellor at the end of 1962, the chairman of the UGC made clear that there would be a single block grant for each University, instead of the special schools being separately funded, as had been the case since 1925. The UGC would calculate the amount of the block grant, but without divulging their calculations to the university, which now had the responsibility of allocating a proportion to any special school. The rationale for the secrecy was to increase the budgetary flexibility and responsibility of the university councils.[18]

When the UGC visited Otago in November 1963 the Medical and Dental Deans expressed their anxiety about the new system. Dr Llewellyn was immovable, although he acknowledged the possibility of hard feelings when what he referred to as 'the rampant special school' had to argue its case with its own University Council, instead of negotiating directly with the UGC.[19] The Otago University Council had no objection to the principle of a single block grant, but when the quinquennial grants for 1965–70 were notified, it found it simply had too little to carry out its obligations to the Medical School without penalising other faculties, which were already under pressure from increasing student numbers. The Chancellor wrote to Llewellyn explaining the need to put resources into remedying deficiencies in clinical training in the Medical School. He warned, 'We can no longer carry out our own responsibilities for the efficient training of the nation's medical practitioners, having regard to the standards which obtain overseas and which should obtain in New Zealand.' Llewellyn refused to come to Dunedin to discuss the issue and did not reply to further correspondence on it from the new Vice-Chancellor.[20]

It is likely that Llewellyn's confrontational style exacerbated the disagreement. He has been described by someone who knew him as 'very forceful – [with] good ideas, but a bit too sure he was right and his arrogance built up unnecessary opposition.'[21] He was not the only person to fit that description. It so happened that the disagreement between the UGC and Otago University coincided with the arrival of a new Vice-Chancellor, in January 1964. Arthur Beacham, formerly Professor of Economics in the University College of Wales, Aberystwyth, and known for his analytical mind, persuasive tongue and great energy, was a strong champion for Otago. He was also, it seems, even more abrasive than Llewellyn and, in the words of one colleague, 'could not see a hornet's nest without wanting to stir it up.'[22]

The Dean of the Medical School and the Vice-Chancellor of the University fell out over the Medical School's share of the 1965–70 quinquennial grant and remained at daggers drawn until Beacham's departure in 1966. According to Gould, 'After extensive scrutiny of financial and statistical information supplied by the university, the UGC came to the conclusion that Otago had no case for an addition. On the other hand, the University had not targeted as much of the grant to the Medical School as the UGC's calculations had suggested.' These calculations were not known to the Otago administrators. 'Is it necessary', wrote Beacham in his 1965 Annual Report, 'for the University Grants Committee to remain so detached from the Universities, participating in most important decisions but accepting little responsibility for the upshot?' There was not much doubt, he added, that the main cause of Otago's difficulties was the very high cost of running a modern medical school. The intense and acrimonious nature of the quarrel was due,

in some part, to the personalities of Beacham and Llewellyn but the issues at stake were real and of the greatest moment.[23]

If the inadequacy of the Medical School share of the University's government grant could have been blamed on the UGC rather than the Vice-Chancellor, the other bone of contention between the Dean of the Medical School and the Vice-Chancellor in these years could not. It related to the crucial matter of the selection and appointment of staff. There had been a Standing Committee on Staffing and Promotions, for the Arts, Science and Commerce Faculties, at the University since 1955. Beacham made two changes to this Committee: he extended its scope to include all Faculties, including Medicine, and he excluded all Faculty Deans from its membership, on the ground that no person should be both advocate and judge. The enhanced powers of the reconstituted staffing committee, which advised on the academic staffing needs of all university departments and made recommendations on all appointments up to professorial level, were approved at a special meeting of Senate on 1 September 1965. Morrell comments that it was unfortunate that so fundamental a change should in effect have been imposed upon the special schools by an arts and science majority. The exclusion of the special school Deans from the staffing committee weakened their position when they were already reeling from blows to their financial independence.[24] John Hunter maintained that the fact the committee could approve or advise on staff appointments without having to accept the advice of the Faculty Dean inevitably undermined the Dean's authority and led to open conflict between the Dean of the Faculty of Medicine and the Vice-Chancellor. The next Vice-Chancellor, Dr Robin Williams, believed the staffing committee served its purpose well and chose to retain it. Under the chairmanship of the Pro-Vice-Chancellor, Dr Hugh Parton who, as Professor of Chemistry, was also a member of the Faculty of Medicine, the committee developed sound judgment, born of experience and detailed work, and Williams thought no one had cause for complaint. Leaders of the Medical School did not share this view.[25]

The Medical School in Crisis

The acrimonious atmosphere of the early 1960s was partly relieved in 1966–67 by changes among the key players. Llewellyn left the UGC in June 1966 and Professor Alan Danks, of the Economics Department at the University of Canterbury, took his place.[26] In the same year, Beacham resigned the vice-chancellorship, after less than three years. He kept up his determined fight for Otago University and especially the Medical School to the end, firing his last broadside on the very eve of his departure. Despite a similar growth rate to other universities, he pointed out, Otago's grant over the last five years had not kept pace. 'Our inability to meet the needs of the Medical School, especially on the clinical side, and the whole question of University/Teaching Hospital relations continue to be a particular source of anxiety.' Beacham fought hard and consistently for the Medical School and the hostility of some of its members towards him was seriously misdirected.[27] Robin Williams, an outstanding mathematician with a background in the State Services Commission, and an open manner, became Vice-Chancellor early in 1967 and for the few months until Sayers' retirement at the end of the year, relations between the Medical School and the University registry settled into an unaccustomed cordiality.[28]

Nevertheless, the basic problems of the Medical School remained, although there were some positive developments in the direction of expansion and greater specialisation. Some new departments, with energetic younger leaders, were emerging as offshoots of the established disciplines. When Norman Edson took early retirement for health reasons in 1967, Biochemistry was split into two: George Petersen succeeded Edson as Chair and J.G.T (Sam) Sneyd returned from the United States to head a new Department of Clinical Biochemistry. Both these professors were local graduates in their early thirties, with extensive overseas training. Generally, however, staff were pushed to the limit during what John Hunter bluntly calls a 'crisis in teaching'. Financial constraints were tightening, there were further delays in the planning for the

urgently needed library, staff recruitment was difficult and morale was plummeting.[29]

Simmering discontent boiled over when John Hunter, returning in September 1967 from five months' leave in the United States and Britain, decided to go public. 'I led a revolt, really,' he affirmed later. The period overseas had given him the chance to see new trends in medical education and he had been appalled at what he found on his return to Dunedin. 'In staff, budget, everything was rock bottom and we were headed for disaster.'[30] He gave an explosive interview to the *Otago Daily Times*. Under the front-page headline, 'Medical School Status at Stake', he told the reporter that his visit overseas had confirmed his worst fears about the Medical School. With medical knowledge developing as rapidly as it was, the School simply could not maintain the standards of medical education the public expected unless radical steps were taken fairly urgently. It was what both the Medical School and the University had been telling the University Grants Committee and the Department of Health for some time, but it was now brought into the full glare of public view. 'Our teaching hospital situation is worse than that in any medical school I visited,' Hunter said. 'Nowhere in the United States or Britain did I find a teaching hospital staff which was expected to train more than a hundred students a year in a hospital of less than a thousand beds and with clinical facilities as abysmally poor as ours.' In every clinical school he had visited the number of clinical staff had been at least three or four times greater and there were often fewer students. 'Here in Dunedin we are expected to achieve miracles on a "string and sealing wax" budget in what is virtually a second-rate provincial hospital.' In spite of the efforts of a well-informed University Council and a sympathetic Hospital Board, the Ministers of Health and Education could not seem to grasp the situation. It was high time they stopped 'duck-shoving their responsibilities' and thought in terms of modern medicine instead of 'horse and buggy' health services. Hunter had no problem with the establishment of a medical school in Auckland. However, he believed it was being done for the wrong political reasons and that the Government should consider quality as well as quantity in medical education. According to Hunter, there were several specific steps the Government should take:

- Approve a properly set up Teaching Hospital administration, as promised by the Minister of Health, Hon D.W. McKay
- Treble the clinical teaching staff of the Medical School
- Build urgently needed teaching and research facilities in our hospitals
- Expedite the building of the new Hospital ward block
- Allow a reduction in the number of medical students.[31]

The *Otago Daily Times* endorsed Hunter's comments in the next day's editorial, under the heading 'It Had To Be Said', pointing out that his views also reflected those of the Dean Sir Edward Sayers and of Sir Horace Smirk. The editorial identified the fact that the Medical School was not financed as a special institution as one of the causes of the difficulties it was facing.[32]

Although he had approved Hunter's decision to speak to the press, when the Dean saw the newspaper report he was horrified. In March 1967, at a special meeting of the Sub-Deans of the Branch Faculties and Heads of Departments, Professor Hunter, with the strong support of Professor Gus Fraenkel of Surgery, pushed for the opening of a clinical school in Christchurch, to compensate for the limited resources in Dunedin for clinical training. (Fraenkel's own suggestion was to move the whole Medical School to Christchurch, where the old university buildings near the hospital were vacant, but he was not taken seriously.) The Dean vetoed further discussion of the matter. The old problem, Hunter commented bitterly, was simply swept under the carpet, its existence denied by the current Dean as it had been by the previous one.

Sayers' retirement at the end of 1967 provided an opportunity for action. 'When we set about looking for his successor', Robin Williams recalled, 'we soon became aware that it would be difficult.' One potential candidate is said to have declined an approach with the comment that he thought the problems of the Medical School were insoluble. The Vice-Chancellor quickly came to the decision to relax the quest for a Dean and, instead, set about solving some of the so-called insoluble problems. He identified these as being of three kinds: the size of the School and of Dunedin, the School's structure, and a series of questions relating to staffing, buildings and curriculum. He thought the last group could be left for the incoming Dean, but the size and structure of the School had to be resolved before the Dean's job could even be defined. Williams remembers the suggestion of inviting Professor Ronald Christie to review the School as coming from Hunter. The idea appealed greatly. 'Looking back,' he commented, 'we were ... very lucky in the availability of Christie, but the initiative in selecting him clearly lay with John Hunter and a few of his colleagues.' It is likely that Christie's name had been suggested by his colleague David Bates, who spent some time at the Otago Medical School during this time.[33]

The Debate in the *New Zealand Medical Journal*

In October 1967, the Dunedin reporter for the *New Zealand Medical Journal* wrote that the Otago University Council had decided not appoint a replacement for Sir Edward Sayers when he retired at the end of the year. Instead, Professor Ronald Christie, Dean of the Faculty of Medicine at McGill University, Montreal, was to come for three months early in 1968 to assist in a review of the problems facing the Medical School. Professor W.E. Adams would be Acting Dean for the year and Professor John Hunter, as Acting Associate Dean, would assist in the administration of the clinical departments.

Professor Christie, a graduate of Edinburgh University, had been Professor of Medicine at St Bartholomew's Hospital, London, before moving to Canada. During his long career, he had served as an adviser on medical education in a number of countries.[34]

The concise, factual tone of the report contrasts sharply with that of the editorial in the same issue of the journal. Under the heading 'Medical Education', the writer launched a broadside against the Otago Medical School, contrasting its prospects with those of the new school due to open in Auckland in 1968. Auckland, the writer affirmed, had the supreme advantage of starting with a clean slate, ample clinical resources and up-to-date educational advice from Britain. Indeed, the only thing that could 'emasculate its promise [was] the lagging of funds and buildings as dogged Otago's steps'. There followed a damning indictment of Otago. '[I]t is no secret' wrote the editor, 'that the medical school in Dunedin has run out of steam.' There was increasing difficulty in filling chairs, lack of competition for hospital appointments and an unsuccessful quest to find a Dean. In the editor's opinion, Dunedin had always had 'too few resources chasing too many students'. The development of the Branch Faculties in 1938, excellent as they had been, had only postponed the inevitable breakdown, which had come when the intake had been increased to 120 in 1943. The clinical resources at Dunedin were probably the least of any Medical School in the world. The solution was not to develop the Branch Faculties. It was for the Otago School to reduce its student intake to fifty, while Auckland built up, over the next few years, to take 120. As a matter of urgency, the Government should invite two members of the General Medical Council of Great Britain, at the same time as Dr Christie, to delineate the overall future of medical education in New Zealand in relation to resources and to determine a common entrance policy.[35]

The editorial drew a long response from Sir Edward Sayers, which ran to three pages in the next issue of the journal. Its careful, measured tone was very different from the hostile polemic of the editorial and it is worth considering in some detail. Before he retired as Dean, Sayers wrote,

he felt he should make some comments which, although not underestimating the difficulties and failings of the School, would show how they arose and why they were difficult to remedy. There were four fundamental problems: too many students, too few staff relative to student numbers, not enough patients and insufficient finance. Sayers dealt first with the question of staff and student numbers and the alleged lack of patients. It was the failure of Dunedin to grow that had hindered the recruitment of new staff, not the quality of the school. Most staff would welcome fewer students, but there had been a constant clamour for more house surgeons and doctors. He denied that students were disadvantaged in their clinical training, because they had excellent clinical experience, in very small groups, in the Branch Faculties. There was no better alternative to the present system, at least until Auckland was in a position to take 150 students. The planned building of additional wards in Dunedin Hospital would attract more patients and help solve the problem of a shortage.

The question of finance was crucial. Quite simply, the Medical School was not provided with sufficient money to carry out its functions. The cost of medical education had risen steeply over recent years and, unless good research facilities were also provided, potential applicants for chairs were not interested. The School had insufficient funds to provide accommodation adequate to its needs. Its splendid collection of medical books and journals was wretchedly housed and it had been pleading for a new library for years. Pharmacology was taught in a disused Sunday School. The only new building in recent years was owed to the generosity of the Wellcome Trust. The Dunedin Hospital was old and, in many ways, inadequate but a new clinical services block was due to open the next year, with excellent outpatient facilities, new operating theatres, laboratories, an x-ray department and auxiliary services. Sayers placed the responsibility for the problems of the Medical School squarely on the University Grants Committee. The University of Otago had made the strongest representations on behalf of the School, but without success.

Sayers denied that the Medical School had

'run out of steam'. In spite of the acknowledged problems, it was fundamentally sound. He referred to the new Chairs in Psychiatric Medicine, Paediatrics and Clinical Biochemistry and the strengthening and extension of the School's clinical teaching. A most vigorous Department of Preventive and Social Medicine had been built up, with extensive postgraduate commitments. Many departments had upgraded laboratories and the Pathology department had been redeveloped and altered. The School had first-class facilities for electro-microscopy. Research was flourishing, with staff, even excluding the Medical Research Council Units and the Branch Faculties, producing 144 papers over the previous year. The quality of the School's graduates was its true test and Otago's were highly regarded.

Although there were no formal changes to the curriculum, there had been significant developments in the teaching of every part of the course. The future of the Medical School depended on the University of Otago, the Otago Hospital Board, the Grants Committee and the Department of Health. It was up to these four bodies to get together to decide how many graduates they wanted, what facilities and staff were required and who was going to pay.[36] Sayers' assessment was sober and balanced and showed clearly that the problems Christie would identify the following year were already known in the School.

In other letters, N.H. North, expressed the dismay of graduates of the Medical School, who had noted its gradual decline in status, and Robin Irvine offered a robust rebuttal of the claim that the School had run out of steam. In spite of being 'grossly short of staff and money' and facing many difficulties, it had attained and was still attaining high standards. 'One would have hoped', he wrote, 'that Sir Edward Sayers' retirement would not have been accompanied by such harsh criticism of the Otago school as appears in the editorial, but by acknowledgment of better teaching, better research and a better spirit than existed in 1958.'[37]

In September, the *Otago Daily Times* joined in the debate, calling for 'heavier artillery' against 'entrenched positions' which threatened the future of the School. Referring to John Hunter's interview a year earlier, it noted that while he had found support among his colleagues, Wellington remained immovable. The paper considered 'Departmental stupidity on such matters … a phenomenon of remarkable and incomprehensible consistency.'[38] The call to have Professor Christie act as a one-man review team must have seemed like a final desperate attempt to break the deadlock. He proved exactly the right man for the job.

The Christie Report

Professor Christie's Report on the Otago Medical School marked a turning point in its history. This was not because it identified the School's problems for the first time, but because an overseas expert of Christie's standing described them trenchantly and suggested bold solutions, which the University, the Otago Hospital Board, the University Grants Committee and the Department of Health all agreed to implement. Even before Christie arrived in Dunedin, on 8 February 1968, he sent word that his office in the Medical School would be open to all members of Faculty, including those from the Branch Faculties. He had also arranged discussions with the Chair of the UGC.[39]

Consulting widely during his weeks in Dunedin, Christie also maintained regular contact with the committee set up to assist him. Alan Clarke, at the time a senior lecturer in surgery, remembers the visit as an exciting time. His own contact with Christie was through the curriculum committee. Christie engaged with their ideas with evident interest and, although Clarke thought him quite traditional in his approach to medical education,

'In effect, what the Council of the University of Otago is doing in engaging a Canadian expert adviser, is calling up heavy artillery for use against entrenched positions which threaten the future of the Medical School.'

Editorial, *Otago Daily Times*, 16 September 1967.

he remembered some 'marvellous meetings' in the Medicine seminar room. 'One felt there was great excitement in the air ... the problem was overload of students in a small hospital. We got to know George Rolleston [Sub-Dean of the Christchurch Branch Faculty], very well, as he came down again and again to be included in the discussions.'[40]

Christie's Report, dated 13 April 1968 and presented to Council on the 23rd of that month, pulled no punches. As he explained at the outset, he saw a Medical School which was 'struggling to maintain its considerable reputation' and a Faculty which had 'become discouraged and despondent because of lack of support and opportunity'. While the quality of many of the staff, both in teaching and research, was up to the standard of the better medical schools, unless something was done soon, the ranks of what amounted to a skeleton staff would be depleted and the University faced with a difficult crisis. Drastic changes were required if the Medical School was not to lose the respect it had gained over almost a century of endeavour. Rehabilitation would be expensive, he warned, and only effective if associated with changes in administration.

Christie and the Curriculum

That more than half of the Report was given over to the medical curriculum reflected growing dissatisfaction with its content and delivery throughout the 1960s. Staff and students had long agreed that change was desirable, but it was impeded by financial constraints and large student numbers. Dissatisfaction with the course and positive ideas on how to improve it run as a strong theme through the *Digest* during these years. The 1960 issue set the tone. 'The system set over eighty-five years ago', the editor maintained, 'has scarcely changed to meet the pressing needs of medicine today, nor have the methods employed in teaching its disciplines altered greatly.' Sayers reported on innovations in medical education in the United States, covering admission policies, curriculum (a four-year course), emphasis on general culture as well as vocational training, and a mode of instruction

that included fewer lectures and a good deal of free time for students. Other staff contributors addressed the need to change medical training to fit a changing environment and John Hunter derided the kind of student the current system produced. They were known at home and abroad, he said, for their 'superb, inoffensive inarticulateness'.[41]

While the occasional article expressing the need for change appeared after this, the momentum was not maintained. However, in 1967, on the eve of the Christie review, the *Digest* featured a whole section on medical education, which demonstrated the depth of student and staff dissatisfaction. The students produced five quite detailed reports criticising both the preclinical years, for confusion over aims and poor presentation, and the clinical years, as lacking 'active learning' and leading to a 'decreasing sense of direction'.[42] From the staff and graduate side, Professor Trotter explained recent changes in the selection of students. Drs Howie and Emery emphasised the need to put teaching above research or service to the public, affirming that 'the primary obligation of a teacher is to teach'. Professor Fraenkel lambasted the Medical School, its teaching and its students. In his view, the basic problem of medical education at Otago was trying to educate 120 students in a small town, with restricted and under-funded hospital facilities and in a school with inadequate grants and endowments. He held that a medical school should simply supply the facilities to enable the student to learn, without didactic teaching, but he did not think Otago students were of the calibre to work in this way. According to Fraenkel, they expected 'to be pushed and dragged along by the instructors almost up to the end of the course'. He believed the course should be shortened and the subjects integrated and that the students should be allowed contact with patients early in their training.[43]

Using his acute critical judgment and broad knowledge of up-to-date practices and trends, Christie reinforced what local reformers were advocating and suggested some new directions and changes of emphasis. He advocated fewer lectures, more integrated teaching and block courses, the incorporation of electives for students and allocation of research time for staff. Some of his recommendations would be implemented quite promptly, others provided guidelines for a more distant future.

The Preclinical course

For the preclinical years, Christie placed emphasis on the teaching of scientific method rather than knowledge of facts, but he was also quite specific in his recommendations on the space allocation and staffing levels of each department. In regard to the curriculum, he welcomed the robust discussion and energetic activity already in progress. Admission regulations had just been modified, to allow a fourth 'free' subject in the Intermediate examination and to permit students who had done very well at school in chemistry and physics to substitute other subjects for these in their Intermediate year. A committee, convened by Professor Douglass Taylor, to conduct a detailed investigation of the second- and third-year programme, had consulted with all Heads of Department and made a preliminary report to Faculty.[44] Christie attended two of the curriculum committee's meetings and warmly approved its plans for second and third year. These included a substantial reduction in the teaching of anatomy at second year, from 960 to 600 hours, and more formal instruction in statistics. He recommended reducing the time given to anatomy by a further hundred hours. 'I know of no medical school where anatomy has not surrendered time in the curriculum', he wrote. 'It is now only the extent of this sacrifice which is debated.'[45]

Before commenting on the individual departments, Christie suggested the Medical School experiment with integrated teaching across disciplines. Biochemistry staff, he noted approvingly, were already planning a drastic revision of the teaching in their department, though he warned that they would need a considerable sum of money to bring their teaching equipment up to date. He found Physiology the most 'precarious' of the preclinical departments. 'Only the loyalty of its members to Otago University has allowed it to survive, and unless something

is done its viability will be in considerable doubt', he wrote. Its staff were disheartened and lacked adequate research time. Although the subject was increasingly important in the medical curriculum, and also had a teaching commitment to the Faculty of Science, the department was operating in less space than ten years ago.[46] In their third year, students should learn to apply the anatomy, physiology and biochemistry taught in second year to the problems of medicine, and should advance to study pathology, microbiology and pharmacology. Christie also supported the curriculum committee's proposal to introduce a course on human behaviour at third year. He singled out Biochemistry and Microbiology as particularly active departments. Pharmacology and Pharmacy were in difficulties because of haphazard growth, which left them scattered over six buildings.

The Clinical Years

Christie reserved his sharpest criticisms and boldest recommendations for the clinical years of the course. Reforming the clinical curriculum, something considered overdue in medical schools on both sides of the Atlantic, was a 'delicate task', to be approached with circumspection. A Faculty committee, chaired by a senior academic, should consider integrating the curriculum and designing block courses, in which students would devote all their time to a single subject for a short period. This had the added advantage that the final examination could be done away with. He advocated establishing electives to develop the students' approach to self-education as a lifelong learning process.[47] In relation to individual departments, Christie noted that Medicine, which carried the greatest teaching burden for the clinical course and which had a tradition of strength in one or two highly specialised areas, had recently diversified. However, it needed more staff at all levels to enable it to build up its special units in cardiology, respiratory and renal medicine, gastroenterology and neurology, develop graduate training and retain promising junior staff. The weakest area, in his view, was endocrinology. He was scathing about the Hospital, where poor facilities were forcing staff into obsolete teaching methods, with 'too many lectures, and too little clinical instruction, too much poorly supervised clinical apprenticeship and too little scientific tuition.' Immediately needed were more staff, more beds and many more teaching rooms. Dunedin needed a metabolic ward, such as was provided in Auckland, Wellington and Christchurch, and investigative laboratories alongside the ward areas. He found it remarkable that few staff, either full-time or visiting, had hospital offices for their clinical work.[48]

Other clinical departments operated under similar constraints. Surgery, for example, lacked teaching space and staff, especially at junior level, suffered from 'grossly inadequate' teaching facilities in the Dunedin Hospital and lacked provision for research. Plans for the development of genito-urinary and plastic surgery should be implemented and a cardiac surgical unit set up. Facilities for teaching and research were better in Obstetrics and Gynaecology but there was a serious lack of beds for Paediatrics

and Child Health. Psychological Medicine was developing strong undergraduate and graduate teaching at Wakari Hospital, but suffered from its geographical isolation. Preventive and Social Medicine won commendation as a young department making social medicine 'a subject rather than an outlook'. The thesis it required of fifth years was seen as a step to an elective educational pattern that was the trend in most medical schools.[49]

All the clinical departments suffered from too few staff, too few patients and poor hospital facilities. Recruitment of staff was difficult because salaries were far below the rest of the English-speaking world and this had resulted in a vicious circle of under-staffing. Dunedin Hospital simply did not have enough patients to train more than a hundred clinical students a year to international standards and its facilities, although fairly good in some specialties, were worse in general medicine and surgery than in any of the teaching hospitals he had seen in Europe or North America. What could be done? One solution would be to

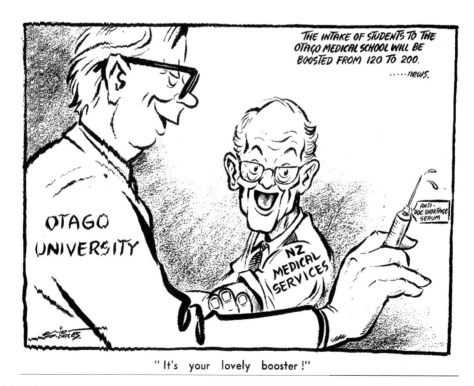

"It's your lovely booster!"

Sid Scales' cartoon celebrates the increased intake of medical students, as recommended by Professor Christie.
Otago Daily Times, 30 July 1970.

reduce the student intake to sixty or seventy a year. However, Christie was against this option, because it would be politically unpalatable and would not greatly reduce the overall running cost of the School. Besides, New Zealand needed more, not fewer doctors. He recommended, instead, that a full clinical school be established, either in Wellington, or preferably, on grounds of proximity, in Christchurch. He noted that excellent medical schools overseas used two or more teaching hospitals, although admittedly none of these were two hundred miles distant from the base school. If such a clinical school were opened, the graduate class, rather than being halved, could actually be increased, to 120 or even 130 a year. To look to expansion rather than contraction as a solution to the Medical School's problems was an exciting new take on an old, apparently intractable problem and the chief novelty of the Christie Report.

Administrative and Other Matters

Concerning the role of the Dean, which had exercised Faculty on the retirement of both Hercus and Sayers, Christie was decisive. The responsibilities of a medical Dean were heavier than those in other faculties and he needed the authority to carry them out. He had to hold the loyalty of clinical staff, who were paid little or nothing by the University and yet played an essential part in its teaching. The Dean was involved in the complex relations between the Medical School and the Department of Health, the Hospital and the University, and also had to represent the University on a number of professional bodies. In addition, he had to meet the challenges of change, at an unprecedented rate, in the practice of medicine and the techniques of medical education. At Otago, two recent changes had undermined the Dean's traditional authority: the abandonment of a separate financial grant for the Medical School had set the needs of the School in direct competition with those of other parts of the University, and the lines of communication between the Medical School and the University had become tangled. Christie maintained that these lines should be clearly established, running from Head of Department to Dean to Vice-Chancellor, so that in staffing matters (appointments, promotions and sabbatical and conference leave) the Dean should be responsible for presenting the case to the Vice-Chancellor. The Dean, he added, in evident reference to the University's staffing committee, should not have to defend his case before an advisory committee that contained a member of his own Faculty.

On other issues, Christie endorsed the views of the Faculty. For example, he acknowledged the need for closer relations with the Hospital, finding it 'unbelievable' that the University was not represented on the Hospital Board. A single Joint Planning Committee was needed immediately to plan the proposed new hospital ward block. There was room for more development in postgraduate work and, while quality research was being pursued in the School, staff needed more time and more money for it. A new library was urgently needed.

Christie saved his final broadside for finance. 'The Faculty of Medicine in Otago University', he wrote tersely, 'must be one of the most economical in the English-speaking world.' Financial restraint had been carried to the point where the whole future of the Medical School was in jeopardy. Urgent action was needed – it could not be left until the present quinquennium ended in March 1970. Authority had to be sought at once from the UGC to advertise an additional twenty positions at lecturer, senior lecturer and associate professor level, funded by a special addition to the block grant.[50]

Christie had one final task to perform before he left New Zealand. It took place on 10 April 1968, a date etched in the memory of New Zealanders as the stormy day the inter-island ferry *Wahine* sank in Wellington harbour. Accompanied by Robin Williams, Christie travelled to Wellington to meet the Chairman of the UGC, Sir Alan Danks, and the Director-General of Health, Dr Douglas Kennedy. He impressed both men by his astute observations and practical proposals. Williams believed that by the end of the two-hour meeting they had accepted the principles of the Report.[51] Reaction from the medical community and the general public was not slow to follow.

The Christie Report: Reaction and Action

Promptly published by the University of Otago, the Christie Report ran to a thirty-page booklet. It also appeared in its entirety, in the May 1968 issue of the *New Zealand Medical Journal*, accompanied by an editorial, 'Medical Education in Crisis'.[52] While the editorial rightly found little in the Report that had not been in Sayers' assessment of the previous year, it expressed support for one of Christie's two major recommendations, increased government finance, and opposition to the other, expansion into Christchurch. The editor readily agreed that the Otago Medical School had two overriding problems, a lack of finance and 'an accident of history', which had put it 'in a place without much developmental potential'. The issue of finance was important, he went on to argue, in case the new Auckland school was treated as scurvily as Otago. The two medical centres must combine to insist on a return to special financing from the UGC, separate from the universities' block grants. However, the editor was unsympathetic towards Christie's solution to the other major problem of the Otago School, Dunedin's shortage of hospital beds for teaching. He argued for economies of scale, noting that Auckland had the capacity to expand in the foreseeable future, to an intake of two hundred students a year, the economic size of a medical school, according to recently published findings of a British Royal Commission on Medical Education. He took a gloomy view of Otago's future, recommending that Otago 'cut its losses' and simply transfer the whole school to Christchurch or Wellington. Such a move would make economic sense, because the cost of Dunedin Hospital's new ward block (which would not be needed other than for teaching purposes) and the planned new Medical Library would not be much under $20 million. The editorial ended with a plea for a royal commission on medical education in New Zealand, to project the number of doctors needed through to the end of the century and to recommend the best means of producing them.[53]

Surprisingly, the 1968 *Digest* did not comment on the Christie Report. The editor explained that, because staff were too busy with internal politics and preparation of the quinquennial budgets, articles of a medico-social nature had been solicit-ed from people outside the Medical School. Nevertheless, there was little doubt that 1968 was one of the most important years for medical education in New Zealand since classes first commenced in 1875: the Auckland Medical School opened, the findings of a British Royal Commission on Medical Education were published after three years' research and Professor Christie reported on the Otago Medical School.[54]

The Dunedin press was supportive of the Report. The *Otago Daily Times* of 3 May carried a detailed summary of it under the heading 'Medical School's Future in Jeopardy'. In the same issue, it reported approvingly the Vice-Chancellor's call for a combined and systematic approach, by the Otago Hospital Board, the UGC, the Health Department and the Government, to tackle the two basic needs of the Medical School: adequate finance and better arrangements for the teaching hospitals. The Vice-Chancellor ridiculed the suggestion of moving the entire School north as an 'appalling idea', a 'gold-plated herring' and claimed the estimated cost of the ward block and library was grossly misleading.[55]

From Wellington, Keith Eunson of the *Otago Daily Times*, described the reception of the Christie Report in the capital. Early in May, he portrayed this as 'cagey' and commented that, although the 'power-packed punch' of the Report had provoked little official reaction, unofficially several people considered it to be 'hair-raising'. Eunson warned that political pressure was needed in the cause of the Medical School, in view of Otago and the South Island's rapidly diminishing leverage, through a population shift which would see three times as many people in the North Island as in the South by 1988. The future of the Medical School depended on both the UGC and the Government and although the Christie Report might be seen as a blueprint in Dunedin, it had a steadily declining impact the farther north one travelled. A good case, without political pressure, he stressed, was no case at all. By July, however, Eunson was able to quote a statement in Parliament by the Minister of Education that the Christie Report would be assured of urgent treatment.[56]

In fact, the momentum was impressive. On 1 August, the *ODT* reported that members of the University had joined the Hospital Board, a week later it announced salary increases for medical and dental staff and, in late October, it stated that $100,000 had been promised to fund additional staff for the Medical School. By mid-December, it was able to display a model of the proposed Medical School Library, already approved by the University Council and, at the time, being considered by the UGC.[57] Much later, Hunter accounted for the speed of action in terms of personalities. He thought that the circumstances for implementing the Report had been uniquely favourable. Vice-Chancellor Robin Williams was fully supportive of Christie's recommendations, as his predecessor might well not have been, and the change of chairman at the UGC also helped. Williams himself agreed that, if the Otago negotiators had had to argue the Christie increases with Llewellyn instead of Danks, they would have had a more difficult task. He also believed the restructuring of the School would not have been possible under Sayers. Williams took the credit for suggesting the team to carry out the reconstruction and expansion, Professor Bill Adams as Dean and Dr Robin Irvine as Clinical Dean. He believed the integrity and leadership of the one, and the skill in planning and negotiation of the other, were valuable complementary qualities.[58]

In the University context, there was less resentment of the benefits to the Medical School – major additions to buildings and staffing in the middle of a quinquennium – than might have been expected. With the Medical Library receiving a much-needed boost, and buildings such as Biochemistry, the rest of the University, as Williams put it, 'might have [had] the feeling that Christmas had come early for the Medical School'. However, because other university buildings were also in train, this was generally accepted with good grace. Indeed in late 1967, at a time when student numbers were exploding in New Zealand as elsewhere, the University had three major buildings under construction and another ten at various stages of planning.[59]

Revisiting the Christie Report in 1998, John Hunter singled out for special comment three significant changes that resulted from its recommendations. One was the increased influence of the Medical School on the Dunedin Hospital, through the appointment of University representatives to the Hospital Board. This settled an old issue. In 1949 and again in the mid-1960s, the University had been unsuccessful in its attempts to secure representation, although in 1966 the Hospital Board did agree to a Joint Advisory Committee and the Minister of Health designated the Dunedin Hospital a teaching hospital. Because its criticism of the Medical School's facilities for clinical teaching reflected on the Hospital Board, the Christie Report provided the needed spur to action. The Minister of Health pushed through the necessary legislation to allow five University nominees to be appointed to the Hospital Board: the Dean, the Clinical Dean, the University Registrar, the Vice-Chancellor and a University Council member. The status and experience of the appointees made them a force to be reckoned with, from the Hospital Board's viewpoint increasing the already substantial weight the Medical School had in its affairs. From the School's point of view, the new arrangements set in train a refreshing period of greatly improved cooperation between the Medical School and the Hospital Board, exemplified in the joint planning of a new ward block for the Hospital, on the basis of the close integration of its service and teaching functions.[60] The other elements of the Christie Report that Hunter chose to emphasise were the development of a clinical school at Christchurch and an increase in the student intake, to 150 a year. Within a year both of these recommendations would be taken up and dramatically extended.

The Irvine Report

Much of the detail of implementing the Christie proposals was entrusted to Robin Irvine, in his role as Clinical Dean, but he went further than mere implementation. In a lengthy report to the

Vice-Chancellor, dated 1 May 1969, he detailed the developments at the School that had resulted from the Christie Report, others that were still in the planning stage, and the future of the Medical School in respect to student numbers and the utilisation of clinical facilities outside Dunedin.[61]

The 'recent developments' section told a story of satisfyingly prompt achievements. It included the changes proposed by the committee revising the preclinical curriculum, which had come into effect in 1969. Faculty had established a standing curriculum committee to keep the medical course under constant review and to take responsibility for revising the content of the clinical years. The UGC had supported the University's request for twenty additional positions, for which the Government allocated a special block grant. Their distribution among the departments closely followed Christie's recommendations: Medicine received five, Surgery three, Physiology two and eight other departments one each. The University was represented on the Hospital Board. The duties of the Dean were shared with a Clinical Dean, who was responsible for clinical matters relating to Dunedin Hospital, supervision of the Branch Faculties in Auckland, Wellington and Christchurch, the curriculum and postgraduate activities. A remodelled joint planning committee was planning the new ward block as a combined Hospital Board/University exercise.[62]

The 'planned developments' section included a miscellany of items on which action had been initiated or was pending. The Medical Faculty had agreed to the lengthening of the fourth-, fifth- and sixth-year courses. This should be possible with the increased staff and reduced student numbers in these years, while still allowing time for staff research. It would necessitate an increase in student bursaries to compensate for loss of earning time on holiday jobs. The selection of students at the end of the Intermediate year was retained, in spite of Christie's recommendation against the scheme, with guaranteed entry to very high achievers in the secondary school scholarship and bursary examinations. The clinical curriculum was being reviewed by a new committee. It reported in April 1969 that the six-year course should be retained and there

should be a combined examination at the end of fifth year, but in the fourth or sixth years the examination should be replaced by continuous assessment. Discussions were in progress about the academic rank to be given to research workers employed by the MRC and other bodies, and about the possibility of awarding a degree at the end of the third year.

There was satisfying progress on buildings. Final approval for the new library was expected shortly. It would have greatly improved facilities and space for a hundred and fifty readers. The Departments of Biochemistry, Physiology and Pharmacology were looking forward to the completion of the biochemistry building. Plans for the new hospital ward block were progressing, and it was expected that the academic wing would give greatly improved facilities for Medicine, Surgery, Obstetrics and Gynaecology, Psychological Medicine and Paediatrics. Immediate improvements were needed, however, in clinical lecture theatres and student amenities.[63]

Of broader significance and more controversial nature was the 'future of the Medical School' section, which took up most of the report and boldly extended Christie's recommendations. Irvine argued that the twenty additional staff had done no more than fill gaps and lift staff morale. The Medical School was still in danger and needed more staff and a new curriculum for the new decade. The recent British Royal Commission on Medical Education had shown the need for a better ratio of staff to students, to produce a new type of doctor. 'The doctor of the future must be educated for a world in which everything, the content of medicine, the organisation of medical care, the doctor's relationship with his colleagues and the community, and indeed every feature of his professional life and work, is on the move.' The changes to the medical curriculum that Irvine proposed were aimed at producing graduates able to cope with a professional life of continual change.

That there were too few patients at Dunedin Hospital to give a broad clinical training to medical students was the most intractable problem. Whereas Christie had recommended developing the Branch Faculty in Christchurch

Sir Robin Orlando Hamilton Irvine, 1929–1996

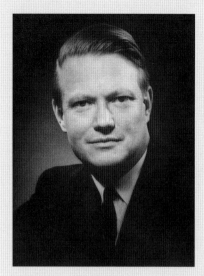

Robin Irvine.
Registry, University of Otago.

ROBIN IRVINE was the youngest Vice-Chancellor to be appointed to the University of Otago since the office became an executive one in 1948, the first to have been born in Dunedin and the longest-serving, his tenure lasting from 1973 to 1993, twice as long as any other Otago Vice-Chancellor before or since. His influence on the Otago Medical School was deep and lasting: he persuaded the University to open a clinical school in Wellington and Christchurch and he oversaw the establishment of what became the University of Otago Schools of Medicine and Health Sciences in those two centres.

Born in Dunedin, but educated at Wanganui Collegiate School when his family moved to the North Island, Robin Irvine returned to study medicine. He graduated in 1953, winning the Marjorie McCallum medal for theoretical and clinical medicine. After a house surgeon year in Auckland, he returned to Dunedin, as part of Sir Horace Smirk's research team, and to a position in the Department of Medicine. He gained his MD in 1958 and travelled on a Nuffield scholarship to Britain, where he worked in London hospitals until 1960. Back in New Zealand, he and his wife – he married fellow medical graduate Elizabeth Corbett in 1957 – came to Dunedin in 1963. Irvine rose quickly through the ranks in the Department of Medicine, to become Associate Professor by 1968 and Clinical Dean, then personal Professor, from 1969 to 1972. In this decade, he published more than seventy academic papers, many of them dealing with kidney disease and high blood pressure and also gained a formidable reputation as an administrator and negotiator.

As Vice-Chancellor, Irvine headed a capable administration and effectively represented the University in the community and abroad. With his intimate knowledge of the Medical School, he adopted a hands-on approach which was not always appreciated by the Dean of the day, but his expertise was universally acknowledged. He served on a myriad of educational and medical bodies. He chaired the Vice-Chancellors' Committee and the Council of the Association of Commonwealth Universities. He served on the Otago Polytechnic and Dunedin College of Education Councils and the Otago Hospital Board, the Selwyn College Board of Governors and the New Zealand Red Cross Foundation. In 1970, he acted as assessor for New Zealand's medical aid programme in South Vietnam. He chaired discussions on Pacific regional cooperation in medical education and, in 1971, convened a review on the future of the Fiji School of Medicine. He received numerous honours, including an honorary degree from the University of Edinburgh, in 1976, and a knighthood, for services to the University and the community, in 1989. His retirement, in 1993, was recognised by his admission to the degree of Doctor of Laws, honoris causa. Sir Robin died in 1996.[64]

into a full clinical school, Irvine went further. He argued that Wellington should also become a clinical school. The number of staff in the clinical departments of medical schools, his argument ran, depended on the clinical work available. This, in the end, was determined by the size of the local population and was the factor limiting Dunedin. But New Zealand needed more doctors. Irvine set out the numbers involved. The combined intake of the Auckland and Otago Medical Schools was 180 students, but should rise to at least 300 by 1986. If Auckland gradually increased its intake to 150 and Otago to 200, this target would be more than reached. In Dunedin, the target figure of 150 in 1972 could be achieved by additions to staff (he suggested eight) and space. The new Biochemistry Building and Medical Library would free up teaching space elsewhere, a fourth floor could be added to the Wellcome Building and there would be a new ward block at the Hospital by 1976, but these additions would still not meet the need for extra clinical facilities. Adding a clinical school in Christchurch would not provide enough either: it was necessary to look to Wellington as well. Irvine suggested that in their fourth and fifth years, seventy students might remain in Dunedin and seventy go to Christchurch. In their sixth year, thirty-five would remain in each of Dunedin and Christchurch and the other seventy would go to Wellington. Auckland would not be able to take Otago students after 1972, but Christchurch should be ready to take fourth years by 1973. Irvine made it quite clear that neither clinical school was to be regarded as the seed of a full medical school. Indeed, with this plan in place, there would be no need for a third medical school in the foreseeable future.

The rest of the report dealt with the consequent developments that would be required if the main recommendation was accepted. Additional staff would be needed for the clinical schools and their facilities expanded – both Christchurch and Wellington Hospitals had hospital buildings at the planning stage. The status of the new schools, as well as their relationship to the Otago School and to their local Hospital Boards, would also have to be determined. In relation to the Medical School, he recommended they should enjoy 'a reasonable degree of autonomy' with 'well-defined lines of communication' and, to the Hospital Boards, a 'well-defined' relationship achieved through strengthened Joint Relationship Committees.[65]

If Christie's response to the shortage of clinical material in Dunedin had been to increase rather than decrease student numbers and to upgrade the Christchurch Branch Faculty to the status of a clinical school, Irvine was prepared to go much further and he won support for his bold concept from Faculty and Council. It marked a new era for the Otago Medical School, now to be spread over three sites on two islands.

CHAPTER 18

Building a 'Three-Legged Stool':
The Christchurch and Wellington Schools

'In the decade that followed Christie's influence', John Hunter wrote from a vantage point thirty years on, 'the medical faculty was revitalised.' He went on to describe the rapid construction and staffing of clinical schools in Christchurch and Wellington, which stimulated fruitful debate on medical education and positive changes in curriculum and examination procedures.[1] The early 1970s were characterised by a mood of confident optimism, that peaked in 1975 when the School celebrated its centenary. There were substantial additions to staff and a New Zealand-wide university building boom benefited the Medical School in Dunedin as well as the new clinical schools. In the second half of the decade, however, reduced resources, the expectation of a cut in the number of medical students and tensions among the geographically separate units of the School created a quite different atmosphere.

The change reflected what was occurring in the wider New Zealand society. Historian Michael King describes how the excitement of the late 1960s and early 1970s, which seemed to come to fruition under the Third Labour Government, ended abruptly with Prime Minister Kirk's sudden death in 1974. The election of the following year brought National's Robert Muldoon to power. 'The warm positivism of the Kirk era', King wrote, 'was replaced by defensive negativism' and, quoting political journalist Colin James, '[t]he New Zealand way of life became antagonistic, mean and grudging.'[2] It was not merely a matter of politics. The first of two massive and unexpected rises in the price of oil struck New Zealand in 1974, just after Britain entered the (then) European Economic Community, which signalled the weakening of Commonwealth ties.

In this new environment, the University Grants Committee found its recommendations to Government being challenged, or their implementation repeatedly delayed, on Treasury advice. The University building programme stalled. The early 1970s perception that New Zealand was short of doctors gave way to a belief that the country was training too many. At the end of the decade, as the National Government cut student numbers by a quarter at both the Otago and Auckland Medical Schools, Otago had to face the hard question of whether spreading clinical training over three campuses was the best use of its limited funds.

The Years of Expansion, 1969–1975

The Dean who guided the fortunes of the Medical School in the years of expansion and optimism after 1968 was Professor Bill Adams. Acting Dean after Sayers' retirement and during Christie's visit, he was persuaded to accept the post permanently in 1968. However, because the deanship had such a large clinical component, he insisted that a new post of Clinical Dean be created. This was filled by Robin Irvine. Supported by Vice-Chancellor Robin Williams, and with the cooperation of Sir Alan Danks of the UGC, they worked harmoniously to bring in a new order.

William Edgar Adams, 1908–1973

Professor of Anatomy, 1944–68, Dean 1968–73

IT IS striking, in what people have written about Professor Bill Adams, how often the word 'integrity' occurs. After his sudden death in May 1973, his colleagues remembered his 'intellectual integrity', his 'courage and integrity' and 'impeccable integrity, with an instinctive sympathy for the under-dog'. His successor as Dean, John Hunter, believed his 'absolute integrity and lack of any suggestion of medical pretentiousness' were important in ensuring the recommendations of the Christie Report were accepted by the university community. Adams was also a warm friend, an outstanding researcher and a superb, although undeniably fierce, teacher.

Born in Foxton, where his father was in general practice, Adams developed a close bond with his forthright schoolteacher grandfather, with whom he lived for some years. He completed an MSc Honours in zoology, before studying medicine, graduating MB ChB from Otago in 1935. Adams served three years as senior tutor in anatomy under Gowland, before joining the Department of Anatomy at Leeds University, where he gained his PhD. He married Ena Mathewson in 1937 and the couple would have four daughters.

Back at Otago as Professor of Anatomy, Adams aimed to build on the strengths of Gowland's anatomy course, which he believed had been ahead of its time. The department won a fine reputation and research, which focused primarily on the nervous system, flourished. Of Adams' own research, his successor Professor Bill Trotter singled out two important papers on the blood supply to the peripheral nerves, which were of relevance to surgeons in World War II, and a series of papers and a book on the *Carotid Body and Carotid Sinus*, which won him international acclaim.

Throughout his career, Adams served on the editorial boards of journals in his area of expertise, and he was an active member of many learned societies, a number of which honoured him with life membership or fellowships. Among these were the Anatomical Society of Great Britain and the Anatomical Society of Australia and New Zealand, of which he was founding member and first President (1963–65). In 1958, the University of New Zealand awarded him the DSc for his scientific work and, in 1962, the Royal Australasian College of Surgeons, for which he was an examiner, made him an honorary Fellow. He was a member of the Medical Council and the Medical Research Councils of New Zealand, the Otago University Council and the Otago Hospital Board. In 1970, he visited Nigeria to advise on medical education.

Reluctant to take on the deanship, Adams combined his administrative capacity with tenacity, directness and sound common sense and made an important contribution to the resurgence of the Otago Medical School after 1968.[3]

Changes and additions to the staff from the end of the 1960s brought a new, younger group of men to the fore. In 1969, Bill Trotter was promoted to Adams' former Chair in Anatomy and, in 1970, Alan Clarke replaced Gustav Fraenkel as Professor of Surgery. The next year, John Blennerhassett succeeded Alun Wynn-Williams as Professor of Pathology. When Professor Horace Smirk retired from the Wellcome Medical Research Institute in 1968, however, his research Chair was not filled. New positions were also created around this time. In 1972, a Department of Orthopaedics separated out from Surgery, with Alan Alldred as foundation professor, and John Hubbard was appointed to a new Chair of Neurophysiology within the Department of Physiology. When Hunter became Dean in 1974, David Stewart replaced him as Mary Glendining Professor of Medicine. All these new professors were former Otago students with British postgraduate qualifications who would make their careers at the Medical School. The passage of the old order was symbolised by the death of Sir Charles Hercus in 1971, and the advent of the new by the opening of the Auckland Medical School in 1968. In addition, between 1971 and 1976 a whole raft of foundation professors were appointed in the nascent Christchurch and Wellington clinical schools: seven in Christchurch between 1971 and 1973, and six in Wellington between 1973 and 1976.[4]

A prompt start was made on preparations for coordinating the clinical training at Dunedin, Christchurch and Wellington. The Faculty Standing Curriculum Committee considered the degree of uniformity in teaching and examining that would be required. It was an opportunity for innovation and the thrust of its first report, in 1969, was towards reducing examinations. The Committee recommended having all three schools participate in a combined examination at the end of fifth year, but no examinations at the end of either the fourth or sixth years, because the smaller student numbers in each school would permit progressive and continuous assessment instead. The fourth- and fifth-year courses would be expected to include both topic teaching and block attachments and the fifth-year exam would serve as a formal confirmation of the student's achievement, as assessed by each department, over the preceding two years. The sixth year would be entirely vocational and, with the exception of some compulsory clinical attachments, the courses would become elective.[5] These recommendations were implemented over the following years. Formal written Faculty Professional examinations were dropped for fourth years in 1971, and for sixth years in 1973. An integrated clinical science course was introduced in 1971 for fourth and fifth years, with an examination at the end of the latter year.[6]

It took some time before the extent of the changes that occurred in the wake of the Christie Report became evident to the student body and the dissatisfaction with the medical course that had been expressed earlier in the *Digest* was not immediately dissipated. In 1969 the Intellectual Affairs representative on OUMSA, under the provocative heading 'Medical Education at Otago – revolt, cooperate or give up?' asked, 'Is student frustration over poor lecturing, hysterical ward sisters, crowded clinics, bad facilities and no patients heading towards a remedy?' He hoped a new staff/student curriculum committee might provide the solution. When Fraenkel left Otago in mid-1970 he wrote back to the *Digest*, repeating his opinion that Dunedin was too small to support a medical school. He also warned that, now government funding was to be stretched over two medical schools, academic standards may not be able to be maintained in either. Recent advances in medical knowledge were so rapid that only small-group teaching could produce graduates with the built-in flexibility required. He added that he had enjoyed his thirteen years at Otago and had done his best to 'sabotage the didactic teaching of facts which will be fallacies in the future and to encourage a spirit of critical assessment and enquiry in all aspects of the theory and practice of medicine.'

The next year's editors echoed the now familiar criticism of the style of Otago teaching. 'In five years', they said, 'we have not only been taught innumerable facts (an unfortunate necessity) but also not to question knowledge.'[7] Senior staff responded with a whole section on medical education in the 1972 *Digest*. The centrepiece, titled 'Trends in Medical Education', was by Robin Irvine. Divided into two sections, Irvine's article summed up changes to the delivery of health care and the likely effect they would have on undergraduate medical education. He foresaw the changes as being wide-ranging and comprehensive, and requiring a more careful definition of objectives, a reduction in the length of the course, more integrated teaching both horizontally and vertically, new subjects such as behavioural science, biostatistics and genetics, computer science and management and communication skills, a problem-solving approach, early patient contact and an attempt to ensure 'relevance'. It was a final fling. By the early 1970s, the *Digest* was faltering and, when it ceased publication before the end of the decade, a useful forum for staff-student debate was lost.[8]

The Medical School had a very good relationship with the *Otago Daily Times* during this period. It gave unqualified support to the School in 1972, when a major row erupted between the Otago Hospital Board, with the strong support of the Medical School, and the North Canterbury Hospital Board. At issue was the siting of a cardiac surgery unit to service the South Island. Prime Minister Holyoake had given an undertaking that Dunedin would get the unit, and this had been a factor in enabling John Hunter, then Professor of Medicine, to assemble a fine cardiac team. When news came through that the South Island unit was to be located in Christchurch instead, there was an outcry in Dunedin and the Hospital Board and Medical School joined in a determined campaign to achieve what they had been promised. In August, the *ODT* devoted an entire page to the Otago case, letters to the editor were uniformly supportive and, early in November, the Government backed down and announced that the Dunedin cardiac unit had been given the go-ahead. Professor Pat Molloy was appointed Director at the end of the year and the unit was formally opened the following June. The repercussions of the dispute lingered, however. Christchurch heart surgeon Sir David Hay commented in his autobiography that although Holyoake's promise had been kept, it had 'fuelled the controversy which soured relations between Dunedin and Christchurch for decades'.[9]

Among the routine announcements in the press of arrivals or resignations of Medical School staff, or deaths of former staff, was the occasional stuff of tragedy or drama. In February 1974, the press reported an horrific plane crash at Pago Pago, in which Associate Professor Peter Lewis, his wife and three of his children were among the ninety-two people killed. Lewis had been a pioneer in child psychiatry in New Zealand.[10] At the end of 1974, the resignation of Dr Donald Malcolm who, as Associate Professor of Paediatrics and Child Health and neo-natal paediatrician to Queen Mary Hospital, had built up a world class special-care baby unit, roused public indignation. There had been a crisis the previous year, when Malcolm had resigned through frustrations connected with

his work, but had been persuaded to reconsider. This time, the threatened loss of sixteen maternity beds in Queen Mary proved too much for him. His resignation was accompanied by expressions of the highest praise from representatives of the Hospital Board and the University and from correspondents to the press.[11]

In the early 1970s the stability in the leadership of the Otago Medical School, which had seemed assured with the announcement, late in 1970, that Irvine would replace Adams as Dean at the end of 1973, was shattered.[12] The team that had worked together so effectively on behalf of the School since 1968 suddenly broke up. When Robin Williams was appointed Vice-Chancellor of the Australian National University, in November 1972, the University Council appointed Dean-designate Irvine to succeed him. The post of Clinical Dean lapsed and the work was covered in the meantime by three part-time Assistant Deans.[13] The Dean's own retirement had been deferred until February 1975, to enable him to preside over the celebrations planned for the centenary of the Medical School in that year, but events overtook this plan. Bill Adams died suddenly, after an illness of only a few days, on 19 May 1973. It would be John Hunter, so influential in setting up the Christie review, who would oversee the early development of the two clinical schools that resulted from it.

The Building Programme: Dunedin

As well as the provision of new buildings for the clinical schools in Christchurch and Wellington, the expansion of the Otago Medical School necessitated an extensive building programme in Dunedin. It was badly needed. Since 1948, the sole additions to the School had been a temporary, single-storey building, constructed in 1956 to house the Departments of Surgery and Obstetrics and Gynaecology, and the Wellcome Institute in 1963. The first of these had been financed partly from salary savings, while the second was gifted by the Wellcome Trust. The Medical School had repeatedly been frustrated in its requests to government for new, up-to-date accommodation. Faculty and departmental annual reports are

Professor John Hunter, 1925–2003

**CBE MB ChB MD (NZ) FRACP FRCP (Lond),
Faculty Dean, Otago Medical School, 1974–77 and 1986–90,
Dean Christchurch School, 1982–85**

'A RADICAL and a firebrand in a way [but] intensely conservative in professional areas'. Professor John Hunter would probably have appreciated the first part of this comment from a former colleague more than the second. He was always proud of his part in the agitation of 1967 that led to the Christie review of the Medical School and its consequent dramatic expansion. However, his purpose throughout had been to maintain the standards of medical training at Otago.

John Hunter, J.D. to many, suffered deprivation in his early childhood. Born in 1925, he was left homeless five years later when his mother died and his father disappeared. He and his older brother spent six harsh years in orphanages. Then, in an extraordinary turnaround, their uncle took the two boys to his palatial Auckland home and sent them as boarders to King's College, from where each in turn embarked on a medical course at Otago. Hunter won the Travelling Scholarship in 1948, and was seconded to a cardiology course at Green Lane Hospital in Auckland, where he stayed for three years and found his professional direction. In 1950, he married fellow university student Heather Cornish and set off for London to study cardiology at the Royal Postgraduate Medical School and the National Heart Hospital. Three of the couple's five children were born in London.

A lecturer in medicine at Otago from 1956 and Professor from 1962, Hunter first served as Dean of the Faculty of Medicine in the mid-1970s, when the post-Christie expansion was over and government money was tight. From 1978 to 1981, he worked in Sydney as the foundation Director of Continuing Education for the Royal Australasian College of Physicians. The College later awarded him its medal for outstanding services. His next post, as Dean of the Christchurch Clinical School in the early 1980s, gave him an insight into the concerns and priorities of the northern schools. An outstanding administrator, he resumed the deanship of the Medical Faculty in 1986, from 1989–90 adding the newly established position of Assistant Vice-Chancellor Health Sciences to his portfolio.

Hunter's work stretched well beyond the Otago Medical School. He helped develop the Cardiac Society of Australia and New Zealand, served as its President from 1976 to 1978, and was made a life member in 1989. He was on the founding Council of the Heart Foundation in 1968, chaired its scientific committee from 1985 to 1989, and was made a life member. He served on numerous national health-related committees, including the Medical Council of New Zealand and the Medical Research Council.

Outgoing in personality, Hunter enjoyed entertaining and he and his wife were known for their hospitality. Their retirement was spent largely in Wanaka, where he could indulge his pleasure in fishing. However, it was marred by his ill-health, which necessitated their return to Dunedin. He died in 2003.[14]

full of tersely worded complaints about teaching and research space. 'Sub-standard, cramped and unhygienic' were the words Sayers used in his first annual report, in 1959, to describe the rooms in the Knox Church Sunday School buildings occupied by the Department of Medicine. He described the Medical Library as being 'grossly inadequate and inconvenient' and the student common room 'woefully inadequate'. Four years on, he was making the same complaints, sometimes in the same words. The Library was still 'grossly inadequate in space and design' and, by this time, he claimed the weight of the books was affecting the very structure of the building. It was a 'source of deep disappointment that nothing had happened in response to our requests to the Grants Committee for urgent consideration of the problem.' In his first report in 1964, the new University Vice-Chancellor, Dr Beacham, was equally scathing. About 22 per cent of the gross space occupied by the Medical and Dental Schools, he pointed out, was in converted attics, basements or old houses. Conditions in some departments were congested and even dangerous. He described the situation as intolerable.[15]

Acceptance of the Christie Report, in Irvine's expanded form, finally broke the logjam. Irvine explained that if 150 students were taken into second year in 1972 a new Medical Library and Biochemistry Building were an absolute requirement. If the intake were to rise to 200, another new building would be needed, including a lecture theatre to hold 250.[16] The year 1972 saw the opening of the Sayers Building to house the administration and a fine library, with study space for 150 and a three-storey building for Biochemistry in the science area of the campus. The following year the Adams Building opened. As well as Pharmacology and Pharmacy, which occupied two floors, it housed Preventive and Social Medicine on the specially designed ground

floor and provided space elsewhere for the Medical School's artists, Surgery and the Higher Education Development Centre. New lecture theatres, ready for occupation in 1974, and the clinical services block formed part of a massive redevelopment of the Hospital that was carried out in conjunction with the University. In 1975, a seven-storey Microbiology Building, with the same internal design as the Adams Building, was opened on the northern part of the campus. At the same time, building was going ahead for the clinical schools in Christchurch and Wellington. Vice-Chancellor Robin Williams paid tribute to the drive of the University's Planning Officer, Ted Dews, in running the building programme.

The Otago Medical School's remarkable growth in these years was part of a New Zealand-wide university expansion. For most of the 1970s, four or five major university buildings were completed each year. Gould has graphed the annual appropriations of the university works programme (in 1985–86 dollars) between 1962 and 1985, when it rose from $40 million in 1962 to a peak of $111.2 million in 1973–74. Thereafter, there was a steady decline to just $27.8 in 1985–86, only a quarter of the peak period. The Otago Medical School, on all three campuses, did strikingly well out of the boom. It was fortunate in its timing. From the mid-1970s, the National Government

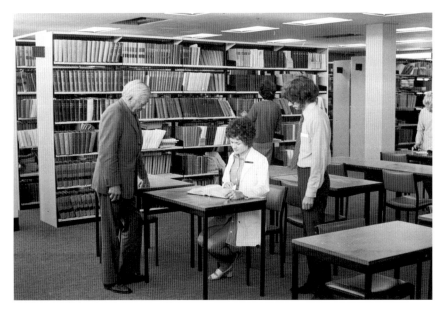

The Medical School gets its new library at last. Mrs J. Gillies, seated, is assisted by the Dean, Professor W.E. Adams, and the medical librarian, Mr D.G. Jamieson.
Otago Daily Times, 7 March 1972.

embarked on determined measures to reduce its budget deficit. The 1975–79 quinquennium was a setback for the universities, as reasoned argument and negotiation in determining funding seemed to give way to arbitrary political decision. The *Otago Daily Times* reported in July 1977 that, for the first time in fifteen years, the University of Otago's building programme had virtually come to a standstill, with several planned projects 'stacking up' and the government unwilling to commit to new ones.[17]

Construction proceeded during the late 1970s, however, on what was perhaps the most important building of the era for the Otago Medical School, the new ward block of the Dunedin Hospital. Work on the building had begun in 1974, after years of planning, and when it opened in 1980 it was hailed as 'the largest and most important single community building authorised by a New Zealand government up to the present time'. A public asset worth $45 million, ten storeys high and connected at each level to the clinical services block, the new ward block boasted some half million square feet of floor space, five hundred beds and the most modern facilities of any New Zealand hospital. It was intended to house a working population of about 3000 nurses, doctors, university and other staff. An entire wing was given over to the Medical School and its associated teaching. As the booklet printed to mark the opening of the block put it, 'The essential and historic role played by Dunedin Hospital within the teaching function of the University of Otago Medical School will be strengthened by the inclusion of an academic and clinical teaching wing in which each discipline is positioned adjacent to the beds it services': an ideal integration, achieved for the first time in Australasia.[18]

The building was the culmination of years of work since 1956, when the Australian firm of Stephenson and Turner, specialists in medical architecture, had been asked to draw up an overall development plan for Dunedin Hospital, but instead recommended its demolition and replacement. The Medical Superintendent of Dunedin Hospital and the Dean of the Medical School had each chaired committees to determine the needs of their respective institutions and

the resultant documents were combined into a brief, approved by both the Hospital Board and the University in 1969 and then accepted by the Government. Once sketch plans by the architects were approved, a Detailed Planning Committee considered the design, floor by floor and room by room, consulting widely at each stage. Buildings on site had to be demolished with as little disruption as possible to either patient care or the medical course. Fletcher Development, appointed as the main contractor, began work in April 1974. A commissioning unit prepared the building for occupation and use (furniture, fittings, equipment and staffing) in conjunction with some sixty departments in the Medical School and Hospital. The whole operation was a splendid example of the Hospital/University cooperation recommended by Christie. The new ward block was opened by the Duchess of Kent in November 1980.[19] It won high praise from an overseas expert, familiar with the School, who visited in 1981. 'The educational resources provided for learning in the clinical setting', wrote David Bates, 'which were non-existent in 1967, are now superior to those in most medical schools with which I am acquainted.'[20]

Setting up the Clinical Schools

Christchurch

In seeking the origins of the Christchurch Clinical School (later the Christchurch School of Medicine and Health Sciences and now the University of Otago, Christchurch) the historians of its first quarter-century looked back to the very beginning of the colony, a meeting in London in 1850 at which members of the Canterbury Association expressed their intention to found a medical school. The school did not eventuate, but the idea did not die. When the University of Otago 'upstaged Canterbury' by adding a medical course to its curriculum in 1875, the Canterbury Provincial Council responded by gazetting its own school and voting to put aside £300 and 5000 acres to support it. It proved an empty gesture, and medical education did not begin in Canterbury until much later, when the first batch of sixth-year

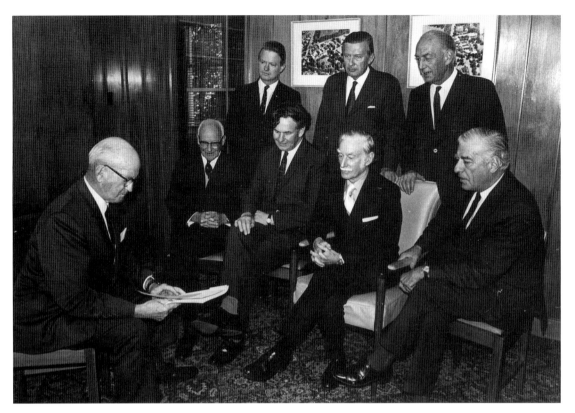

Acceptance of the constitution of the Christchurch Clinical School, 28 April 1971.
Standing, left to right: Professor R.O.H. Irvine (Clinical Dean, University of Otago), Professor G.L. Rolleston (Dean, Christchurch Clinical School), Dr J.W. Hayward (Registrar, University of Otago).
Seated: Mr L.A. Bennett (Deputy Chairman, North Canterbury Hospital Board), Dr R.M. Williams, Mr T.K.S. Sidey (Chancellor, University of Otago), Professor W.E. Adams (Dean of the Faculty of Medicine, University of Otago).
Facing the group is Dr L.C.L. Averill, Chairman, North Canterbury Hospital Board.
University of Otago, Christchurch.

students from Otago were sent up for clinical training in 1924. The scheme proved successful, was extended to Wellington and Auckland and was formalised in 1937. Branch Faculties were set up in the three centres, each with a Sub-Dean to deal with academic issues. Joint Relations Committees, with equal representation from both the University and the Hospital Boards and the requirement to report to both, were also established to deal with administrative matters.[21]

From the point of view of staff at the Christchurch Branch Faculty, the system worked well. However, their satisfaction was challenged when, in 1947, the Senate of the University of New Zealand undertook a broad review of medical education, and recommended the eventual establishment of a second medical school, in

Auckland. Canterbury objected to a proposal from Auckland that it take all sixth-year Otago students as the first stage of planning for the new proposed medical school, and in the 1950s the Christchurch Branch Faculty was expanded. It won a ten-year reprieve for the status quo. Medical and surgical tutors were appointed to supervise the teaching programmes and student and staff facilities were improved. The top floor of St Andrew's Sunday School was leased as a lecture theatre and, as in the other Branch Faculties, plans were made for a full-time teaching and research unit, which was established in 1960 at Princess Margaret Hospital. Under Dr Don Beaven, the unit of about a dozen people developed research expertise in endocrinology and metabolism, achieving an impressive publication record. In

1962, a new stage was signalled when Professor George Rolleston, whose energy and style would profoundly influence the Christchurch School, became Sub-Dean.[22]

This was the situation when, in 1966, the Government approved the prompt establishment of a medical school in Auckland. This would mean the closure of the Branch Faculty there, probably in 1972, and a consequent doubling of the numbers of sixth-year students going to Christchurch, from twenty to about forty. As a result, the Christchurch Branch Faculty prepared to add to its academic unit in medicine, units in surgery and obstetrics and gynaecology, as well as a medical centre with a library and teaching space. About the same time, John Hunter lashed out in the Dunedin press about the inadequate resources at the Otago Medical School and, at a meeting of the Sub-Deans of the Faculties, floated the idea of a clinical school in Christchurch to take half the students in their fourth and fifth years. Although Sayers was against proceeding along these lines, the groundwork was laid for accepting the idea when Christie recommended it in 1968. The recommendation was not initially popular in Dunedin. Only after intense and lengthy debate at special meetings of Faculty was it accepted and the way cleared for the development of the Christchurch Branch Medical Faculty into a clinical school of the University of Otago.[23]

Detailed planning for the Christchurch Clinical School began in 1969 and, by February 1973, the School was ready for its first intake of fourth-year students. It was an extraordinary achievement, in the face of daunting administrative, academic and building problems. How big should the proposed Christchurch Clinical School be and what facilities and staff would it require? Christie's view was that it should be able to compete with Dunedin on equal academic and clinical terms. However, Irvine seems to have envisaged something more modest. Debate was heated on this issue when, 'to everyone's surprise and delight', as Rolleston put it, Christie himself returned to New Zealand on holiday and took time out from trout fishing to hold discussions in Christchurch with the Sub-Dean, the Joint Relations Committee and the four-man working party. Christie affirmed the need for space. He was dismissive of the mere 10,000 square feet proposed for research accommodation. Even doubling that, including office space, would still be inadequate, he said. 'If you trebled it, you would be getting into a fairly good figure for a clinical school.'[24]

Negotiations followed between the North Canterbury Hospital Board, the Otago Vice-Chancellor, the University Grants Committee and the Department of Health. A meeting of all parties in Wellington in mid-July 1970, chaired by Sir Alan Danks of the UGC, to determine how the costs should be apportioned, was driven by the demand for more doctors and, therefore, the importance of Christchurch being ready to receive its first intake of fourth-year students on schedule, in 1973. It was agreed that a nine-storey medical centre for essential services, including teaching facilities, student accommodation, library, research laboratories, animal house and school administration, would be constructed on the site of Christchurch Hospital. Temporary teaching facilities at Christchurch Hospital, Princess Margaret Hospital and Christchurch Women's Hospital would also be needed. The University would be responsible for the construction of the medical centre and the temporary facilities, and alterations to existing and future buildings would be the responsibility of the Hospital Board. It was agreed that 'he who builds equips'. Ted Dews produced the required justification document for the medical centre within a matter of days and this was accepted by the Grants Committee in August. The way was clear to proceed and time was pressing. The first students, due in Christchurch in a little over two and a half years, had already begun their medical course in Dunedin. From this point, Dews' role became critical. He pushed the project along, his abrasive energy counterbalanced by the diplomacy and administrative skills of John Riminton, the School's academic secretary. They worked through a Detailed Planning Committee, chaired by Rolleston, to which a number of more specialised sub-committees reported. When the Auckland architects, Thorpe, Cutter, Pickmere and Douglas, presented their design report in

November 1970, the user committees could begin. Speed was of the essence and committee minutes were often posted to the Detailed Planning Committee on the very day the meeting had taken place. The tricky question of research facilities was resolved, although controversially, by the creation of shared research space on two floors of the medical centre for thirty-two fully serviced and versatile laboratories. Problems with the foundations involved some delay at this stage, but by August 1971 the Committee was ready to recommend that the University engage Fletcher Construction to build the medical centre, for $3,120,664. The building was still not complete when the first student intake arrived in February 1973, but a system of staged occupancy was put in place and construction and equipment were completed halfway through the year.[25]

There were no Otago precedents for this 'first offshore base' of the Medical School and, just as the components of the building to house it became the subject of ongoing negotiation, so did the administrative structure. Although, geographically, the new School was distant from Dunedin, legally it was not an independent entity. The way forward had to be trodden carefully. In 1970, the University and the Canterbury Hospital Board agreed to invite George Rolleston to become Dean, offering him at the same time a personal Chair in Radiology in the University of Otago. He took up the position the following February. Rolleston was clear about what had to be done. To create a centre of excellence in patient care, medical education and research, he would require staff and facilities comparable with those at the clinical school in Dunedin. To develop the necessary close relationship with the North Canterbury Hospital Board, he would also require

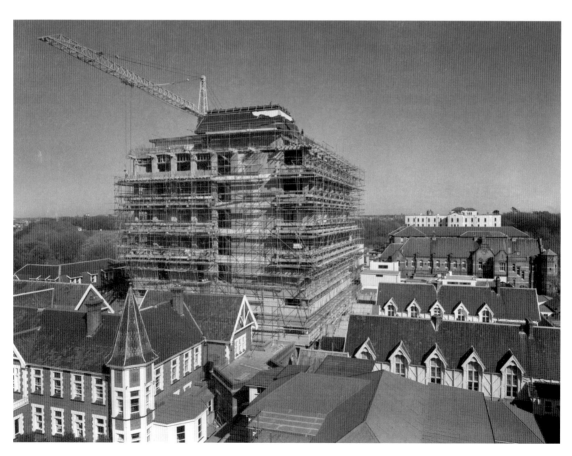

Christchurch School under construction, September 1972.
University of Otago, Christchurch.

a fair degree of independence from Dunedin. Both advisory and executive authority were vested in a new body, a twelve-member Council, representing equally the University and the Hospital Board, to which various sub-committees, such as those for finance and appointments, were responsible. The School was formally brought into existence on 28 April 1971, when the University of Otago and the North Canterbury Hospital Board ratified the constitution of the Christchurch Clinical School Council.[26]

Rolleston worked with Don Beaven, Fred Shannon and senior surgeon Pat Cotter, in what was popularly known as the 'gang of four', to lay solid foundations for the School. Each would serve the Christchurch School long, loyally and often with flair. Don Beaven, who was appointed to the Chair of Medicine in 1971, already had considerable experience in the Otago Medical School's Christchurch operation. An Otago graduate of 1948, he spent two years' residency in Christchurch and a year as a general practitioner before going to London, where he held various registrar posts, becoming MRCP in 1954 and MRACP in 1956. He returned to New Zealand that year, was appointed medical tutor at the Christchurch Branch Faculty and in 1960, after a time at Harvard University Medical School, took up the position of physician-in-charge of the Medical Unit at Princess Margaret Hospital. He was elected FRACP in 1965, FRCP (Edinburgh) in 1966 and FRCP (London) in 1971. His research interests included adrenaline-pituitary relationships, obesity and diabetes. Fred Shannon, the new Professor of Paediatrics, who spent his early life on Stewart Island and in Temuka, studied medicine at Otago, where he won a blue for fencing, and graduated in 1951. After further training and research in paediatrics in London, he returned in 1958 to take up the position of visiting paediatrician, later senior paediatrician and head of department, with the North Canterbury Hospital Board. In 1964, he was elected to the fellowship of the Royal Australasian College of Physicians. Active in research into juvenile arthritis and childhood urinary tract infection, he also set in motion the acclaimed Christchurch Child Development Study, to investigate the influence of social demographic and economic factors on child health.[27]

Apart from its administrative centre, the Department of the Dean, the new Clinical School was made up of seven academic departments. Surgery was headed by Professor Bill Macbeth, who completed his undergraduate and early postgraduate training in Adelaide, South Australia, before gaining further qualifications and experience in London and at the Harvard University Medical School. He became FRCS (Edin) in 1958 and FRCS (Lond) in 1959. He came to the new Chair, which included Anaesthesia and Orthopaedics, from an associate-professorship at Otago University. The new Professor of Obstetrics and Gynaecology was Donald Aickin. Graduating from Otago in 1958, Aickin had gained extensive practical and research experience in Melbourne, where he took his MD, and in Belfast and Glasgow. At the time of his appointment, he was Head of the Obstetrics and Gynaecology Department at Christchurch Women's Hospital. Roy McGiven, Professor of Pathology, also an Otago graduate of 1958, stayed on to join the Pathology Department and completed an MD in 1963. He then took up a lectureship at Monash, where he completed a PhD in the area of his research interest, immunopathology.[28] These foundation professors were already in place when the students arrived. Others soon joined them. From 1974, until he returned to Britain in 1979, Kurt Schwartz headed Preventive and Social Medicine. Ken Adam, a Canadian medical graduate with a background in psychodynamic psychiatry, was appointed to Psychological Medicine. He built well for the future. Insisting that his department should be based in Christchurch Hospital, he set up in the St Andrew's Outpatient building, formalised the Christchurch Consultation Liaison Psychiatry Service and formed a Crisis Team. Family circumstances necessitated Adam's return to Canada in 1979.[29]

That the first fourth-year student class could walk through the doors of the Christchurch Clinical School on 26 February 1973 was an achievement to celebrate. The resolution of all the administrative, academic and building problems the planners had come up against since they began work in 1969 was due in large part to the degree of cooperation between the University and the North Canterbury Hospital Board, which was a good portent for the future. Prime Minister Norman Kirk did the honours at the formal opening of the School on 11 September, in a colourful ceremony attended by representatives of the University, the Hospital Board, the Christchurch City Council, local Members of Parliament and national bodies connected with medical education. Speakers welcomed the new School as a focus for medical education and a centre to serve the medical needs of the community. Rolleston described the new 'partnership of service and education' in Christchurch as 'the most important single event that has occurred in our medical community.'[30]

Professor George Rolleston, 1916–2001

CBE MB ChB DMRD FRACR,
Founding Dean, Christchurch Clinical School, 1971–81

GEORGE ROLLESTON, founding Dean of the Christchurch Clinical School, was a Cantabrian through and through. His father was the MP for Timaru and his grandfather the last Superintendent of Canterbury province, in which capacity he had supported the unsuccessful bid to set up a medical school in 1876. Educated at Christ's College and the Otago Medical School, Rolleston graduated MB ChB in 1940 and served in World War II with the Army Medical Corps in the Pacific, North Africa and Italy, attaining the rank of major. At the end of the war, he undertook postgraduate training in radiology in London, returning to Christchurch in 1948 as Director of Radiology to the North Canterbury Hospital Board. Rolleston built up a fine department and, in 1949, established a School of Radiology at Christchurch Hospital. His work in paediatric radiology and radiology of the urinary tract was recognised internationally. In 1956, he was elected a Fellow of the Royal Australasian College of Radiologists and, in 1969, an Honorary Fellow of the Royal College of Radiologists, only the second New Zealander (after Lord Porritt) to be so honoured.

Rolleston's association with the Christchurch School of Medicine began in 1962 when he was appointed Sub-Dean of the Christchurch Branch Medical Faculty of the University of Otago. When the Christchurch Clinical School was in its planning stage, his superb administrative ability made him an obvious choice as Dean. He was also appointed Professor of Radiology. From 1971 his role was crucial in overseeing the development of the School's facilities and its three-year clinical teaching programme. He was described by someone who worked with him as 'an elder statesman and … a gracious and benign presence', with an unimpeachable trustworthiness and highly developed planning skills, and whose seriousness of purpose was lightened by an endearing sense of humour.

In his ten years as Dean, George Rolleston established the Christchurch School as a centre of excellence in clinical teaching and oversaw the establishment of a number of outstanding research groups. The historians of the Christchurch School of Medicine and Health Sciences pay tribute to his pivotal role in 'translating a fragile vision into a concrete reality' in educational policies, clinical practice and administration. Rolleston had many interests outside the School and the Hospital. He served on the Board of Governors of Christ's College for twenty-five years, played tennis into his eighties and was a skilled woodworker. He was awarded the CBE in 1980 and the next year, the year he retired, he was honoured with the gold medal of the Royal Australasian College of Radiologists. For some years after this, Rolleston continued to chair the National Children's Health Foundation and work part time as a radiologist at Burwood Hospital. He died in 2001.[31]

Wellington

The earliest plans for the Wellington settlement, like those for Christchurch, included sites for medical services. Plans dating back to 1839 include a 'College of Surgeons and a College of Physicians', as well as hospitals. While these intentions to establish facilities to teach medicine were never fulfilled, the Wellington School of Medicine eventually rose on the site of a hospital that opened in Newtown in 1881. The development of the Wellington Clinical School paralleled, or was modelled on, that of Christchurch in many ways but the process was often less smooth. In the 1920s, the Otago Medical School had called on Wellington Hospital, as well as those in Christchurch and Auckland, to share in the clinical training of its sixth-year students. As Hercus put it in a letter to the Wellington Hospital Board, it was invited to become 'a recognised hospital of the University National Medical School'. Teaching duly began in 1926, when eight of the 1925 class, who lived in the Central Districts, were seconded to Wellington for their sixth year. Dr John Cairney was appointed Sub-Dean and part-time lecturers were appointed in clinical medicine, clinical surgery and clinical pathology.[32] The next stage came in 1937, when the Wellington group, like those in Auckland and Christchurch, was recognised as a Branch Faculty of the University of Otago, with Dr John (Jo) Mercer as Sub-Dean. However, whereas Auckland and Canterbury University Colleges were content with these arrangements, Victoria University College was not. Founded in 1899 and conscious of its lack of a special school to attract students New Zealand-wide and provide prestige and funding, it had ambitions for a fully-fledged medical school, which emerged strongly from time to time. That the University's Chancellor, Duncan Stout, had taught surgery for a time from 1927 was seen by some as a first step in this direction.[33] The possibility that the Wellington Clinical School would break with the Otago Medical School and join Victoria University ran as a persistent theme through relations with the parent institution over a number of years.

Dr Brian Corkill, a senior obstetrician and gynaecologist at Wellington Hospital, later Assistant to the Dean and, at times, Acting Dean, was an astute observer of the development of the Wellington Clinical School. In the postwar period to about 1953, he reports, there was little enthusiasm to extend medical teaching and research. Pressure on the Wellington Hospital Board by the Dunedin Faculty to set up a thirty-bed medical unit, headed by a full-time physician, met with a cool response from the physicians at Wellington Hospital. In 1959, a twelve-bed medical unit, jointly administered by the University and the Hospital Board, was established. It was headed by Dr Ian Prior until 1971, then briefly by Dr Ken North, until his departure to the United Kingdom in 1972. Attempts to set up an equivalent surgical unit failed.[34]

A letter from Mercer to the Wellington Hospital Board, at the end of 1965, changed the mood. In Corkill's view, it was the single most important stimulus to advance Wellington's claim to be a centre of medical education. Mercer, who had been Sub-Dean of the Branch Faculty for twenty-four years until 1962, director of Pathology and chairman of the Medical Council, was a man of influence. He had been on the 1953 Committee, which had recommended Auckland as the site of the second New Zealand Medical School, and he was aware that the question of a third school was already under discussion. 'Clearly a third medical school will be established in New Zealand in the foreseeable future', he wrote, and suggested that a 'preliminary body from our staff' should, with Hospital Board approval, prepare a first approach to the Victoria University Council.'[35] A six-person working committee, which included Corkill with Dr Ken North as secretary, was set up 'to consider the future of Wellington as a regional medical centre and teaching hospital'. The committee met fortnightly in the first half of 1966, reporting in June that if a medical school were to be established in Wellington it would need the support of Victoria University and land adjacent to the hospital for premises for preclinical teaching. Victoria was interested but had its own demands. It would consider taking on a medical school only if the basic sciences were taught on its own campus. It wanted further justification of the need for a third school, as well as more detailed information on the proposed site, curriculum, student numbers, land needs and residential requirements. The committee duly produced its detailed case in December 1967 – a matter of weeks before Professor Christie's visit to Otago.[36]

With such discussions in train, many in the Wellington medical community felt aggrieved at the manner of Christie's visit and its outcome. They believed it was a mistake to investigate the particular problems of the Otago Medical School rather than consider more broadly the most efficient way to produce the doctors New Zealand needed. They regarded the fact Christie visited the capital for less than a day as a slight. When his report came out, they interpreted it as promoting the interests of Christchurch at the expense of Wellington. The issue was particularly sensitive because the Auckland Medical School took in its first students in 1968 and the Wellington Branch Faculty saw itself being threatened from two directions. Victoria University College shared these concerns. Its quinquennial submission to the University Grants Committee in June 1968 included the comment that it was time to begin planning for a third medical school. It added that, as Wellington had the best developed hospital in the country and Victoria had a strong science faculty and sociology department, the capital was its logical site. The response from the Grants Committee was cautious. It was prepared to agree that if a third medical school were to be established, it should be in Wellington, but it would not be drawn on the probability or timing of this. On the other hand, the Wellington lobby had a powerful ally in the Labour Party, which openly favoured a Wellington medical school.[37]

It may have been at least partly to forestall the possibility of a medical school being approved for Wellington that Irvine proposed developing the Wellington Branch Faculty into a Clinical School of the University of Otago. Medical staff at Wellington Hospital responded by urging the Hospital Board and the University jointly to prepare a case showing that a Wellington Medical School was in the national interest. The working committee already in existence took a cautious view of the Irvine report. It approved the proposal

that Wellington should be the main centre for sixth-year training and a postgraduate medical centre, but the committee resented the fact that the report had been accepted by the UGC without adequate reference to bodies outside Dunedin. It found little evidence to support Irvine's statement that there was 'no real case for a third medical school being established in the foreseeable future'. Prompt action of some sort was required, however. Even without the addition of a clinical school to teach fourth- and fifth-year students from Otago, Wellington Hospital would very likely have to deal with sixty sixth-year students from 1973 onwards, when Auckland ceased taking them. Accordingly, increases in staff, accommodation, teaching and other facilities would have to proceed without delay.[38]

Despite this sense of urgency, uncertainty dragged on, with a powerful group on the Wellington Hospital staff pressing for a full medical school. The Wellington Hospital Board equivocated, most of its members convinced that the Irvine report served the interests of Otago rather than the nation. At last, early in 1970, it instructed North, the secretary of the working committee, to prepare its case for a third medical school, despite the UGC having warned Victoria that it would not fund such a development. In October, North's report duly set out the case for a full medical school in Wellington, to open in 1975–76. The report argued that a full medical school would be no more expensive than a clinical school and would be preferable to separating preclinical and clinical training, as the Irvine plan proposed. Victoria could easily accommodate a medical school within its current site development plans. The UGC remained unconvinced, even after a deputation appealed to it and to the Prime Minister. In December 1970 the Wellington Hospital Board agreed to a clinical school, which was formally constituted on 1 April 1971. Corkill gained the impression that the Board was still not firmly behind the proposal. It was left with a slim ray of hope, in the form of a promise from the UGC to consider, at the appropriate time (probably the early 1980s), the transfer of financial and academic responsibility for the clinical school from Otago to Victoria.

'The whole question of the clinical school versus third medical school over the previous three to four years', wrote Corkill, 'had increased passions in many of the staff and of the Board.'[39]

The Dunedin papers kept a watching brief on the developments in Wellington through Press Association reports. In July 1970, for example, under the headline 'Medical School Claim Pressed by Wellington', the *Otago Daily Times* reported that if there was to be a third medical school, it should logically be placed in Wellington. In December, both the morning and evening papers carried a report along similar lines and the following February the heading 'Wellington Wants Medical School' introduced an item about the deputation to Prime Minister Holyoake from representatives of the Wellington Hospital Board and Victoria University College.[40] There followed a report that Dr North had challenged the Minister of Education over the estimated cost of a new medical school in Wellington.[41] However, these reports of rumblings from Wellington were clearly subordinated to local success stories relating to the Otago Medical School, such as government approval of a $643,000 grant for a new library and the University Council's approval of the clinical schools plan, which were both announced in September 1970, and the opinion of the Regius Professor of Surgery at the University of Glasgow that the Otago Medical School was 'undergoing a renaissance'. From April 1971, there was a series of articles on plans for making Dunedin Hospital a fully integrated teaching hospital.[42]

In the meantime, arrangements to set up a clinical school in Wellington, modelled on Christchurch, were going ahead. The Joint Relations Committee was reconstituted as a management committee for the School and a Wellington Clinical School Council, with equal representation of Otago University and the Wellington Hospital Board, was established. The appointment of Dr Frank Hall as Dean, in October 1971, marked a new stage. A leading Wellington physician and medical administrator, he was to advise the Wellington Hospital Board and the University on the appointment of clinical professors and other academic staff, oversee the conversion of Wellington Hospital to a teaching hospital and generally prepare for the first intake of fourth-year students from Otago in 1977. He was expected to work closely with the Otago Dean, the Clinical Dean, and the Dean of the Christchurch Clinical School on the curriculum and matters of medical education. Frank Hall was a man of broad interests and outstanding probity, and was kind, courteous, and conscientious to a fault. He had been involved in the teaching of final-year medical students for many years.[43] If, as has been suggested, he was appointed for his tact and willingness to listen to all, the strategy was a sound one. He established a tradition of solidly based cooperation between the Clinical School in Wellington and the Medical School in Dunedin.[44]

The provision of suitable accommodation for a clinical school in Wellington was an immense task, which involved not only building the School itself, but also rebuilding obsolete facilities in the Wellington Hospital. Many of the buildings in the hospital complex were sub-standard and had acknowledged earthquake risks. A total

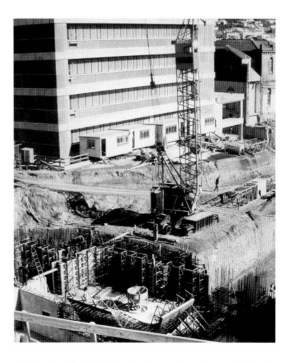

Wellington Clinical School under construction, early 1970s.
University of Otago, Wellington.

Professor Graham Francis Hall, 1914–1979

Dean, Wellington Clinical School, 1971–76

'A Christian and a gentleman, who never pursued even his own interests for his own gain', is how one of Frank Hall's friends described him. The description has an old-world flavour which reflects the traditional values to which Hall adhered.

Frank Hall was born in Dunedin in January 1914, the son of a doctor. He completed an MA with Honours in French before entering Medical School. He graduated MB ChB in 1941 and at once joined the Medical Corps of the 2NZEF. He served in the Middle East and Italy, was mentioned in dispatches and achieved the rank of major. After the war, Hall returned to Dunedin and, in 1949, married Winifred McQuilkan, the brilliant young principal of Columba College, who was already (as Clare Mallory) launched on a career as a writer of girls' school stories. The couple went to Britain, where Hall embarked on postgraduate study in London and Edinburgh. He became MRCPE in 1952 and would later gain FRACP in 1960, FRCP (Edin) in 1966 and FRCP (London) in 1970.

In 1953 Hall was appointed visiting physician to Wellington Hospital, a position he held until a few months before his death. He was always prepared to take on heavy administrative duties and his devotion to his patients was a byword. Hall also served, until 1971, as physician (from 1967 senior physician) at the House of Compassion Hospital. As secretary to the Dominion committee of the Royal Australasian College of Physicians for many years, he kept up a vast correspondence with members, arranged examinations and scientific meetings, organised public appeals for funds and handled the detail of visits for guest speakers. He later became the New Zealand Vice-President.

Well qualified for his role as founding Dean of the Wellington Clinical School, Hall and his wife were also generous in their hospitality to colleagues. Hall gave himself wholeheartedly to the work, but it took a heavy toll. Never robust – he suffered from diabetes – he faced intractable problems over the new building and the new staff. In September 1973, he was rushed to Wellington Hospital in a coma. Hall's health deteriorated seriously from this point, and he had to take leave on more than one occasion before he retired in 1976. He retained a position at Silverstream Hospital for two more years. Soon after he suffered a second stroke, which left him severely disabled, and he died in March 1979.

Hall's contribution to the Wellington School is remembered in its most prestigious award, the Graham Francis Hall Prize, awarded annually to the top student over the fourth, fifth and sixth years of the undergraduate medical course.[45]

redevelopment of the Hospital, with embedded clinical departments, library and medical facilities, meant scrapping existing plans for its upgrading, some of which had been under discussion for years. Ted Dews took a hard-line approach, pushing to change the Board's architects in favour of the firm who had the contract for the Christchurch Clinical School. It was a slow process. Only in July 1972 did the Board decide to go with the Christchurch School architects, and the clearing of the building site did not begin

until 1973. When Ted Dews moved to Australia in that year, there were further delays while the new director of works at Otago University, Roger Dodd, familiarised himself with the project. From 1973 until the School opened, Brian Corkill bore the main administrative responsibility, either as Acting Dean when Hall was ill, or as Assistant Dean with special responsibility for the building programme.[46]

Staffing of the new Clinical School went ahead. In 1972, Ken North, who had recently succeeded

Ian Prior as head of the Medical Unit, moved to Britain. He was not replaced, but a Chair of Medicine was advertised, to which Thomas O'Donnell was appointed. He brought to the position a depth of local knowledge and relevant experience. Born and educated in Wellington and a 1949 graduate of the Otago Medical School, O'Donnell had undertaken research under Professor Smirk before studying at the Postgraduate Medical School in London and at the University of California's Cardiovascular Research Institute in San Francisco. He returned to the Department of Medicine at Dunedin in 1960 and was appointed to a personal chair in 1970. His clinical and research interests were in cardiovascular and respiratory medicine. Having been involved in assessing sixth-year students in Wellington, he was well known to hospital staff. A long-time colleague considered that his particular strength was his ability to communicate effectively with staff, students, the hospital administration and the general community, while his clinical skills gave him a high profile with the hospital and medical staff. O'Donnell took up his position in December 1973 and, as the only departmental head at this time, worked closely with Hall and Corkill over the years until the School opened, the beginning of a long apprenticeship for his later role as Dean.[47]

The other foundation professors, some New Zealanders, some from overseas, took up their posts over the next three years. First to arrive, early in 1974, was William Stehbens, to take up a dual position as Professor of Pathology and Foundation Director of the Wellington Cancer and Research Institute (now the Malaghan Institute of Medical Research), which occupied one floor of the Academic Block of the School. Born in Sydney and educated there and at Oxford University, Stehbens had held academic appointments in Australia and the United States. He came to Wellington from a Chair in Pathology at the Albany Medical College of Union University, Albany, with a high reputation for his research on atherosclerosis and the pathology of the cerebral blood vessels.[48]

Most of the other professors took up their posts in 1975. As Associate Professor of Obstetrics and

Gynaecology at the Auckland Medical School, Richard Seddon had played a major part in designing the Auckland School's undergraduate course. An Otago graduate of 1954, his research interests were in endocrine aspects of gynaecology. Professor Jeffray Weston, an Otago graduate of 1950, had gained local knowledge working as a senior paediatrician for fifteen years with the Wellington Hospital Board. He also had overseas experience at the Postgraduate Medical School in London and the prestigious Hospital for Sick Children at Great Ormond Street. The Professor of Surgery, William Isbister, trained in Manchester and Edinburgh, came to Wellington after three years as Senior Lecturer at the Royal Brisbane Hospital and the University of Queensland. He was a specialist in colorectal surgery, with research interests in abdominal inflammation conditions and colorectal diseases. Professor John Roberts, Psychological Medicine, also came from Britain. His first qualification was from London and he had others from Durham, Bristol and Edinburgh. He had been Senior Lecturer in the Department of Mental Health at Bristol and consultant to the British Samaritans since 1965. The team was completed when Kenneth Newell, an Otago graduate of 1948, with a Diploma in Public Health from London and a PhD from Tulane, New Orleans, arrived in 1977. He had held senior posts, since 1958, with the World Health Organization.[49]

While progress was made on a number of fronts, it was not all smooth sailing. Cordial relations were established between the University representatives and the Wellington Hospital Board. Corkill worked effectively with the contractors and the University's building authorities to develop the School's facilities, curriculum planning went ahead, Sir Arnold Nordmeyer accepted the chair of a new School Council and the Department of Medicine recruited some talented young physicians, several of whom had academic experience in prestigious overseas institutions.[50] However, delays in the building programme held up the settling in process for the new Heads of Department. The Academic Block was not completed until 1977, then cutbacks in government spending meant a reduction in the extent of the proposed hospital building and further delays in achieving satisfactory departmental space. Obstetrics and Gynaecology were well provided for on the top floor of the new Women's Hospital, but it was some years before Paediatrics achieved adequate space in a new Children's Hospital. Equipment was a problem, as the UGC grant for this was much less than expected – $1.5 million instead of $2.374 million – and priorities had to be set. First came shared teaching facilities, the library, audio-visual equipment for lecture theatres and seminar rooms and equipment for practical classes in pathology, but resources for research were limited. Stehbens, who required space for sheep on which he was surgically creating arterial-venous vascular connections, was especially frustrated. Both he and Isbister resented the fact that their departmental space and provision for academic staff compared unfavourably with the Department of Medicine, which was well provided for because it was also responsible for applied physiology, clinical methods and clinical pharmacology. Both professors also encountered difficulties with Hospital staff in their disciplines. Friction between the academic staff in Pathology and corresponding senior Hospital staff led to the resignations of some recently appointed senior lecturers. In Surgery, there were disagreements over the number of beds available for a professorial surgical unit and adequate operating theatre times for the professor and his staff.[51]

The difficulties the new School was facing were compounded by Hall's deteriorating health. In August 1975, and again from May 1976, Corkill had to take over and it became his responsibility, as Acting Dean, to oversee the final stages in the setting up of the School. The careful plans of the Otago Medical School, which would have seen the foundation Dean of the new School in place and providing academic leadership and guidance for six years before the first students arrived, were thrown into disarray. A new Dean, Ralph Johnson, would take up his appointment just a fortnight before the students began classes.

CHAPTER 19

Interlude:
A Year to Celebrate, 1975

I T WAS fitting that the centennial year of the Otago Medical School, 1975, occurred at a fortunate conjunction of circumstances, before the economic stringencies New Zealand endured in the late 1970s cut too deep. Much of the impressive building programme was complete, staffing levels had risen sharply in Dunedin and key appointments had been made in Christchurch and Wellington. In Christchurch, students from the first fourth-year class were in their final year and the Wellington Clinical School was on track to accept its first intake in 1977. A new curriculum had been developed, with larger preclinical and smaller clinical classes, fewer examinations and a trainee intern year as the final stage.[1]

In the Foreword to *An Historical Sketch,* written by Gordon Parry to mark the centennial, the recently appointed Dean, Professor John Hunter, could write that the storms of the past two decades, which had reached their peak around 1967–8, had been weathered and the School was embarking on a fresh course in readiness for its second century. 'Today', he concluded, 'we have more than a School. It is a major resource for education and research, built on solid foundations.' By the beginning of its centennial year, the Otago Medical School had graduated 4623 students and the expectation was that, with the planned increase in intake to two hundred in 1979, the number would double over the next twenty-five years. Most of the Otago-trained doctors practised in New Zealand, 'the backbone of one of the finest health systems in the world'.

Academic staff across the three bases numbered 486 and there were many support staff as well.[2]

The centenary of the Medical School was celebrated in several ways and events continued throughout the year. It centred on 17–21 February, when the School hosted five hundred doctors and a number of distinguished overseas guests, at the biennial conference of the New Zealand Medical Association. In February, an entire issue of the *New Zealand Medical Journal* was dedicated to the centenary and it was proudly covered, in some detail, in the local press. Coverage began with a splash in the *Otago Daily Times* of 6 February, with a picture of a commemorative postage stamp and a double-page spread, generously illustrated and entitled 'A Place of Honour after Early Struggle'. The article was informative and entertaining, and included anecdotes about some of the more colourful characters, staff and students, who had been associated with the School.[3]

The February programme began with an interdenominational Sunday service at Knox Church, at which Professor Angus Ross, of the History Department, gave the oration in honour of members of the medical profession who had lost their lives in the two world wars.[4] The Vice-Chancellor opened the conference itself on the Monday morning. In keeping with his own background as a medical academic, Irvine took as his theme 'Medical Education in a University Setting'. A medical school, he said, should take the broadest view of education. As well as producing vocationally trained experts, it should reach out into the community, offering its knowledge and skills to promote national welfare and development. It should help to produce informed citizens, 'to create an alternative society based on self-fulfilment for the individual and a caring community'.[5]

The conference featured plenary sessions each morning, addressed by distinguished former staff of the School: Sir Michael Woodruff from Edinburgh, Professor Archie McIntyre from Monash, Dr H.D. Purves and Sir Horace Smirk. The scientific programme was broad in scope and rich in content, focusing on research or clinical work with a direct bearing on the Medical School. On the first day, for example, the morning session dealt with the surgery of vascular diseases, immunology, dermatology, neuroanatomy and cardiology. In the afternoon, respiratory diseases, neurophysiology, electron microscopy and immunology were covered. In the final plenary session, Sir Horace Smirk described the research he had initiated and led at the Otago Medical School on the management of hypertension.[6] The topic of medical education was a strong theme of the conference. It was acknowledged as being an urgent issue, because of the rapidity of socio-economic change and alterations to traditional patterns of health and disease. Continuing education was discussed in a symposium and the Dean picked up on the subject in his closing address. He announced the School's intention to expand its role in postgraduate study and in the training of non-medical students. Medical schools of the future, he maintained, would have a part to play as health-science resource centres for teaching scientists, pharmacists and dentists.[7]

The conference was only one element in the celebrations of the centenary week, which attracted congratulatory messages and gifts from places as far away and as varied as the United Kingdom and the Middle East. The intervals of the conference programme and the evenings were filled by decade reunion dinners and private parties. Members of New Zealand clubs which had reciprocity with the Dunedin (Fernhill) Club, were invited to become honorary members for the week. It was typical of the time, when the great

majority of doctors were male, that there was a special programme of entertainment for their accompanying wives. Between three and four hundred women were offered a variety of lectures, a champagne luncheon, a visit to Glenfalloch Gardens, a tour of the local Art Society exhibition and an excursion to Otago Peninsula to see the seals and albatrosses. The scrapbook put together to commemorate the centenary celebrations contains dozens of appreciative letters and cards sent by women who had taken part in the programme.[8]

The Centenary Assembly for the Conferment of Honorary Degrees, February 1975

The spectacular showpiece of the celebrations was the Assembly for the Conferment of Honorary Degrees, which took place in the town hall on the Monday evening. At a colourful, dignified ceremony, the honorary degree of Doctor of Science was conferred on seven distinguished medical graduates. They were Wellington physician and cardiologist Sir Charles Burns, Emeritus Professor Eric D'Ath, the Professor of Endocrinology at the University of London Post-graduate Medical School Thomas Russell Cumming Fraser, Sir Edward Sayers, Sir Horace Smirk, the former Nuffield Professor of Obstetrics and Gynaecology at the University of Oxford Sir John Stallworthy and Mr Stanley Wilson, a Dunedin consulting surgeon and Medical School lecturer. Sir John Stallworthy delivered the centennial oration, in which he warned that medicine was at the crossroads and the ethical codes taught and practised by Hippocrates and the early fathers of medicine were being challenged as never before. That, he said, was the immediate challenge to the practice of medicine and those who taught it, as the Otago Medical School entered its second century.[9]

The Orators of the University of Otago are noted for the perception and wit of their citations for recipients of honorary degrees from the University, but the challenge facing the Orator on this occasion was surely beyond the usual. He needed to pay appropriate tribute to the achievements of seven candidates, all medically

Celebrating the Centenary, 1975

Centenary Photograph Album, Otago Medical School

At left, Sir John Stallworthy receives the degree of Doctor of Science, *honoris causa*.

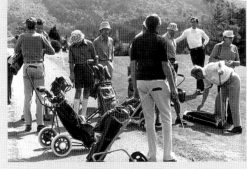

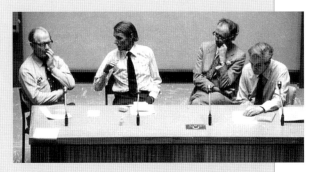

Panel discussion, Barnett Theatre. Left to right: Russell Fraser, Don Beaven, J.A. Kilpatrick and Alec Turnbull.

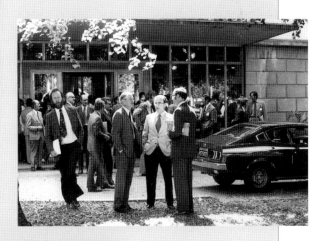

An afternoon of golf.

Delegates outside the museum after a plenary session.

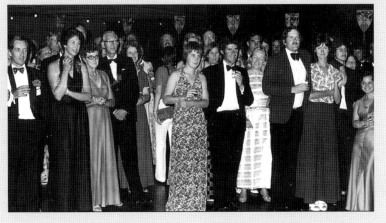

A group at the centennial ball listen to the University Quintet.

qualified, keeping each entirely distinct, but honouring them equally. He accomplished his task with concision, insight and humour.

As a group, the men had several things in common. Their ages, in 1975, ranged between sixty-seven and seventy-seven and, while officially all were retired, they were all still deeply involved in medically related activities. Almost all had been associated with teaching Otago medical students. All but one had been a student at Otago in the Lindo Ferguson era, graduating between 1922 and 1932. Most had put their careers on hold during World War II, to give their services to the war effort. All had strong personalities and a prodigious capacity for work, finding extra hours for their pursuits either late at night or early in the morning. All thrived on their self-imposed regimes to live into their eighties, in most cases their late eighties.[10]

Sir Charles Ritchie Burns (1898–1979)

The first full-time physician in the Auckland Hospital, Sir Charles Burns was subsequently consulting physician and consulting cardiologist to the Wellington Hospital. 'In his tireless devotion to his patients, his relentless search for precise diagnosis, his intolerance of anything that fell short of his own exacting standards [he] gave to those who worked with him a distinct idea of the excitement and the interest of practising good quality medicine – and of the sheer hard work that made this possible.' He was known to call staff conferences at 6 a.m. Determined to serve overseas in the war, despite his age, Burns became O.C. Medicine at No. 3 General Hospital, Bari (and was reprimanded for organising a mule race on the beach on VE Night) and went to Japan as Deputy Director, Medical Services. He was an examiner in medicine for the Otago Medical School, and served on the Medical Council, the Council of the Wellington Medical Research Foundation, and the New Zealand Censors' Board of the Royal Australasian College of Physicians, of which he was Vice President in 1956–58. He supported voluntary organisations, such as the National Society on Alcohol and Drug Dependency. In

his retirement, he gave a great deal of time to the treatment of alcoholics, both in Invercargill, where there is a Charles Burns Medical Centre named for him, and at Hanmer Springs, the former residential care facility.[11]

Thomas Russell Cumming Fraser (1908–94)

'His impetus, his tirelessness (he never seemed to need sleep), his phenomenal ability to get people to work as a team, his restless pursuit of problems, his fertility in ideas, his unending patience and kindness, these all made up an experience which none of the many New Zealanders who passed through the Department of Medicine at the British Postgraduate School, Hammersmith, have ever been able to forget.' An Otago graduate in physics and chemistry in 1926, Fraser moved to medicine, graduated with distinction, and went to Britain, where he promptly took the prize for top place in the primary examination of the Royal College of Surgeons. Following this, a Rockefeller Travelling Scholarship took him to the Massachusetts General Hospital and, on his return to Britain, he set about gaining experience in psychiatry. During the war, he investigated the way bombing affected civilians and the incidence of neurosis in factory workers. In 1945 Fraser returned to endocrinology at Hammersmith, to engage in his life's work. One of the first clinical endocrinologists in Britain, he researched thyroid diseases, diabetes, pituitary function and growth hormones and led a team which extended his already varied activities into a number of other fields. He was a 'pioneer of endocrinology and a trainer of its pioneers elsewhere.'[12]

Sir John Stallworthy (1906–93)

John Stallworthy graduated in 1931, winning the Travelling Scholarship and the Batchelor medal in obstetrics, and set off for Britain, where he remained, but always keeping in touch with his Otago roots. In 1939, he was appointed obstetrician and gynaecologist to the Radcliffe Infirmary, where he was charged with developing the Area Department of the United Oxford Hospitals, which he did to a high standard. Training posts at the Radcliffe were highly valued by people from all over the world wishing to specialise in obstetrics and gynaecology. Weekly discussions, where cases for which the final diagnosis and treatment were still undecided, were presented to the Director, and were famously stimulating and frightening. 'Out of all this came the most extraordinary increases in the knowledge of such conditions as infertility or carcinoma of the cervix, along with a remarkable lowering of the figures for morbidity and mortality in, for instance, vaginal hysterectomy.' In 1967 Stallworthy was invited to occupy the prestigious Nuffield Chair at Oxford, a recognition of his eminence and a responsibility that required 'appalling stamina and ceaseless compassion'. Other high distinctions showered on him were overshadowed by Stallworthy's influence as a teacher in Oxford.[13]

Stanley Livingstone Wilson (1905–90)

'Consummate in the quietness of his work with his own hands', Stanley Wilson used his skill as a surgeon in a lifetime of service to Dunedin, broken only by four years with the New Zealand Medical Corps in World War II. A graduate of 1929, Wilson held resident appointments in hospitals in London and Dunedin before joining the visiting staff of Dunedin Hospital from 1937 to 1940. In Egypt with the Third Echelon he treated casualties in front-line positions, sometimes working for forty-eight hours without rest. He introduced new methods for the management of abdominal wounds, together with techniques of intravenous nutrition. He was awarded the DSO, promoted to Lt. Col. and, in 1943, transferred to Guadacanal as the CO of 2 Casualty Clearing Station (Pacific). After the war, Wilson resumed his hospital work and private practice and took up a senior lectureship in surgery at the Medical School. He retired from both institutions in 1965 but remained in private practice for a further seventeen years. Wilson insisted on the then novel procedures of confining his practice to surgical patients, having the same anaesthetist for all his cases (thus helping to establish anaesthesia as a discipline in its own right) and grouping like operations together in operating lists. Wilson

served as president of the Royal Australasian College of Surgeons in 1961–62.[14]

The other three recipients, *Emeritus Professor Eric D'Ath (1899–1979)*, *Sir Edward Sayers (1902–85)* and *Emeritus Professor Horace Smirk (1902–91)*, who had all served on the staff of the Medical School, have already appeared in this narrative.

A Commemorative Issue of the New Zealand Medical Journal

The *New Zealand Medical Journal* that appeared on 12 February 1975 honoured the centenary with a collection of essays on the theme of medical education. The editorial set the tone with the statement that the Otago Medical School had been able to 'evolve a system of medical education that fitted the local scene and had international acceptance.' It drew attention to the crucial significance the extension of sixth-year teaching to Christchurch, Auckland and Wellington in the 1920s had for the whole future of medical education in New Zealand. The solid base of teaching experience in those centres had smoothed the path towards the establishment of the Auckland Medical School in 1968 and had led to the establishment of clinical schools in the other centres. To keep its place in the world, a medical school had to continually modernise its course, to keep it interesting and relevant to changing professional needs and give an equal emphasis to continuing education.[15]

While a few essays looked back on the history of the Otago Medical School, its context and its achievements, most commented on trends in the modernisation of medical education. Together with a small number from abroad who had Otago connections, the contributors made up something of a *Who's Who* of medical academics in New Zealand. Dunedin-based staff did not generally take part in this tribute to the School, but the Vice-Chancellor's conference address on 'Medical Education in a University Setting' was included. Academics from Auckland, Christchurch and Wellington joined with graduates from other locations and areas of expertise to create a collection notable for its combination of educational philosophy and direct experience. The Christchurch Clinical School was represented by Professors Donald Aickin, Don Beaven and Fred Shannon,[16] the yet-to-be-opened Wellington Clinical School by Professor Tom O'Donnell, the Auckland Medical School by Professors E.M. Nanson, J.B. Carman and J.D.K. North, Sir Douglas Robb, and Associate Professor P.J. Scott.[17]

Among prominent New Zealand graduates, Dr Neil Begg, Director of Medical Services for the Plunket Society and current President of the Medical Association, put in a plea for physicians and the public to work together for child health. Dr John Hiddlestone, Director-General of Health, discussed the 'Prospects for Medical Education in New Zealand'. Dr Geoffrey Brinkman, Medical Superintendent of Waikato Hospital, argued the need to inculcate in medical students the desire to participate in lifelong medical education and urged the tempering of scientific skills with compassion and humility. The Assistant Medical Superintendent at Waikato Hospital, medical historian Rex Wright-St Clair, explained the 'Historical Background of New Zealand Medicine'. In 'The Medical School and the Problem of Relevance', Alan Clarke floated ideas he would later put into practice as Dean of the Christchurch School of Medicine, to make the course 'relevant' to students.[18]

Overseas contributors included Professor L.W. Cox from Adelaide, who described trends in medical education in Australia in terms that would later be at the heart of curriculum debates at Otago: the integration of disciplines (both vertical and horizontal), problem-solving approach teaching methods, more free time and electives for students, fewer examinations and a shift in emphasis from traditional subjects towards newer ones, such as behavioural science, community medicine, clinical pharmacology, genetics and geriatrics. Professor J. Ludbrook looked ahead to what medical schools might be like in the Year 2000 and T.G. Hawley, formerly Principal of the Fiji School of Medicine, considered medical education in the South Pacific. Former students now at the top of their profession, Derek Denny-Brown, Emeritus Professor of Neurology at the

Harvard Medical School, D.G. Potts, Professor of Radiology at Cornell Medical College and Sir John Stallworthy from Oxford, were all represented.[19] The commemorative issue of the *Journal* took a variety of approaches to a rich theme.

The Medical Education Trust and the Alumnus Association

There were two permanent legacies of the centenary. One was the Medical Education Trust, for the promotion and encouragement of postgraduate medical education. Planning for the Trust had been set in motion two years earlier. In June 1973, Governor-General Sir Denis Blundell accepted the role of patron and some 250 people, including the Prime Minister, the Dean of the Auckland Medical School and the Director-General of Health, attended an inaugural dinner. The Trust aimed to raise the sum of $1 million, of which $67,000 had already been given or promised. The fund was to be administered by a Trust representing the two medical schools, the clinical schools, the Postgraduate Federation, the Medical Association and the Health Department. It was intended to support postgraduate medical education in the widest sense, with a special emphasis on the needs of general practitioners. The Medical Education Trust held its inaugural meeting during the week of the centenary, and a general practitioners' representative was added to its membership. Of the $500,000 target for 1975, $338,489 had already been raised.[20]

The second legacy was the Otago Medical School Alumnus Association. Shortly before the February celebrations, John Hunter sent an open letter to all graduates of the School, extending an 'enthusiastic personal invitation' to form such an association. At an inaugural meeting in the Colquhoun theatre on 20 February, the main objectives of the Alumnus Association were agreed to be:

To stimulate interest in the historical and cultural background of the Otago Medical School and its progress.

To disseminate information regarding the School and its graduates.

To hold meetings, social and otherwise, to further its objects.

To coordinate with similar existing bodies.

To collect and spend monies for these purposes.

Membership was not intended to be a financial burden. Ordinary members would pay a token $2 a year and life members $40. All graduates aged sixty-five years or over would be honorary members.

Among the activities suggested at the inaugural meeting were the collection of artefacts for a medical historical museum, the organisation of social arrangements for alumni visiting Dunedin and the distribution of a newsletter. Associate Professor John Borrie was elected president and Dr Rosalie Sneyd was co-opted on to the small committee to represent women graduates. The Association settled in well. By the end of 1976, it had 262 ordinary, 104 honorary and 49 life members. Its first newsletter, an informal document, reported progress on the School's collection of medical instruments, a project dear to Borrie's heart, and a pleasing attendance at a sherry party after the December graduation. Mention was made of an award in memory of former Dean, Bill Adams, to recognise 'an especially meritorious contribution by a preclinical medical student' to further the student's special interest. It also included the first of what would become a regular and valuable feature of the annual newsletter, a report from the Dean of Faculty.[21] Over the next few years the Alumnus Association initiated a luncheon for graduands and a welcome, with a tour of the School and afternoon tea for second years and their parents.[22]

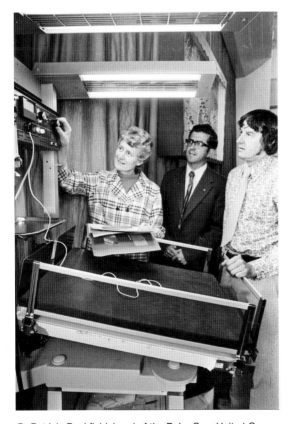

Dr Patricia Buckfield, head of the Baby Care Unit at Queen Mary Hospital, explains to visitors the working of a new neonatal unit, donated by the Kiwanis' service organisation. Otago Daily Times Collection, February 1975.

The Medical School and the Community

For the public, the most interesting part of the Medical School's celebrations was an open day on 4 December. The first for fifteen years, the open day was intended to demonstrate teaching aids and techniques and show the range of disciplines that made up medical education. Medical School staff were on hand to explain displays, most of which had a bearing on life and health, such as the relationship between smoking and lung cancer. All the main Medical School buildings and the Medical Research Council laboratories were open to visitors. A printed programme gave directions as to the location of the various departments and introduced the displays, which often featured work by students. The Audio-Visual Learning Centre and the Medical Illustration and Photographic Unit were open to visitors, the library displayed works from the Monro Collection and the School's glassblower demonstrated his skill. Both local newspapers sent reporters and photographers to record the enthralled reactions of the 3500 visitors who took advantage of the open day. The *Evening Star* called the array of equipment 'mind-boggling'.[23]

While the centennial celebrations were extensively covered in the press, another Medical

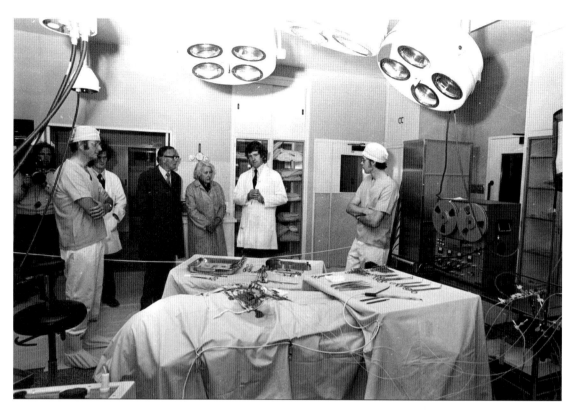

Open Day, December 1975. Professor Alan Clarke explains to Sir John and Lady Walsh the operation of some of the machinery used in experimental animal surgery. At left is senior technical officer Nelson Redshaw and, to the right, surgical technician Ross Christie.
Otago Daily Times, 5 December 1975.

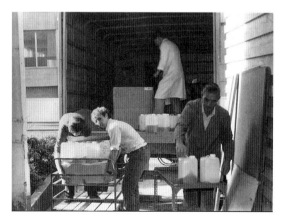

The Milton Survey. Loading the truck with samples to take to the Medical School in Dunedin for analysis.
Photograph, Janet Ledingham.

School activity in 1975 also involved members of the public and caught the popular interest. This was a large-scale, multi-purpose medical survey in Milton. Led by Professor Olaf Simpson and Associate Professor Ted Nye, the survey involved more than 1200 subjects, about 82 per cent of the town's population aged sixteen and over. Over a five-day period in May, St John's Church hosted what was, at the time, the largest medical survey of its type in New Zealand. Eleven researchers took part, including staff from the Wellcome Medical Research Institute and the Departments of Medicine and Preventive and Social Medicine, a representative from the School of Physical Education and the Dunedin Medical Officer of Health. They administered questionnaires on the personal and family history of the subjects and took data on any family medical history of hypertension, diabetes, cardiovascular, thyroid and liver disease and gout. They asked a range of questions on the subjects' medical history and current medication, and carried out an exhaustive series of tests: measuring height, weight, blood pressure and heart rate; taking electrocardiographs and mass miniature x-rays of the chest; and testing respiratory function, cholesterol and blood sugar through a twenty-four hour urine test, audiometry (for those aged forty-five to fifty-four) and thyroid function. It was a challenging logistical exercise to keep the volunteers moving, following their individual timetables around the different points of the survey, including the mass miniature x-ray van and caravans for dietary recall and audiometry parked outside the Church hall. Precise organisation was also required to distribute, collect and deliver the bottles for urine samples to the Medical School for testing. The whole survey proved a rich source of information. Interviewed by the *Evening Star* soon after, Nye said it was providing information on heart disorders, high blood pressure, thyroid diseases, abnormalities connected with diabetes and people's dietary patterns. No other survey in New Zealand had covered such a range and it would provide the basis for reports in scientific journals over the following two years. There were benefits for the participants, too. More than a hundred Milton residents had abnormal electro-cardiograms,

and 3–5 per cent of these were urgently notified through their family doctors. In mid-1978, there was a follow-up to the study.[24]

At the end of the year, staff of the Medical School held their own centennial celebrations, for past and present members. It took place over the weekend of 5–7 December, just after the open day. The programme was relaxed, with plenty of free time to catch up with old friends. There were sports fixtures on the Friday – golf, tennis, cricket, squash, sailing – followed by a reception in the Lindo Ferguson building. On Saturday there was a chance to view the open day displays and, in the evening, a banquet-ball in the University Union. According to taste, Sunday was given over to a bush walk, a car rally or a picnic at Bethunes Gully.[25]

At the December graduation ceremony, Ronald Christie was awarded an honorary degree and the year was rounded off by an attractive piece of symmetry. The first graduate to be capped, as the second century of the Otago Medical School began, was Dr Richard Hugh Acland, great-grandson of Millen Coughtrey, the School's first Professor.[26]

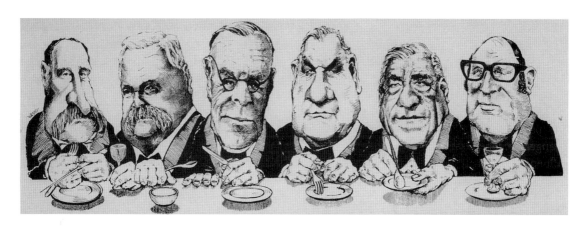

Medical School Deans, 1875–1975. From left, in chronological order, are Scott, Ferguson, Hercus, Sayers, Adams and Hunter. With the caption '50% of the Last Supper', the caricature appeared on the menu of the 1975 centennial dinner.
Otago Medical School.

CHAPTER 20

Times of Tension, 1975-1981

IT COULD hardly be expected that the excitement of the centenary year would be maintained, but the latter half of the 1970s was a period of more than mere anticlimax. It was characterised by considerable tension for the Otago Medical School and, at times, acrimony among its component parts. Money was at issue. There were three levels of potential conflict: the amount of the block grant from the Government to the University of Otago, the proportion that would be allocated to the Medical School and the division of this among the three campuses. The first two sums were resented by the Medical School as inadequate, the third was seen by the Christchurch and Wellington Clinical Schools as inequitable.

The financial environment in which the new Schools had to work out their relationships with the parent University was both difficult and changeable. John Gould has traced the increasing influence of Treasury in the process of allocating government funding to the universities through the University Grants Committee. In the first two quinquennia, 1965–69 and 1970–74, the UGC formulated its proposals without formal discussion with Treasury. In each case, the proposals were accepted by the Government. However, in the chillier economic climate of 1975–79, the UGC was required to discuss its proposals with Treasury in detail. The process was much slower and the UGC had to reduce its bid (which was already an underestimate) substantially to secure approval. In the planning for the 1980–84

quinquennium, Treasury was involved from the start and, after nine months of almost-weekly meetings, no agreement could be reached. Eventually, two separate proposals were put to the Government, which simply compromised on a global figure. Gould blamed the 'ever more intrusive and carping participation by Treasury' and the increasing concern to reduce government spending for the deadlock. Although finance was not the only point of disagreement between the University and the new clinical schools, it was fundamental to others, such as the University's inability to bring staffing at the new schools up to the promised level. The lack of transparency in the University's budgeting process also aggravated their suspicion and discontent.[1]

Despite the high point of the centenary, John Hunter found little satisfaction in his four years as Dean, from 1974 to 1977. Certainly there were achievements. In the Dunedin School, a new Department of Anaesthesia and Intensive Care separated out from Surgery, with Professor Barry Baker as head. Frederick Fastier (already a personal professor) was appointed to a Chair in Pharmacology. Ophthalmology, which had not had a professorial head since Lindo Ferguson, reached a new stage when John Parr, an Otago graduate of 1945, who had been in the department as senior lecturer since 1961, was promoted to a personal chair. He proceeded to reform undergraduate training, write a textbook, and initiate a postgraduate programme, as well as playing a major role in the more general administration of the Medical School. Microbiology gained a fine new building. There were major changes in the preclinical curriculum. However, Hunter felt trapped between the Otago University authorities, themselves suffering budget cuts, and the two northern schools, which were trying to complete their establishments and introduce innovative programmes. 'I took on the deanship', he said 'but within four years I felt it was becoming impossible for me to take on any role that involved any innovation or any independence.' In 1978, he accepted a position as inaugural Director of Continuing Education for the Royal Australasian College of Physicians, which took him to Sydney until 1982.[2]

The new Dean, Geoffrey Brinkman, was an Otago graduate of 1944 who had returned a few years before from a long and successful career in the United States. In 1976, he moved from an appointment as Chairman of the New Zealand Council of Postgraduate Medical Affairs to a post as Associate Dean for Postgraduate Affairs at the Otago Medical School. It was not an onerous position, since postgraduate students were traditionally a departmental responsibility and departments showed no interest in giving up this aspect of their work, but he was also Hunter's deputy and was called on as Acting Dean on several occasions before taking office in 1978. Like Hunter, Brinkman found some aspects of his role frustrating. His authority as academic and administrative leader of the Otago Medical School seemed 'more in name than in function'. The lack of autonomy was especially galling in the two vital areas of resources and staffing. He was not consulted about the Otago Medical School budget as a whole, or the apportioning of resources among the three component schools. Money was tight throughout his deanship. Financial cuts reduced the income of the Dunedin School by approximately a million dollars a year, which meant the cancellation of twenty registrar posts the University had funded at Dunedin Hospital. His hands were also tied in relation to staffing. Although he was a member of the University's staffing committee, he had no greater say on medical appointments than any other member. He was not consulted about the

promotion of professors. Well aware that the two Clinical Schools believed Dunedin dominated them, he acknowledged that the belief had some substance, because the Faculty Board, the main liaison committee representing the three Schools, had a majority of Dunedin members. In addition to his responsibilities in relation to the three Schools, and the day-to-day running of the Dunedin School, which took most of his time, Brinkman also handled a great deal of committee work. He served on the Otago Hospital Board and its various committees, the New Zealand Medical Council, the Medical Research Council and various Department of Health committees. He calculated that he averaged forty-five working days a year out of Dunedin attending to these duties. He also visited every department annually and made time to support student activities.[3]

In Dunedin some professorial appointments of long-term significance were made. A new department was established in 1978, when Radiology separated out from Surgery, and Stuart Heap, born in the West Indies and trained at the Charing Cross Medical School, University of London, was appointed to the Chair. Professor John Loutit, already a personal professor, succeeded John Miles as head of Microbiology. In 1980, David Skegg, an Otago graduate, Travelling Scholar and Rhodes Scholar of 1972, returned from study and teaching at Oxford to succeed Cyril Dixon as Professor of Preventive and Social Medicine. In the same year, Tony Macknight succeeded James Robinson as Wolff Harris Professor of Physiology and Richard Laverty took over from Frederick Fastier in Pharmacology.

After the new Dunedin Hospital, with its fine teaching facilities, opened in 1980, pressures on space were relieved elsewhere in the School. The decade ended, however, with the expectation that the Government would slash the intake of medical students. Faculty Board minutes illustrate the tension. Members were critical of the UGC, which they believed lacked an understanding of the requirements of a medical school, contrasting it with the United Kingdom, where there was a special medical subcommittee. The introduction of population-based funding for hospital boards was greeted in Otago with the utmost apprehension.[4]

Furthermore, at the beginning of 1980, the Medical School and the Otago Hospital Board were stunned to learn that the Government intended to install the CT (computerised tomography) body scanner, promised to Dunedin three years before, in Christchurch. Indignation at the decision, which was part of a country-wide, high-cost technology package that gave Otago only an upgrade of its cardiac equipment, also involved the scaling down of the established and highly regarded Neurological Unit, putting its entire future in jeopardy. A new unit would be set up in Christchurch to serve the South Island. Indignation was compounded by the fact the decision had been made without local consultation or any consideration of its effect on medical education. Scanning, the Dean explained to the press, was an essential procedure used not only by neurosurgeons, but by physicians and surgeons in a wide range of disciplines. The community rallied behind the Board and the School and the *Otago Daily Times* kept the issue to the fore throughout February, in a series of bold-headline, front-page articles. At a special general meeting, Medical School staff voted their unanimous support for the Hospital Board. Brinkman, neurologist Martin Pollock and the retiring head of the Unit, Professor R.G. Robinson, were outspoken in their public comments. The southern members of parliament and the Dunedin and Invercargill mayors gave strong support, and the Hospital Board and the Medical School jointly drew up a well-argued submission to the Prime Minister to persuade him to reverse the decision. This having failed, the next step was to raise money locally for a scanner. Within weeks a Scanner Steering Committee, various service groups and Radio New Zealand combined in an energetic campaign, to which the Medical School and individual staff members, as well as the people of Otago and Southland, contributed generously. The appeal succeeded well beyond its target.[5] By August 1981, the *ODT* could announce proudly that the Otago Southland body scanner (commonly called the CAT scanner) was in operation, that 'people in the region now have

access to a complete range of the most up-to-date imaging equipment it is possible to muster' which would enhance diagnostic ability in a whole range of areas. Within weeks the scanner was in full use, serving up to ten patients daily. It was a notable example of cooperation among the Hospital Board, the Medical School and the public.[6]

Christchurch

In Christchurch, the years from the graduation of the first class in 1975 to the end of George Rolleston's deanship in 1981, after a decade at the helm, were a time of consolidation. Rolleston's personal style, characterised as consultative, with a 'scrupulous search for consensus rather than confrontation and pragmatic policies rather than flashy insubstantialities', protected the young Christchurch School from much potential turmoil. Nevertheless, questions of space and finance inevitably caused controversy.[7] The Christchurch School was fortunate in that it had achieved its University building before the economic downturn, but in 1978 the Hospital Board failed to provide the academic accommodation it had earlier promised, because of delays in the rebuilding of Christchurch Hospital. The School, its administrators claimed, had begun life some 1300 square metres short of requirement. Negotiations dragged on for years, until academic space was at last provided in the Hospital's Stage Three development. Accommodation for students was created by the conversion of four conveniently located properties, transferred to the School by the Department of Education. Some departments were housed separately. The Department of Preventive and Social Medicine was located in a property in Cambridge Terrace. Another, in Cashel Street, housed the Board's Blood Transfusion Service (in exchange for another site for Psychological Medicine) and a long-term Child Development Study being developed under the Department of Paediatrics.

Financial questions were always to the fore, not least because the UGC had allocated a substantial block grant to the School (£750,000) for a multitude of purposes, from office furniture

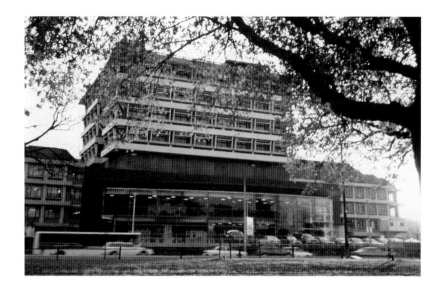

The Christchurch School in the Rolleston years.
University of Otago, Christchurch.

to laboratory equipment and library books, leaving the decisions of the detail of spending to the people on the spot. The decision to share facilities added complexity to attempts to divide the funding equitably and debates continued within the School, and between the School and the University Registry, until 1978, when the grant had been expended. Debate over the allocation of the block grant was nothing compared to the annual furore over the School's budget. From 1975, the Dean was required to travel to Dunedin each year to submit a detailed budget proposal and, each year, the Vice-Chancellor simply told the Dean what would be allocated. It was invariably less than requested and no negotiation on the amount was permitted. The Dean then had to return to Christchurch to face his outraged Heads of Department and to work with the Finance and General Committee to allocate the limited funding as fairly as possible.[8]

In contrast, academic and research questions were not in dispute. Rolleston had the loyal support of an experienced team of senior academics and administrators who were united in their commitment to excellence in teaching, research and clinical practice. The basic lines of a curriculum common to fourth- to sixth-year students in all three centres had been agreed on, on the basis of recommendations of a Dunedin curriculum committee in 1969–70. Formal examinations were replaced at fourth and sixth

years by continuous assessment and clinical tests, and at fifth year the departments in all the schools combined to produce a common examination. Faculty was divided into three 'divisions', one for each centre, and its work was coordinated by a Faculty Board, made up of the three Deans and representatives from each division. While the requirement to work within a Faculty-wide examination system which included the two Clinical Schools as well as the Dunedin Medical School, and also adhere to calendar prescriptions, imposed some limitations, setting a full clinical curriculum in place, with such a high proportion of internal assessment, was still an exciting prospect. There was also room for innovation in teaching methods and Christchurch staff were eager to experiment. The specific fourth-year programme, consisting of clinical attachments in medicine, surgery, psychological medicine and paediatrics, together with an interdepartmental clinical science course (which would be continued in fifth year) was a Christchurch innovation. The Christchurch School was also the first Otago centre to trial a trainee intern programme at sixth year. Under this scheme, which had been introduced in Auckland in 1972, final-year students became 'apprentice House Officers', with both educational and service components to their work. They were employed by the Hospital Board, but their assignments were rotated according to educational requirements and their salaries (about 60 per cent of the earnings of a first year House Officer) came from the education budget. In Christchurch from 1975, under the efficient supervision of Associate-Professor Barry Coll, the system proved very successful. By the time Rolleston retired, in January 1981, the Christchurch School was strongly established.[9]

Wellington

In Wellington, pressures mounted as the date for the commencement of fourth-year classes approached. The schedule was very tight and the level of activity over the six months before the first students arrived was nothing less than frantic. The contractor advised that the library, student facilities, administration area, lecture theatres, cafeteria area and pathology accommodation would be ready by 14 February 1977, the very day the students were expected. There were times, however, when this seemed impossible. Towards the end of 1976, Isbister recommended that, unless items required for teaching could be guaranteed by mid 1977, fourth-year students should not be accepted that year. Amazingly, as the deadline approached, it all came together. Some of the fourth years arrived a week early to assist in the move into the new premises and, over the final weekend, in

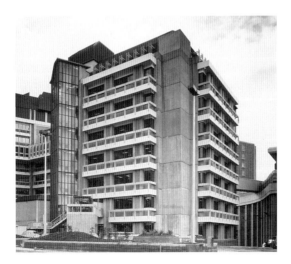

The Wellington School, ready for the students, 1977.
University of Otago, Wellington.

an extraordinary exercise, a rugby team raising funds for an Australian tour transferred the entire contents of the library. The Hospital Board senior administrative staff showed support where they could, by refurbishing relevant ward rooms for small group clinical teaching. The academic staff, Corkill wrote, 'did magnificently in getting their programmes in order'. When the students arrived on 14 February, they had to negotiate puddles and tarpaulins to get from one part of the site to another as construction continued. Even so, the Wellington Clinical School was open for business.[10]

The new Dean had just arrived, as Dr Ralph Johnson reached Wellington on 28 January and began work the next day. A senior lecturer in neurology at Glasgow at the time of his appointment, Johnson had an impressive academic record and the advantage of being a complete outsider. When he came for his interview from Tasmania where he was on leave, he showed himself to be assured and articulate, although he lacked high-level administrative experience. He faced a challenging situation. Tensions among the staff, primarily over space and resources but exacerbated by issues of personal incompatibility, had intensified after Hall's departure. Unfortunately, the arrival of the new Dean did nothing to resolve them. He was met with a barrage of complaints, from the Medical Research Council about the lack of research facilities, from Stehbens about the cramped accommodation for Pathology, and from a group of professors about the inadequacy of teaching and research facilities in general.[11]

The question of the relationship of the Wellington Clinical School with Victoria University College soon resurfaced. When it approved the establishment of the Wellington School, the UGC had agreed that when a third medical school was required it would be attached to Victoria. It also suggested that 1980, the beginning of a financial quinquennium, might be the appropriate time to consider the transfer of financial and academic responsibility. Victoria took the matter seriously, retaining a standing committee on the Medical School. In October 1977, however, the UGC informed the Wellington School that discussion on this subject would be deferred for another

Professor Ralph Hudson Johnson, 1933–1993

Dean, Wellington Clinical School, 1977–86

RALPH JOHNSON was born in 1933 in Sunderland, County Durham, and educated at Rugby, St Catherine's College, Cambridge and University College Hospital, London. He graduated MB ChB in 1958. His career from that point falls into blocks of roughly a decade. The first was in Oxford, as research registrar in the Neurology Department at the Radcliffe Infirmary and included four years as Dean of St Peter's College. He achieved further academic qualifications in this period, an MD from his old College at Cambridge and a DM from Oxford. He took part in scientific expeditions, for example as medical officer to the Oxford University mountaineering and ethnology expedition to Ecuador and as leader of an expedition to Jordan. He also conducted a study of medical services in Israel. Johnson then moved to Glasgow for eight years, as senior lecturer in neurology, consultant neurologist to the Western Regional Hospital Board and Warden of Queen Margaret Hall. He fitted in a fourth doctorate, from Glasgow in 1975, and published extensively. Over his career, he would produce four books, more than 150 papers and various chapters.

Johnson arrived in Wellington, with his wife Gillian and two young children, in January 1977. During the decade he served as Dean of the Wellington Clinical School, he was also consultant neurologist to the Wellington Hospital Board, a member of the Board of Management of the Wellington Medical Research Foundation, chair of the Medical Advisory Committee of the Multiple Sclerosis Society of New Zealand and, for a time, a member of the Medical Education Committee of the NZMA. He continued an active clinical research programme relating to the sympathetic nervous system and published frequently in international scientific journals. Nevertheless, his time in New Zealand proved frustrating. Hoping to head an independent Medical School, he chafed at direction from Dunedin. Relations with the Faculty of Medicine were tense and often confrontational. He also failed to win the loyalty of his colleagues in the Wellington School. A.W. Beasley summed up judiciously that, while he gave dedicated service to what he identified as the needs of the School and the region, 'his perceptions were not shared by the more conservative of his colleagues and … his time in Wellington did not do justice to his talents.'

Johnson returned to Oxford in 1987, as Director of Postgraduate Medical Education and Training for the University and a Professorial Fellow of Wadham College. He became consultant neurologist to the Oxford Regional Health Authority and the Oxfordshire Health Authority, a member of numerous committees and of the General Medical Council. He added to his fine collection of antiquarian books and spent his leisure landscaping the property around the family's elegantly restored barn. By a shocking irony, a swarm of bees from his own hive stung him to death in 1993.[12]

five years. The Heads of Department complained to the School Council that they had not been adequately consulted.[13]

Building continued throughout 1977 and 1978 while teaching was going on and new appointments were made, although these did not happen quickly enough for Professor John Roberts. Frustrated by repeatedly deferred promises about space and facilities for his Department of Psychological Medicine, he returned to Bristol. In July 1977 Corkill resigned to resume full-time work in his specialist field with the Hospital Board and subsequently became its Medical Superintendent-in-Chief. The Clinical School recorded its warm commendation for his contribution towards the building of the new School facilities.

The students settled in quickly. The fourth-year

class of 1977 is remembered as outstanding, with 'some great young leaders who were enthusiastic about their roles in the new clinical school' and both staff and students coped well with the incomplete and sometimes fairly primitive accommodation. The 1978 fourth years showed their mettle and 'made an indelible impression', as one reported in the *Digest* that year, by sending a letter critical of 'staff-student-patient relationships and communication' to all teaching staff. Student social life developed, though limited in the first two years by the lack of their own facilities. In 1978, a group of fourth and fifth years, accompanied by staff and their families – some eighty in all – spent an unforgettable weekend on a marae at Otaki, as guests of the Ngati Raukawa tribe, and later hosted a return visit. There were the usual smokos and sports fixtures and one group of fourth years made a nostalgic trip to Dunedin for the annual medical revue. At last, on 29 November 1979, the Wellington School could celebrate, in a ceremony that combined the graduation of the first intake of fifty-four students and the formal opening of the new School buildings by the Governor-General, Sir Keith Holyoake. By that time the University had agreed to a name change from the Wellington Clinical School to the Wellington Clinical School of Medicine, to improve community understanding of the work of the School. In 1981, the Hospital Board showed its appreciation of the work of the School by granting the Dean attendance and speaking rights at Board meetings. The main academic building was now fully occupied, the link block completed and ample laboratory space was available. There was a justifiable sense of achievement, no doubt tempered by the knowledge that in the previous month the Ministers of Health and Education had announced a 25 per cent reduction in student intake to both the Otago and Auckland Medical Schools over the next two years.[14]

The Bates Report

By the late 1970s, the Otago Medical School was threatened by the general economic recession and the Government's perception that there were too many doctors. In a 1977 discussion document on the future of the Dunedin division of the Medical School, Hunter included among major new factors affecting it the probability of a government decision to reduce the student intake. He also drew attention to the reduction in the School's clinical resource base, because of the region's static population, and pointed out that the Government was making decisions in these areas, without engaging in a proper discussion of their implications for the Medical School in staffing and research funding. In June 1979, in an editorial headed 'A Basis for Medical Manpower Cuts', the *New Zealand Medical Journal* reminded readers that, for more than a decade, there had been discussion as to whether the country was headed for a 'glut of doctors'. The Department of Health's advisory committee on medical manpower had just made its first report, which took into account not only the number of doctors being trained but also the cost of training them. Warning that the 'buoyant days of unjustified expansion' were gone, the committee recommended a 25 per cent cut in the student intake and made the sobering comment, 'We have at least one-and-a-half clinical schools too many'.[15]

Within the University of Otago, there was an expectation of harder times. In 1977, the Vice-Chancellor distributed to all staff a confidential document, entitled 'Planning for the Future of the University of Otago', as a basis for a comprehensive series of planning meetings. For the Medical School, Brinkman and a small team of senior academics put together a discussion paper, 'Planning for the Future'. In its final version, after Faculty discussion, it accepted that the current recession, which could be expected to last for several years, was restricting programmes and would limit further expansion. At the same time it was acknowledged that openings overseas for Otago graduates (currently 30–40 per cent took these up) would decrease. The report was born of crisis, but its recommendations deliberately focused on how to maintain and enhance the quality of the medical course. They included broader criteria for the selection of students and procedures for excluding and redirecting those who proved unsuitable, greater student involvement in curriculum planning, a more organised programme of postgraduate education, support for research and increased autonomy for the two Clinical Schools, including local administration of a pre-determined budget. The 1980–84 quinquennial grant provided no significant increase in Otago's funding and the Wellington School's budget committee was faced with the prospect of severe financial limitations, even before its departments were fully staffed. The Government cut numbers entering second year in 1981 from 180, which was already 20 below the intake of 200 on which the Clinical Schools were predicated, to 150. Ironically, there had been a record number of applicants that year.[16]

This was the background to the decision to invite Professor David Bates, Dean of the Faculty of Medicine at the University of British Columbia, to visit in 1981 to review the working of the Medical School. Bates had been a close colleague and protégé of Ronald Christie, the designer of the blueprint for dispersed clinical teaching at the Otago Medical School. Bates had spent some months in the Department of Medicine in 1967, had probably helped persuade Christie to undertake his review and was deeply interested in its outcome. He was now asked to advise on two matters:

> The most appropriate allocation of scarce and limited resources between the three divisions of the Faculty of Medicine in the eighties, bearing in mind the likely economic situation of the University in the period 1982–84 and the need to ensure the best possible conditions, in the circumstances, for teaching, research and the care of patients.

and

> The most appropriate development of the Faculty in the light of the possible distribution of these resources.

Bates' visit was brief. Beginning on 3 October, he spent six days in Dunedin and then fitted both Christchurch and Wellington into the next six, before returning to Dunedin to write up his findings. He reported verbally to the Vice-Chancellor on 19 October. Bates was impressed by the 'remarkable development' of the Faculty

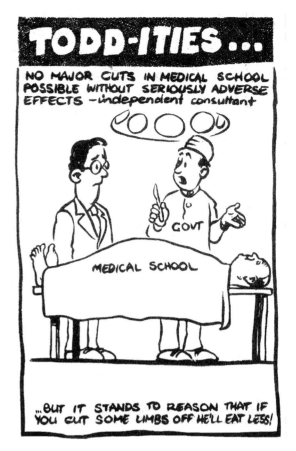

Cartoonist Hugh Todd comments on the warning in the Bates Report.
Otago Daily Times, 21 December 1981.

of Medicine since his earlier visit, reporting favourably on the facilities for clinical teaching (he was not concerned with the preclinical years) on all three campuses. In Dunedin, he praised the close integration of the School and the community, which compensated in areas such as obstetrics for the smaller population base. In other areas, such as medicine or surgery, the small population base restricted student opportunity and he identified this as the major problem of the Dunedin School. In Christchurch, too, the collaboration of the School and the local community was strong. Particular problems were the ongoing difficulties in the organisation of obstetrics, the lack of manpower in epidemiology and community health and the small staff available in sub-specialties of medicine and surgery. In Wellington, Bates admired the planning that had gone into constructing buildings on a constrained site. He saw the School's research in epidemiology and its undergraduate programme in community health as particular strengths, and noted the opportunity to develop a programme in health service administration. Problems that he identified included the late development of academic strength in pathology and the difficulties in developing certain areas, such as clinical pharmacology, medical genetics and psychiatry, on a slender base of funding.[17]

Looking at the student programme as a whole, Bates was positive. 'Otago has every reason to be proud of its medical school', he wrote. He drew attention, however, to the balance of components in the curriculum, querying the unusually high number of hours given to the basic sciences and the strong emphasis on neurophysiology and neurology. He found that little attention was being paid to medical genetics, psychiatry and family practice. If budgets had to be cut, he thought it would be an appropriate time to re-examine the values underlying the balance of the curriculum. More specifically, if a staffing freeze had to be applied for several years, he recommended it should be applied first to the clinical departments and possibly also to the preclinical departments in Dunedin. Bates noted the 'ambiguous nature of the responsibility of the dean' in relation to the budget and staffing, where his lack of autonomy ran directly contrary to Christie's recommendations. He urged more openness and flexibility in the process and believed each clinical school should be allowed to develop along its own lines. The Wellington and Christchurch Schools were already an essential resource within their respective communities. In summary, Bates was firmly convinced that each of the three schools provided such a well-based facility for medical teaching in New Zealand that no individual sector should be regarded as in any sense 'negotiable'. 'The present medical school', he said, 'consists of a three-legged stool, with each leg essential to the balance of the whole.'[18]

CHAPTER 21

Student Life:
A Change of Direction

WITHIN the Medical School, student interests continued to be served by their Association. As the 1950s give way to the 1960s, the minutes and annual reports of OUMSA show a stable pattern of day-to-day activities, of which social occasions were an important element. Departing or retiring staff were farewelled and newcomers welcomed, meetings of the Medical History Society and the Clinical Society were held, with variable attendance, and the medical ball was always described as a 'great success', although it was sometimes a cause of anxiety to the Executive. After the 1958 ball, two of its members were summoned to morning tea with the Vice-Chancellor and, as a consequence, the Executive decided it would not, in future, put a bottle of whisky in the middle of the dance floor and would also 'tactfully try and fence off the official party'. Class bashes and smokos could be problematic, often requiring an apologetic follow-up from the Executive. In 1959, the President reported that, although the venue for the Third Year Drinking Horn had 'benefited from us by the installation of a new toilet', medical students would not be allowed to use the building again. The following year, a 'rousing farewell' to a popular professor resulted in a ban on future medical student smokos in the Rose Pavilion at Carisbrook. The embittered Rugby Football Union suggested White Island as a suitable alternative.[1]

Money matters were never far from the surface for OUMSA. The canteen was an ongoing worry. In 1959, the President described it as the 'major financial concern of the Association' and the 1961 Executive began the year with £200 in hand and a canteen debt of £210, amid fears that the new Student Union and the Dental School canteen would permanently take away their trade. These fears proved groundless and within a year or so patronage had increased to the extent that more chairs were needed and the Association could embark on renovations. In 1963 OUMSA gained its own room and, at the end of the decade, student facilities were transformed by the addition of a seminar room, coffee room, reading room, kitchen and showers in the former X-ray basement.[2] The secondhand book exchange for medical books, taken over by OUMSA in 1961, proved a welcome source of revenue. Its profit of £100 that year doubled the next and continued to rise. With the help of the Dean, the 1961 Executive also raised an impressive £1345, mostly from the University Council, to embark on a complete renovation of the canteen and common room. In 1966, the Association engaged a qualified accountant as treasurer, to advise them on what had become a £9000 turnover from the canteen and the book exchange.[3]

In the 1970s, the word 'apathy' was much bandied about by medical student leaders. 'During the last five years', wrote OUMSA President Roger Wilson in the 1975 *Digest*, 'the steady downward trend in medical participation in extra-curricular activities has become something of a nosedive'. According to Wilson, the average medical student was 'about as interested in student affairs as a post-pubescent boy is in toy trains.' Most portfolio holders on the OUMSA Executive were elected unopposed, no medical student had been president of OUSA since 1969 and the 'traditional Rabelaisian presence' of medical students in Capping was no more. Why these changes? Wilson put them down to the reduced percentage of medical students in a greatly expanded university and the fear of failure inculcated by continuous assessment.[4]

Wilson's comments remain pertinent. There has still been only one medical OUSA president since 1969, continuous assessment has become embedded and the University has grown mightily. However, there were other reasons for medical students turning away from general student politics. Changes in OUSA made participation in its activities less attractive. From the late 1960s, the University was caught up in an increasingly widespread and radical wave of student unrest, which challenged the postwar consensus. Traditionally a steadying influence, OUSA itself became a focus of controversy, with meetings of the Student Council and even the Executive often degenerating into chaos. In 1970, student

discipline was an issue throughout the University, including the Medical School. A third-year medical student was arrested for possessing marijuana and unprescribed tablets and the OUMSA President unwisely attended a notorious post-tournament reunion in the Student Union. The University authorities drew up new discipline regulations and, in 1971, some two thousand students took over the registry in protest.[5] At the same time, the responsibilities of the President of OUSA were becoming more onerous and did not easily fit around the demands of a medical course. New portfolios were added to the Executive and in 1972 the extent of the President's responsibilities was acknowledged by a $1000 honorarium. As well as running the Logan Park facility and the Student Union, OUSA took half shares in the University Book Shop in 1975. In 1980, after years of fundraising and planning, it opened the million-dollar Clubs and Societies Building.[6]

At the same time as its ties with OUSA were loosened, OUMSA was increasingly drawn into Medical School affairs. In this development, as in so many others, the 1968 Christie review was a turning point. It marked the beginning of the

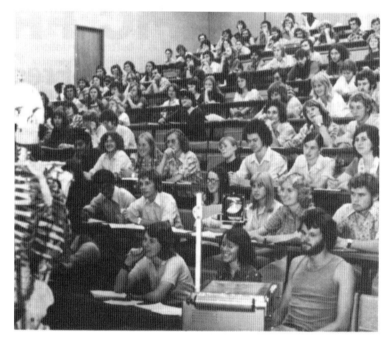

Class of second-year medical students, 1972.
Digest 1975, p. 23, j. Hocken Collections, Uare Taoka o Hakena, University of Otago.

'My own impression of modern senior medical students is that they are more eloquent, more knowledgeable, more inquiring, less inhibited and much more promising than their counterparts of 1945. Their general appearance, demeanour and dress improves as they advance through the course.'

J.F. Gwynne, 'The Medical School Then and Now (1945–1975)'. A second-year student in 1945, Gwynne was on the staff of the Pathology Department when he wrote in 1975.

≈ Anatomy of a Medical School ≈

regular consultation of medical students about their own education. In July 1968, at a special general meeting of three hundred students, President Bill Sugrue reported that the Vice-Chancellor would keep him informed on any actions resulting from the Christie Report and was keenly interested in student opinion. The meeting 'heartily endorsed' the report, agreeing that drastic steps were required if the Medical School was to keep its century-old reputation. This was not the first general meeting of students (there had been several in recent years, for example, to work out a scheme for the provision and laundering of clinical students' white coats) but it was certainly the largest and most significant in recent memory. Over the following months, students came to be included in Medical School policy-making. In 1969, five students were added to the Medical Faculty and a Staff Student Curriculum Committee (SSCC) was formed. OUMSA had already signalled its interest in the curriculum by setting up an Education Committee, under an Intellectual Affairs Representative, at the end of 1967. In 1970, its chair, Sue Wilson, who was a member of the SSCC, reported to the *Digest* on 'Student Power at Otago Medical School'. She said that, while most medical students expected to 'sit back and function as receptacles of facts and wisdom', others wished to participate as mature members of the university body, but she was also critical of the tactics of those students who demanded 'immediate alteration to the course' to give them greater access to patients and more responsibility for their care.[7] From this time, medical students were routinely included on Faculty committees. Acceptance of the recommendation of the Christie Report to increase the student intake had another direct benefit. In July 1970, the Dean wrote to the OUMSA that Faculty had agreed to 'substantial increases in the student amenities', including a better canteen.[8]

The Medical Students' Association was also finding common ground with other medical students' associations in New Zealand and Australia. The opening of the Auckland Medical School changed the dynamic of Otago's medical student politics, especially as it coincided with

a disagreement over fees between the medical students and OUSA, which at times looked as if it might lead to secession. In 1968, OUMSA put a detailed case for the reduction of its fees to OUSA – as it had done in 1951, 1953, 1958, 1961 and 1965 – on the grounds of its low use of OUSA facilities and the need to finance its own activities, such as running the medical canteen, publishing the *Digest* and paying for visiting lecturers. As usual, it received a cool response.[9] A medical student organisation in Auckland, which might well have similar problems, must have seemed worth cultivating. Relations with Auckland were not automatically cordial, however, and in the Auckland School's early days there was a good deal of North/South trading of insults. Otago proclaimed the Auckland students juvenile, while Auckland considered Otago students stodgy. The headline of an Auckland medical student publication summed up the northern attitude, 'Auckland Medical Students have Sex, Otago Medical Students have Hot Water Bottles'. Nevertheless, common interests dictated common action. In mid-1972, the Otago President visited Auckland where, despite finding 'even more student apathy than at Otago', he negotiated the setting up of a New Zealand Medical Students' Association.[10] OUMSA also forged links with the Australian Medical Students' Association (AMSA). From 1967, increasingly large groups of Otago delegates attended the annual AMSA convention, at first as associates but, from 1970, as full members. The Australian Medical Students' Association renamed itself 'Australasian' in recognition. In 1975, in conjunction with the centenary celebrations of the Medical School, Otago hosted an AMSA convention. It was a great occasion: seven days and nights of lectures, meetings, seminars and socialising, 182 hours, of which, it was rapturously reported in the *Digest*, only five of every twenty-four were wasted in sleeping. Some four hundred Australian students flocked to Dunedin but, disappointingly, only a handful of local fifth years joined them.[11] It was the high point of Otago's association with the AMSA and also its farewell. The Otago Association chose to put its energy into NZMSA, which aimed to

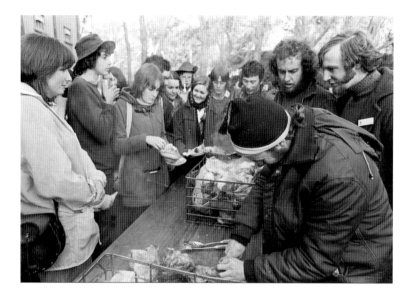

Medical students attending the AMSA conference in Dunedin enjoy a hangi at Logan Park.
Otago Daily Times, 26 May 1975.

represent the interests of New Zealand medical students by facilitating communication among them, studying and speaking out on medical education, keeping medical students informed about political issues that affected them and generally promoting their welfare. The New Zealand Association held its first convention in May 1976.[12]

In sport, medical students continued to make a name for themselves. In 1960, the *Digest* ran an article on international sportsmen, all medical students, who were touring overseas. Mark Irwin and Tony Davies were going to South Africa with the All Blacks, John Cullen to the Rome Olympics as the only Otago member of the hockey team, Duncan McVey to Tahiti with the New Zealand soccer team and Michael Gill to climb with Sir Edmund Hillary in the Himalayas. With a BMedSc in physiology, Gill had leave of absence to study at Oxford physiological techniques that he would employ in gathering data on the body's need for oxygen at high altitudes. Gill also shared the record for the fastest ascent of Mount Cook.[13] In his annual report for 1966, the Secretary of OUMSA used a headline from the local press to describe his President: 'Peter Welsh, the enigma, student and athlete extraordinary'. Welsh had won gold in the 3000 metres steeplechase at the Commonwealth games at Kingston that year. At the same games,

Dave Gerrard won the 200 yards butterfly. Gerrard, who would later develop a career as a specialist in sports medicine at the Medical School, was an outstanding butterfly swimmer in the 1960s, winning the New Zealand title in the 200 metres butterfly ten times consecutively from 1960, and the 100 metre title six times.[14] Such students excelled individually, but overall medical dominance in University teams was less striking. In 1976, Gwynne noted the changed pattern. Whereas, just after the war, thirteen of the first rugby fifteen had been medical students, the predominance had passed to students from the main campus, especially Phys Ed students. Most medical students played social rugby, although Gwynne thought they took it more seriously than in the past, when the social Med Boozers had been noted for their disdain of training and preference for a five-gallon keg on the sideline instead of oranges. In 1964, the inter-class rugby competition for the Nichol Cup resumed after more than a decade.[15] University cricket flourished in the 1960s, which Griffiths calls the 'years of triumph'. Two pharmacists turned medical students, in turn, captained the team with great success: John Barry, who had led the New Zealand under twenty-three team against the West Indies in 1956, and Lindsay Green. The team took the senior title in both the 1967–68 and 1969–70 seasons.[16]

OUMC to UMU

The Otago University Medical Corps underwent a number of major changes in these years. The Government abandoned Compulsory Military Training at the end of the 1950s, in favour of a volunteer system and, in 1961, this was supplemented by selecting trainees through a ballot based on date of birthday. Not many medical students volunteered. The OUMC reporter to the *Digest* in 1966 bemoaned the fact that the Corps was 'gradually becoming a national service training unit', but could find no reason for the slow decline in the number of volunteers, other than the general unwillingness of medical students to engage in any extra-curricular activities. 'At the moment', he wrote, 'OUMC is in the somewhat paradoxical situation of being a Unit consisting of Volunteer Territorial Officers commanding students who have been balloted into serving.' Service in the OUMC was an attractive option for those whose names had come up in the ballot. If a second-year student joined the OUMC within three months of entering Medical School, he could do his Compulsory Military Training in 'divided doses' over five years. This obviated the need to spend a stretch of fourteen weeks, or of two seven-week periods, in camp over the summer vacation. Instead, he could take part in twenty training days a year, six in term time and fourteen at Burnham Camp in May. Moreover, he would be paid. Interestingly, the rather dejected tone of the anonymous writer of the 1966 'OUMC Notes' has disappeared by the time the next year's 'Notes' came to be written. At this time, OUMC was said to be enjoying 'enormous popularity', with a membership of over a hundred. The reporter enthused about the May camp, the highlight of a year which itself had been a 'rewarding and enriching experience', thanks in large part to the new commander, Lt. Col. Irvine.[17]

The part-volunteer, part-ballot scheme lasted until 1973. There were a number of positive changes in this time, such as the decision to camp at Burnham in May rather than February, when students wanted to work at holiday jobs, and the introduction, in 1967, of a well-designed three-year training scheme which coincided with the second, third and fourth years of University study. Some students took their student electives with the Services Medical Team in Vietnam. In 1973, OUMC, which had been part of the 3rd Infantry Brigade Group, was transferred to Home Command. The reasons for the change are unclear, but the effect was unfortunate as it effectively isolated the corps. At the same time, a name change to the University Medical Unit (UMU) was adopted, in recognition of the fact

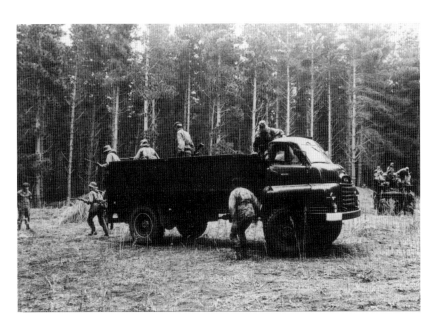

The University Medical Unit training in the Kaipara Forest, north of Auckland in 1980.
Medical Alumnus Association Collection.

that students from the Auckland Medical School were now able to join, and that most senior Otago students would soon be located in Christchurch and Wellington. In 1975, the Whangaparaoa army camp, near Auckland, was adopted as the camp site for the new Unit and women were recruited from 1976.[18]

While the Unit's function was to train officers for Defence Medical and Dental units, it also gave night assistance to St John Ambulance drivers (students were on duty from 10.30 p.m. to 7.00 a.m. two nights a week) and helped with community projects, such as the Coronary Care Club. Students could join in the first year of their course and progress through a three-year training programme, at the end of which they would be posted to other units. Sixty or so joined each year but fewer than ten stayed long enough to be posted. The annual training programme consisted of a fortnight at Whangaparaoa and six days' out-of-camp training. Three accounts of the 1977 camp appeared in the *Digest*, one from UMU B company, which consisted of sixty-three 'new Otago Troopies', one from A company, made up of ten men and six women, and one from the Officers' Training Group, which had twenty-three members, but only six Otago medics among them – 'an indication of the way in which UMU is being overrun by Otago dentists and Auckland medics.' They all claimed to have enjoyed themselves, in spite of incessant rain, which fell during the camp for the third time in three years.[19]

There were various attempts to increase the cohesion of the medical student community through written communications. The *Digest* was faltering by the early 1970s, in spite of a high proportion of advertising. The 1975 issue, at seventy-one pages, including advertisements, was only half the size of the 1967 edition and a fraction of the quality. Grateful for small mercies, the 1977 President expressed his relief that it had 'not made a huge loss'. The last issue, in 1978, was a mere nineteen pages, with all the signs of having been hastily thrown together. The 1981 Executive, investigating the failure, concluded it was due to 'insufficient editor potential'. Increased printing costs also made the *Digest* too expensive for most students to buy. The Executive decided not to resuscitate it but to try instead more informal, cheaper newsletters, such as *Litterhoea*, which comprised a few cyclostyled sheets, that had already been launched in 1971. The Dean offered a cautious welcome. 'I understand', Adams wrote, 'that you are embarking on a courageous venture to produce a racy – but not, I gather, scandalous – magazine of interest to the staff and students of the Medical School.' He warned, 'No apocryphal stories, please.' Short of contributions within these guidelines, it did not survive beyond 1972. The OUMSA newsletter *Borborygmi* proved longer lasting. It first appears in the Executive Minutes in September 1979, when a suggestion that the medical students should produce their own news sheet was enthusiastically received.[20]

The loss to Dunedin of first half, then two thirds of senior medical students, as they left to complete their training in the new clinical schools in Christchurch or Wellington, was unsettling to the parent School. It reduced the pool of those who might take a leadership role in student affairs in Dunedin, as medical students had done over the decades. There was much talk of medical students opting out of University activities. With hindsight, however, it is clear that what was happening in the 1970s was not an effect of apathy, but a change of direction, a turning away from the University towards a closer engagement with the Medical School and the medical community. Two initiatives of the later 1970s demonstrate the new orientation: the Med Camp, where third-year students welcomed the incoming second-year class with a heady mixture of lectures and socialising, and the Med Revue, where the exuberance, wit and bawdiness for which medical students were once renowned in Capping concerts found a new outlet.

PART V

Decades of Challenge and Opportunity
1981–2000

CHAPTER 22

The 1980s:
Economic and Political Pressures

'Learning to Roll with the Punches', 1981–1985

'Despite problems associated with reductions in the budgets of the University and Hospital Boards in Dunedin, Christchurch and Wellington, the Medical School is learning to roll with the punches and boxes on with vigour.'

Geoffrey Brinkman, 'Letter from the Dean' in *Alumnus Association Bulletin,* 1982.

David Bates' affirmation that all three Schools making up the Otago Medical Faculty were essential to its operation and that each also had a vital role to play in its own community was welcome, but it did not resolve the practical problems the School faced in the early 1980s. Financial stresses and inter-School acrimony were sometimes intense in these years, with frequent rumours that one or other of the Schools was to be closed. Furthermore, the impact on the Faculty of the far-reaching changes to the health system that began in 1983 was all-pervasive.

Geoffrey Brinkman was the Dean of the Medical School through the stormy years of the early 1980s. Reporting to the Alumnus Association in 1980, he summed up the situation in sombre tones:

The expansive years of the 1970s, when the student intake increased to 200 per year and both staff and facilities increased dramatically, are over. Instead the 1980s will require our ingenuity to maintain

the quality of the School in face of a falling budget and decreasing student numbers – 180 this year and probably 150 in 1981.

Already all vacant staff positions have been disestablished and new appointments must await vacancies created by retirement or resignation. The only exceptions are the two Clinical Schools in Wellington and Christchurch, which will receive some special consideration as they are still in the process of building up their staff, but there is little likelihood that they will reach the establishments originally planned. The problem is further compounded by the simultaneous reduction in the teaching hospital budgets.

Brinkman laid out some options. The Otago Medical School could develop particular strengths in each of its component schools rather than duplicating expertise. However, this would require students to move from one centre to another, and would weaken the schools through the absence of one or more major disciplines. Another option, frequently proposed, would be to close one of the clinical schools, but with at least 180 students in each until 1984, two schools would not be able to cope. Yet another option would be to relieve the staff by reducing the intake still further, to 120. Brinkman's own view was that no radical changes should be made in the immediate future and that the various options should be reconsidered if there was no improvement in the situation by the mid-1980s.[1] As he wrote in 1982, despite the problems associated with the budget reductions, the Medical School was 'learning to roll with the punches.'[2] Given the weight of some of the punches, the determination and vision that Brinkman brought to his deanship are impressive.

The weightiest blows came from government. The reduced intake of students and consequent reduction of staff were followed by major changes to the whole New Zealand health system. In 1983, the twenty-seven Hospital Boards were restructured into fourteen Area Health Boards, financed on a population-based formula which did not take into account the extra expenses associated with a teaching hospital. The change was implemented over the next six years, and the public health functions which had formerly been the responsibility of the Department of Health were decentralised. The replacement of Robert Muldoon's National Government by Labour, under David Lange in 1984, made little difference to the process.[3]

Brinkman's annual reports to the Alumnus Association from 1980 to 1985 enable us to trace

Professor Geoffrey Brinkman

MB ChB MD MRCP (Ed) FRCP (Edin) MRACP FRACP FACP DCH (Lond), Dean, Otago Medical School, 1978–85

'DO NOT be fooled by Professor Geoffrey Brinkman's conservative appearance and polite manner', the *Otago Daily Times* warned its readers in December 1985. It went on to describe the innovative ideas and imaginative guidance that Professor Brinkman had given the School through the previous eight difficult years. Some of his former colleagues, looking back with the benefit of twenty years' hindsight, were similarly struck by the contrast between their Dean's outward conservatism and his capacity to think outside the square.

Brinkman was born in Wellington in 1921 and, although the family lived in a number of locations in New Zealand and Australia, he had all his secondary schooling at Wanganui Collegiate. He came to Otago to study medicine in 1939. Theoretically under army control throughout his course, he and his fellow medical students spent long weekends and vacations in camp or barracks. He enjoyed his student days, in spite of the 8 a.m. to 5 p.m. timetable, and the class, together in vacation as well as during term for six years, bonded firmly. After serving his internship at Christchurch Hospital, Brinkman spent three years on postgraduate work in London, returning in 1949 as registrar to Sir Horace Smirk. He married Ngaire Macalister that year. They would have six children.

Brinkman's professional direction was determined by an unexpected occurrence. The Director of TB services – that is, the sanatoria at Wakari and Pleasant Valley and a clinic, some one thousand patients in all – suddenly disappeared overseas. On the basis of six months' training in chest disease in London, Brinkman was called on as Acting Director. He became absorbed in the field, first moving to Cashmere Sanatorium, then, funded by scholarships, to the United States. The American sojourn developed into a twenty-year-long career. After experience at various specialist centres, Brinkman spent twelve years at the Henry Ford Hospital in Detroit, during which he published on physiological, epidemiological and electro-microscopic research. A move to Wayne State University Medical School in Detroit, as Professor of Medicine and Assistant Dean, took him into high-level administration.

Returning to New Zealand for family reasons, Brinkman moved from Waikato Hospital to the Otago Medical School in 1976 and became Dean two years later. Despite the pressures of the position, he ensured that he spent time with his family at Wanaka and kept up his fitness with fishing and hiking. In retirement, he chaired the Advisory Committee on the Medical Workforce from 1986 to 1989. The Brinkmans retired to Waikanae, which has proved a suitable base for an active life style in which golf features prominently.[4]

both the problems and the achievements of this period. Thanks to the generosity of a former student, Dr Elaine Gurr, Dr Campbell Murdoch, senior lecturer in General Practice at Dundee, was appointed to the first Chair in General Practice in New Zealand. The former Dean, John Hunter,

A Friend of General Practice

BORN in Wellington, Elaine Gurr graduated from the Otago Medical School in 1923. After a year as a house surgeon in Timaru, she travelled to Britain for postgraduate experience in gynaecology, midwifery and antenatal work, gaining her licentiate in midwifery at the Rotunda, Dublin, and antenatal experience at the Royal Free and Chelsea hospitals, London. Back in New Zealand, Gurr was invited to become officer in charge of antenatal clinics in the Department of Health. From late 1924, with the assistance of Sister Winifred Wise, she travelled the country, setting up the first antenatal clinics, attached to St Helen's and other maternity hospitals, and instructing the nursing staff in up-to-date antenatal practice. She then set up in general practice, at first on the East Cape then, in 1933, in central Auckland, where she practised for thirty years, specialising in obstetrics and gynaecology. Gurr served as an anaesthetist to Auckland surgeons and had a long association with St John Ambulance, the hospice movement and a Salvation Army geriatric home. After World War II, she travelled to Scandinavia to study the new specialty of endocrinology. Firm in her belief in the value of general practice and holistic medicine, she endowed in perpetuity a Chair of General Practice at the Otago Medical School in 1983 (the same year she was made an Honorary Fellow of the New Zealand College of General Practitioners) and a Chair of Community Health at the Auckland Medical School in 1988. Elaine Gurr has been described as 'the most generous benefactor New Zealand general practice has ever had'.[5]

had initiated negotiations for this Chair and Brinkman was able to bring the arrangements to a satisfactory conclusion. He also made sure that general practice got what a colleague called 'a place in the sun in the curriculum'. It was the only new examinable subject introduced during this period.[6]

In 1983, an attempt was made to require all prospective medical students to take their Intermediate year in Dunedin. This would have enabled part of the overcrowded second-year curriculum to be transferred to first year. The attempt failed, but scheduled teaching in second year was reduced from 814 hours to 660 hours, which allowed more time for independent study. Teaching staff were also making more use of computer-assisted learning. The number of women students entering the Otago Medical School jumped from 33 per cent to 48 per cent in 1983 (in Auckland it went from 40 per cent to 52 per cent) and there was concern that this would have an adverse effect on medical manpower in the future. The year was difficult, Brinkman reported, because reduced University and Hospital Board funding had forced the curtailment of some activities. Nevertheless, it was satisfying that the Chair of Experimental Medicine in the Wellcome Institute, which had been vacant since the retirement of Professor Smirk seventeen years before, had been filled by Dr Vincent Chadwick, head of gastroenterology at Hammersmith hospital in London. Once again, this had been achieved through bequest money, underlining the importance of sources of funding beyond the declining government allocation. Research was also being well supported by outside funding agencies, and was enhanced by the contribution of the Clinical Schools.[7]

The next two years' reports show continued innovation, despite adverse circumstances. In 1984, John Campbell was appointed to a foundation Chair of Geriatric Medicine, which had been established with financial support from the Perpetual Trustees. An Otago graduate of 1969 and widely published in the epidemiology of old age, Campbell would later take on the responsibility of Dean of the School. The curriculum committee reviewed the third- and sixth-year courses, working towards increasing teaching in a community environment. The fifth-year examination was modified to accommodate a 50 per cent local component (usually an OSCE or objective structured clinical examination) as well as a common examination. Closer relations were established with Southland Hospital and an exchange programme was set up with, and funded by, the Cleveland Clinic in Ohio. At the same time, the Medical School's problems were compounded by a reduction in hospital budgets, especially in Dunedin and Wellington. That teaching standards and research were being maintained, the Dean wrote, was due to greater efforts from the reducing numbers of staff. He pointed out that the staff/student ratio at Otago was 1:12 in preclinical classes and 1:7 in the clinical years, whereas in North America and Britain the ratio was 1:1. He warned that any further reduction of resources would make it hard to maintain standards.[8]

In his last letter in 1985, Brinkman could report another first: a residential conference involving Faculty from all three centres, at Lincoln College. It was the first time the Schools had met since they had been established twelve years earlier. Planning was under way to introduce formal teaching in medical ethics and to increase vertical integration between the preclinical and clinical years of the medical course. Moves were also being made to facilitate greater interchange of staff between the Schools and to enable teachers within specific disciplines to meet, in order to enhance the coordination of the teaching programmes of the three Schools.

There were developments specific to the different centres. In Dunedin, the Medical School joined with the six Hospital Boards south of the Waitaki in planning a regional health service. This was an exciting development which would give the School access to the 300,000 people in the region and offset problems associated with the declining number of patients in the Dunedin area. In Christchurch, plans were under way for a distance-learning course on musculo-skeletal medicine. In Wellington, discussions were in train regarding the possibility of integrating the Wellington Clinical School with Victoria

University, although it was expected to be some time before a final decision would be reached on this matter.[9] More immediately, the School was preparing to contribute to a new nursing degree at Victoria University, an initiative promoted by the Department of Health to provide graduates who could take leadership roles in nursing practice, management, teaching and research. A Professor of Nursing was appointed to the Wellington School in 1983 and early enrolments to the course exceeded expectations. Brinkman's final comment as Dean was that the School was in excellent heart and was not stagnating, despite financial restrictions. 'In the last few years', he wrote, 'it would have been easy to sit back and contemplate the past and ignore the future. Instead the School is planning for the future.' That this was so, was in part a tribute to his own farsightedness.[10]

Tension between the Clinical Schools of Medicine in Christchurch and Wellington and the Faculty in Dunedin was passed over lightly in Brinkman's generally upbeat reports in these years, but it was not insignificant. Because of the abrasive style and separatist aims of the Dean, Ralph Johnson, the tension was sharper with Wellington. Personalities aside, however, there were important basic differences of opinion over academic programmes, resource allocation, appointments and promotions. Johnson was frustrated by the negative reactions from Dunedin to his ideas for potential academic developments at Wellington, in areas such as nursing and pharmacy. When he and Professor Newell presented innovative proposals to establish the subsequently successful diploma and masters degree courses in Public Health, they met opposition to their being based in Wellington rather then Dunedin. In 1982, Johnson 'led a charge' to set the Wellington Clinical School free from Otago and attach it to Victoria University. 'In these times of cutbacks of regular resources', a Faculty Board valedictory minute would run, in April 1986, in masterly understatement, 'Ralph Johnson has ensured that the needs of the Wellington School have been represented.' He had some, perhaps limited, support in the Wellington School, and from

Victoria as well, during the three years, from 1982, that Dr Ian Axford was Vice-Chancellor. In 1984 a working party, set up by Axford to explore closer relations, recommended full integration, but the Vice-Chancellor's precipitate departure, in mid-1985, was a blow to the cause. Although a poll taken towards the end of that year showed that 90 per cent of senior clinical staff at Wellington Hospital favoured closer relations with Victoria, the University's Professorial Board was not convinced.[11]

The view Christchurch staff took of the Otago Medical School was not always cordial, but it lacked the sharp edge that Johnson's style of leadership seemed to generate. When the gentlemanly and diplomatic George Rolleston retired as Dean at the beginning of 1981, staff were delighted that John Hunter, widely regarded as the 'godfather' of the School, was prepared to return from Australia to take on the deanship. His friend, Fred Shannon, wrote to him from Christchurch that, 'It's the first time we've heard of a rat swimming back to a sinking ship'. He must have welcomed Hunter's return. Reluctantly serving as Acting Dean for 1981, Shannon faced, as the historians of the School briskly put it, a somewhat rancorous debate with the Dean in Dunedin over reimbursement for trainee interns, a student confrontation about a scurrilous broadsheet and a major confrontation with two Heads of Department.[12]

Established earlier, and therefore less vulnerable than the Wellington School to economic pressures, the Christchurch School seemed in good heart when Hunter took over in 1982, but he soon identified worrying problems of finance and staffing. A number of academic posts were unfilled, having been frozen before agreed staffing levels had been reached. Student intakes at fourth year were declining and would decline further, with the reduction of the second-year intake to 150. Medical Research Council funding to the School had been severely restricted. Several departments were geographically isolated, which strained relations with the North Canterbury Hospital Board. On the other hand, the Bates report ended rumours that the School was about to close and endorsed its role, beyond the teaching of medical students, as an essential resource in the community.[13]

Hunter's wish for the School was that it would become a 'more free-standing enterprise, without being continuously over-regulated by the University on the one hand and the Area Health Board on the other'. This hope, and the obstacles in its path, form a dominant theme of his deanship. Hunter resented the low level of funding allocated to the Christchurch School and the secrecy surrounding its allocation, but he could do little about it. He was frustrated from two sides in his attempts to remedy the acknowledged shortfall in space at the Christchurch School: the Otago Medical School needed to refurbish its preclinical departments in Dunedin and the North Canterbury Hospital Board's fear that government approval to increase the School's space might prejudice approval of its own planned ward block extensions. Frustrations aside, however, Hunter was a careful and diplomatic Dean and he oversaw a number of clear achievements. All forty-nine approved staff positions were filled (although some only temporarily) and curricular innovation and research were encouraged. Hunter worked for greater independence for the Christchurch School and led the move, achieved in 1984, to rename the two Clinical Schools as Schools of Medicine to reflect this. Although his relations with the Dean of Faculty in Dunedin were sometimes tense, as the Christchurch School sought to have more control over its own curriculum and examinations, he still believed firmly in the value of the Otago connection. He accepted variation in teaching methods at fifth year, for example, but fully supported a common examination. He also gave no encouragement to staff who wanted to secede from Otago and join the University of Canterbury. He argued that it was preferable to be part of a powerful Faculty at Otago University than a small element at Canterbury, whose Vice-Chancellor did not want the School anyway. It was a balancing act that he managed with great skill.[14]

Anxieties about the future of the Medical School reached a crisis point in mid-1985. Brinkman described the situation tersely in a paper he circulated in June. The financial implication of the 25 per cent cut in student intake was a probable 5 per cent cut in the academic budget and a fall in other components of the Medical School budget. In negotiations for the present quinquennium, the Vice-Chancellor had quoted Christie's 1968 prediction that, unless something was done at once, the ranks of what was already a skeleton staff would be depleted and the University would face a difficult crisis. Christie had said, 'Drastic changes will be required if the Medical School is not to lose the reputation it has gained over almost a century of existence'. Brinkman commented, 'Many of us feel we have already reached this situation'. Since 1981, when the Bates report warned that there was no 'elbow room' anywhere in academic staffing, the academic budget had been reduced. This had resulted in the loss of more than ten full-time staff positions in Dunedin and the planned establishments for the Christchurch and Wellington Schools having to be put on hold. The problem was compounded by the introduction of population-based funding for hospitals, which led to a reduction in funding for the Wellington, Christchurch and Otago Hospital Boards, all of which were forced to reduce their support for patient services. This placed an increased burden on their clinical staff, who had to assume a heavier service load.

On 18 July 1985 Brinkman called the Dunedin Faculty together to debate options for the future of the Medical School. The University Grants Committee had recognised the extra costs of having three centres for the School, but if it was to receive continued preferential funding it had to justify this structure. The meeting

---

The Gavel (Toki-Poutangatai)

Early in 1985 Professor David Cole presented an ornately carved gavel to the School, on behalf of friends and colleagues in the Faculty of Medicine, University of Auckland. Of Maori design and carved in kauri, its edge was described as 'quite sharp, expressly designed to cut short Faculty waffle.'

Otago Medical School Alumnus Association, 1985

---

considered ten options for a sustainable future, including maintaining the status quo, increasing student numbers, disestablishing Chairs in some disciplines or closing one of the schools. Faculty saw no alternative to closing one of the schools (which one was not specified), unless funding was increased to a level equivalent to that for two hundred students. The student paper *Critic* had already come to the same conclusion. Two days before, it had published a double-page spread, based on the Faculty options paper and an interview with the Dean, entitled 'The Squeeze is On'. While Brinkman would not be drawn as to his own preferred option, *Critic* had no doubt that one of the schools would have to go. Within a fortnight, however, the whole picture was altered. No one had taken seriously the option of increasing medical student numbers, but on 2 August the *Otago Daily Times* reported the Minister of Health had announced just that, an increase to 170. The Vice-Chancellor hinted that there had been informal talks on the issue, but the Dean of the Medical School had not been involved. 'Ironically', the *ODT* pointed out, 'the boost to intake comes within five years of two substantial cuts'. The following day, under the heading 'Doctor Shortage', the paper criticised the extent to which official attitudes on how many doctors the country needed had 'wavered rather wildly' in recent years.[15]

As Brinkman's retirement approached, the University requested his views on the future of the deanship. He advocated separating out the positions of Dean of Faculty and Dean of the Dunedin School. Aware that the two northern schools felt dominated by Dunedin, he believed that the change would remove any perception the Dean of Faculty was primarily interested in Dunedin.[16] Brinkman's colleagues expressed their appreciation of what he had managed to achieve in unpromising circumstances. 'In contrast to previous years', ran a valedictory minute at the December meeting of the Faculty Board in 1985, the eight-year period from 1978 had seen 'an enforced cut in student intake, the concomitant withdrawal of financial support, the freezing of many posts, the attendant repercussions on medical education of the Government's population-based funding of teaching hospitals, as well as a reduction in funding for medical research.' The Dean had not only battled on in this frustrating climate, he had 'found extra time and energy to improve the profile of the Otago Medical School, to further the School's standing in the community and in the political scene and

... make several important innovative thrusts.' It was noted that he was leaving his post just as the School's future was beginning to look rosier again. A similar minute at the Divisional Board also stressed Brinkman's personal commitment to the promotion of moral and ethical standards in the profession.[17]

Keeping the Wheels Oiled

THE TRANSFER of authority from one medical Dean to another always marks a point of change. However, the end of 1985 marked another change of some significance, the retirement of Sheila McKellar, personal secretary to five Deans over a period of thirty-five years. Indeed, the long-service achievement of the first three Otago Deans, eighty-one years from 1877 to 1958, may be matched by the sixty-five years' service of the two Deans' secretaries, Misses Thomson and McKellar, from 1920 to 1985.

The unflappable and supremely efficient Miss Thomson, appointed by Lindo Ferguson early in his deanship, 'kept the wheels of her department oiled and revolving so smoothly', wrote Carmalt Jones, 'that it was taken as a matter of course. Which it was not.' Hercus and Bell sketch a vivid picture of the dignified Ferguson pacing to and fro, and pausing from time to time for careful cogitation and the choice of a right word or phrase, as he dictated one of his many and voluminous reports to his faithful secretary. Miss Thomson stayed on to serve Sir Charles Hercus,

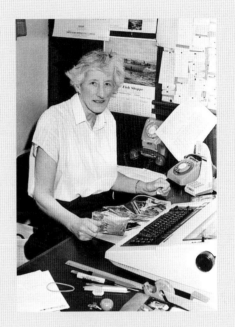

Sheila McKellar, 'Secretary with a special faculty'.
Otago Daily Times, 10 December 1985.

retiring in 1948 after twenty-eight years. By this time, the administrative work had increased to the point that a Medical School secretary was required (a role to be filled for many years by John H. Scott, grandson of the first Dean) and, later, three clerical assistants.

Sheila McKellar became confidential secretary to the Dean in 1948. Brought up in London, she had joined the WRENS in 1939 when she was eighteen years old, and served in South Africa, Egypt and England, before coming to New Zealand after the war. She soon knew the names of all the medical students, and kept an eye on the standard of their dress and hair. She also knew which were in need of help. Her concern for them was maintained after they left the School: she kept up the graduate file, adding information – employment, postgraduate qualifications, an up-to-date address – to each person's page as it came to light. Sheila McKellar was protective of her Deans, in turn, Sir Charles Hercus, Sir Edward Sayers, and Professors Bill Adams, John Hunter and Geoffrey Brinkman. If the time was unsuitable, the query if she could make an appointment for someone to see the Dean, might elicit the response, 'I could, but I wouldn't advise it.' Sheila McKellar died in 2005.[18]

'A Working Relationship' in a Difficult Environment, 1986–90

The Labour Government which took office in 1984 at once embarked on change radical enough to deserve the term social revolution. Upheavals in both the health system and the tertiary education system deeply affected the Medical School. At the same time, with new people in positions of authority in all three centres, there was some easing of tension between the Otago Medical School in Dunedin and the Schools of Medicine in Christchurch and Wellington.

Although, in its first term from 1984 to 1987, the Labour Government focused mainly on economic and fiscal policies, the controversial health system reforms begun under the previous Government proceeded apace. The Area Health Boards struggled to come to terms with their extensive responsibilities. It was indicative of the thinking of the day that in response to more expensive doctors' visits, increased hospital expenses and longer waiting lists, government advisers recommended giving a larger role to private and voluntary agencies, as well as making fundamental changes to hospital management and administration. When Helen Clark became Minister of Health in 1989, she added an emphasis on public health, which required Area Health Boards to negotiate public health goals with the Minister. Slowly the new hospital management system, which used professional administrators, settled in.[19]

There were equally rapid and far-reaching reforms in the tertiary education sector. Treasury had given an indication of its plans for education as early as 1984, when it made clear that it regarded education not as a public good but private capital, to be traded in a competitive marketplace. In 1988 the Hawke Report recommended the application of market liberalism to the universities. Through the State Sector Act the following year, Vice-Chancellors were brought into closer alignment with Chief Executives in the Public Service. Appointed for five-year renewable terms, they were expected to work with smaller Councils and were accountable to government according to individually negotiated charters. Competition

and private funding were encouraged, the University Grants Committee was disestablished and the allocations for teaching and research partially separated out. The medical Deans took over financial responsibility for their schools, in essence becoming general managers responsible to the University of Otago. As a consequence, the Schools' Councils, which lost some of their reason for existence, had to be restructured and Joint Relations Committees re-established with Hospital Boards.[20]

The mid-1980s saw an extensive change of personnel in the upper administrative ranks of the Otago Medical School. When John Hunter, who returned to Dunedin as Dean of Faculty, chaired his first meeting of the Faculty Board in April 1986, he welcomed newly appointed Deans from all three Schools. The Dean of the Dunedin School was David Stewart, a graduate of the School and the Mary Glendining Professor of Medicine from 1974. Stewart had already embarked on an outstanding career in academic administration in 1983, when he was appointed Brinkman's deputy. Hunter's place as Christchurch Dean was taken by another Otago graduate, Alan Clarke. Professor of Surgery in Dunedin since 1970, Clarke was energetic, innovative and clear on the direction he intended to take the School. In Wellington, the transition was less smooth. When Ralph Johnson's contract came up for renewal late in 1985, a three-person committee elected by staff to sound out opinion on his reappointment unexpectedly reported that a strong majority were against renewal. A brief visit by air to Wellington by the Vice-Chancellor and the Registrar saw the contract quickly terminated and Tom O'Donnell, who had been Deputy Dean, was appointed. No one knew the Wellington School better. Not only were all four Deans graduates of the Otago Medical School, they all knew each other well, in some cases for well over fifteen years. There was some rivalry involved but, as David Stewart commented, 'There was an enormous amount of history among the four of us … you now had a group of people who were well used to working with each other.' Johnson retained a full-time position with the Wellington Hospital Board, where he led his neurological research group

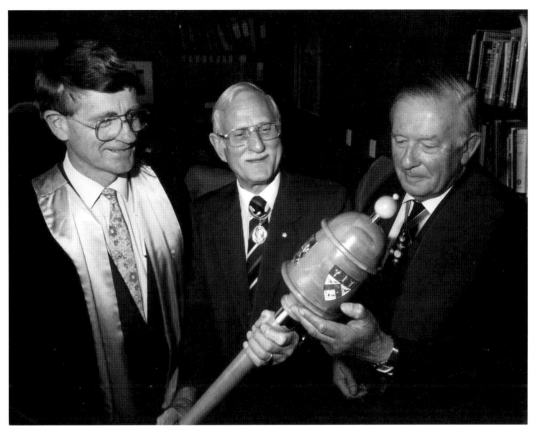

The President of the Canterbury Medical Research Foundation, Sir Lawrence Govan (centre), hands over a ceremonial mace, carved by the first Dean of the Christchurch School (Professor George Rolleston, right), to the current Dean, Professor Alan Clarke. The mace, intended for use on official occasions, such as the academic inauguration ceremony, inaugural lectures and prize-givings, carries four crests: of the Canterbury Province, the University of Otago, the Medical Staff Association and one representing the union between the Canterbury Hospital Board and the University of Otago from which the School was formed in 1972.
The Press, 16 December 1985.

and continued in clinical neurological practice for almost two years, before he returned to England.[21]

Some of the issues that had been worrying the northern schools for years were resolved quite quickly. One was the approval of the name change from Clinical Schools to the Christchurch and Wellington Schools of Medicine, a 'hugely symbolic political issue'. David Skegg remembered Hunter making this a condition of his taking on the deanship of Faculty. Of more practical importance was a change in the procedures around funding allocation. As Stewart described it, 'John opened the box and all of us sat down and looked at the size of the cake.' Until then, the income

of the Otago Medical School in Dunedin had been boosted by funding for a number of extra positions, specifically for its clinical departments, agreed to by the University Grants Committee. Stewart took the figures home, analysed them and, at the next meeting, proposed dividing all government funding equally, in a 'transparent funding carver' among the three Schools. Over the next two to three years, a formula was worked out which removed this 'significant aggro point'. While the medical sciences departments had to relinquish money to the Schools, their heads were both generous and pragmatic about this. 'Wellington and Christchurch', one of them said, 'are important to us.'[22]

By this time, all three schools were establishing their place in their own communities, and working towards good relations with their Area Health Boards. During Alan Clarke's deanship, the Christchurch School became closely linked to the local community and developed an identity distinctive to Canterbury. In 1987, the School held a three-day workshop, 'the Mission Conference', which helped clarify its identity and community responsibilities. Aided by the conference facilitators, the Dean and Administrator of Flinders University School of Medicine, the workshop identified the School's goals as providing excellence in patient care and health care. These goals were identical to those of Christchurch Hospital and their common mission was stressed. They agreed that the presence of medical students tended to improve health care and research, and led to a better outcome for patients. The workshop advocated the acceptance of more non-medical students, in a School of Health Sciences, and the provision of ongoing professional development for graduates. The obverse of this emerging Canterbury identity was the occasional expression of resentment towards the ties that bound the school to the University of Otago. Giving up on the possibility of affiliating with the University of Canterbury, the School toyed with the options of joining Lincoln College or becoming a fully independent institution, with graduate entry and its own basic science course provided by local medical scientists.[23]

In Wellington, O'Donnell enjoyed a good working relationship with his Area Health Board, in spite of the pressure the Board was under to provide health services to the region. Facilities the School shared with the Hospital, especially the Medical Library, benefited from a generous annual budget provision. O'Donnell met regularly with the Chief Executive to discuss budgets and joint staffing, had speaking rights at meetings of the Board and its committees, and experienced no difficulty in finding a consensus on appointments. On the other hand, he found the University staffing committee in Dunedin unhelpful about the promotion of staff with joint University/Hospital appointments. He believed they were disadvantaged by the emphasis the committee placed on research and thought the committee too ready to ignore the recommendations of both the Dean of the Faculty and the Dean of the School.[24]

In his first report to the Alumni in 1986, Hunter obliquely acknowledged the tensions by emphasising the need to maintain cohesion, understanding and mutual support if the Faculty was to progress in a time of political and economic pressure. While the increased student intake was helpful and there was evidence of some easing of the severe financial constraints of previous years, the clinical departments in all three centres, especially Dunedin, were suffering because of the inadequacy of the supplementary funds granted to the major teaching hospitals associated with the schools. The shortfall was an 'unfortunate by-product of the so-called equitable distribution of hospital funding based on population-based criteria', which ignored the pursuit of excellence in teaching centres. It was essential that the community, as well as the politicians, had a clearer understanding of the several roles of the medical schools. Preoccupation with the curriculum and the undergraduate medical course should not diminish the appreciation of the Schools' other roles. These included providing resource facilities and teachers for postgraduate and continuing medical education, teaching students of other faculties, assisting in health-related courses, upholding high standards of medical practice in the region and country and, most importantly, providing a major institution for the pursuit of medical and scientific research. 'Our medical schools', he wrote, 'are national resources for many purposes.'[25]

If the lines of accountability from the University to the Government had been sharply altered by the end of the 1980s, major changes to the University's own administrative structure also affected the Medical School. The Faculty of Medicine was joined with the Faculty of Dentistry in a new Division of Health Sciences, headed by an Assistant Vice-Chancellor. In 1989, Hunter added this responsibility to his role in the Medical Faculty and set about preparing the strategic plan required to fit in with the University's new charter. When he wrote his Alumnus report in 1989, he

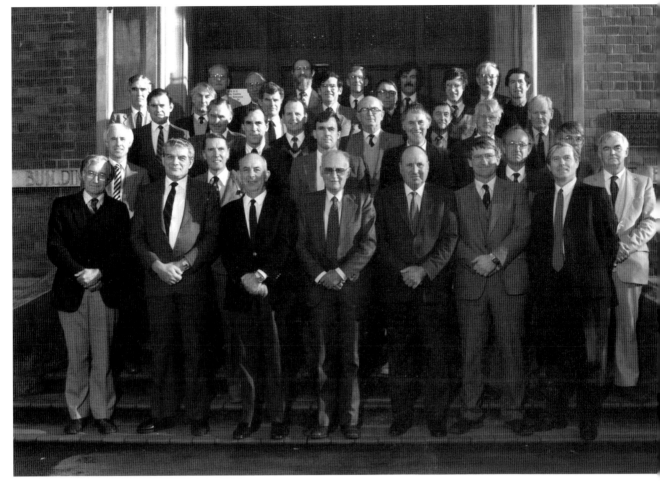

Faculty of Medicine Joint Heads of Departments meeting, Dunedin, 1–2 July 1987.
The group photo of professorial and associate-professorial Heads of Departments (thirty-nine, if the absentees are included)
illustrates the growth of the Medical School under the three-site model.

Otago Medical School

Back row, left to right: Professor J.B. Blennerhassett, Professor F.T. Shannon, Professor A.B. Baker,
Professor W.J. Gillespie, Professor M.S. Roberts, Professor G.B. Petersen.

Fourth row: Associate-Professor R.D. Gibson, Professor R. Laverty, Associate-Professor A.R. Hornblow,
Professor A.K. Jeffery, Associate-Professor J.M.B. Smith, Professor A.M. van Rij, Professor E.W. Pomare.
Third row: Professor J.D. Hutton, Professor D.R. Aickin, Professor J.G. Mortimer, Professor J. Campbell Murdoch,
Professor H.J. Weston, Professor G.O. Barbezat, Professor J.M. Gibbs, Professor W.A.A.G. Macbeth.

Second row: Professor G.W. Mellsop, Professor D.W. Beaven, Professor P.R. Joyce, Professor P.E. Mullen,
Associate-Professor R. Fraser, Professor W.H. Isbister, Professor W.H. Stehbens.

Front row: Professor L.A. Malcolm, Professor R.J. Seddon, Professor T.V. O'Donnell, (Dean, Wellington),
Mr C.A. Monroe (Secretary to the Faculty), Professor J.D. Hunter (Dean of Faculty),
Professor A.M. Clarke (Dean, Christchurch), Professor R.D.H. Stewart, (Dean, Dunedin).

Absent: Professor V.S. Chadwick, Professor J.I. Hubbard, Professor D.G. Jones,
Professor D.C.G. Skegg, Professor J.G.T Sneyd.

was just beginning the process. 'What sort of a plan this will be and how the future of the School will be affected', he wrote, 'will become clear in the next few months.'[26]

The strategic plan was not the only documentation required of the Dean at this time. Indeed, Hunter's last years in office seem to have been dominated by the production of a series of lengthy and complex reports. The longest was the information for the Medical School's accreditation by a review committee of the Medical Council of New Zealand. This was a new procedure. For many years, the General Medical Council of the United Kingdom had made periodic assessments of the University of Otago medical course, as it did for many other schools in the Commonwealth. Accreditation was always achieved for the MB ChB (Otago) to be recognised for full medical registration in the United Kingdom. The last on-site visit had been in 1974 and since then recognition had been granted annually, after written information was provided in response to specific questions.[27] In 1988, the Medical Council of New Zealand informed the University registrar that it wished to introduce a more formal accreditation procedure. The Council would send a committee of eight to visit the Otago and Auckland Medical Schools over several days, between May and July 1988. The preliminary information Hunter provided about the Faculty of Medicine describes the School, its history, administrative structure, staff, students, courses, examinations and research. It includes a section on what he saw as the 'Strengths, Weaknesses and Problems of the Otago Faculty of Medicine'. The document is the forerunner of the increasingly massive databases of 1994, 1999 and 2004, which were prepared for accreditation visits by the Australian Medical Council and, like them, it offers a sharply focused picture of the school at a particular moment.

In his assessment of the School's weaknesses, Hunter drew attention to the problems facing medical education that had resulted from the introduction of the Government's Vote Health policies and allocations. He pointed out that the level of supplementary funds for teaching granted to hospital boards with medical school connections fell far short of the allocations made in Britain and Australia. He argued that, while the academic staffing levels established through current University Grants Committee allocations could be regarded as satisfactory relative to those of other faculties, they were still 'sub-optimal'. As a consequence, growth was restricted in several areas of increasing relevance to future medical practice needs. Full Departments of General Practice and Geriatric Medicine, for example, were needed in the Christchurch and Wellington Schools.

Hunter was positive about the three divisions of the School. 'Although the separation of the three divisions is a definite disadvantage geographically and administratively, and limits the exchange between staff', he wrote, 'the presence of the Christchurch and Wellington Schools in their respective regions is now of great importance to the standards of medical practice maintained in those regions.' Moreover, the wider input into the Faculty from three regions, instead of one, enlarged its horizons.[28] In his last Dean's report, in 1990, Hunter noted with satisfaction the accreditation of the courses and curricula leading to the degree in medicine at the University of Otago, in this first formal procedure adopted by the Medical Council of New Zealand.[29]

At the turn of the century, Hunter looked back over his nine years as Dean of Faculty. In his first tenure, from 1974 to 1977, his primary task had been to work for the coordination and integration of the Faculty. On his return in 1986, he aimed to improve the cooperation among the three schools and ensure the equitable distribution of resources. He believed that, while greater stability had been achieved by 1990, the financial problems would eventually reappear. When he wrote, he was far enough removed from the day-to-day anxieties of the position to view them simply as part of the repeating pattern of the peaks and troughs of the Medical School's history.[30]

CHAPTER 23

The 1990s:
A Decade of Upheaval and Expansion

The Medical School and the Health Reforms

There is no intrinsic reason why the beginning of a new decade should be taken to mark the beginning of a new era but there is a good case that, for the Otago Medical School, the year 1990 did just that. When a National Government surged into power after six years of Labour, it brought in far-reaching changes to the education and health sectors which affected the Medical School directly and deeply. It was the responsibility of David Stewart, as Dean of Faculty for the first half of the decade and Assistant Vice-Chancellor Health Sciences for almost all of it, to meet the challenges and take advantage of the opportunities of a very different environment in both tertiary education and the health sector. He worked very effectively in this, leading the School through an initial period of stress, to the restructuring of its Dunedin component into the Dunedin School of Medicine and the new Otago School of Medical Sciences. He oversaw the expansion of staff and postgraduate student numbers and the introduction of new health-related courses in all the schools. He initiated innovative curriculum changes at all levels and fostered a research environment. Stewart also oversaw preparation for the first accreditation review by the Australian Medical Council in 1994 and the preliminary work for the second review in 1999.

Stewart called the '90s a 'decade of expansion', pointing to underlying factors in the external environment and facilitating factors in the internal environment to justify the description. He identified the following as the principal external factors: the abolition of the University Grants Committee, with its rigid quinquennial funding grants, and its replacement by funding based on annual student numbers; open and flexible arrangements for the accreditation of new courses; the opening of the tertiary sector to external full fee-paying students; and changes in research funding, especially the establishment of a contestable Public Good Science Fund, but also more commercial investment in research and the acceptance of the principle of full cost funding of research by the Health Research Council. Within the University, Stewart noted with approval the trend towards financial devolution, with clear incentives to increase revenue, the relative autonomy of the Clinical Schools, changes to the first-year health sciences course and the growth of other health science programmes aligned to the medical course, such as Pharmacy and Physiotherapy, the Bachelor of Medical Laboratory Science course, bachelor and doctoral degrees in medical science and various paramedical programmes.[1]

Under his leadership, the Faculty of Medicine responded to these changes by participating willingly in the new health science programmes. The Faculty also benefited from an increase in student numbers, justifying the establishment of new chairs and expansions to accommodation, either by the construction of new buildings, such as that for Physiotherapy, or extensive upgrades, for example, to the Hercus and Biochemistry Buildings and the Christchurch School. Research flourished in all the centres. The period was viewed less positively, however, by clinical staff of the School, who were caught between conflicting demands from the hospitals and the University.

The Political Environment

In both the education and health sectors far-reaching changes, initiated by the Labour Government in the late 1980s, were brought into full operation under National in the 1990s. The recommendations of the 1988 Hawke Report on post-compulsory education and training, with its across-the-board approach to tertiary institutions, business model of administration and user-pays funding, had created a furore in University circles. While the Government held back from implementing the recommendations fully, it did bring in major funding changes and a new fees regime in what has been called a 'Treasury triumph' in tertiary education and made changes to the universities' administrative structure. Vice-Chancellors were put on five-year contracts and, although these could be renewed, the twenty-year record of Sir Robin Irvine (as he became in 1989) was unlikely to be challenged by any successor after he retired in 1993. National went further, giving the Hawke recommendations legislative form in the Education Amendment Act of July 1990. The universities strenuously opposed certain elements of the Act. The Vice-Chancellors waged a lengthy and ultimately successful battle to maintain their academic freedom against the threat of 'quality control' by a new Qualifications Authority. They were less successful in their attempts to save the University Grants Committee which, despite numerous disputes over financial allocations, had served them well as their advocate before government. The old system of quinquennial grants, which had permitted the security of longer-term planning, was replaced by one in which the universities were bulk funded on annual estimates of student numbers.[2] For the students, there were also dramatic changes. Because tertiary education was now classed as a private privilege, students were expected to contribute a higher proportion of its cost through increased course fees. Entitlement to the Study Right student allowance was reduced from five to three years and the amount, which was also reduced, set at a low threshold and based on the parental income of the student, up to the age of twenty-four. A state-funded student loan scheme was introduced, with the loan to be repaid once the student had graduated and was in paid employment. Because of the length and expense of their course, the impact of the new arrangements on medical students was especially sharp.[3]

Changes to the health system were equally far-reaching and occurred with disconcerting frequency during the decade. Robin Gauld, the historian of New Zealand health policy, wrote in 2005 that 'Since 1989 New Zealand has had four completely different systems for the delivery of publicly funded health care'. These comprised an area health board system in 1989–91, a competitive internal market system from 1993 to 1996, a central planning and purchasing system from 1996 to 1999 and, from 2000, a district health board system.[4] Although the Labour Government had decided not to implement the sweeping structural changes to hospital management and administration recommended by the 1988 Gibbs Taskforce on Hospitals and Related Services, it did make a number of significant changes. It restructured and streamlined the Health Department, required Area Health Boards to become more accountable to the Government and introduced a business model system of general management to hospital administration. Initially unpopular, these changes were providing increased efficiency by the end of 1990 when the government changed. National's 1991 budget signalled something much more radical. To implement a concept of separating purchasers and providers, the fourteen Area Health Boards were replaced by four Regional Health Authorities, headed by government-appointed commissioners who contracted for health services. The larger hospitals became Crown Health Enterprises, with appointed Chief Executives and Boards of Directors. As they

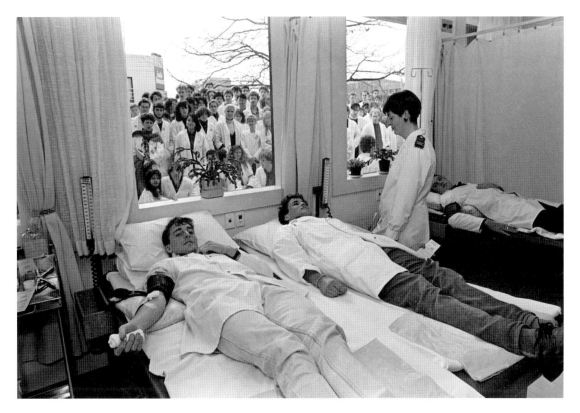

A 'Bleeding' Protest.
More than three hundred medical students in white coats line the footpaths outside
Dunedin Hospital to give blood in protest at the 'bleeding' of the health system.
Here third-year students (left to right) Blair Leslie, Grant Christie and Matthew Reid,
with charge donor attendant Margaret Budge, are watched
by fellow students through the window.
Stephen Jaquiery, *Otago Daily Times*, 25 July 1991.

were expected to make a profit, part-charges for hospital services were introduced. A Public Health Commission was established to advise government.[5] The new system was hurried into place by July 1993.

A new Dean faced the challenges that these arrangements posed to the Medical School. John Hunter, as Dean of Faculty and foundation Assistant Vice-Chancellor, Health Sciences, had led the School into the new age of market liberalism and enhanced accountability, of accreditation reviews and strategic and corporate plans. It would be his successor, Professor David Stewart, who developed the role of AVC Health Sciences and who set his mark on the 1990s. When he took over in 1991, Stewart was well prepared for his dual role as AVC and Dean of Faculty. Most recently,

as Dean of the Dunedin School since 1986, he had worked closely with Hunter and served on the Otago Hospital Board. He had the experience and the skills to guide the Medical School through an unsettled and unsettling period and take advantage of the opportunities offered by the new arrangements. He appreciated the fact that bulk funding allowed the School more control over spending and that there was also active encouragement to search for additional non-government income, an exercise in which the Otago Medical School had already shown considerable initiative. He found fewer obstacles in the way of setting up new courses.[6] It was on the clinical staff of the Medical School, whether in Dunedin, Christchurch or Wellington, that the repeated upheavals in the health system had the most direct and sharpest effect. Early in 1994, Stewart pointed out the potential threats posed by the change of ownership of the teaching hospitals. A range of issues were involved: the employment of joint clinical staff, conditions of access for staff and students to clinical training and research, provision of accommodation within the teaching hospitals for School of Medicine staff and students, the supervision and teaching of students and trainees by hospital staff and the provision of services, such as library access.[7] The attitude of Healthcare Otago (as the new Dunedin Crown Health Enterprise was called) was not reassuring. In August 1993, the local press reported Healthcare Otago's estimate of what the School's teaching and research cost it annually, under the headline 'Medical School costs CHE $1m'. Early the next year, Healthcare Otago warned it might cut some specialist tertiary medical services linked to the University.[8]

The Health Reforms, Clinical Teaching and Accreditation

It was unfortunate timing that in 1994, while the new health system had not settled and its effect on the Medical School was still in doubt, the School was reviewed for the first time by an accreditation team from the Australian Medical Council (AMC). This was an immensely significant development. One of the first acts of the AMC when it was set up in 1985 had been to establish a process to ensure that new Australian medical graduates were 'competent and responsive to the health needs both of individual citizens and communities.' It began by assessing the teaching at the Australian medical schools, using guidelines provided by the General Medical Council of Great Britain, but after reviewing six Australian schools, it developed its own guidelines in 1992. By an agreement with the Medical Council of New Zealand, the AMC extended its accreditation process to include the two New Zealand medical schools, so that their graduates had the right to practise in Australia. The Accreditation Committee was expanded to include two members appointed on the advice of the Medical Council of New Zealand (MCNZ)

and it was agreed that assessment teams visiting New Zealand would include at least one assessor suggested by MCNZ. The visit to the Otago School, from 31 July to 5 August 1994, was the first in New Zealand. In advance of the visit, the School was required to provide extensive documentation, which was followed up by a full schedule of interviews, with faculty, graduates and students in Dunedin, Christchurch and Wellington, staff of the hospitals providing teaching facilities and government offices such as the Ministries of Health and Crown Health Enterprises: more than three hundred persons in all. The team of seven was led by Professor Richard Larkins, Chairman of the Department of Medicine at the Royal Melbourne Hospital, University of Melbourne. The New Zealand member was Professor Peter Gluckman, Dean of the Auckland School of Medicine.[9] The report of the 1994 accreditation team, and those of subsequent teams in 1999 and 2004, have not only provided expert assessment of the school's activities but also required certain changes to be made in its practices within a given time frame, if accreditation was to be granted. The reports have thus given, and continue to give, direction and impetus to the overall development of the Otago Medical School.

Included in the written material prepared for the committee were comments by the Dean of Faculty and the Deans of the three schools on the relations between the new Crown Health Enterprises (CHEs) and the Medical School. David Stewart was guardedly optimistic. He summed up that after a 'frustrating beginning' in 1993, the three schools were each developing effective relationships with the new owners of the major teaching hospitals. The school Deans were also cautious. The Dunedin Dean, Graham Mortimer, went into most detail, raising issues that affected the northern schools as well. There were many uncertainties, he believed, in the relations between the School in Dunedin and Healthcare Otago, which administered the Dunedin and Wakari Hospitals. The former joint relations agreement and the Joint Relations Committee, at which matters of common interest had regularly been discussed, had been discontinued in July 1993 and had not been replaced. Both hospitals were staffed by a mix of clinical staff and CHE specialists with joint appointments, but arrangements for student and staff access to the hospitals, for clinical training and clinical research, were unclear. He was awaiting with some anxiety the results of 'unbundling' exercises then in train to ascertain the respective additional costs incurred by these activities. An understanding was being negotiated about the joint employment of University clinical staff, on a 50/50 basis, and for rental of academic space in the Hospital ward block. However, it was worrying that the Otago Medical School had little input into the Healthcare Otago boards or committees. In Christchurch, Andrew Hornblow reported, the scale and complexity of the issue was compounded by the fact that five urban hospitals, Christchurch, Burwood, Christchurch Women's, Princess Margaret and Sunnyside, were involved in the teaching and research activities of the Christchurch School, and that their services were controlled by two separate CHEs, Canterbury Health and Healthlink South. Relationships were still being negotiated. In Wellington, Eru Pomare explained that relations were still not formalised with the principal teaching hospitals, Wellington Hospital, operated by Capital Coast Health, and Hutt Hospital, operated by Hutt Valley Health Corporation. The Wellington School had had very little time working with the CHEs but there was a firm intention on both sides to maintain a close relationship under the new system.[10]

The AMC team recommended that the Otago Medical School be given accreditation for five years, rather than the maximum ten, and that this was subject to certain conditions. The first of these was that 'urgent discussions' should be held with the relevant Regional Health Authorities and Crown Health Enterprises, to resolve the uncertainties and problems identified in the report. Satisfactory progress was to be demonstrated within twelve months. In its 'Conclusions and Recommendations' the report pulled no punches. The Faculty, it stated baldly, was 'faced with a number of major threats which in some areas had already affected the educational process and which would need decisive action from within the Faculty and University, as well as strong support from all tiers of the health and

education systems, from the Minister down, to overcome.' The first of these threats came from the health reforms and the unresolved nature of the relations between the Medical School on its three sites and the RHAs and CHEs. Without wishing to comment on the merits or otherwise of the reforms, or the 'unbundling' exercise that was attempting to separate out the costs associated with teaching and research, as opposed to service, the team believed it was 'entirely counterproductive' to attempt to separate the time spent in the delivery of undergraduate teaching, postgraduate training and service delivery by an individual, on a day-to-day basis. The team found the different approaches taken by different CHEs a cause for concern. It also noted the general exclusion of University staff from business planning procedures and the continued insistence on breaking down activities for contractual and funding purposes.[11]

Over the next few years, in Christchurch and Dunedin, relations between the CHEs and the schools remained tense, with clinical staff holding joint appointments caught in the middle. There were various attempts to resolve the differences. Memoranda of Understanding were signed between all three schools and their respective CHEs late in 1994, which formalised the setting up of Joint Relations Committees. While the annual reports of that year noted a resultant improvement in relations, meetings of the Committees revealed the two bodies had fundamental differences in attitude.[12]

At the end of the year, the Government announced that the Public Health Commission, which had been set up to give independent advice to government, was not an appropriate principal policy adviser and it was disestablished. It was generally believed that the Commission was axed because its advice tended to contradict the Government's market-oriented policies and that it had fallen foul of the powerful food, alcohol and tobacco industries. Professor David Skegg, who had chaired the Commission, argued strongly that some replacement body should be set up to give independent advice to government.[13]

The CHEs themselves were under acute financial pressure. They were not funded for teaching and research and threats that they might 'exit' these activities polarised academic staff and CHE management in Christchurch and Dunedin. The disputes were acrimonious and were fully aired in public. When Canterbury Health's Chief Executive Officer was quoted in the press as saying that managing doctors was like herding cats, the Dean of Faculty and the Dean of the Christchurch School joined in a strong response. The *Press* headline ran 'Culture change is not the problem – a rigidly authoritarian style is', beneath which the Deans demanded a fundamental change in management style. In August 1996, the Chief Executive resigned, followed a few months later by the Chair of the Board. The medical staff complained that management decisions were putting patients at risk and passed a vote of no confidence in Canterbury Health management. This led to an investigation into the Hospital's practices and a scathing report by the Health and Disability Commissioner. The Christchurch School's relations with Healthlink South, which

had responsibility for mental health, women's health and health care of the elderly, were more amicable.[14]

In Dunedin, financial pressures on both sides, and the confrontational style of Healthcare Otago CEO John Ayling and his team of three general managers, exacerbated disputes between Healthcare Otago and the Medical School from 1995. There were some high-profile departures among the academic staff. Pathology was especially hard hit. In April 1996, as Healthcare Otago was moving to a joint venture deal with a private company for use of the Dunedin Hospital laboratory, the highly respected Professor John Blennerhassett took early retirement. Two of his senior staff in the Pathology Department left at the same time. In June, Alistair Campbell, the high-profile Professor of Biomedical Ethics and foundation Director of the Bioethics Research Centre, established in 1990, resigned to take up a position in Britain. Before he left, he fired a parting salvo at the health system. In a lecture

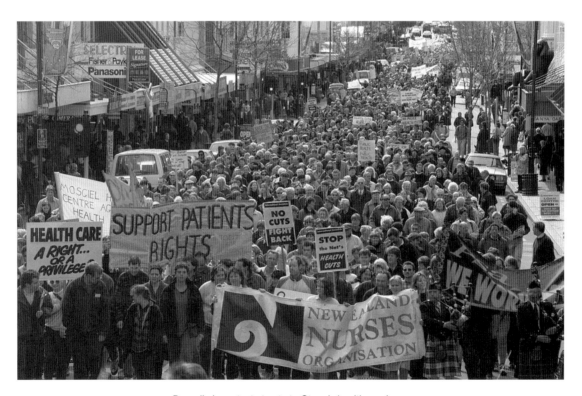

Dunedin in protest at cuts to Otago's health services.
Otago Daily Times, 20 September 1997.

entitled 'Dangerous Liaisons: ethics, politics and health care', he slated the booking system for hospital treatment, the increase in private surgery in public hospitals, the disbanding of the Public Health Commission and the push for a more commercially driven health system.[15] Early in 1997, the *Otago Daily Times* reported that relations between the CHE and the Medical School were at a low ebb, with the two parties locked in dispute over who should pay an agreed 3 per cent salary rise to about fifty joint clinical staff. Other CHEs had met this cost, but Healthcare Otago refused.[16]

Dunedin, with its limited population and traditional pride in its Medical School, was strongly opposed to funding hospitals on a population-based model that did not take into account the extra costs (and benefits) associated with clinical teaching and appeared to threaten medical education in the city. This was reflected in the local press. An editorial early in 1997 put it bluntly: 'If the population-based funding model is retained, then the Dunedin Medical School is clearly doomed, as is the scale of medical and surgical services at Dunedin hospital.'[17] A few weeks later a lengthy, anonymous article was given prominence in the paper. Headed 'Inefficiency in delivering medical teaching', it argued that the only way to cut the costs of the Otago Medical School was to close the clinical school in Dunedin. Faculty Dean John Campbell, given right of reply on the same page, lambasted the article as 'simplistic and inaccurate'. He was supported soon after by an open letter from the Dean and an Associate Dean of the Auckland Medical School. They affirmed that New Zealand needed two medical schools, arguing that the bulk of the costs in teaching hospitals did not

arise from medical education and so could not be laid at the door of the Medical School.[18]

By this time, action was under way to end the impasse between Healthcare Otago and the Dunedin School of Medicine. In December 1996 the two institutions jointly commissioned Suzanne Snively, of Coopers and Lybrand, to assess the 'clinical, service and financial impacts of their association with each other.' The position of each of the parties was clear. Healthcare Otago was required to provide health and disability services while operating as a successful and efficient business. Increasingly specific Regional Health Authority contracts had led to a more defined focus on health care services, and the CHE's new management structure and responsibilities reduced the traditional role of Heads of Department of the Dunedin School. The School required access for its students to various medical services and experiences traditionally supplied by Healthcare Otago. Both parties wanted to ensure that they were not bearing additional costs because of the relationship. A four-person project team carried out detailed research and reported, in September 1997, that there was direct, quantifiable added value in the joint relationship, as well as certain indirect costs and benefits. The key issue, and the most complex, involved staff costs, which the team assessed by dividing staff into three categories. Joint clinical staff were perceived to be a cost to the Dunedin School of Medicine because the clinical demands on their time prevented them fulfilling the services required of them by the School. Clinical lecturers in some departments were perceived as a benefit, because their level of service exceeded remuneration. Junior medical staff, practitioners and registrars, employed by Healthcare Otago, provided the benefit of unpaid teaching services to the Medical School. Overall, the report found the School bore a cost, but it was 'insignificant'. The report rejected the option of separating the two institutions, recommending instead that they add further value by defining and developing their relationship.[19]

The Snively Report was welcomed by those clinicians of the Dunedin School who had felt increasingly pressured by the burden of hospital work. They saw it as marking a significant turning point. The Chief Executive of Healthcare Otago was less pleased and it is possible the report may have been one of the factors which prompted him to resign, after less than four years in the job, in April 1998. At a press interview in June, he openly discussed his unpopularity, the price he had paid, he said, for heading a CHE which had been constantly forced to restructure (the workforce had been reduced by 10 per cent under his management) and deal with funding pressures. Within a few weeks and in the wake of a ten-day strike by junior doctors, the three senior managers he had appointed in September 1995 also resigned.[20]

An immediate change of tone and policy followed the change of personnel, supporting Stewart's contention that it was not the health reforms as such that had been the problem, but the people implementing them. The Chairman of the Board of Healthcare Otago, Ross Black, took over as a conciliatory and efficient Acting Chief Executive, until Dr Bill Adam was appointed at the end of 1998. Adam was medically qualified and saw the school as an ally, not an opponent. In a Faculty Newsletter, in April 1998, Campbell noted pleasing changes to the Healthcare Otago Board, including the appointment of Stewart as adviser, to become a full member when he retired at the end of the year.[21] In December, Ross Black wrote encouragingly to Healthcare Otago's 3200 staff that, 'We have firmly left behind a time and culture that was not an Otago culture'. He congratulated staff on their impressive level of efficiency and affirmed that the Board was 'totally committed to providing an open and inclusive

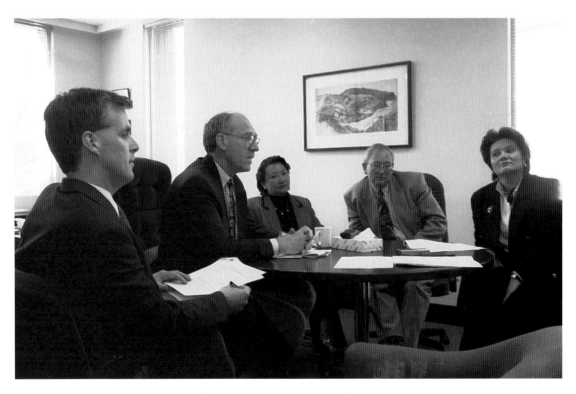

In July 1998, in what the *Otago Daily Times* reported as a 'corporate clean-out', the last three senior managers of the team appointed by Healthcare Otago's Chief Executive John Ayling three years earlier resigned. It marked the end of a period of extreme tension between Healthcare Otago and the Medical School. Cooper had resigned in October 1997 and Ayling in April 1998. The others all left in July. The *ODT* printed this photo with the word 'Left' in bold at centre top and arrows pointing to each person with their date of resignation.

From left to right: Donovan Wearing, John Ayling, Susan Law, Nic Cooper and Dr Coralee Barker.

Otago Daily Times, 29 July 1998.

environment.' The good news continued. The *ODT* could report, in July 1999, that Healthcare Otago had outperformed its 1998 budget and was likely to break even for the first time. This achievement was attributed, in large part, to a reduction in ongoing non-medical costs of running the hospital.[22]

The friendlier local atmosphere in Dunedin mirrored broader changes in health policy, what Gauld calls the 're-reforms' of the National/ New Zealand First Coalition Government, which assumed power after the country's first proportional representation (MMP) election. Under a revised scheme, announced in the 1998 budget, the four Regional Health Authorities were combined into a centralised Health Funding Authority, intended to ensure equity and standardisation in service access and funding. Vote Health funding was increased. The Crown Health Enterprises were renamed Health and Hospital Services (HHS), with a stress on cooperation rather than competition. They were expected to be business-like, but were not required to make a profit.[23]

Whether the health reforms of the early 1990s were misguided, as most clinical staff of the Medical School believed – and some were disenchanted enough to depart – or simply gave authority in certain cases to people without the skills or sensitivities to handle it, as others maintain, the tension between the Otago Medical School and Healthcare Otago attracted a considerable amount of media attention. It also runs as a disturbing theme through the report of the 1994 Australian Medical Council accreditation team. The Medical School, as the Dean of Faculty reminded the next AMC accreditation team in 1999, had been 'operating in an environment which was at best indifferent and at worst hostile', to which the School had adjusted only slowly. By 1999, however, the 'rigid and naïve' philosophy behind the first wave of health reforms had been tempered by experience and reality, with competition giving way to cooperation, and the requirement for hospitals to make a profit softened to recommendations for a business-like approach. It was possible to engage in medium- to long-term planning. Whereas in the early 1990s

teaching and research had not been considered the core business of the teaching and tertiary hospitals in New Zealand, this had changed in 1998, with the Ministry of Health requiring the Health Funding Authority to formalise access arrangements for students with education providers. On the Joint Relations Committees at each of the main teaching hospitals, the Chair of the Board and the Chief Executive would typically sit with the Vice-Chancellor, Dean of Faculty and Dean of School. Informal working relations were also good. The financial pressures on the HHS remained, but were being met with greater understanding. Students were also able to gain clinical experience in smaller hospitals and through community contact weeks organised from Christchurch, Dunedin and Wellington.[24] The crisis of the 1990s was over.

The report of the 1999 AMC accreditation team confirmed this positive view. Otago had opted for a limited review, that would add another five years onto the period for which accreditation had been granted in 1994. The team which visited in March 1999 gave special attention to relationships between the Medical School and the health services. It echoed the Dean's view, noting with approval that there had been a 'widespread and significant change in the ethos of the healthcare system' in its structures, policies and personnel. The AMC team singled out for favourable comment the evolution of policies emphasising cooperation rather than competition, good business practice rather than profitability and explicit recognition, in strategic and business planning, of the contribution of teaching and research to their goals.[25] The team also considered issues specific to each school. In Christchurch, for example, disputes between the Department of Psychological Medicine, the CHE and Sunnyside service had been settled. Team members were especially impressed with the Christchurch School's recently completed teaching facilities and approved the extent to which academic activities were embedded within the hospital services. Tensions between the Wellington School and the HHS had also largely been overcome and there was close cooperation between the Dean and the Hospital's Chief

Executive Officer. In Dunedin, where a change of personnel went with the change in government directives, strong leadership was contributing to a significant improvement. The Dunedin School was also less reliant on Dunedin Hospital for students' clinical experience, because it was using smaller hospitals in the region and developing an innovative plan for rurally-based clinical teaching.[26] All in all, the problems identified five years before had been resolved as far as was practicable.

It would be tidy to end there, but the topic is not tidy. Once again changes in the health sector were followed almost immediately by a change of government and further, initially disruptive, change. The Labour-led Coalition Government that took power in 1999 had included health restructuring in its election promises and at once set about implementing a system of District Health Boards along the lines of its 1989–91 scheme. The aim, as Gauld summed up, was for democratised, locally controlled decision-making over planning, resource allocation and services configuration, and a focus on service integration and collaboration. This meant reasserting the overall responsibility of the Ministry of Health as chief policy adviser, planner and funder of public health and creating twenty-one regionally based District Health Boards (DHBs) responsible for planning and purchasing services in consultation with their communities. The DHBs, which were mainly elected, with various specialist sub-committees responsible to them, were to be run by a full-time chief executive. The HFA was abolished, and its functions divided between the Ministry of Health and the District Health Boards, a complex exercise. A series of health strategies were signalled, in areas such as Maori health, child health, diabetes, cardiac disease and the reduction of alcohol, drug and tobacco use. Some elements of earlier systems remained in place, such as Pharmac, the pharmaceutical purchasing agency, the nurturing of 'by Maori, for Maori' health care and the controversial clinical scoring criteria for prioritising non-urgent surgery. Gauld's assessment of the successive health reforms is that they were disruptive and expensive and that New Zealand needed to be

'Through the restructuring period, when key changes corresponded with general elections and a change of government, planning and purchasing responsibilities have been decentralised, marketised, centralised, then decentralised again, while service providers have been required to compete and then collaborate with one another.'

Robin Gauld, 'New Zealand', in *Comparative Health Policy in Asia and the Pacific*, 2005.

protected from further politically motivated restructuring.[27] It is likely that the Medical School clinicians of the day would agree.

By the time of the next accreditation report, in late 2004, the relationship between the Medical School and the health sector had ceased to be a significant concern. The Faculty and its Schools were considered to have 'very good constructive relationships' with the District Health Boards and the administrations of the major health units. The Faculty was strongly represented on appropriate bodies in the health sector and had a good working relationship with the Ministry.[28]

'A Decade of Expansion': Staffing and Restructuring

The clinical staff of the Otago Medical School might well have found the 1990s the most stressful period of their professional lives, and the press certainly found the confrontations between the CHEs and the Medical School excellent copy. However, the overall picture of the decade for the Medical School, in all three centres, was one of expansion in staffing, innovation in teaching and distinction in research. It did not start well, however. When David Stewart took over as AVC, he was confronted by reduced budget allocations for medicine as well as for dentistry and pharmacy.' He responded by freezing all new and replacement staff positions. The financial pressure was caused by two events: the change to funding in the University based on student numbers and the transfer of staff superannuation costs, which had previously been borne by registry, to cost centres.

The Dean of the Otago School, Graham Mortimer, believed that although the freeze was brief, its effects lingered on. Immediately, the effects were certainly sharp. The Chair of Paediatrics, which Mortimer had relinquished to become Dean, remained vacant until 1999. Overseas applicants for some posts, who were going through the appointment process, had to be told there was no job after all. In Anaesthesia, the loss was particularly serious. There was no professorial replacement when Barry Baker, who had been appointed from Queensland as the Foundation Professor in 1975 and led the department from strength to strength for seventeen years, accepted a position in Sydney at the end of 1992. It marked the end of the 'golden years' of the department in the late 1980s and early 1990s, when staffing had been built to an appropriate level, research in well-appointed laboratories had flourished and the impact of the health reforms had not yet hit home. Added to the loss of professorial leadership, was the disestablishment of some lecturer positions and a number of staff departures. Even in 2006, there was evidence that the department had failed to regain the 'collective strength and wellbeing' of those years.[29] As it happened, the freeze coincided with the retirement of some senior academic staff of many years' standing. Wellington was especially hard hit, with the loss of four of its foundation professors. Tom O'Donnell, Professor of Medicine since 1972 and Dean since 1986, Bill Stehbens, Professor of Pathology, and Jeffray Weston, Professor of Paediatrics, all retired and Richard Seddon, Professor of Obstetrics and Gynaecology, transferred to the Dunedin School. Although a new Dean, Professor Eru Pomare, was appointed, professorial appointments were deferred. O'Donnell registered his personal protest by absenting himself from the Senate dinner in Dunedin, at which he was to have been the principal respondent to the toast to retiring professors.[30] In Wellington, the retirements were given front page coverage in the *Dominion* newspaper when a large gathering of school staff, students and friends, including the Vice-Chancellor, the Mayor of Wellington and the Chairman of the Wellington Hospital Board, came together to pay tribute to the professors' role,

over fifteen years, in establishing the Wellington School on a firm basis.[31]

The stay on appointments did not last long. By April 1992, David Stewart could assure the *Otago Daily Times* that the Medical School was not under threat of closure and that the School would soon be recruiting, not shedding staff.[32] By the end of the year, all the schools were indeed reporting new appointments, as well as sometimes disgruntled departures. In Dunedin, Sarah Romans was appointed to the Chair of Psychological Medicine and there were several appointments to associate-professorships and associate-deanships. Some long-serving members of staff retired, including Professor Pat Molloy of Cardiac Surgery. As well as Barry Baker, Dunedin lost David Palmer, who retired from a personal Chair in Rheumatology and Campbell Murdoch, who left the Elaine Gurr Chair of General Practice. Murdoch, New Zealand's first Professor of General Practice, was typically outspoken about his reason for leaving: inadequate funding for health care. Professor Paul Mullen and eight staff from Psychological Medicine departed about the same time, leaving a disturbingly high workload for those who remained. Nevertheless, the approval to fill vacant posts was 'morale-boosting'. Murray Tilyard was appointed to the Chair of General Practice and several other positions were advertised in 1993.[33]

The Wellington School was buoyed by the appointment of its new Dean, who was universally admired and liked. As an outstanding Maori graduate and leader Eru Pomare was, as his colleague and successor Linda Holloway put it, 'a Dean whose time had come'. But it was not easy. Wellington took rather longer to recover from the staffing freeze than the other centres. In his first annual report, in 1992, Pomare wrote that the staffing situation remained precarious, with three key chairs still unfilled. When cost-cutting by the Wellington Area Health Board was added to the restrictions on the school's budget, staff found themselves 'stretched to the limit'. In 1993, he reported another 'difficult' year in the Wellington School, with the majority of departments still without professorial leadership. He welcomed the appointment of Richard Beasley as Professor of Medicine, but noted that Psychological Medicine

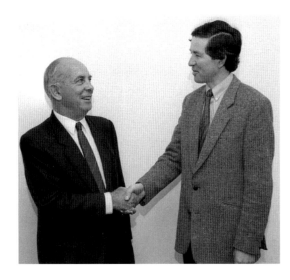

Retiring Dean of the Wellington School, Professor Tom O'Donnell (left) hands over to his successor, Professor Eru Pomare.
University of Otago, Wellington.

'I want Maori people to reach their full potential. We are proud of many achievements. We look forward as Iwi and as a people to where we want to go. It can be an exciting future where leadership and clear direction will be essential ...'

Eru Pomare, in the Maori newspaper *Kia Hiwa Ra*, April 1994, cited in *Tihei Mauri Ora!* The Maori Health Commission 1999, p. 8.

Professor Eru Woodbine Pomare, 1942–1995

MB ChB, MD, FRACP,
Dean, Wellington School of Medicine 1992–95

ERU POMARE came of a distinguished family. Of Te Atiawa, Ngati Mutunga, Ngati Toa, Ngati Kahungunu, Rongomaiwahine, Rongo Whakaata, Te Aitanga-a-Mahiki descent, he was the grandson of Sir Maui Pomare, the first Maori medical graduate, Minister of Health and Minister of Internal Affairs, who did much to benefit Maori health in the 1920s.[34] Educated at Wanganui Collegiate, Eru Pomare entered Otago Medical School with a Ngarimu VC Scholarship and graduated in 1966. He did his specialist training at Wellington Hospital, becoming a member of the Royal Australasian College of Physicians in 1970 and a fellow in 1975. A Commonwealth Scholarship enabled him to undertake advanced study in gastroenterology at Bristol, where he took his MD, and in Canada. He published on nutrition and gastroenterology and was recognised for his work on dietary fibre.

Returning to the new Wellington Clinical School in 1975, as senior lecturer in medicine, he championed Maori health. In 1981, he published the first edition of *Maori Standards of Health*, which contained accurate data for the years 1955 to 1975. It was the basis for his future research. He chaired the Maori Health Committee of the Health Research Council and set up the Maori Health Research Unit, Te Hotu Manawa Maori, at the Wellington School of Medicine. He chaired the ministerial Maori Asthma Review. He held many other positions in national health organisations, such as the Cancer Society of New Zealand, the New Zealand Drug Foundation, the Royal Australasian College of Physicians and the Medical Council of New Zealand. Linda Holloway, his friend and successor as Dean, called him the 'ultimate multi-tasker'. He became Professor of Medicine at the Wellington School in 1986 and Dean in 1992.

Eru Pomare was just fifty-two years old when he died. A colleague wrote of him, 'His instantly engaging manner, gentle compassion and open and honest friendship were a unique blend of qualities rarely found in someone who reaches the top of his chosen profession'. More simply, another said he was a 'marvellous guy'. His premature death robbed New Zealand medicine and Maoridom of a special leader. The Maori Health Research Unit at the Wellington School of Medicine is named in his honour.[35]

had been badly hit by the resignation of three senior staff, including Professor Graham Mellsop, and the small Obstetrics and Gynaecology department was finding it hard to manage with the resignation of Professor Hutton. The chairs of Psychological Medicine, Paediatrics and Pathology were all under advertisement. There were achievements, however. The most significant was the establishment, in 1992, of Te Manawa Hauora, the Maori Health Research Centre, to be funded for three years by the Health Research Council under Pomare's directorship. The Asthma Research Group also gained HRC funding, for five years. By 1994 new Heads of Department had been appointed in Pathology, Psychological Medicine, Public Health and Obstetrics and Gynaecology, as well as some senior lecturers.[36]

Over the summer break, in January 1995, tragedy struck. Eru Pomare died suddenly while on a tramping holiday. Professor Linda Holloway, Acting Dean while he was away, found herself continuing in the post and was then appointed to it. Holloway, the School's first woman Dean, was Scottish by birth and a graduate of the University of Aberdeen. She had come to New Zealand with her Kiwi husband, a forest scientist she had met when he was studying in Aberdeen, in 1970. She spent some time in rural practice in Central Otago and as a pathologist in Dunedin Hospital, before joining the Pathology Department of the Wellington School in 1979. By 1996, she could report that the staffing situation at the school was improving. Professor Brett Delahunt had taken up his position as Head of Pathology during the year, Professor Keith Grimwood would arrive in 1997, to head Paediatrics, and Anthony Dowell would fill the new ACC Chair in General Practice. There had also been a 'large number' of new academic staff appointments. The Maori Research Centre, now named for Eru Pomare, was progressing under the direction of Dr Papaarangi Reid. The School had held its first Open Day, a celebratory occasion when 2000 people visited to view the facilities, listen to the annual Nordmeyer lecture and the Dean's inaugural lecture, and attend the trainee intern prize-giving, addressed by Professor John Campbell, Dean of the Faculty of Medicine. The Mayor of Wellington was among the guests. Linda

Holloway's term as Dean did not prove to be long. In 1998, she moved to Dunedin as Assistant Vice-Chancellor Health Sciences.[37]

In Christchurch, Alan Clarke's eight innovative and controversial years as Dean ended in 1993. Three years before, spinal injuries sustained in an accident had left him wheelchair-bound, without appreciably diminishing his drive and vision for the School. He now decided to take up a new challenge, as Director of the Christchurch Spinal Injuries Unit at Burwood Hospital. His determination to raise the profile of the Unit led to the establishment of the Burwood Spinal Trust (later the New Zealand Spinal Trust), he spearheaded the Allan Bean Centre for Research and Learning and set up the Burwood Academy for Independent Living. His own example was an inspiration to patients and, in 1995, his contributions to medicine were recognised by the award of the CMG. Alan Clarke died in January 2007.[38]

Professor Alan Clarke described himself as a 'surgical consumer and survivor'. His *Cancer Consensus Manual* **(1984) was born of his own experience with cancer. His outlook on life was epitomised by a comment he put at the end of his cv: 'In December 1991, eight months after my accident, an old lady said to me, "At your age, you are very lucky to become a paraplegic – you can start your life all over again."**

Otago Bulletin, 23 February 2007.

Andrew Hornblow, Professor of Community Health, and Deputy Dean for the previous four years, replaced Clarke. The first non-medically qualified Dean of a Medical School in New Zealand, Professor Hornblow had a background in psychology, experience in public health and extensive experience in a range of national and regional health organisations. He too would serve for eight years, taking the Christchurch School through into the new century. Hornblow's appointment signalled a change of focus. His aim was to add to the school's established role as a provider of medical education and research, that of a provider of advanced training for a range of other health professions. As he put it,

> We ended up, by the conclusion of my deanship, having a range of programmes, with the Master of Health Science/Postgraduate Diploma in Health Science structure, which could allow nurses and other health professionals – with nurses being the biggest group – to pick up a postgraduate degree or a Master's degree. The School became a fairly major provider of advanced training for people who were moving into leadership positions, other than those who were medically qualified.

Eventually the new programmes attracted more resources, but the programmes had to be in place before the money flowed. Not all departments were equally involved in the initiatives. Medicine and Surgery remained at the core of medical education, but the Departments of Public Health and General Practice, and Psychological Medicine moved into extensive postgraduate activity, with the number of their postgraduate students far outnumbering undergraduates.[39]

Hornblow had to deal, not only with the problems created by the health reforms, but also ongoing tensions with the Medical School and the University administration in Dunedin. There was a strong push by a number of influential Christchurch people for an independent Christchurch Medical School with graduate entry. He favoured this but he believed 'Dunedin' saw it as a move to secede from Otago and accordingly blocked it. There were disagreements on staff appointments and the general question of the degree of autonomy of the Christchurch School again came to the fore.[40]

The teaching at the Christchurch School continued to achieve a high satisfaction rate with medical students throughout the 1990s. There were also many staff changes during this time. Some of the foundation professors, whose capacity and length of service had provided admirable stability to the school, reached retirement. Fred Shannon left the Chair of Paediatrics in 1990 after eighteen

years, and was replaced by David Teele. Donald Aickin, appointed to the Chair of Obstetrics and Gynaecology in 1972, happily remained in place through the 1990s, but Bill Macbeth retired from the Chair of Surgery in 1993, after twenty-one years. Justin Roake, who had been a fourth-year student at the school in 1979, became Professor and Head of Department in 1997. Roy McGiven, Professor of Pathology, died suddenly in 1987, and Ross Boswell ('Ross the Boss') headed the department until 1996, when Robin Fraser took over. Psychological Medicine went through some stormy times in the early 1980s. However, there was a new beginning when Peter Joyce became Professor in 1986. At thirty-four, he was the youngest professor in the University of Otago at the time and the first Christchurch graduate to gain a chair in the School. He at once set about raising its research profile. Bill Gillespie was appointed Foundation Professor of Orthopaedic Surgery and Musculo-skeletal Medicine in 1981 and, when he moved on, was succeeded by Alistair Rothwell in 1990. In Public Health and General Practice Andrew Hornblow had been Acting Head, then Professor in 1988. When he became Dean, Jane Chetwynd was appointed, the School's first woman Professor and Head of Department. It was an expanding department, and it proved possible to establish a new Chair of General Practice in 1997, through a guarantee of five years' external funding. Les Toop became the first professor.[41] Looking back on his years as Dean, Hornblow took satisfaction from the fact that the School had worked as a team in a very turbulent period, that postgraduate education and research had grown strongly and that the School building had been completed in time for the twenty-fifth anniversary in 1998.[42]

In his report on staffing to the AMC accreditation team in 1994, David Stewart explained the University's staffing procedure. Posts were not 'frozen' but whenever a vacancy occurred, through retirement or resignation, a decision was made whether or not to maintain the position and a review of staffing in each department was part of every budgeting round. At the time he wrote the report, a number of chairs were vacant. The Chairs of Paediatrics and Pathology in the Wellington School of Medicine, Surgery in the Christchurch School of Medicine, and Anaesthesia and Intensive Care and Pathology in the Otago Medical School had been advertised, but no appointment had been made. Advertisement of the Otago Chairs of Obstetrics and Gynaecology, and Paediatrics and Child Health had been deferred. The University was seeking to fill three more chairs, Obstetrics and Gynaecology and Public Health in Wellington, and Public Health in Christchurch, but had decided not to maintain the Otago Chair of Experimental Medicine.[43] This less than satisfactory staffing position had been fully rectified by 1999. The accreditation team noted that, whereas five years before there had been a worryingly large number of unfilled positions and the Medical School had not been recruiting to fill all of them, in 1999 it had not only filled all senior posts but also established a number of new leadership positions. It noted approvingly the establishment of Chairs in General Practice in Christchurch and Wellington, and the development of a strong academic General Practice presence in all three schools. It believed there could be a greater emphasis on Maori health, especially in Christchurch. The team also raised two matters that would recur in the 2004 report, the relative absence of women in senior academic posts and a salary differential between hospital and medical school clinicians, which was likely to act as a disincentive to young clinicians considering an academic career.[44]

Administering the Faculty

The management structure of the Faculty of Medicine was one of the main issues the 1994 accreditation team considered required urgent attention. They found it 'difficult to develop a clear picture of the decision-making pathways' and commented on the 'widespread confusion, diffusion of responsibility and lack of Faculty-wide direction'.[45] The system had in fact grown piecemeal. In the mid-1980s, the Dean of the Faculty of Medicine had relinquished his role as Dean of the Otago Medical School, in order to remove any perception that his interests

were primarily focused on Dunedin. Towards the end of the decade, the Dean of Faculty was also made Assistant Vice-Chancellor of Health Sciences at Otago. As a result, oversight of Dentistry, Pharmacy and a growing number of health-related courses on the Dunedin campus were added to his responsibilities in Medicine. By 1990, a number of interdisciplinary research centres had been established in the Health Sciences, in neuroscience, drug development, bioethics, genetics and injury prevention. David Stewart added Physiotherapy to his portfolio as AVC Health Sciences, as well as new courses, such as the Master of General Practice and the Postgraduate Diploma in Aviation Medicine. Once again, it was possible to view the Dean of Faculty, who also served as the AVC, as having predominantly Dunedin interests, as well as an immense workload.[46]

The University reviewed the Faculty's administrative structure in 1995 and made two important changes. It separated the position of Dean of Faculty from that of Assistant Vice-Chancellor Health Sciences and divided the Otago Medical School in Dunedin into a clinical school, the Dunedin School of Medicine, and a preclinical school, the Otago School of Medical Sciences. The term 'University of Otago Medical School' was inclusive of both of these, as well as of the Wellington and Christchurch Schools. The new Dean of Faculty, with oversight over all four schools, was John Campbell, Foundation Professor of Geriatric Medicine in Dunedin from 1984. The former Dean of the Otago Medical School, Graham Mortimer, became Dean of the Dunedin School of Medicine, which was made up of the clinical departments, as well as Pathology and Preventive Medicine. The status and role of the new school were the same as those in Christchurch and Wellington, but it also maintained a close relationship with the School of Medical Sciences, based on their common obligations in teaching, scholarship and research. The Otago School of Medical Sciences was a new creation, made up of five departments – Anatomy and Structural Biology, Biochemistry, Microbiology, Pharmacology and Physiology – together with a number of research centres. Each

DIVISION OF HEALTH SCIENCES MANAGEMENT STRUCTURE

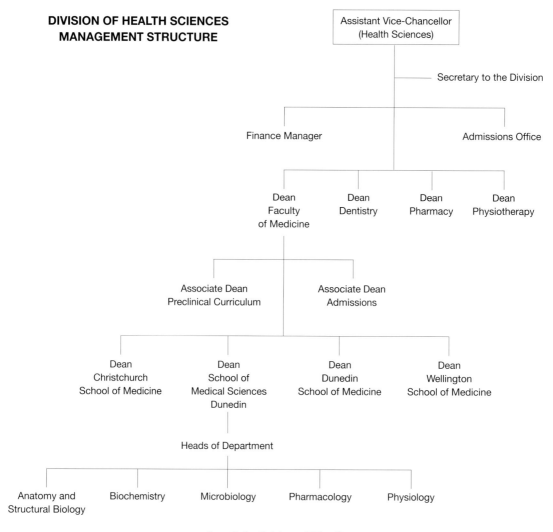

Accreditation Database, 1999, p. 9.

department was large, with most of its teaching being outside the medical curriculum and, under the new scheme, each remained a separate cost centre. The Dean of this new School was David Jones, Professor of Microbiology, who had come to the chair from South Africa in 1989. The School of Medical Sciences had responsibility for teaching part of the extensively remodelled health sciences first-year course which, after 1998, all students intending to proceed to any second-year health professional course were required to take. It also had an important role in the integrated second- and third-year courses, introduced in 1997 and 1998 respectively. The new

scheme appeared to work well. In 1999, Campbell reported that it gave Medicine a clearer voice within and outside the University, made internal funding allocations more transparent, facilitated the development of coordinated programmes in the biomedical sciences and generally improved cohesion in the Faculty. The 1999 accreditation team also approved the reorganisation of the Faculty, noting that it had been uniformly well received at all sites. It had allowed the School of Medical Sciences to achieve a corporate identity and to develop supra-departmental courses, scholarships, teaching and research facilities. Student numbers in the departments that made up the School had grown by an average of 8 per cent annually over the five years of its existence, which enabled it to contribute to the resource demands of medical curriculum reform. Medical Sciences was seen as a Faculty-wide resource by all three schools and offered possibilities for vertical integration of course material, although its major teaching responsibilities in undergraduate and postgraduate science programmes as well as service responsibilities to dentistry, medical laboratory science, pharmacy and physiotherapy were constraining factors on this.[47]

There was one further piece of restructuring in the 1990s, relating to the clinical disciplines in Dunedin. Graham Mortimer retired at the beginning of 1998, after seven challenging years as Dean in Dunedin, at first of the Otago Medical School, and then at the Dunedin School. Bill Gillespie, a graduate of Edinburgh University, returned from the Chair of Orthopaedic Surgery in Edinburgh to become Dean of the Dunedin School. Gillespie knew the Otago Medical School well, as he had been lecturer in Orthopaedic Surgery at the Wellington School of Medicine from 1977 to 1981 before becoming Professor at the Christchurch School of Medicine. He amalgamated the nine small clinical departments under his jurisdiction into four larger ones, while retaining Pathology and Preventive and Social Medicine as separate departments. His reasoning was pragmatic. 'In changing times when money is tight', he wrote in the Alumnus Association Newsletter of 1999/2000, 'it becomes difficult to cling to traditional departmental structures as new specialties emerge and the boundaries between old ones shift'. The Departments of Anaesthesia, Medicine, Orthopaedic Surgery, Ophthalmology, Surgery and the Bioethics Research Centre were joined to form a Department of Medical and Surgical Sciences, under Professor Rob Walker, and the Departments of Obstetrics and Gynaecology, and Paediatrics and Child Health formed a new Department of Women's and Children's Health, with Professor Don Wilson as the first Head of Department.[48]

Throughout the 1990s, the Schools of Medicine in Christchurch and Wellington continued to establish a secure place in their respective communities. They also developed their own areas of research expertise, postgraduate programmes, particular teaching philosophies and curricular experiments, the last held in check by the requirements of the AMC for comparability of the clinical courses at the three centres. Each of the Deans established a small group of Associate Deans to share administration. Financially, they enjoyed considerable independence.

In this complex and decentralised structure, care had to be taken to counterbalance the autonomy of the schools by maintaining regular contact among them. In the 1990s the AVC Health Sciences, the Dean of Faculty and the four School Deans met monthly as a Faculty Board, and the School Deans acted as an Executive Committee to advise the Dean of Faculty. The Deans and all the Heads of Department in the Faculty met annually. Teleconferencing was regularly used to supplement personal meetings. The 1999 accreditation team believed that, in facing the challenge of a 'necessarily complex and decentralised structure', the Faculty had 'the potential to become a model of best practice in the management of a decentralised medical school'.[49] In the new century, there was further restructuring with the Assistant Vice-Chancellor, Health Sciences, renamed Pro-Vice-Chancellor, resuming the role of Dean of Faculty. And there was yet another name change for the northern schools. Reflecting pride in the Otago connection, they became the University of Otago, Christchurch, and the University of Otago, Wellington.

CHAPTER 24

New Ways of Teaching and Learning

THE LAST TWO decades of the twentieth century saw rapid changes in the techniques of teaching and learning at the Otago Medical School. Students embarked on new areas of study, with new professors, in general practice, geriatric medicine and biomedical ethics, and found a new emphasis in their courses on acquiring skills of communication with patients and sensitivity to their cultural differences. They were exposed to different techniques of study, through problem-based, small-group, cooperative and self-directed learning, in a course that was more integrated, both between disciplines and between the preclinical and clinical years. As major examinations slowly gave ground to continuous assessment, they were tested by new methods which, by the mid-1990s, were often self-administered by computer, and aimed less to check recall of factual detail, than the understanding of principles. Although not going as far as some of the proponents of change wanted, it amounted to a quiet revolution in teaching.

The 1980s: Curriculum by Conference

In the 1980s a number of staff, inspired by overseas trends in medical education, pressed for the introduction of problem-based and self-directed learning and received support from a series of professional conferences and workshops. When three of the reformers, Peter Schwartz, Chris Heath and Tony Egan, came to write up the experience a decade later, they entitled their book *The Art of the Possible*, and focused on the

politics of negotiating radical change in a large, old-established medical school with strong traditions. They took 1985 as their baseline, on the ground that there had been little modification of the curriculum for more than ten years before that date. They did acknowledge some more recent changes, such as the reduction of teaching time for anatomy, biochemistry and physiology and the introduction, at second year, of courses in first aid, in 1978, and epidemiology and public health, in 1981. There were also hints of things to come. In the preclinical years, there had been early trials of computer-assisted learning, some inter-departmental cooperation in the third-year Abnormal Structure and Function course, the use of videotaping for case presentations in preclinical neurology and the introduction of problem-solving exercises in various courses. In the clinical years, both the organ system-based clinical science course at fourth year and the trainee-intern sixth year were innovative. In Dunedin, the sixth-year programme was already being modified to give more time to general practice, both rural and urban, and a module was shared between a community-based specialty and a group health care evaluation project.[1]

In the early years of the decade, debate was lively in the curriculum committees. Chris Heath, as Associate Dean with several roles in curriculum development, chaired no fewer than five committees, which sometimes resulted in his having to report to himself. In medical schools overseas, especially new ones such as McMaster in Canada, Limburg in the Netherlands and

Newcastle in Australia, problem-based learning was being introduced on a large scale. Newcastle was particularly influential because it was so close to home. Staff exchanged ideas, visited centres of interest when on leave and made contacts. A series of seminars on medical education was held in 1980, books and papers were circulated and the annual conference of the Australasian and New Zealand Association for Medical Education, which was held in Dunedin in 1984, further raised awareness.[2] This was the background to a series of conferences and workshops on medical education that were held in New Zealand between 1985 and 1987.

The Lincoln Conference, February 1985

The first and largest of the conferences took place over three days in February 1985, when staff and some students from all three Otago Medical School campuses converged on Lincoln College to consider the question: 'Are we making the optimum use of our educational resources to train doctors for the 21st century?' It marked a new stage in the debate on medical education. The Lincoln conference was the brainchild of Geoff Brinkman. Heath recalls that, when the Dean had casually mentioned the idea to him, it seemed 'utterly ridiculous'. Taking a hundred people away and making them spend a weekend together sounded like 'something one might be contemplating in the Middle East at this time.'[3] But the conference was a success beyond everyone's expectations, as he wrote later in the conference report. 'We worked together, talked together, argued together with an accord that augurs well for the future of the Faculty.'[4] The conference participants, numbering almost a hundred staff and a small number of students, worked through discussion groups, with regular plenary sessions, to debate medical ethics, continuing education, the examination system, student boredom, curriculum models and curriculum overload. Inter-school differences were set aside and people worked well together as colleagues and also simply enjoyed each other's company. Dunedin staff, who went up to Lincoln together by bus, even relished standing

talking in the country sunshine, when they had a flat tyre on the way home.[5]

In the month after the conference, Chris Heath circulated a summary of its proceedings. All had agreed that the medical curriculum was too crowded and too reliant on formal teaching. There was anxiety about the scale, timing and purpose of the examination structure and concern that techniques of self-directed learning were not being taught. There was too little staff–student contact. The curriculum needed to be integrated, both vertically between the preclinical and clinical years and horizontally between disciplines. There was support for the introduction of problem-based learning in some sections of the course and further exploration of the teaching of ethics.[6] The purpose of the Lincoln conference was to debate and exchange ideas not plan change, and it did not have immediate, tangible results.

The Role of the Doctor Conference, October 1985

Most of the pressure for curricular change came from within the Medical School. Later in 1985, however, there was something quite different: a national conference on the role of the doctor in New Zealand. This was not a professional conference, but a new style of meeting. With consumers of health services represented as well as providers, it was intended to produce well-informed recommendations for change. This reflected the open political climate of the first months of the Labour Government, which encouraged discussion and criticism of established institutions such as the health system. Once again, Brinkman was the instigator, this time in cooperation with the Dean of the Auckland Medical School and the Deputy Director General of Health. The aim of the conference was to review the role of medical practitioners in New Zealand society and assess how effectively the training of medical students fitted them to fulfil that role. There were forty-one participants, equally men and women. Half came from outside the medical profession and four were Maori. The medical schools and the Department of Health, who were allocated a total of eleven representatives, selected those with a special interest in curriculum. The World Health Organization provided a consultant. For four days, participants worked in groups on assigned tasks, with frequent plenary sessions and regular written updates on the conclusions reached.[7]

It immediately became clear that New Zealanders expected a great deal from doctors. Before the conference opened, the organisers received some 230 public submissions, strikingly consistent in their content. They criticised doctors for their inadequate communication skills and lack of a holistic approach to healing, as well as cultural insensitivity and sexist attitudes. They maintained that doctors needed to focus more on health promotion, including a willingness to suggest alternatives to drugs, knowledge of nutrition and an understanding of mental illness. Conference participants reinforced these views. They signalled a changing environment in which

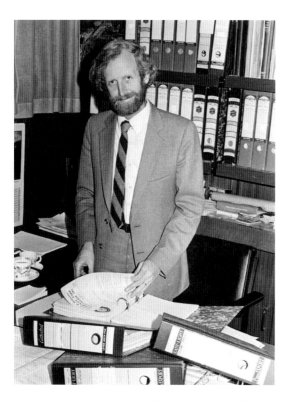

Dr Chris Heath, convenor of the planning committee for the Conference on the Role of the Doctor, is surrounded by submissions from community groups, agencies and individuals, three months before the conference is due to open.
Otago Daily Times, 2 July 1985.

doctors needed to be dynamic, flexible and accountable to their community. They insisted that the traditional role of the doctor, working largely in isolation, must be replaced by a team approach, with other health professionals and with the patient. Doctors should provide 'holistic care', which involved open communication with patients and going beyond treating illness, to fostering health and advising on the prevention of disease. They should also be committed to their own ongoing education.[8]

To train future doctors to meet these high and varied expectations, the conference recommended more elective periods and special projects, and the development of skills in critical analysis, problem-solving, counselling and communication. Attention should be paid to multi-cultural issues, with special emphasis being given to the indigenous Maori culture. Delegates voiced the dissatisfaction that women felt with the health system. They criticised sharply the style of teaching in the medical schools, describing it as 'dictatorial' and over-reliant on the acquisition of facts. They advocated a problem-solving, competency-based approach, with the use of innovative teaching and assessment methods, to encourage self-directed learning and teamwork among different disciplines. Students, they said, should be taught to regard multi-professional teamwork as the norm in the provision of health services and should be encouraged to move more freely out of the Medical School into the community.[9]

The conference report, written in both English and Maori, was produced very promptly and sent to every member of the teaching staff in New Zealand medical schools. A decade on, Schwartz and his colleagues maintained that the conference had been valuable in providing cogent statements about the pressing need for changes to medical education, but that 'massive inputs' of time and energy were necessary if they were to be acted on. The real influence of such a conference, in their view, would only be expressed in the long term and was unlikely to be overt.[10]

In some areas, especially in relation to the dissatisfaction of Maori and women with the health system, the Role of the Doctor Conference signalled issues that would grow in importance. In June 1986, Eru Pomare published a leading article in the *New Zealand Medical Journal*. In 'Maori Health: new concepts and initiatives', he explained that Maori criticised the Pakeha public health system for its omission of a spiritual component from its health practices and its failure to acknowledge the role of the extended family. He described recent Maori health initiatives and urged Maori and Pakeha to work together to tackle Maori health promotion and disease prevention, warning that neither one could succeed in this without the other.[11] In 1987, an inquiry into an 'unfortunate experiment' at National Women's Hospital where, since 1966, some doctors had been following the progress of women with major cervical abnormalities without treating them, validated the complaints of women about their treatment within the health system and recommended sweeping changes to patients' rights. More than twenty-five years on, Dame Silvia Cartwright, who presided over the inquiry, looked back on it as a catalyst for change, partly because 'it was such a dramatic event, with doctors being lined up against the wall for the first time ever'. Two of Judge Cartwright's medical advisers were Dr Charlotte Paul (from the Department of Preventive and Social Medicine) and Dr Linda Holloway (from the Department of Pathology in Wellington). Both later became influential professors in the Medical School.[12]

The Teschemakers Workshop, April 1986

The full influence of the Role of the Doctor Conference might have been longterm and indirect but the clear, concise statements of the report soon proved their value in debates on curriculum development. The conference was acknowledged as a 'powerful, intelligent and articulate group, which had to be taken seriously.'[13] In April 1986, when the Faculty Board Curriculum Committee arranged a three-day workshop, they took the conference recommendations as the basis for discussion. 'As Medicine moves rapidly towards the challenges of the 21st century', they explained, 'medical teachers must identify those attitudes and curricular issues

needed to meet these challenges.' A group of forty or so academic staff from the three schools and some students assembled at Teschemakers, a former Catholic girls' boarding school in North Otago, on 18 April. Co-ordinated by John Hunter, the new Dean of Faculty, they worked in small groups on the same tasks, reporting back regularly to plenary sessions. Unlike the two previous conferences, this workshop was intended to make decisions to be acted on, rather than explore ideas and make recommendations.[14]

The workshop consisted of three sessions, on attitudes, curriculum and propositions, the last covering 'novel ideas that may not have had an airing elsewhere'. The session on attitudes included the integration of health promotion into existing subjects, teamwork between departments and with other health providers, communication skills, women's health and women in medicine, and sensitivity to cultural differences. The curriculum session focused on 'developing scholarly practitioners' and looked specifically at problem-based learning and a curriculum to take the Medical School into the twenty-first century. Introducing this session, Stewart asked participants, 'How should change be introduced, and how much?'[15] There was extraordinary unanimity: problem-based learning would correct the defects in the current curriculum and should be introduced into the preclinical curriculum as early as 1988.[16]

An Attempt at Self-directed Learning, 1986–88. The preclinical course

It was a daunting undertaking and an extraordinarily tight time-frame to bring in problem-based, self-directed learning by 1988. The Faculty Board Curriculum Committee (FBBC) began immediately, setting up a series of working parties on Problems, Objectives, Early Clinical Contact, Learning Materials and Specialist Credits (on electives). Although some staff were already using problem-based techniques in their teaching, it was evident that the proposed changes would need widespread staff support and the careful selection and training of a considerable number of tutors. The FBCC warned that it was 'not aware of any other large medical school with our traditions which has made the transfer to problem-based self-directed learning to the extent proposed'. Nonetheless, it proceeded to chart a plan of action, from April 1986 through to the implementation date, 1988.[17] Confident that the efficacy of problem-based, self-directed learning as a method of tertiary education had been 'well proven in many other settings'[18] and buoyed by the support at the Teschemakers workshop, the FBCC concentrated on detailed planning, rather than spending time trying to persuade colleagues. A Medical Education Development Unit (MEDU), which consisted of two senior academics, half-time, a part-time secretary and a full-time researcher, was set up in May 1987, to provide liaison among the various committees and keep full records.[19]

In July 1987, the FBCC issued a discussion paper on self-directed learning. It set out the now-familiar case for reviewing an overcrowded curriculum that had not seen a major change of direction in many years, which failed to train students for lifelong self-directed learning and did not give staff teaching satisfaction. The paper listed basic questions for debate and decision: the primary purpose of the undergraduate medical curriculum, the best mix of problem-based and traditional learning, the optimum use of staff if problem-based learning was introduced on a large scale, the management of the curriculum and the role the departments would play in this, and whether change could be made with the resources available. A number of departments, such as Clinical Biochemistry and Physiology, had already introduced elements of self-directed learning and case-based learning days were being trialled in the abnormal structure and function course at third year.[20] In an appendix to the paper, Dr Terry Crooks, of the Higher Education Development Centre, summed up the arguments for and against problem-based learning. The arguments in favour have been covered. The arguments against proved decisive. Staff believed lectures were an economical means of transmitting factual knowledge, as they could be sure their students had been exposed to knowledge they deemed important. Changes to long-established assessment methods raised doubts about standards. The new approach would require adaptation on the part of students. Some staff would have less student contact. On the other hand there could be problems in finding and training the tutors required for increased small-group work. Some lecture facilities would become redundant, while more small rooms would be needed. There would be extra pressure on library and audio-visual resources.[21] The focus in the paper on self-directed learning, rather than course integration, meant that the determination of individual disciplines to continue to teach and examine their own subject without outside interference did not feature on the list. That determination was, nevertheless, of great practical importance.

The result of all this intense activity was limited. Early in 1988 the FBBC abandoned its attempt to introduce a fully problem-based, self-directed curriculum. Some departments were already setting in place innovative courses of their own and they hoped that the Otago Faculty could 'evolve towards this ideal gradually'. The conveners of new programmes at second and third year were interviewed late in 1988 and the students were surveyed in 1989. Both groups responded positively. Staff enjoyed small-group teaching and students generally found working on problems in small groups stimulating. Departments were willing to consider revising their assessment practices, so long as they retained their autonomy.[22] In 1989, the Faculty Board adopted a revised set of Goals and Objectives, which addressed Knowledge, Skills and Attitudes in some detail and emphasised the application of the principles of scientific method, teamwork, communication skills, lifelong learning, health promotion and ethics.[23] It was the only tangible outcome from all the work of the energetic and conscientious committees that were set up to give form to the enthusiasm for curricular reform that had been expressed at the Teschemakers conference.

Reflecting on these attempts at preclinical curricular reform in the 1980s, the authors of *The Art of the Possible* asked, 'Why, in spite of the apparent enthusiasm evident at the 1986

Teschemakers Workshop, did the Faculty Plan to introduce problem-based self-directed learning fail?' They concluded that the supporters of the reforms had failed to recognise the extreme difficulty of making such a major change in a long-established medical school. They had overestimated the degree of staff enthusiasm and underestimated known obstacles, especially the fear of loss of control over assessment by departments and a staff promotion structure that rewarded research over teaching. There had not been enough incentive for change, adequate resources to implement it, or much pressure to do so from outside the school. They also recognised the positives, however, such as the discipline-based initiatives, a list of objectives for the preclinical course, and a set of problems that could have formed the basis of a workable problem-based preclinical course. There was also a programme of early clinical contact, which the authors considered 'ambitious and novel even by international standards' and the fact some teachers were acquiring the skills needed in a problem-based learning curriculum. Moreover, increased teacher satisfaction and more student enthusiasm indicated an educational atmosphere vastly different from that of 1985. 'On the whole', they summed up, 'the School can be reasonably proud of its accomplishment, given its organisational structure, long history, faculty and resources.'[24]

The Clinical Course: Three Interpretations

There was less pressure in the 1980s to change the clinical years of medical teaching. Most teaching took the form of a series of clinical attachments, where the relevance to the student's future career of what was being taught was self-evident and where problem-solving skills, self-directed learning and small group work were already at the heart of the process. From the early 1970s, however, fourth-year students in all three schools also took a course in clinical sciences, intended to integrate pathology, the basic medical sciences and related disciplines, with clinical teaching. The didactic style in which this course was taught came under intense scrutiny. While all three

schools opted to change the clinical sciences course, each had a different plan.

In Wellington, a committed group of teachers set up a pilot programme in problem-based learning in 1987, with a small group of volunteers. The student participants were enthusiastic and in 1990 a ballot had to be held to select eighteen out of the thirty-nine (the majority of a class of fifty-seven) who wanted to join the problem-based learning group. In 1991, under pressure from students, Wellington moved to full problem-based learning for the course.[25]

In the Christchurch School, the changes were more drastic and made in a sometimes turbulent environment. In 1986, Alan Clarke, a long-time advocate of curricular reform, proposed simply to discontinue the clinical sciences lecture course. Although the resulting furore caused him to defer his plans, he succeeded in 1988. Announcing the change in the student handbook the next year, Clarke explained:

> In past years the course was not well attended by students and to some extent it impeded appropriate learning in clinical medicine. You will have more opportunity to work with patients and for contact with staff.

After a brief introductory course, students were plunged into five-week blocks of clinical attachments, plus half a day of pathology each week. Some reacted angrily, claiming they were being made educational guinea pigs and that their parents had paid taxes to have them 'taught in traditional ways which had established the school's reputation'. When in their examinations the next year the fourth-year class of 1988 outperformed students from the other two centres, some of them put it down to the terror factor. The Christchurch School also made all fifth-year assessment internal. The new system was bedded in, with minor adjustments, in the 1990s.[26]

In Dunedin, the clinical course was changed less than in the other schools, despite originally ambitious aims. In 1986, a working party was set up to advise on removing the clinical sciences course from fourth year and, more generally, to consider problem-based learning in all the fourth- and fifth-year courses. A year on, the working party presented their ideas to another three-day workshop at Teschemakers. This one was a southern region affair, with staff and a few students of the Dunedin School and clinical staff from hospitals in Balclutha, Invercargill, Oamaru and Queenstown. There were two representatives from each of the Wellington and Christchurch Schools.[27] Over six sessions, the participants debated various practical issues: an alternative to the clinical sciences course, the teaching of particular subjects such as pathology, clinical pharmacology and ethics, the relationship of continuous assessment to self-directed learning, how to assess clinical and communication skills, the role of out-of-town attachments and strategies for using the community as a resource. The replacement of the clinical sciences course was the most contentious issue, but they agreed to go ahead with more detailed planning for this.[28] Then, just seven months before the changes were expected to come in, the Dunedin clinical teachers rejected the entire proposal. A frantic round of consultation followed, before staff agreed to have the clinical sciences course reduced, from 143 sessions to 122, and an introductory clinical competencies course brought in. Over the following years, the course was further contracted, down to 110 sessions in 1992, and case-based teaching and small group work was increased, although a large didactic element remained. The experience showed that even wide consultation and apparent general approval of an innovative course were no guarantee of success in the final vote for its adoption.[29]

When the New Zealand Medical Council accreditation team visited in 1988 they endorsed the changes made and asked for more. 'Methods of teaching,' they reported approvingly, 'are rightly seen in relation to course objectives and curriculum content, to library and other resources for individual learning and to methods of evaluation and examination.'[30] They encouraged the School to press ahead towards a mode of undergraduate teaching aimed at developing critical analytical skills and frameworks of understanding that would enable students to organise, evaluate and use information in an appropriate manner. They advocated further reductions in formal teaching and more time in tutorial groups, more teaching and assessment based around medical problems encountered inside and outside hospitals, more problem-based learning, fewer examinations, more self-directed learning and more comprehensive methods of assessment.[31]

Curriculum in the 1990s: Systems Integration and Self-Directed Learning

In the early 1990s, the Medical School shared in the rapid growth of the Otago University student population, but not by training more doctors. The departments of Anatomy, Physiology, Biochemistry and Microbiology taught an ever-higher proportion of non-medical students. The Bioethics Research Centre attracted staff from disciplines other than medicine, the Medical School offered a new degree, the Bachelor of Medical Laboratory Science (BMedLabSc), and combined with the Otago Polytechnic to offer the degree of Bachelor of Physiotherapy. It was thus in an environment of change that the Faculty Board drew up General and Intermediate Objectives to be achieved by the end of the medical course. The document was intended as a checklist for students to monitor their progress through the course and a guideline for their subsequent careers. It covered the traditional, inter-related domains of knowledge, skills and attitudes, with fourteen pages of general objectives, each supplemented by detailed intermediate objectives.[32]

Course objectives had to be achieved through an appropriate curriculum. In 1992, the Faculty Board set up a working party to make recommendations on the courses to be taught and skills to be acquired in each semester of second and third year. It was expected to go into detail for each course, advising on the number of teaching hours, the nature and timing of major examinations and the appropriate time for the division of the class among the three schools for the clinical years. The working party was instructed to ensure that the course had a substantial component of self-directed learning, fewer timetabled hours, and a greater degree of vertical integration (between preclinical and clinical years) and horizontal integration (between courses in any year). To help ensure this, the working party contained representatives of departments teaching second and third years, and also representatives of the fourth, fifth and sixth years of the course, as well as a recent graduate or senior student and a non-medical person who was not a member of Faculty.[33]

By 1993, in spite of concerns expressed about the reduced power of departments in an integrated system, the overloading of teachers, the potential for a crowded and disorganised course and the timing of the introduction of a new curriculum, there was a growing awareness of the need to create a coherent second- and third-year course.[34] The Faculty Board endorsed a series of principles, including that:

– The course structure, teaching and assessment should be consistent with the agreed general and intermediate objectives.

– There should be horizontal and vertical integration to ensure that the relevance of the learning was apparent.

– Teaching and assessment should focus on principles rather than factual detail.

– The course should foster independent learning skills.

– Teaching should be evaluated and recognised in the Faculty's reward system.[35]

An Implementation and Development Committee was set up to develop an integrated second- and third-year course along these lines. David Loten was appointed to the new position of Associate Dean for Preclinical Education, to oversee changes to the curriculum, which was envisaged as being a single structure lasting four semesters. The detail of what has been described as a 'change from a discipline-based course to an integrated system-based course' was put in place between 1994 and 1997. The course was made up of overlapping modules, typically based on an organ system and integrated across disciplines by a convener responsible to a Board of Studies. Clinical staff from all three schools were involved in the design and teaching of the modules to ensure vertical integration. Teaching methods were varied, including traditional lectures, clinical demonstrations and practical laboratory classes as well as small group tutorials, with some using a problem-based format.[36]

Describing the new system for the accreditation review committee of the Australian Medical Council in 1999, Loten commented specifically on the two integrating modules, which ran through both years. The Patient, Doctor and Society course related to attitudes and skills, such as critical appraisal, communication, ethical reasoning and awareness of professional development. It also included a component of early clinical contact, through clinical and community contact weeks. The Systems Integration course, which was entirely case-based and taught in small groups, enabled clinically relevant material from the modules to be highlighted and revised as the course progressed. It included ethics, legal issues and personal and professional development and was assessed through a 30 per cent in-course test, much of which was administered by computer. The remaining percentage was made up of three examinations, one for Doctor, Patient and Society, the other two for a combination of the rest of the course.[37]

As the first cohort of students completed third year at the end of 1998, the new curriculum was subjected to a detailed review. The review committee examined relevant documents and course evaluations, interviewed some thirty staff, including the heads of department involved, on the basis of a questionnaire, and considered the balance of the course as a whole. In March 1999 the committee reported that the integrated course gave students a greater appreciation of the relevance of the basic sciences to clinical practice, earlier clinical contact and a higher proportion of self-directed learning. Systems Integration was highly regarded by students, who responded enthusiastically to some modules, but criticised the teaching in some sections of all of them. Students acknowledged the need to 'learn and practise skills of information retrieval and manipulation' and the committee recommended that this should form part of the curriculum at all levels. The senior lecturer in Maori health was satisfied with teaching in this area and third-year students were pleased with the programme of Humanities electives.[38]

The preclinical programme won plaudits from the 1999 Australian Medical Council review team and was reported in international journals. The team congratulated staff on its development and noted its favourable reception by students, while encouraging even further integration and less didactic teaching. The 2004 AMC team would express similar views, this time suggesting more vertical integration could be introduced into the programme.[39] In *Academic Medicine* in 1999, Schwartz, Loten and Andrew Miller, all keen proponents of the new style of teaching, described the programme as the successful introduction of a modern systems-based preclinical curriculum. They emphasised two components which they believed were 'innovative by any standards': systems integration and a large-scale programme of computerised in-course assessment. The following year, the same trio published an article in *Medical Teacher*, the title of which summarises its content, '"Systems Integration": a middle way between problem-based learning and traditional courses'. They commended systems integration as an attractive alternative that would enable teachers at traditional medical schools to gain many of the advantages of problem-based learning without accepting it in full.[40]

The criteria for entry to Medical School were also modified. In 1998, a new health sciences first-year course, with several new or redesigned papers, was introduced. The intention was to devise a first-year course tailored to health professional requirements as a prerequisite for all students aiming to study medicine. That the Intermediate year could no longer be taken at any other university caused an outcry in other centres. However, there were good academic reasons for the requirement, not least that some of the material from the overcrowded second-year course could be transferred down to the first year. It was also proving impossible to ensure an equitable selection of medical students based on grades achieved in 'equivalent papers' at different universities. The new health sciences first year provided an introduction to the biomedical sciences, and also contained an English paper and a paper on biostatistics and research design. Students were selected for Medical School on the basis of their examination ranking, the top 120 being offered places. The course was too new to be assessed by the 1999 AMC accreditation team, but they did query the use of academic ranking as the sole entry criterion. Over the next few years, more students were accepted by revised methods. For most (130 by 2004), entry was based partly (66 per cent) on a grade average in first year and the remainder on an Undergraduate Medicine and Health Sciences Admission Test (UMAT), an aptitude test designed by the Australian Council for Educational Research and used by most Australasian medical schools. Sixty places were reserved for special categories of candidates, those of Maori or Polynesian ethnicity, graduates or applicants from rural areas.[41]

The next stage was to tackle the clinical course. In the late 1990s, a new fourth- and fifth-year programme was developed by the Faculty Curriculum Evaluation and Assessment Committee, which had representatives from each of the Schools of Medicine and the School of Medical Sciences. Consultation with Heads of Department and staff resulted in a programme which had a common core curriculum, common objectives and common examinations, but was delivered in a different way in the different schools. It emphasised professional development and aimed to leave students more time to gain clinical experience and to pursue special interests. They would be exposed to a greater diversity of clinical experience, including provincial hospital experience, community and rural practice and longitudinal case studies, and would be assessed on their clinical skills and attitudes as well as knowledge. The programme was intended to strengthen teaching in Maori health, rural health and the use of medical information. Using integrated rather than discipline-based modules, the new curriculum aimed to strengthen the threads of professional development, communication skills, and biomedical ethics.[42]

In Dunedin, the new course was reviewed when the first cohort of students had completed it. Under the direction of Emeritus Professor

Keith Jeffery, the review team considered a mass of written material, including detailed course evaluations, drew up questionnaires for staff and students, interviewed thirty-seven staff and met with the fourth- and fifth-year classes. In June 2001 the team reported that the aims of integration had generally been achieved well, although not equally in all areas. There was some feeling that the changes had been rushed. Both staff and students expressed doubts about the effectiveness of self-directed learning. Student evaluations suggested there were problems with the thematic 'threads', which the committee thought could be resolved if each thread had its own convener. The use and value of information technology was still unresolved. The committee recommended that a Clinical Board of Studies should be set up and an annual Medical School Education Forum be held, to discuss undergraduate medical teaching at the Dunedin school.[43]

Over recent years the Faculty has been careful to involve students in curriculum planning and discover student opinion about curriculum change and different methods of teaching and learning. Not everyone took it seriously. The Fourth Year Rep wrote in *Enema 1999* that 'The biggest mystery ... remains to be the whole concept of self directed learning. Every afternoon of every day was timetabled as "self-directed learning". More often than not I had no idea what to do, so I self-directed myself home to bed. After all, I'd probably been there since 8.00 am.'[44]

On the other hand, a fifth-year student wrote to the Jeffery committee:

> I understand that organising and running a course like medicine is a very complex process and I would like to take this opportunity to thank all of the people who have been involved in conducting and organising the new curriculum during the past five years. The new curriculum is not perfect but is improving and is changing for the better. The University of Otago has done a superb job in training doctors and will do so in the future under the nearly new curriculum scheme.

While it would be tempting to conclude that, on the eve of the millennium, the Medical School was moving steadily in the right direction in what it was teaching and how, curriculum development does not have an end point. Perfection could never be agreed on, let alone achieved, and would probably be considered unacceptably static if it was. As well as changes in the selection of medical students, new courses have been introduced and broader proposals have come and gone. When John Campbell was appointed Dean of Faculty in 1996, he brought with him experience in the AMC accreditation process for Australian and New Zealand universities. This led to his proposal for a radical 'New Pathway' for Otago medical students, with earlier clinical contact and the division of the class among the three schools at the end of second year. In 2000, together with Chris Heath of HEDC, he set up the Intercampus Network for Educational Development (INED), now the Medical Education Group, to provide for curricular development in all the Schools of Medicine. Joy Rudland was appointed Director of Educational Support and Development, to assist curriculum development, especially the New Pathway. After several years' work, the University put the scheme on hold in 2004 as unaffordable. In the view of the Dean of Medical Sciences, it had perhaps been too revolutionary to achieve an unequivocal 'buy-in' by staff.

A more evolutionary style of curriculum reform, however, which includes some of its concepts, is progressing strongly. The aim is to ease the transition from basic sciences to clinical training. In 2007 a new Health Science First Year, which included material formerly covered in the second-year medical course, provided an opportunity to make changes to the programme for the second and third years. The School responded to students' requests for earlier learning of clinical skills, earlier patient contact and clinically related basic science teaching. The revised course has an emphasis on community-based health and independent learning. While the role of lectures has been reduced, they remain an important element. It is a carefully balanced programme, but no doubt will not be the last word: curriculum development, in the apt phrase of the 2004 AMC report, is about 'continuous renewal'.[45]

CHAPTER 25

The Research Culture

I
N HIS introduction to the *University of Otago Magazine* of February 2007, the Vice-Chancellor refers with pride to a new report from the Ministry of Research, Science and Technology, which describes Otago as the most research-intensive university in New Zealand. This was important, wrote Professor Skegg, because teaching is more effective in a research-rich environment and the advancement of knowledge is one of the key functions of a university.[1] The Otago Medical School has long held a dominant position in the research profile of the University, for the quality of its work and its success in attracting external funding. Furthermore, the community perceives medical research as being valuable to ordinary people, in a way that most academic research is not.

The front-line researchers Hercus appointed, with the aim of creating a research-intensive Medical School, had a lasting influence. It is not surprising that Sir Horace Smirk, after twenty-seven fruitful years at the Medical School, left a well established research group at the Wellcome Institute. On the other hand, it is striking that Sir John Eccles and Sir Michael Woodruff (as they became), who stayed at Otago for much shorter periods, also made a lasting impression. In each case, people they attracted to work with them remained and the lines of research they initiated continued. An excellent collection of essays on medical research in Otago between 1922 and 1997 was compiled to mark the seventy-fifth jubilee of the *Proceedings of the University of Otago Medical School*. One of the interesting features of

this collection is that it traces networks, almost genealogies, of researchers whose work stretches from the 1950s to the present.[2]

Smirk's Dunedin Hypertension Research Group was well placed to carry on after he retired. Led by F.O. Simpson from 1968 to 1989, the group built on the work begun under Smirk. A remarkable number of its researchers moved to positions of responsibility in the Medical School. Among these were John Hunter, later Professor of Medicine and Dean, Tom O'Donnell, Foundation Professor of Medicine and later Dean of the Wellington School, and Robin Irvine, who became Vice-Chancellor of the University. Others included Frederick Fastier, Smirk's long-time collaborator, who became Foundation Professor of Pharmacology, and his successor, Richard Laverty, Associate-Professor Gary Blackman and Garth McQueen, Professor of Clinical Pharmacology, who came to New Zealand in order to work with Smirk. D.G. Palmer became Professor of Rheumatology in Dunedin, A.M.O. Veale, Professor of Community Health in Auckland, Ted Nye Associate-Professor in Medicine, and D.G. Rayns Associate-Professor in Anatomy. There were also several who gained prestigious chairs overseas.[3]

Other networks were on a smaller scale. When Eccles left the Otago Physiology Department in 1951, the 'small but very active school' he had gathered round him and the momentum in neurophysiological research he initiated were maintained by his successor, Archie McIntyre. 'Neurophysiology, Phase I', as the next Professor of Physiology, James Robinson, called it, lasted through McIntyre's tenure, to 1961. 'Phase II' began in 1972, when Professor John Hubbard, a former BMedSc student of Eccles and McIntyre, was appointed to a new Chair in Neurophysiology. Although his work had a different emphasis, after a period of study at Oxford, Hubbard had completed a PhD under Eccles at Canberra and was thus 'grounded in the same tradition' as his early mentors. This phase ended with Hubbard's untimely death in 1995.[4]

In Surgery, Professor Woodruff left a not dissimilar legacy. During his few years at Otago, he established a transplantation research group, which Norman Nisbet, Associate Professor in Orthopaedic Surgery, took over when he departed in 1957. Barbara Heslop joined that year and kept the group together when Nisbet unexpectedly left in the mid 1960s. A later Professor of Surgery, Andre van Rij, described her as 'without doubt the most influential non-surgeon investigator within the department of surgery'. The group moved to the Adams Building when their temporary accommodation was demolished and, when Pharmacy took over the laboratories in that building, some of them joined the Pathology Department as the Immunology Group. Margaret Baird, one of Heslop's PhD students, and the outstanding technician, Pam Salmon, were the 'direct intellectual descendants of the original transplantation team'.[5]

The Sinews of Medical Research

Government Funding

The prerequisites for such continuities in research are obvious – researchers, space and money. There was seldom a lack of talented people eager to do research and from 1948 the Hercus Building accommodated most of the Medical School research, together with the temporary Surgery and Obstetrics Building from 1956 to 1972, and the Wellcome Institute from 1963. The cluster of new buildings that opened in the early 1970s, Microbiology and Biochemistry on the main campus in 1972, and the Adams and Sayers Buildings in Great King Street, housed further research groups or freed up space elsewhere. The money requires fuller comment.

The Medical Research Council played a crucial role in funding research at the Medical School. In 1950, it became an autonomous body, financed by government grant. As John Hunter noted, in a statement he prepared for the Medical School's first accreditation review in 1988, for many years the MRC was virtually the only major research funding body and, until the Auckland Medical School opened in the late 1960s, most of the grants went to Otago. In 1956, for example, the MRC received a government grant of £60,000, as well as a separate grant of £3700 for Island Territories research. By 1964, the amount had increased to £150,000 and this was supplemented by funding from such bodies as the Dairy Board, Meat Producers' Board, Wool Board and Golden Kiwi lottery, which brought the total to more than £200,000. The growth in funding was impressive, although the total amount seems minuscule compared with more recent research funding.[6]

The 1960s was a decade of financial pressure for the Medical School, but MRC money still seemed to flow easily through the Dean's office to the departments and then on to the researchers. 'It seems scarcely believable now', wrote Barbara Heslop, 'that until the 1970s we were not troubled by the necessity to write grant applications.' There was also generous lottery funding. Heslop recalls, almost with awe, one occasion when her department was offered a lottery grant simply because it was deemed to be their turn. The high international profile of hypertension research attracted support from a variety of sources: the University of Otago, the Medical Research Council of New Zealand, Life Insurance Medical Research Fund, US National Institutes of Health, Lottery Funds and, to a lesser extent, pharmaceutical firms.[7] The external funding, separate from the Medical School's share of the University's block grant, cushioned the research activities of the School in this difficult decade.

From the end of the 1960s, the task of the Medical Research Council became more complex. Its Director from 1968 to 1990, Dr Jim Hodge, understood medical research well. He had been one of Smirk's team at the Wellcome Institute and had, in fact, briefly taken over its leadership between Smirk's retirement and his own appointment to the MRC. In the 1970s, the Council had to spread its funding over both the Auckland and Otago Medical Faculties, including the developing research programmes of the Christchurch and Wellington Schools. The Council worked through a series of expert committees, on all of which senior Medical School staff were represented. These included assessing committees for preclinical, para-clinical, clinical and social medicine, an awards committee, a South Pacific committee and a standing committee on therapeutic trials. The Council's 1977 report illustrates its activities. It was the twenty-sixth report since the MRC had become independent, so its systems were well established and in spite of inflation, another year of steady progress was reported. The Council had received a $300,000 increase in its base grant to enable it to meet its research commitments, but it still had to fund many projects below the optimal level. Overall grants totalled almost $3.5 million and the same amount would be available the following year. Fifty-eight new grants had been made during the year.[8]

The significance of Medical Research Council support to the Otago Medical School can be precisely demonstrated by listing the grants made in 1977 for long-term research in special fields. Unless otherwise indicated, the named directors were from Dunedin: the Immunopathology Research Unit (D.D. Adams), Toxicology Research Unit (E.G. McQueen), Virus Research Unit (J.A.R. Miles), Biostatistical Sciences (C.W. Dixon from Dunedin and G. Rolleston from Christchurch), Epidemiological Services (A.M.O. Veale, Auckland), Electronics and Engineering (A. Annand) and Animal Services (Dunedin and Auckland). In addition, there were programme grants for long-term research at Otago for Endocrinology (D.W. Beaven, Christchurch), Autoimmune Diseases (J.B. Howie), Body Fluids and Renal Physiology (A.D.C. Macknight and J.R. Robinson), the Christchurch Child Development Study (F. Shannon, Christchurch) and the Dunedin Multidisciplinary Child Development Study (J.M. Watt). The lengthy list of individual projects includes many from staff of the Otago Medical School.[9]

In 1981, with the New Zealand economy in trouble and the medical schools reeling from a reduced student intake, the MRC Director's report is imbued with a sense of anxiety, even though a supplementary grant from government had allowed the growing needs of the medical research community to be met at 'near normal levels'. There had been a reduced level of new initiatives and only one round of applications and awards had been possible. As the decade wore on, the world's stock markets slumped and the New Zealand economy went into a tailspin. Accordingly, the funds continued to fall far short of the level of applications.[10]

In 1988, in line with growing government and public concern for health promotion, the Council published its concept of a 'more broadly based Health Research Council'. This new council 'would give greater prominence to research of public health importance, while preserving the quality control systems developed in relation to more traditional fields of biomedical research'. In a period of tight funding, where only one third of applicants might expect to be successful, the Government required medical research to be more aligned to its own health priorities. These included women's health, epidemiology, Maori and Pacific Island health, the health of the elderly and the very young. The committees on Asthma, Diabetes, AIDS and Ethics in Research were retained. The committee on major equipment had a reduced grant. In 1990, the Medical Research Council was duly replaced by a Health Research Council with a mandate for a broader spectrum of research. The Government explained that the current strong predominance of biomedical research was not appropriate in a time of restricted funding, when there was a clear need to increase research into public health areas, including Maori health. A change of government occurred just after the new Council was set up. On 17 October 1990, on the eve of the general election, Health Minister Helen Clark reminded the first meeting of the new body that it was required to support research aligned with the Government's Health Charter. After a landslide National victory, it was a new Health Minister, Simon Upton, who attended the next meeting, on 23 November. He affirmed the need for more research in public health areas, but also stressed the need to protect biomedical research and the careers of trained biomedical scientists.[11]

With this last point, Upton addressed one of the chief anxieties experienced researchers held about the new regime. Professor George Petersen, for example, initially saw little point in the change and believed that setting up an entirely new committee was 'reinventing the wheel'. He was especially concerned that researchers would lose their security of tenure, effectively going on to short-term contracts and that the MRC fund for capital equipment had disappeared. Within a short time, however, it became clear that the HRC was proving its worth. By July 1991, the *Otago Daily Times* was able to announce that medical researchers had received $3 million in funding in the first round of allocations. Over the next few years, the annual reports of the three Otago Schools acknowledge the receipt of very substantial grants from the HRC, as well as from international bodies, drug companies and private sources. In 1993, for example, the total research income of the Otago Medical School was just over $11 million and, in 1994, it had risen to close on $19 million.[12]

Medical Foundations

Commenting on research for the Medical School review in 1988, John Hunter drew attention to the increasing importance, from the late 1960s, of research funding by bodies other than government. As well as the Lottery Board, he singled out various charitable foundations and Medical Research Foundations. The charitable foundations did much more than simply fulfil a funding role and the efforts of the Otago medical graduates who helped set them up, and who gave their time and skills towards guiding their activities, have been impressive. Sir David Hay, for example, was Medical Director of the National Heart Foundation (NHF) for almost two decades. His vivid description of its establishment and of the work it undertook illustrates the role of such foundations. The National Heart Foundation began in the 1960s, when a group of cardiologists and surgeons from the Australia

and New Zealand Cardiac Society, motivated by the successful launch of the Australian National Heart Foundation in 1958, met to consider setting up a similar body in New Zealand. Lay volunteers joined and, by the end of the 1960s, the group had adopted a constitution and raised $450,000 through a major fund-raising appeal. It was the Foundation's only door-knocking effort, that form of fund-raising subsequently being replaced by large-prize lotteries. A Scientific Committee, chaired for its first ten years by Sir Edward Sayers, was responsible for awarding fellowships and research grants. '[Sayers] used to say', recounts Hay, 'that it was the best committee he had ever served on and we enjoyed his leadership.' John Hunter chaired a hardworking Coronary Committee to assess the significance of factors claimed to be involved in the causation and prevention of coronary disease and to make appropriate recommendations. It produced a comprehensive monograph. Support for cardio-vascular research had been the primary reason for setting up the NHF and it remained the top priority. In 1985, the Foundation decided to further this cause by establishing a Chair of Cardiovascular Disease at Auckland. The first Professor, Wilhelm Lubbe, was appointed by the University and, when he retired in 1996, the NHF chose Otago as the host institution for the next professor. Mark Richards, of the Christchurch School of Medicine, a world leader in medical research, was appointed. The Foundation also conducted publicity campaigns, aligned with the World Health Organization's recommendation for a population strategy to prevent coronary disease. The idea was to persuade the whole community to modify its behaviour in terms of diet, smoking and exercise. The Department of Health contracted with the NHF to initiate the Heartbeat New Zealand prevention programme. From 1989, the special problems of Maori cardiovascular health were addressed through Te Hotu Manawa Maori in Wellington, under the guidance of the gifted and hugely respected Professor Eru Pomare and Dr Papaarangi Reid, whose lectureship in Maori Health was partly funded by the Foundation. Hay recalls a host of smaller initiatives, some with

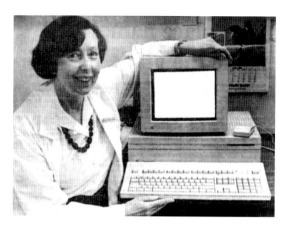

Professor Norma Restieaux, Head of Cardiology at Dunedin Hospital, welcomes the arrival of a second Macintosh computer in her Department. Gifted by the scientific committee of the National Heart Foundation, the computer was expected to make information more readily available to staff, thus enabling them to spend more time with patients.

Otago Daily Times, 12 April 1989.

large consequences, such as the success of Heart Weeks, the campaign to Jump Rope for Health, and the 'Pick the Tick' campaign, which began in 1991, to enable shoppers to choose healthier foods at the supermarket. By 2005, over nine hundred products had been approved. Writing in that year, after thirty-seven years' association with the Heart Foundation, Hay believed it had contributed to improved cardiovascular mortality figures and increased life expectancy over the period. However, he also warned against complacency.[13] Other foundations with a similar mix of medical and lay people and dedicated to fundraising for research and education are the Asthma and Respiratory Foundation, the Cancer Society and the Neurological Foundation.

In the 1980s and 1990s, regionally based Medical Research Foundations flourished. The first had been set up in Auckland in 1955 and in his report on the Medical Research Council in 1959 its chairman, the Director General of Health, Dr Turbott, noted that similar bodies were being set up in Palmerston North, Wellington and Christchurch to encourage local research projects. He hoped for 'close and sympathetic collaboration' between the regional Foundations and the Council. In Christchurch, at least, this was unlikely. Don Beaven and his

team at the Medical Unit had followed the Auckland example because they were convinced that Dr Turbott was unsympathetic to medical research based on hospitals outside Dunedin. The Canterbury Medical Research Foundation sought broadly based community support, with a goal of two thousand subscribing members in five years. By the time Alan Clarke became Dean in 1986, lean times had arrived for research. His response was to form a Canterbury Research Committee, representing the Hospital Board and the University, which could work with the Foundation to raise the standards of health care in Canterbury through research. It took the issue of medical research to the community in a sophisticated publicity campaign that included Medical Expos. New for New Zealand at the time, they were held in Christchurch, and also toured outlying districts. Money flowed into the Foundation, which was widely recognised as an outstanding regional health research funding agency. The Otago Medical School also benefited from the support of the Otago Medical Research Foundation, founded in Dunedin in the late 1970s by members of the Otago Medical School staff, the Dunedin Heart Unit Trust, and various residents and corporate bodies of Dunedin. It solicited subscriptions, donations, subsidies and bequests in order to provide research grants, bursaries and scholarships for persons engaging in medical research and funds to appoint lecturers and demonstrators in medical and allied subjects. By March 1993, its assets were in excess of $2.3 million. The Wellington School benefited in the same way from the Wellington Medical Research Foundation and Malaghan Research Trust.[14]

'Research, untrammelled by near reference to practical ends, will go on in every properly organised medical school', wrote the great American medical educator, Abraham Flexner. If there was a problem with some of the funding from the HRC, and money from the charitable foundations devoted to one particular health problem, it was that it was not 'untrammelled by near reference to practical ends'. Since 1994 the Marsden Fund, which is administered by the Royal Society on behalf of the Minister of Research, Science and Technology, has supported 'blue skies' research, with no specific practical end in mind – the kind of research, it has often been pointed out, that has led to many of the greatest scientific discoveries. The research is specifically not subject to priorities set by the government and allows the 'sometimes serendipitous aspects of research which may lead to profound or unexpected discoveries'. In 2007, it had $33.88 million at its disposal However, it can still fund only a small proportion of applications. The Government has also put funding into the Public Good Science Fund (PGSF), its major strategic research fund which, in contrast to the Marsden Fund, is concerned with general outputs of future benefit to New Zealand.[15]

Research at the Otago Medical School

The number and variety of research projects at the Otago Medical School over recent decades make it impossible to treat even a selection of them in any detail in a general survey. The trend has been from the individual to the team; from the departmental to the multi-disciplinary; from research fitted in by heavily committed teachers to the employment of a proportion of full-time researchers, attached to departments but often funded by outside bodies. In the meantime, research-related paperwork has grown exponentially, with elaborate grant applications for contestable funding and detailed and regular reports on progress.

Traditionally, staff members' research was something private and separate, that took place in the evenings and the summer breaks from teaching and which medical students knew very little about. In 1966, a fourth-year student, J.W.G. Tiller, attempted to correct this 'anomalous situation' in a long article in the *Digest*. He reproduced, without comment, information given him in a series of interviews with staff of the different departments. The resulting descriptions vary in style but they are a useful summary of the research of the day. Tiller dealt in turn with Anatomy, Anaesthetics, Biochemistry, Cancer Research, Endocrinology, Genetics, Medicine, Microbiology, Nutrition Research, Obstetrics and Gynaecology, Pathology, Pharmacology and Pharmacy, Physiology, Preventive and Social

Medicine, Psychological Medicine, Surgery, and the Wellcome Medical Research Institute. Overall, while the brief, factual statements do not make for easy reading, Tiller's article described a flourishing departmentally based research programme.[16]

More helpful, in that he was prepared to comment on what he saw as especially important projects, is an unpublished paper by Associate-Professor Ted Nye on 'Research at the Otago Medical School'. After dealing with earlier research at the School and its inevitable limit-ations, Nye considered aspects of the discipline-based research in the Medical School from the 1950s to the 1980s.

In Microbiology, there was a steady output of research papers in increasingly sophisticated areas of microbial metabolism. Original work on viruses was appearing. Professor Miles and his team isolated the Whataroa virus, which appeared to be unique to New Zealand. By the 1980s, Otago microbiologists were publishing in international journals on a wide range of topics, including bacterial molecular biology.

In Medicine, Professor Smirk and his team achieved a position of world leadership in the investigation of hypertension.

In Pharmacology, which became a separate department in 1962, researchers were moving into studies of agents active on the nervous system, as well as some basic investigations into naturally occurring toxic substances peculiar to New Zealand.

In Anatomy, from the 1950s, there was a movement away from early studies of species unique to New Zealand, such as the tuatara or the kiwi, into collaborative work with other departments, especially taking the opportunities offered by the advent of electron microscopy.

In Physiology, where earlier work had been on nutrition, Professor Eccles took a new direction into neurophysiology and Professor Robinson, in the 1960s, into renal metabolism.

In Preventive and Social Medicine, research had grown beyond earlier studies of infectious diseases. The emphasis was on the community problems caused by infectious diseases, degenerative diseases and malignant disease, with specific focus on New Zealand problems and with the results being made available to health planners in government. Preventive and Social Medicine had developed into a strong research department, with a whole series of sub-areas.[17]

The volume on *Medical Research in Otago, 1922-1997* provides much more detail. The fifteen authors, most of them heads of departments, were asked to review significant publications in the *Proceedings of the University of Otago Medical School* over the fifty-year period. At this stage, the *Proceedings* appeared three times a year and consisted of collections of brief, two-page articles on original research presented at the meetings of the Research Society. Between 1951, when this format of the *Proceedings* began, and 1997, the number of papers ranged from thirty-five to fifty annually. The final two chapters of *Medical Research in Otago, 1922–1997*, summarise the research being carried out in the Otago School of Medical Sciences and the Dunedin School of Medicine.[18]

Although the memorial volume of the *Proceedings* is restricted to research in the Dunedin-based basic sciences and clinical departments of the Medical School, research was flourishing in this period in the northern schools as well. In a far-sighted move in 1955, Hercus had seeded research in what were then the three Branch Faculties of the School, in Christchurch, Auckland and Wellington. The University Council increased its annual grant to each centre, to enable them each to set up a full-time Medical Unit, with a senior specialist, senior registrar and thirty beds. The intention was to build up a well-staffed and well-equipped Faculty capable of setting a high standard of teaching, research and patient care.[19] Each Unit was headed by a distinguished researcher. In Auckland, the physician-in-charge from 1959 to 1968 was Derek North, back from some years in England as a Rhodes scholar. A fine physician and administrator, his research was primarily in chronic pyelonephritis. In Wellington, cardiologist Ian Prior set up the Unit. Increasingly interested in the different patterns of heart disease among different populations, he moved from investigating cardiovascular disease using epidemiological methods, to directing a separate multi-disciplinary epidemiological unit that worked among Maori and in the Pacific Islands.[20] In Christchurch, Don Beaven established an office and laboratory at Princess Margaret Hospital, for what soon became a strong endocrinology group. By the time the Christchurch Clinical School opened in 1972, there were well-established research teams at both the Princess Margaret and Christchurch hospitals and academic appointments at that time provided further impetus. Based in departments,

'Poised for Poisonings.'

At the National Poisons Centre, set up in 1964 by Professor Garth McQueen, with the help of Associate-Professor Fred Fastier of the Department of Pharmacology and Pharmacy, research and community outreach meet on a daily basis. Initially operating out of the hospital and dealing with serious cases only, the Centre now employs a team of trained toxicologists who provide a free 24-hour phone service every day of the year. It has developed its own massive and growing database, which currently gives access to information on some 160,000 toxins. The Centre is administered by the Department of Preventive and Social Medicine and funded by the Ministry of Health and ACC.

Otago University Magazine, October 2005 and information from the National Poisons Centre, 2007.

the research groups spanned the hospitals, the University of Canterbury and Lincoln College and soon developed important international connections.[21]

A Thematic Approach

'Research has become less individual', wrote John Hunter in 1988, 'with active encouragement for teamwork within an area and collaboration with other disciplines in New Zealand and overseas. Much of it is on a much larger scale and while strictly biomedical research has been maintained, there is a much stronger focus on benefits the community will derive from the research.'[22]

What Hunter described as trends have become entrenched as policy. In the 1990s the University took the lead in the organisation of research through formal, publicly distributed Research Management Plans, the first running from 1997 to 2000. Areas of research strength in the University have been developed into major themes and smaller clusters have been termed 'areas of research excellence'. The University commits itself to provide a level of annual funding appropriate to the management structure, objectives and accountabilities of the research groups. It assesses the progress of research through regular reports and celebrates achievements in a glossy publication of research highlights, *He Kitenga*, articles in the *University of Otago Magazine* and press releases. To qualify as a theme, research must be in an area where the University enjoys national leadership and international recognition for excellence, and is likely to remain a contributor for the next several years. Research might involve active groups, or individuals, from more than one department or division, and should have a demonstrated ability to attract significant funding from outside the University.[23]

These criteria suit medical research admirably and, at an early stage, the Medical School assumed a dominant position in the list of Major Research Themes. Of the ten listed in a published report on the University's *Research Strengths* in 2000, six were based in one or other of the three schools:

- Asthma and Respiratory Disorders (Wellington)

- Cardiovascular Endocrinology (Christchurch)
- Functional Genomics, Gene Expression and Proteomics (Dunedin)
- Immunological Basis of Disease and Protective Immunity (Dunedin)
- Oxidative Stress in Health and Disease (Christchurch)
- Public Health (Wellington)

The other major themes, while based elsewhere in the University, all involved some collaboration with Medical School departments. 'Memory: Mechanisms, Processes and Applications' and 'Neural Systems Structure and Functions' were based in the Psychology Department, 'Oral Microbiology and Dental Health' at the School of Dentistry and 'Spatial Information Processing' in the Commerce Division. Of the nine 'emerging themes' listed in 2000, 'Virology' had achieved full Theme status by 2004, as had 'Pharmacy: Formulation and Drug Delivery'. Both involved collaboration with medical departments.[24]

In 1999, all the major and emerging Theme Groups underwent a comprehensive self and external review of their first years of operation. The result was published in two parts, the first containing the actual reviews and the second bringing together almost 2000 theme-related research publications by about 450 academic staff, together with almost one thousand associated postdoctoral and postgraduate researchers. The review also detailed the external funding of more than $100 million for which theme members had successfully bid.[25]

Consideration of the highly rated Asthma and Respiratory Disorders Theme illustrates the working of the multidisciplinary model. Established in 1997, the Asthma Research Group built on research in all three schools in the 1980s, when researchers and the public were alerted to increased mortality from asthma in New Zealand. Coordinated by Associate-Professor Julian Crane of the Asthma Research Group in the Wellington School of Medicine and Health Sciences, it brought together already established groups in the three Otago schools (the Christchurch group was highly respected for its work on pneumonia caused by air pollution) and the

Malaghan Institute in Wellington. The aim was to understand and quantify risk factors associated with the development of asthma and atopy and improve management and control of the disease for individuals, the community and the workplace. When the review took place, the Asthma Research Group consisted of eleven academic staff spread over the three cities (seven of them in Wellington), thirteen postdoctoral or research fellows, fifteen graduate students and twenty-two full-time-equivalent support staff. There were eleven different research collaborations, several of them long-term, over a variety of areas from immunology and epidemiology to occupational and environmental management. Researchers were also linked to a network of collaborators throughout New Zealand and overseas, in Europe, the United States and Asia. Publications included two books, one hundred refereed journal articles and seventy-nine conference papers and abstracts. As well as University of Otago research funds, financial support came from fifteen external agencies, including the Health Research Council, the Lottery Board, the Marsden Fund, Medical Research Foundations in Wellington, Hawkes Bay and Christchurch and the Asthma and Respiratory Foundation. The external reviewer, Professor Stephen Holgate of the University of Southampton, assessed the group's research as A+, commenting that it was shaping the agenda for diagnosing and managing respiratory disorders internationally. 'This network', he asserted, 'is among the top ranking asthma research groups in the world.' [26]

A similar depth of information and comment was provided for the other Major Research Themes. The Cardiovascular Endocrinology Group, for example, led by Professor Mark Richards of the Christchurch School, reported an unprecedented expansion in funding, staff numbers, and productivity over the period. It comprised nine academic staff, three graduate students and twenty-one technicians, research assistants and other staff, as well as local, national and international collaborators. The Group had been notably successful in gaining contestable funding. It had initiated or completed a broad array of clinical studies and trials during the period under consideration, reporting on its activities under the headings of clinical projects, animal experiments, cell culture, biochemistry and molecular biology. The external reviewer, Professor J.W. Funder, Director of the Baker Medical Research Institute, Melbourne, believed that the impact of the Group on society as a whole was likely to be almost incalculable. Studies in train showed that heart failure patients could be classified by prognostic factors into relative risk groups and that, on the basis of that stratification, much of the care of heart failure patients could be undertaken within the community rather then as inpatients. The implications of this for patients and for the health service were difficult to over-estimate. [27]

The Group researching Oxidative Stress in Health and Disease was coordinated by Professor Christine Winterbourn of the Christchurch School, with regional coordinators from the other two centres. In 1999, the reviewer noted that, over the previous four years, the Research Group had attracted funding amounting to a total of

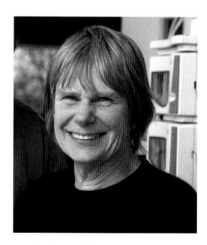

Professor Christine Winterbourn
He Kitenga, University of Otago Research Highlights, 2004.
Marketing and Communications, University of Otago.

'My field is a rather special area of interest; and that's what makes it so intriguing ... We know that free radicals are associated with disease, but what we still haven't found out is whether they're actually critical components of disease development.'

almost $4 million. Oxidative stress, which occurs when the production of damaging free radicals exceeds the capacity of the body's antioxidant defences to detoxify them, contributes to many diseases, such as inflammation, autoimmune disease, cancer, neurodegenerative diseases, heart attack and stroke. Accordingly, those who contributed funds included major foundations, such as the Heart Foundation, the Cancer Society, the Asthma and Respiratory Foundation and the Neurological Foundation, as well as the HRC and the Marsden Fund. The research brought together a wide spectrum of individuals with interests in free radicals, oxidative injury and antioxidants. The 1998 *Research Report* estimated seventy staff and postgraduate students were working on numerous projects across seven departments of the University's three campuses. Since the review, the research has gone on from strength to strength. Christine Winterbourn was the 2004 recipient of the Distinguished Research Medal, Otago University's highest research honour. The Medal recognised the thirty-four years she had given to free radical research, which began when she arrived to work with haematologist Dr Robin Carrell in 1970. That her degree is in biochemistry, not medicine, is another indication of the interdisciplinary nature of modern medical research. Her team includes chemists, biochemists, nutritionists and clinical staff with an interest in heart disease and neonatology.[28]

Areas of Research Excellence

Approximately 130 Areas of Research Excellence were listed in the 2000 *Research Strengths* report. Of these, no fewer than fifty-three were based in the Medical School, twelve in Christchurch, eleven in Wellington and the other thirty in Dunedin, mostly in the School of Medical Sciences. It is impossible to do justice to all of them, but even a brief mention of a few demonstrates their extraordinary strength and variety.

In Christchurch, a cluster of Research Groups in the Department of Psychological Medicine is involved with research into aspects of mental health. 'Affective Disorders', an investigation led by Professor Peter Joyce into depression and manic depression, which together form the single biggest risk factor for suicide, has developed under his leadership into the Mental Health Clinical Research Unit. Ground-breaking work in the Unit has meant that Professor Joyce (now Dean of the University of Otago, Christchurch), Professor Fergusson, of the long-running Christchurch Health and Development Study and Professor Roger Mulder are among the most-cited mental health researchers in Australasia. In 2004, Joyce was honoured with a Fellowship of the Royal Society of New Zealand. Since 2005, the Carney Centre for Pharmacogenomics has added another dimension to the focus on mental health. The Centre is concerned with how people's genetic makeup affects the way they respond to drugs and, under the direction of Associate-Professor Martin Kennedy, it works closely with the Department of Psychological Medicine on the treatment of mental disorders.[29]

Public health is a particular focus of the Wellington School. For example, in 2000 the Sleep/Wake Centre, under the direction of Associate Professor Philippa Gander of the Public Health Department, was undertaking basic and applied multidisciplinary research to understand and reduce the health and safety consequences of shiftwork and to investigate the epidemiology of sleep disorders. A group, He Kainga Oranga, Housing and Health Research Programme, led by Professor Philippa Howden-Chapman, was investigating 'Socio-economic Inequalities in Health' by exploring the relationship between socio-economic factors and health status. Their findings on the health benefits of insulating houses, based on the study of some 1400 homes, investigated by collaborators in seven different areas of New Zealand, had roused public interest and concern. External collaborators on social inequalities have been the Erasmus University, Rotterdam and the Harvard School of Public Health. In an opinion piece in the *University of Otago Magazine* in February 2007, Howden-Chapman described plans to set up a wide-ranging multidisciplinary Centre for Urban Health and Development, with leading national and international collaborators, to carry out solution-focused research on urban health and

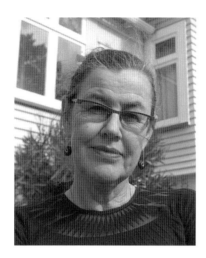

Professor Philippa Howden-Chapman.
Marketing and Communications, University of Otago.

'We see an urgent need for solution-focused research to address complex urban sustainability problems, such as the trend of increasing car travel, despite the need for people to both exercise more and reduce their carbon emissions.'

development problems.[30] Disparities in health between Maori and non-Maori were the research focus of Hauora Maori, which was coordinated by Dr Papaarangi Reid. The purpose of Hauora Maori was to monitor such disparities, examine contributing causes, evaluate interventions and train Maori health researchers. As described in the 2000 report, the research was organised into three portfolios, covering Hauora, Maori standards of health; Mauri Mahi, Mauri Ora, health effects of unemployment and redundancy; and Te Kohanga, examining Maori mortality and morbidity.[31]

In Dunedin, research is spread widely over the School of Medical Sciences, as well as the clinical departments in the Dunedin School of Medicine. Expertise in research into human nutrition dates from the earliest days of the Medical School and is maintained by Professor Jim Mann together with teams of researchers in the Departments of Medicine and Human Nutrition and the recently established Edgar Centre for Diabetes Research. Mann's own research involves the effect of diet on lipids and lipoproteins, antioxidant status and other cardiovascular risk factors, the role of diet in the prevention of diabetes and the health consequences of a vegetarian diet. He also has a long-standing interest in the epidemiology of coronary heart disease and diabetes.[32] The Department of Preventive and Social Medicine is the largest department, and holds a prominent position in the University. It is the home base for a whole range of programmes, from cancer epidemiology to injury prevention, and the multidisciplinary longitudinal study, now some thirty-five years old, of a large group of Dunedin children. In 1998, Professor David Skegg headed the Group for 'Cancer Epidemiology and Control', described as 'a range of studies to investigate causes of cancer and strategies for prevention and early detection.' They included studies of prostate cancer, melanoma, breast cancer, renal cancer and childhood cancer. Also focusing on cancer

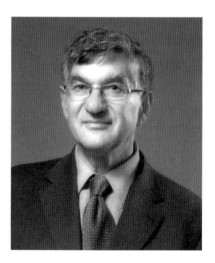

Professor Jim Mann is not only a dedicated researcher, a recipient of the University's Distinguished Research Medal for his work in human nutrition and medicine, but also a passionate campaigner for dietary change to reduce obesity in New Zealand and the consequent risk of chronic diseases, such as diabetes.
He Kitenga, 2006.

'If a sufficient number of individuals were to create a demand for more appropriate food choices, commercial reality would soon ensure availability at reasonable prices.'

research, is the Group led by Professor Anthony Reeve of Biochemistry, who heads the University's Cancer Genetics Laboratory. Research in the Laboratory aims to 'dissect out the genetic events that lead to cancer' and a major focus has been cancers that affect children. Dr Ian Morison and his group have received international recognition for their work on Wilms' tumour, a renal cancer found in young children. Dr Parry Guilford's Group have been working on an inherited stomach cancer in a large Maori family. Professor Michael Eccles and his team are working on the gene PAX2, which is important for the formation and growth of kidneys.[33]

The work on protein synthesis of Professor Warren Tate, who has been in the Biochemistry Department since 1975, also involves genetics. He leads a group researching the 'Regulation of Protein Synthesis' which has used a wide range of technologies to 'understand the molecular signals in protein synthesis, the structures of the decoding factors, their mapping onto the ribosome and the way in which the amount of each protein is regulated, particularly for selenium-containing

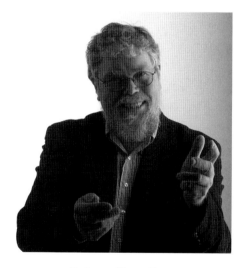

Professor Warren Tate.
University of Otago Research Highlights, 2006, *He Kitenga*.
Marketing and Communications, University of Otago.

'It was one of those moments which you have in a research career if you are lucky – the discovery of a completely new phenomenon.'

protein and the proteins of HIV'. The research had already borne exciting results in 1985, with the discovery of a new type of genetic 'recoding' event during protein synthesis, which is believed to be unique. The group has flourished since, winning funding from the major New Zealand providers and also from the Howard Hughes Medical Research Institute and the Japanese Ministry of Health. In 2006, Tate was awarded the University's Distinguished Research Medal, the latest in a line of high honours, national and international.[34]

'In the nine years of its existence', wrote Professor R.J. Olds in 1997, 'the Bioethics Research Centre has established for itself an enviable reputation as a focus for ethical debate within the Faculty of Medicine, the University and the country.' Professor Donald Evans, who took over that year, leads a team investigating the philosophical and ethical dimensions of clinical practice and research. The topics of 'special emphasis' are daunting in number and complexity: assisted reproduction, resource allocation, care of the elderly, ethical review of human subject research, psychiatry, death and dying, and the nature and limits of medical practice. The Bioethics Centre takes interdisciplinarity to a new level, bringing in expertise from law, philosophy, history, economics, and zoology as well as from a variety of health science disciplines. It also undertakes many consultancies. The 'flagship' publication of the Centre is *Medical Ethics,* which ran into a fourth edition in 2005.[35]

Probably no research emanating from the Otago Medical School has had such a high profile, or captured the public imagination to such an extent, as a pair of longitudinal studies on child development, the Christchurch Health and Development Study and the Dunedin Multi-Disciplinary Health and Development Study. Both began in the 1970s, both have produced an impressive array of significant research findings and publications, and both still flourish. While the studies are not identical, each has followed a large group of young people since infancy: in the case of Christchurch, 1265 children born in the Christchurch region in mid-1977, in the case of Dunedin, 1037 babies born in the city in 1972–73.

Placing great emphasis on the social context of children's development, the Christchurch study has a small research group who visit participants in their homes. The Dunedin study, with a focus on multidisciplinary research, calls individual participants to Dunedin every few years for interviews and physical tests. The founders of the two studies, Professor David Fergusson and Dr Phil Silva, have received many honours. They are the two most cited Australasian researchers in the field of mental health and, in 2007, both were made Honorary Fellows of the New Zealand Psychological Society.[36]

The Christchurch Health and Development Study emerged from the concern of Fred Shannon, Foundation Professor of Paediatrics in the Christchurch School, with the social, demographic and economic factors that influenced child health. David Fergusson has directed the study from the start. Interviewed for the February 2007 *University of Otago Magazine,* Fergusson was of the view that the significance of both the Christchurch and Dunedin studies was better appreciated overseas than in New Zealand. He noted the difficulties securing funding for such long-term, open-ended projects, and steady

staffing, when the norm for science researchers was short-term, three-to-five-year contracts. Nevertheless, the study has been splendidly successful. The 1977 group has been studied from infancy to early adulthood, the researchers have published more than 300 scientific papers, books and book chapters and the research has broken new ground in many social areas, such as the effect of parents' passive smoking on infants and the effect of dysfunctional family situations on children's development. In some cases, official action has been taken on the basis of the findings. The study includes themes of evident social urgency, such as domestic violence or suicidal behaviour in young adults, unemployment and personal adjustment, and the mental health problems of abortion, and alcohol and cannabis use, on young adults. Many of the findings are in sensitive areas and touch off a strong reaction.[37]

The Dunedin Multidisciplinary Health and Development study began as a spin-off from the work done by Dr Phil Silva with the late Associate Professor Patricia Buckfield on the perinatal problems of infants born at Dunedin's Queen Mary Maternity Hospital. Buckfield had been collecting data on all the babies born between 1967 and 1973. Those born between 1 April 1972 and 31 March 1973 were contacted for an assessment at age three years, with the object of finding out whether babies born in adverse circumstances fared less well than those born in more favourable circumstances. After five years, realising that a whole range of health problems were more prevalent than people had assumed, the researchers decided to carry on. The study members were assessed at two-yearly intervals until they were fifteen years old, and then at eighteen, twenty-one, twenty-six and thirty-two years. The most recent assessment was completed in 2005. Of the 1014 of the original group still alive in 2005, 972 took part, a remarkable 96 per cent participation rate – the more remarkable considering that only a minority still lived in Dunedin, and 240 had to be flown in from overseas for their one-day assessment. Professor Richie Poulton, Director since 2000 when Dr Silva retired, told the *University of Otago Magazine* that every aspect of the study members' health and

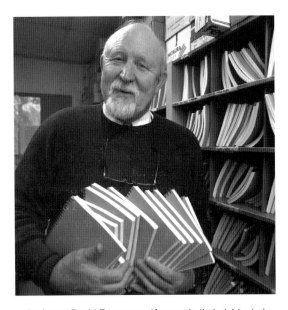

Professor David Fergusson: 'Anyone in their right mind would have to think twice about jumping into one of these studies. They are complex and challenging.'
University of Otago Magazine, February 2007, p. 10.

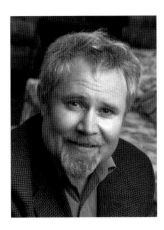

Professor Richie Poulton.
Multidisciplinary Health and Development Research Unit.

Speaking of the Christchurch and Dunedin long-running studies, he has commented: 'Our work challenges people's preconceived notions … In some areas we're answering questions that have been around for thousands of years. For example, we've just ripped the lid off the nature/nurture debate by identifying, in different studies, specific environments and specific genes whose interaction leads to aggression, depression and psychoses.'

University of Otago Magazine, February 2007, p. 11.

development was being tracked, 'their physical and psychological growth, how they negotiated the hurdles life throws up, why they sometimes fail to negotiate them and what health problems they have.' Confidentiality is absolute. The study is based in the Department of Preventive and Social Medicine and funded primarily by the Health Research Council. It does not come cheap: the age thirty-two years assessment cost $1.8 million. However, the high retention rate of study members is a guarantee of the solidity of the findings, and the publications have poured out. In 2007, they added up to over one thousand papers, an average of one every thirteen days.[38]

'Research is an essential ingredient in the proper functioning of a University and a Medical School', Professor John Hunter wrote in 1988, simply stating what for him was a self-evident truth. In 2004, when Professor David Skegg was appointed Vice-Chancellor, he was determined to make research a University-wide priority. So far as the Medical School is concerned, the goal is clearly in view.

Leading by Example

PROFESSOR DAVID SKEGG, the University's Vice-Chancellor since 2004, is an expert on breast and cervical cancer, contraceptive and drug safety, and reproductive health. He chairs an international breast cancer group centred in Oxford and advises a World Health Organisation programme in human reproduction. In New Zealand, he has chaired the Public Health Commission, the Health Research Council and the BSE Expert Science Panel. An outstanding researcher, with more than 150 publications in academic journals, he has been awarded several of the country's highest honours, including an OBE for services to medicine, Fellowship of the Royal Society of New Zealand (1992), the Sir Charles Hercus Medal (Royal Society of New Zealand) (1999) and the University of Otago's Distinguished Research Medal in 2003.[39] 'If I and others leading the University are involved in research and committed to it, then others may follow suit,' he told the *University of Otago Magazine* in 2004.

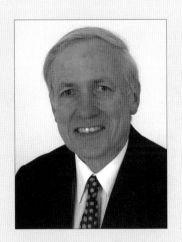

Professor David Skegg.
Otago Daily Times.

He also noted that only two – Sir Robert Aitken and Sir Robin Irvine – of his six predecessors in the office (in its modern form) had been Otago graduates. One might add that both were medical graduates and that for almost half the sixty years since the modern Vice-Chancellorship was established in 1948, the University has been served, at this highest level, by graduates of its Medical School.

University of Otago Magazine, October 2004, pp. 5, 14.

CHAPTER 26

A Rich Diversity:
Medical Students in the Late Twentieth Century

The Medical Student Population

'In the early 1980s', student historian Elworthy writes, 'the Otago campus was divided between two cultures.' The Springbok rugby tour, in 1981, and the actions of the first woman President of the OUSA to change the crude sexism of the Capping concert and Capping book, in 1983, polarised the student population. He argues that the changed composition of the student body created a new environment, one that sharpened tensions and anxieties over gender roles. By the mid-1980s, the proportion of women studying Law and Medicine had risen from a third, at the end of the 1970s, to almost half. The male residential colleges, so long bastions of mateship and leadership in student politics, sport and high jinks, began to accept women in the early 1980s. There was also a new forum for debate. The Student Council, which had been made up of representatives of the various faculties, was replaced by a free-for-all Student Representative Council. At the height of the Springbok tour controversy, between six and eight hundred people would attend Council meetings and the opposing sides would confront one another in noisy and ugly argument.[1] Most medical students were probably pleased to distance themselves from the turmoil and develop their own organisations and traditions.

The medical student population was itself changing during this time. The trend towards a more evenly gender-balanced intake settled and, as women came to make up slightly more than half the class, resentment or disapproval of their inclusion in the course disappeared. A collection of personal and medical memoirs by a group of women doctors, who studied at Otago in the 1970s and who wrote from the mid-point of their professional careers, makes it clear that the warnings of low output from women doctors, common when they were students, have not come to pass. Nevertheless, the difficulties of attaining an acceptable work/life balance was of concern to them all. Only a few mentioned discrimination at Medical School. One recalled two professors agreeing that most of the women in the class were unlikely to complete the course and, if they did, they would become part-time GPs, while their husbands pursued 'proper' medical careers. One Maori woman, who gained special entry to the School, had been verbally abused by a classmate for 'keeping out' one of his friends. For a time in the 1980s, the pendulum swung the other way. With the support of numbers in the classroom and the flourishing feminist movement beyond it, some women insisted on a respect denied their predecessors. Their insistence could go to surprising lengths. Lecturing to a physiology class on sterilisation methods, Professor Sandy Smith showed a slide of an autoclave. The image came from an advertisement and included an attractive technician. Quoting the price of the equipment, he made the throwaway comment that the technician was not included, and was dumbfounded to find himself called to the Dean's office to respond to a complaint of sexism.[2]

Generally, however, an easy companionship prevailed.

Towards the end of the twentieth century, the ethnic composition of medical classes also changed. Maori students had long been encouraged to study medicine through more relaxed entry requirements and effective support networks were well developed. In 1987, the first Maori and Polynesian representative on the OUMSA Executive, the Samoan Tai Sopaoga, explained that her role was to encourage integration and support. Various seminars were arranged on Maori and Polynesian health, attitudes to health and ways of coping with stress and death. A successful dinner united Maori and Polynesian medical students throughout the school and some fifty visited a marae as part of their third-year elective. At a New Zealand Medical Students' Association conference in Dunedin the following year, Professor Eru Pomare spoke on Maori and Polynesian perspectives on health.[3] In 1999, Francie Robbins reported in the medical student publication *Enema* on three excellent huis for Maori medical students held during the year. Nineteen students from Dunedin, Christchurch, Wellington and Auckland had gathered at Waitaia Lodge in the Kaimai Range, for total immersion teaching of the Maori language. This hui had been the highlight of the year for Robbins because, 'as Maori medical students, we want to become Maori doctors who can confidently and competently work in our own communities'. The second hui, at Plimmerton near Wellington, the home of the Pomare whanau, celebrated the centenary of the graduation of Sir Maui Pomare. The third was the Annual National Development Hui at Ohakune, which promoted general practice. Locally, weekly Maori language classes offered by Te Tari Maori were greatly appreciated. Maori medical students have their own association, which arranges a special programme. A freshers' hui is held annually at Otakou Marae, where new second years can get to know more senior Maori medical students from all the Otago Schools. A Maori language weekend and weekly language tutorials have become a regular part of the calendar. For their Early Community Contact in 2006, some Maori

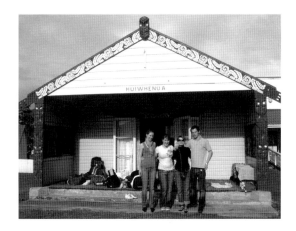

A group of third-year students during their Early Community Contact experience in Gisborne in 2006. Photograph, Fiona Loan.

students found that a week-long sojourn on the East Coast, around Gisborne, billeted at seven different marae, proved an exhilarating chance 'to learn what life is all about … whanau, aroha and happiness'. In 2006, the newly established Pacific Island Health Professional Students' Association also reported on its activities. An impressive contingent of thirty had attended the Pasifika Medical Association conference in Auckland. Nevertheless, the small numbers of both Maori and Pacific Island students is a cause for concern to the student associations. In 2004, Maori were 7.5 per cent of medical students and Pacific students 2.9 per cent, whereas Maori made up 15 per cent of the New Zealand population and Pacific peoples 7 per cent. There is an acknowledged shortage of both Maori and Pacific doctors in New Zealand. The NZMSA is working with government, the University and Maori and Pacific Island stakeholders on strategies to recruit and retain Maori and Pacific Island students. These include putting information into booklets or DVDs and making personal visits to targeted schools.[4]

In the 1990s, the Faculty of Medicine received government funding for 170 students, but had capacity for more, so the Faculty was able to offer about twenty places to Full Cost Recovery students from countries which had agreements with the University. The first group to arrive, in 1992, were from Malaysia. Most were Malays who had been selected by Otago University representatives in Kuala Lumpur. They were required to take a full first-year course and achieve an average of B/B+. English proved to be the main stumbling block for the students and help was arranged through the Otago Language Centre. While the students' reticence also meant they were reluctant to make their problems known, they generally fitted in well. The University has a prayer hall for Muslim students and two of the residential colleges provided halal food. Due to an economic crisis in Malaysia, however, the scheme lapsed and the 1997 intake was the last. In 1998, as the scheme was drawing to a close, international students joined together to write an article for *Enema*. 'A Word on Malaysia' included a description of the lives of the sixty or so Malaysian students sponsored by their government to study at the Otago Medical School. They explained that they

ate, slept, socialised and took up sport as others did, but all within the boundaries of Islam, eating only halal food, abstaining from alcohol and, in the case of women, keeping their bodies, apart from their face and hands, covered when in public. The University replaced its agreement with Malaysia by one with Saudi Arabia. The first group of students arrived in 2000 and, in 2006, when the first four graduated, there were fifty-eight at various stages of the course. The sole woman among the graduates, whose parents had given up their life at home to come with her for the six years, believed she had crossed the gender and ethnic divide with ease.[5]

The cartoon image of the medical student of fifty years ago – middle-class, white, male, hard-drinking, with an easy nonchalance irresistible to women – has little relevance today, if it ever did. There are, of course, continuities in the student experience. Medical students have always been bonded by their specialised coursework and common goals, and they have always enjoyed each other's company. However, today's students are a diverse group of men and women that early lecturers in the Medical School might be hard put to recognise.

OUMSA and Student Activities

Among Medical School activities, the annual revue 'Humour-us', later 'Humerus', which began in 1977, has become firmly established as a social and entertainment highlight. Its proceeds go to charity. An anonymous reviewer of the 1997 'Humerus' explained the never-fail formula, while glossing over the work that went into the show:

> Take a cast of over 40 eager med students, write a script bursting with pisstakes of lecturers and cracks at dent students; practise a couple of times; build a makeshift stage in the Terrace Lounge of the Union; give the cast several casks of wine and quite a few dozen beers and what you end up with is the Med Revue.[6]

Another more recent and less raunchy form of entertainment is the annual Cultural Night, which reflects the ethnic diversity and talent of the modern Medical School. As the 1999 reviewer

---

A day in the life of a typical Muslim medical student

6.00 am	Out of bed. Prepare for *Subuh* (early morning prayer). Takes about 10–15 minutes. Eat breakfast. Get ready for the day's class.
8.45 am	Head to Med School. Spend about 4 hours there. Lectures, tutorials, etc.
1.00 pm	Lunch. *Dzuhr* (midday) prayer. A little rest or afternoon nap.
1.45 pm.	Back to Med School. Another couple of hours there.
5.00 pm	That's it for the day. Home. *Asar* (afternoon) prayer. Time for recreation, sports or gym.
6.30 pm	Prepare for *Magrb* (early night) prayer. Watch news on TV.
7.00 pm	Dinner
8.00 pm	Self studying or complete any homework, etc.
12.00	*Isya* (late night) prayer. Bed time.

From 'A Word on Malaysia',
by the Malaysian Students, *Enema*, 1998.
Otago University Medical Students Association.

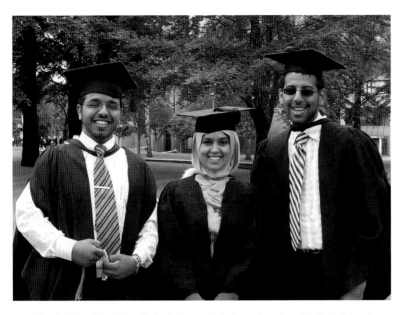

The first Saudi Arabian students to graduate from the Otago Medical School: Drs Abdulrahman Alqahtani, Mai Alshammari and Ali Aisinan. Absent is Dr Jaiai Alsaad. *Otago Daily Times*, 16 December 2006.

'Back home I wouldn't dream of going to the bank and cashing money or filling up my own car with petrol at my age.'

Mai Alshammari, Saudi medical student.

'Transformation is a two-way process. The students have taught us much about their country and culture. We continue to learn.'

Warwick Brunton, Associate Dean, International.

Otago Daily Times, 16 December 2006.

described it, the show is 'a whirlwind magical journey visiting many of the cultures that make up our colourful school'. On that occasion, the student performances ranged from a Korean percussion group, through Indian, Samoan and Sri Lankan dances, to Maori waiata and haka and a Chinese lion dance. There were instrumental performances of all kinds and a wealth of beautiful national costumes.[7]

Since the late 1970s, the welcome from third-year students to second years has established itself as a rite of passage. The 1994 student President explained that the serious purpose of the weekend camp was to enable members of the new class to get to know each other and some of the Executive and thus open channels for discussion and advice if they were needed during the year. Senior staff attending the camp could give the new students an insight into what would be expected of them at the Medical School and the career paths that would be available to them. Informal accounts by second-year students had a somewhat different perspective. They described the getting-to-know-you games, the lack of sleep and the abundance of beer, but they all agreed that the class certainly did get acquainted. Due

to the pressure of numbers the camp has been replaced by an orientation week at the Medical School, but a number of the camp features have been retained. The 2006 orientation included lectures, a cultural lunch, a medieval ball at Glenfalloch and an introduction to the army by a rotation of ten stations of demanding physical activity at Kettle Park.[8]

The role of OUMSA remains central to medical students' extra-curricular life and interests. In the 1980s, it continued to look after the café and student areas, arrange farewells to senior staff, and run the medical ball and class steins, as the former bashes and smokos were now usually called. The uncomfortable tradition of having to apologise and make amends for the damage caused at medical student celebrations was also maintained. In 1983, for example, when the caterer for the medical ball had to pay an extra $300 for cleaning whipped cream from the Concert Chamber curtains, the OUMSA President was reprimanded and the last stein of the year cancelled.[9] In 1985, the University Proctor formally complained to the Dean about medical student pub crawling and 'blatant breaches of the alcohol regulations' at the Med Revue. 'I'm afraid', he wrote, 'that the

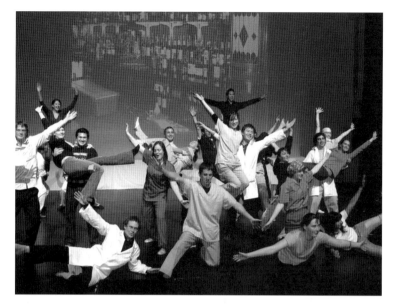

The Med Revue: Finale of 'The Phantom of the Operating Theatre', 2006.
Photograph, Fiona Loan.

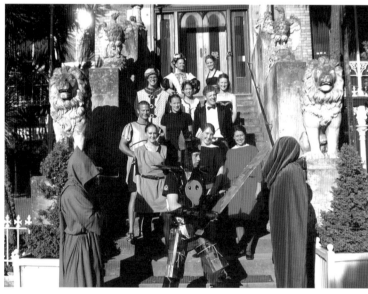

Orientation Week 2006, at Larnach Castle. Third years, in medieval garb, welcome incoming second years.
Photograph, Fiona Loan.

reputation of our medical students is presently at an all-time low.' The University Social Convener banned all medical student social functions for 1986, because under-age children had been admitted to the Med Revue and no permit had been obtained for the after-show party. However, he was persuaded to allow class dinners, at which a 'reasonable number' of staff were present, and carefully controlled steins.[10]

The Medical Students' Association continues to organise a full extra-curricular programme. In 2006, the President listed in his annual report:

'Pot Luck Dinner, Flat Crawl, Easter Picnic, Wine and Cheese, Quiz Night, Ice Skating, Careers Evening, Ski Trip, Med Revue, Grand Ball, Cultural Night, the Forbury Races and various dinners and steins.' A highlight of the year was a new venture, a charity art auction with over a hundred works on sale, which raised more than $38,000 for the Child Cancer Foundation. While the second-hand book sale is no longer held, medical students benefit from a special deal on text books from the University Book Shop. Changes have also been made to the various sporting fixtures.

The men's inter-class rugby competition for the Nichol Cup has gone, but the Medical School plays regular matches against Law and Dentistry. Both sexes now compete for the Ellen Hendry Cup in four sports. Serious sport has been left to individual students and, over the years, they have proved adept at fitting sporting commitments at provincial and even national level into the demands of the medical course. The 1985 Rhodes scholar, David Kirk, represented New Zealand at rugby from 1983 to 1987 and, in the latter year, led the All Blacks to victory in the World Cup. Lesley Nichol captained the successful Southland netball team, the Southern Sting, was a member of the 2003 World Champion Silver Ferns and captained the team in 2004.[11]

There has been change as well as continuity in the narrative of OUMSA. It has recognised the more diverse ethnic makeup of Otago medical students by inviting Maori, Pacific Island and International students on to its Executive. In 2004, the Association revised its constitution and became an incorporated society and, in 2006, it further streamlined its structure by trimming down the Executive and making the Council more widely representative, which also allowed for a broader range of student involvement through focused working groups. Many of OUMSA's activities are costly and corporate sponsorship has become an important consideration. In 2006, a new scheme, promoted through a professionally designed pamphlet, encouraged interested companies to sponsor OUMSA generally, rather than its individual events. The Association offered a number of benefits, depending on the package purchased and the campaign resulted in a sponsorship intake almost triple that of the previous year.[12]

Although the Medical Students' Association remains affiliated to OUSA, the long-held belief that medical students do not get value for money from the parent organisation persists. The Health Sciences representative on the Executive of OUSA does not carry a specific mandate from the Association and medical students do not, as a rule, take office in OUSA. The exception has been Ayesha Verrall, who served on the Executive of OUMSA and, in 2001, became the first medical

student President of OUSA for more than thirty years. First involved in OUSA through the women's group, she moved from being the Women's Rights Officer to the Health Sciences Division representative on the OUSA Executive, before taking a year out to be President. While Verrall's experience as President illustrates the potential for fruitful cooperation between the two student bodies, no other medical student has been willing to take the time required out from a lengthy and demanding course.[13] In the 1999 election year, the issue of student debt brought OUMSA and OUSA together. On 1 June, more than 300 medical students in white lab-coats gathered outside the Lindo Ferguson building and marched along George Street to the Octagon, in a dramatic silent protest at paying interest on student loans. The march was organised by the President of OUMSA, Brandon Adams. OUSA Executive and campaign officers helped by advising the medical students on practical aspects of the protest, such as training marshals for the day. Adams followed up the striking success of the demonstration with co-ordinated media releases from the Deans of the New Zealand Medical Schools, the New Zealand Medical Association and various student bodies. Talkback radio ran hot and Labour's tertiary spokesman raised the matter in Parliament.[14]

Fifteen years elapsed between the demise of *Digest* in 1978 and the advent of the next Dunedin medical students' magazine. *Borborygmi* filled the gap to some extent, but few copies have survived. One from 1988, consisting of five cyclostyled pages, features a report on Humerus '88 and the programme for the approaching NZMSA conference in Auckland. A 1999 meeting of the OUMSA Executive recorded the opinion that '*Borborygmi* was great.'[15] In 1993, medical students began producing an annual glossy magazine entitled *Enema*. Intended as a yearbook, it contained photographs of social occasions, reports of the activities of each class and of special events, such as Med Camp, a number of insider jokes and some interesting interviews with staff members. Although *Enema* began with much less weight (or staff involvement) than the *Digest*, it has developed well and seems firmly established.

In March 2004, *Enema* was joined by a more serious companion publication, thanks to a bold initiative from the Dunedin School. The first issue of an attractively produced *New Zealand Medical Student Journal* offered medical students the opportunity to have their research published, after being reviewed by leading authorities in their field. As explained in the first number, the journal aims to assist students in writing and presenting their work, as well as providing a source of information and opinion for other students. In 2006, a branch of the *Journal*'s Executive was established at the Auckland Medical School and a new writing prize awarded. The *Journal* is justly proud of being the first peer-reviewed medical student journal in Australasia. Its content is varied, well presented and of high quality.[16]

The fourth-year students who moved to Christchurch and Wellington in the mid-1970s promptly set up their own student organisations. Their respective Presidents described their activities for the AMC accreditation review team in 1994. In Christchurch, the fifteen-person Executive of the Canterbury Medical Students Association (CMSA) met weekly, organised social functions, advocated student concerns and facilitated communication between faculty, staff and students. Students at Canterbury were satisfied that they enjoyed a very close and open relationship with the Dean and staff. Education representatives on the Executive provided input into the Curriculum Committee and academic issues were discussed at regular staff/student committee meetings. Regular events were Friday evening steins, an annual ball, a ski trip and an evening at which trainee interns related stories and showed slides on their electives to fourth years. CMSA kept in touch with the Medical Students' Association in Dunedin and sent two representatives to NZMSA. The report from the Wellington Medical Students Association (WMSA) was brief, but along the same lines. The Association had input into the course, represented the students' views on various committees, liaised with other student associations and organised social events, such as sports days, an annual ball, class dinners, conferences, debates and staff/student functions.[17]

OUMC

Since its foundation in 1909, the Otago University Medical Corps has been an important part of Medical School life, for a proportion of the students. The proportion has varied, in response to New Zealand's social environment and overseas military commitments, but has always been significant. Brigadier Brian MacMahon maintains that OUMC put Otago on the military medical map, but adds that, over recent years, the Corps has operated in a very different mode from the halcyon days of 1950, when it was the 'biggest club in the university', boasting some three hundred members. In the early 1970s, many medical students shared the widespread hostility to the Vietnam war and the Dunedin unit was weakened by the loss of most of the senior students to Christchurch and Wellington. Furthermore, the women who have made up half the Medical School's population since the 1980s have shown little interest in military medicine. McMahon believes the military must also take some blame for the decline of OUMC, for not looking after its health professionals adequately. He contends they failed to offer the students formal military training, yet expected them to learn on the job and operate as soldiers. Most of the present Army Medical Corps are not health professionals at all, but soldiers, both male and female, who are trained to a high level as paramedics. Moreover, the combination of medical and military responsibilities has made the position of CO of a military hospital less a position for an ambitious doctor to aspire to than an onerous burden.[18]

The army has also been engaged in repeated and confusing restructurings, which have left OUMC without a clear identity of its own. The University Medical Unit was disbanded in 1983 and its components, OUMC and AUMC, became sub-units of 3 Field Ambulance and 1 Field Ambulance respectively. Then in 2000 both units were disestablished, as part of the Territorial Force Regionalisation, which significantly damaged both the interests and input of medical students. Territorial Force medical personnel became part of either the Auckland/Northland Infantry Regiment or the Otago/Southland Infantry Regiment. After it was absorbed into the Southern Battalion group, OUMC no longer had its own annual camps, its own transport or catering corps. In 2006, responsibility for all Territorial Force medical personnel was transferred from the regional battalions to the new Regular Force Medical Unit, 2 Health Support Battalion and, at the time of writing, there were moves to re-establish the Otago and Auckland medical sub-units under 2 Health Support Battalion.[19]

Nonetheless, there have also been a number of positive developments. Since 1993, the army has offered attractive cadetships to medical students. The cadets' student fees and expenses are paid from fourth year until graduation and they attend camp in the university vacation. After registration, cadets are expected to serve in the army for as many years as they have held the cadetship. The cadetships are open to both sexes and, in the first year, four students, three men and one woman, took them up. All successfully completed their training and three went on to serve on active duty in East Timor. In 2006, three more completed the scheme and a further three were under training. In that year, former cadets were serving in East Timor, Iraq and Afghanistan. The first woman to complete a cadetship was Anna Wyeth. She worked in military medicine alongside her husband, Lt Col Andrew Dunn, an Otago graduate of 1985, who enlisted in the Territorial Force as a student and transferred to the Regular Force in 1996. He commanded the Forward Surgical Team in East Timor in 2001, before taking up the position of Director of Army Health Services. A Fellow of the College of General Practitioners, Dunn completed postgraduate diplomas in Aviation Medicine and Tropical Medicine and was awarded the MNZM for his service in East Timor. Major Anna Dunn also served in East Timor, then combined motherhood with medical practice at Trentham military camp. A reminder of the possibilities now open to women medical graduates in the army, Anne Campbell, an Otago graduate of 1982, went on to become Director General Defence Medical Services and the first woman Brigadier in the New Zealand Army.[20]

OUMSA and the Wider World

Otago University Medical Students' Associations, whether in Dunedin, Christchurch or Wellington, have contributed a great deal to the New Zealand Medical Students' Association. Presidents of NZMSA typically bring to the role experience gained from the student presidency of one or other of the Otago schools. Representing these three centres, as well as the Auckland Medical School, NZMSA has developed into an influential lobby group, able to approach Ministers of Health or Education with confidence and to work with other student or medical organisations on issues such as student debt. The Association regards the Labour Government's implementation of a no-interest student loan policy as a major achievement, in which it had a significant role. NZMSA takes on all kinds of issues, such as a campaign for better funding of rural medical education to ease the shortage of rural doctors. It is especially proud of its Advanced Choice of Employment scheme, which was the culmination of work that began with OUMSA President Chris Jackson in 1996, gained traction from 1998, and was finally achieved under NZMSA President Brandon Adams in 2003. The scheme aims to reduce the stress for new graduates seeking their first hospital post by matching job offers from District Health Boards with a ranked list of trainee interns' preferred employers. Initially, there were teething problems with the scheme, but in 2006 the President was able to report that 83.5 per cent of the 279 New Zealand trainee interns had been successful in getting a position with their first-choice District Health Board.[21] In July 2006, NZMSA mounted an ambitious Medical Leadership Development Seminar for seventy selected members, at which a remarkable group of New Zealand's medical and political leaders contributed to a well-designed programme.

The modern NZMSA also looks beyond New Zealand. The link with the Australian Medical Students' Association has been renewed. NZMSA regularly reports to AMSA councils and New Zealand medical students are eligible to attend the AMSA Convention, which has now grown to cater for 800 students from seventeen medical schools. In 2006, nine Otago students attended, part of a fifteen-person New Zealand team. They were equally 'bowled over' by the world-class academic programme on offer and 'shocked, astounded and delighted' by the 'famous nocturnal programme'. The New Zealand Association has recently gone further in venturing onto the world stage. At the 2006 General Assembly of the International Federation of Medical Students' Associations (IFMSA) in Serbia, NZMSA was voted in as a candidate member. Founded in 1951, IFMSA is the largest student body in the world, with ninety-two member organisations, from eighty-eight countries, representing more than one million medical students. It is officially recognised as a non-governmental organisation within the United Nations and its external partners include the World Health Organization, the UN Educational Scientific and Cultural Organization and the World Medical Association. New Zealand is part of the Asia Pacific IMFSA regional grouping, which meets annually. As Xaviour Walker, the NZMSA representative at the Assembly, put it in the headline of his report, 'New Zealand Medical Students join the World'.[22]

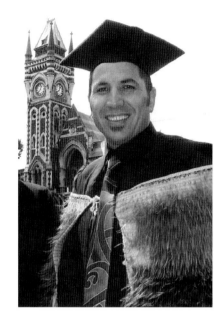

The 10,000th graduate of the Otago Medical School was capped in December 2006. Dr Lincoln Nicholls, of Ngati Raukawa descent, who taught physical education, human biology and Te Reo Maori in Palmerston North before entering Medical School, spoke of his sense of responsibility to uphold the legacy of earlier Maori doctors trained at Otago, and to work especially for his own people.

Otago Daily Times, 11 December 2006.

Postscript

CHAPTER 27

Made at Otago: Some of the Graduates

THERE IS A SENSE in which a medical school is made up of its past, as well as its present students, because they carry its teaching and influence out into the world. The Otago Medical School is proud of its graduates, as they are of the school. Many have pursued remarkable careers, achieving at the highest level in widely differing fields, in New Zealand and overseas, as medical academics, specialist researchers, surgeons and physicians, humanitarian activists, war heroes, political leaders or general practitioners playing a vital role in their various communities. To compile a list of the most outstanding graduates of the School would be an invidious and near-impossible task – someone recently described it as akin to St Peter's role at the pearly gates – but to ignore the achievements of some of them, for fear of omitting others equally worthy, does justice to none. The roles of Otago graduates in staffing the Medical School and in some specific fields, such as military medicine, have been noted already. Here, the bias is towards medical education overseas and research.

The University has itself paid tribute to a number of its former medical students by awarding honorary degrees and this provides a useful starting point. Many of the recipients have already appeared in the narrative. A handful were made honorary Doctors of Laws for achievements outside the strict confines of medicine. In 1962, the first year honorary degrees were conferred at the University of Otago, Sir Charles Hercus received an honorary LLD for his long service as Dean

of the Medical School. Sir Arthur Porritt, who was awarded an Hon LLD in 1968, was a Rhodes Scholar in 1923, captain of the New Zealand team at the 1928 Olympic Games, a Harley Street specialist, Brigadier in World War II and Sergeant Surgeon for a time to Queen Elizabeth, before he returned to New Zealand in 1967, as the country's first New Zealand-born Governor-General.[1] Two of the others awarded the degree served as Vice-Chancellors of Otago University. Robert Aitken (1969) was the first to hold the office in its modern form, from 1948 to 1953, and Robin Irvine (1993) served from 1973 to 1993.[2] Three former medical students who received honorary Doctors of Laws were political leaders. Ratu Sir Kamisese Mara (1973), Prime Minister of Fiji between 1970 and 1992 and then President until 2000, earned the title of 'Fiji's founding father'. Sir Peter Tapsell (1996) left medicine to represent Eastern Maori in the New Zealand Parliament in 1981. He held several ministerial portfolios for Labour before becoming the first Maori Speaker of the House of Representatives, from 1993 to 1996.[3] Sir Thomas Davis (2005) was the first Cook Islander to qualify as a doctor in New Zealand, in 1945. After serving as a medical officer in the Cook Islands, he completed a Master of Public Health at Harvard and worked as a research physiologist in the United States, including time with NASA. He then returned to the Cook Islands, founded the Democratic Party and was Prime Minister between 1978 and 1987.[4]

In 2004, the University celebrated the centenary

of the graduation of its first Maori student, Te Rangi Hiroa (Sir Peter Buck), himself the recipient of an honorary doctorate from the University of New Zealand in 1937, by awarding an honorary Doctor of Laws to East Coast physician Dr Paratene Ngata. A member of a distinguished family (his great-grand-uncle, Sir Apirana Ngata, was one of the outstanding Maori leaders of the first half of the twentieth century) and a medical graduate of 1970, Paratene Ngata helped raise the health status of Maori through his work as a general practitioner and as a medical officer in the Department of Health, as well as through his support for young Maori entering medical school.[5] A sole medical name appears in the calendar list of honorary Doctors of Literature. In 1996, Dunedin physician James Ng was awarded the degree for his definitive four-volume history of Chinese in New Zealand, *Windows on a Chinese Past*.[6]

The honorary degree of Doctor of Science has been linked more closely to achievements in medicine. By the end of 2000, the degree had been awarded to fifteen people connected with the Medical School as students, staff, or both, who had made their names as teachers and researchers. The first recipient, in 1962, was the much-admired Professor of Anatomy from 1914 to 1943, Percy Gowland. Two more staff members followed, nutritionist Muriel Bell in 1968, and full-time researcher Dick Purves in 1972. Of the group of seven honoured at a special assembly for the conferment of honorary degrees during the Medical School centenary in 1975, three had been on the staff of the School, two were clinicians and two were expatriates.[7]

Four of the five remaining on this most select list made their careers overseas. Derek Denny-Brown and Murray Brennan reached the topmost rungs of their profession in the United States, Julian Jack and Ian McDonald in Britain. Denny-Brown went to Oxford in 1924, on a Beit Fellowship, to study under Sir Charles Sherrington. He then lectured at the National Hospital, Queen's Square, the leading centre of neurology and, from 1941 to 1967, was Professor of Neurology at Harvard and Director of Harvard's Neurological Unit at Boston City Hospital. Ian McDonald, himself a Professor

of Neurology, said of Denny-Brown that his work as a doctoral student at Oxford on the physiology of the nervous system had 'become part of our everyday thinking' and that during the middle of the twentieth century he was arguably the most influential neurologist worldwide. By the early 1960s, the chairs of nineteen out of the forty-one departments of neurology in the United States had been largely trained at Denny-Brown's neurological unit.[8]

Murray Brennan (1997) came from a younger generation, graduating from Otago in 1964. He was still in Dunedin in 1970 when one of the American team that had performed the first kidney transplant visited and offered him a residency at Harvard Medical School. He never returned. A surgeon with expertise in soft tissue sarcomas, he was head of the Department of Surgery at the Memorial Sloan Kettering Cancer Centre in New York, the world's biggest cancer hospital, from 1985 to 2006. His clinical trials have produced major findings in the treatment of patients with soft tissue sarcomas, he has authored or co-authored some 800 papers and book chapters and, together with his colleagues, he has created the world's largest database of sarcoma patients. Major awards have been heaped on him, including the highest award of the American College of Surgeons, the Distinguished Service Award in 2000.[9]

Julian Jack began the medical course at Otago, but moved sideways into physiology, completing a first-class MMedSc in 1957 and a PhD in 1960. During his student days at Otago, he was a keen mountaineer and in 1999 the University orator surmised that the team work, resourcefulness and capacity to take infinite pains with the planning and execution of complicated and dangerous manoeuvres at high altitudes required of the mountaineer might well have contributed to his success as a scientist. Jack won a Rhodes Scholarship in 1960 and completed the clinical work for his medical degree at Oxford, graduating BM BCh in 1963 before returning to the world of physiological research. He has gained numerous distinctions for his work in cellular neuroscience, including Fellowship of the Royal Society of London, and rose to become a Professor at

Oxford's Laboratory of Physiology. He has made significant contributions to the understanding of the connectivity subserving motor control and reflexes in the spinal cord and a number of his papers, on such subjects as myelinated nerves, cable models of neurons and the plasticity of synapses, are regarded as definitive.[10]

In 2000, on the 125th anniversary of the foundation of the Medical School, two contemporaries and friends, Professors Ian McDonald and George Petersen, were awarded honorary Doctorates of Science. After graduating in medicine in 1957, Ian McDonald completed a PhD in physiology. He then moved, via posts in New Zealand and Harvard, to the National Hospital for Nervous Diseases in Queen's Square, London, where he rose to become Professor and Chairman of the Department of Clinical Neurology. His research on multiple sclerosis resulted in what the University orator called a 'torrent of publications' and made Queen's Square the leading international centre for the study of the disease. George Petersen's career took a different path, towards research in science rather than medicine. After majoring in biochemistry (the department was new and so small that he was the only third-year student and more or less designed his own course) he went to Balliol College, Oxford, where he completed a DPhil. He spent part of 1964 at Harvard, then returned to New Zealand to the Department of Scientific and Industrial Research, before being appointed to the Chair of Biochemistry at Otago. He held the Chair from 1968 to 1999, most of the time as Head of Department. Petersen established his own research on biochemical aspects of DNA, genes and the genome, and built up an outstanding department in an area which was peripheral when he began, but which is now recognised to be at the heart of the mainstream.[11]

In his graduation address in December 2000, McDonald referred to some of the graduates of the School who had contributed to the welfare of sick people in New Zealand and throughout the world. The first name he mentioned was Fred Hollows, one of a special group who used their skills abroad for the benefit of the impoverished and under-privileged. Hollows was an Otago graduate of 1955 and, after postgraduate training at Moorfield's Eye Hospital in London, he became an Associate-Professor of Ophthalmology at the University of New South Wales, from 1965 to 1992. The work he is remembered for, however, took place well outside the university context. From the 1970s, he visited more than 460 Aboriginal communities, had the eyes of 62,000 people examined, had 27,000 treated for trachoma and arranged 1000 operations. Later, he worked with the World Health Organization to set up training programmes in Nepal, Eritrea and Vietnam, to teach local technicians to examine eyes, prescribe glasses and perform straightforward eye surgery. Through the Fred Hollows Foundation, he later organised the manufacture of artificial lenses at a cheap rate. His work, now continued by the Foundation, restored sight or prevented blindness for thousands of people who would otherwise have had no access to treatment.[12]

A similar practical compassion motivated Dr Reg Hamlin, who graduated from Otago in 1941. Contracted to set up a midwifery school for nurses in Addis Ababa, Ethiopia, in 1959, he and his Australian wife, fellow obstetrician Dr Catherine Hamlin, stayed on to help young women suffering from fistulae. The condition is typically manifest as a hole between the bladder and uterus, that has resulted from a long and obstructed childbirth and which causes pain and incontinence. In 1975, they were able to open a special fistula hospital to provide free operations and treatment. Reg Hamlin died in 1993 but his wife continued the work. In 2000, when the hospital was expanded and upgraded with the help of the Australian Government, it was estimated that 20,000 women had been treated, with a 99 per cent success rate. At the time, the service was being extended to much of sub-Saharan Africa.[13]

A final example of such humanitarian work, in this case recognised by the University with an honorary DSc in 2006, was that of Dr Beryl Howie, who graduated in 1949 and became a member of the Royal College of Obstetricians and Gynaecologists in 1955. Her long-held aim to be a medical missionary became possible in 1959, when she secured a post at the Christian Medical College at Ludhiana in the Punjab, India.

The College had been set up to train doctors and nurses to care for women who would not otherwise have received specialist medical attention. Howie was promoted to the position of Professor of Obstetrics and Gynaecology in 1962, the first woman graduate of Otago University to be appointed to a chair anywhere in the world. She delivered thousands of babies and also trained hundreds of Indian doctors. When she left, in 1982, the entire staff of the Christian Medical College was Indian, many of them graduates of the College. Most graduates remained in India, caring for the needy and training others to do the same. The Christian Medical College has some 2000 health professional students and is recognised as one of the top twelve in India.[14]

Sometimes distinction comes early to Otago students or graduates, as their success in the immensely prestigious Rhodes Scholarship demonstrates. The two to three years' study at Oxford that the scholarship provides and the contacts made there have been a launching pad for many outstanding careers. The University of Otago has an excellent record in the Rhodes. In the century since the scholarship was set up in 1902, Otago won forty-five scholarships, more than a quarter of the New Zealand total. 'If this were an American University we'd be singing these sorts of stats from the rooftops', commented Postgraduate Administrator Margaret Sykes, in an interview for the *University of Otago Magazine* on the centenary of Rhodes' death. In raw numbers, Otago has kept company with the top universities in the United States. Within this Otago total, medical students stand out. There were nineteen over the first century of the award, beginning with Arthur Porritt in 1923 and Robert Aitken in 1924. Between 1970 and 1993, there was a remarkable run when Otago won thirteen Rhodes Scholarships, with no fewer than eleven coming from the Medical School.[15]

Many of the Medical School's graduates have made significant careers overseas in a variety of fields. When the *Encyclopaedia of New Zealand* was published in 1966, it included a brief account of twenty-six distinguished medical expatriates. Some were professors in British universities and a number had distinguished themselves in various branches of surgery: ear, nose and throat, neurosurgery, thoracic, orthopaedic and plastic surgery. They all held, or had held, positions of high responsibility, with a bias towards the academic. All followed careers in Britain, the great majority in London or Oxford. All but one were male. It is an impressive list, representing a period when Britain offered the greatest opportunities and highest rewards for ambitious and able medical graduates from the Commonwealth. An equivalent list today would have to include those women as well as men who chose to follow academic or research opportunities in the United States, Australia or elsewhere.[16]

Among the handful listed in the *Encyclopaedia* who served for a time on the staff of the Otago Medical School before settling in Britain, 1934 graduate Murray Falconer might be singled out, not only for his brilliance, but because of his strong Otago roots. His father, Alexander Falconer, was the first Medical Superintendent of the Dunedin Hospital, serving from 1910 to 1927. Unusually, Falconer came back to the Medical School after postgraduate study and experience, rather than holding a junior position before setting off. Falconer returned as Associate Professor in 1943, after a fellowship at the Mayo Foundation, completing specialised neurosurgical training with Sir Hugh Cairns at Oxford and serving in the RAMC during the war. Supported by special arrangements with the Health Department, which designated Dunedin as the national centre for neurosurgery and arranged dedicated new operating and ward facilities, he quickly established an outstanding neurosurgical department. 'From being a Surgical Cinderella', wrote Hercus and Bell, 'Neurosurgery swung into the van and in a short time Falconer was turning out results of the highest order.' It was an indication of his influence that the 1944 Travelling Scholar, Victor McFarlane, chose not to take up his scholarship because he believed it unlikely he would find 'more valid and exclusive experience abroad' than was obtainable in Dunedin with neurosurgeon Murray Falconer and Professor John Eccles. In 1951, Falconer left to take up a post at the Guy's Hospital-Maudsley

Neurosurgical Unit. McFarlane himself had left New Zealand by then, to become Professor of Physiology at the University of Queensland in 1948. He later held positions at the Australian National University and the Waite Institute, Adelaide. His reputation in Australia is highly regarded and he has been referred to as 'one of the most outstanding figures to have appeared in the Australasian scholastic world.'[17]

Two Otago graduates of the 1950s were appointed to chairs at the University of Cambridge in the mid-1980s. Eugene Paykel graduated in 1956, trained in psychiatry at the Maudsley Hospital in London and then spent five years at Yale, where he became Director of the Depression Research Unit. He returned to London, to a position at St George's Hospital, where he gained a personal chair in 1977. In 1985, he was appointed Professor of Psychiatry at Cambridge. He has published widely, with much of his work being in the biology and treatment of depression. In 2001, he was made an Honorary Fellow of the Royal College of Psychiatrists. Robin Carrell graduated in medicine from Otago in 1959, then in chemistry from Canterbury and in biochemistry from Lincoln, before moving to the United Kingdom in 1965 to study for a PhD in biochemistry at Cambridge. He was associated with some of the early studies of the genetic and structural variants of human haemoglobin. He returned to Christchurch and initiated research which was well established by the time he was appointed to the Chair of Haematology at Cambridge in 1986. He is a Fellow of the Royal Society of London and of Trinity College Cambridge.[18]

The Auckland Medical School, long promoted by Otago graduate Sir Douglas Robb, opened with a high proportion of former Otago students in leadership positions. Cardiothoracic surgeon Professor David Cole served as Dean, as did Professor Derek North. A 1950 Rhodes Scholar, North was head of Otago University's Auckland-based Medical Unit and then served as Professor of Medicine at the School for twenty years before being appointed Dean. For North, establishing the Auckland School was the highlight of his career, but he still felt an affinity with Otago.

'Nearly all the senior professors [had] known each other since med school at Otago,' he commented, 'and at the beginning everyone was from Otago.' In his view, this accounted for the fact that, notwithstanding competitive rivalry, both schools always got on extremely well. Graduates of the Otago Medical School have brought honour to the Auckland School. Sir William Liley performed the world's first fetal transplant. Sir Graham Liggins gave antepartum steroids to women likely to deliver prematurely, a practice that has become established world-wide, preventing death or intellectual disability in tens of thousands of premature infants. The Liggins Institute (2002) at Auckland is named in his honour. Sir Brian Barratt-Boyes used the flawless dexterity that might have made him a concert pianist to take cardiovascular surgery to a new level. In a tribute at the time of his death in 2006, the New Zealand Medical Journal listed his three great achievements: the first, for which he was knighted in 1971, was his pioneering work on replacing the aortic valve of the heart with a homograft valve; the second was his perfection of the technique of hypothermia and circulatory arrest, which allowed surgeons to operate on a still, bloodless heart, thereby enlarging the whole field of paediatric surgery; and the third was his book Cardiac Surgery, which he co-authored with American surgeon John Kirklin and which is regarded as the bible for cardiac surgeons.[19]

Beyond the university context, though with a direct bearing on it, Otago graduates have been influential in New Zealand's public health policy and administration. The influence of Dr Gervan McMillan who, as a member of the First Labour Government, was the chief architect of the 1938 Social Security Act, was unique. Several graduates, however, exercised considerable authority as Directors General of Health. The work of three of them may be cited.

Michael Watt, a graduate of 1910, was the second person to win the School's Travelling Scholarship, which gave him a year gaining experience in London hospitals. He was briefly recruited to the Medical School staff by Gowland, before moving to the Department of Public Health in 1916, as the first New Zealand-trained doctor to become a district field officer. He moved up through the ranks in the 1920s and became Director General at the end of the decade, when retrenchment was the order of the day. As the Depression eased, he embarked on a far-sighted programme, at the same time steering carefully between the medical profession and the Labour Government in their disagreements over social security. He set up the Medical Research Council in 1937, an incalculable boon for the Medical School and medical research. From an extensive overseas study tour in 1938, he developed a clear direction for New Zealand's health system. As summarised by the historian of the Department of Health, Derek Dow, this included an emphasis on industrial hygiene, improved collection and analysis of vital statistics, more focus on health education and dietetics, an intensified anti-tuberculosis campaign and the creation of a national health institute. Delayed by the war, the programme was mostly implemented in the late 1940s.[20]

Watt's successor was Gowland's admired former assistant, John Cairney. He held various hospital posts in Wellington from 1927 to 1950, rising to the position of Medical Superintendent-in-Chief of the Wellington, Hutt and Silverstream Hospitals and advising the Department of Health on several issues. He was also Sub-Dean of the Wellington Branch Faculty of the Medical School from its beginnings in 1937 until 1944. As Director General of Health, he maintained good relations with the Medical School, but he is especially remembered for his extensive reform of the New Zealand hospital system. He also contributed to medical education with text books for nurses and students.[21]

For five years from 1959, the same office was held by Dr Harold Turbott. A 1923 Otago graduate and career health administrator with long experience, he had probably expected to win the position in 1950. Turbott was well known throughout New Zealand for his commonsense radio health talks. He had a special interest in Maori health and children's health. His knowledge of tropical medicine and work in the South Pacific also led to an involvement with the World Health Organization, of which he was elected chairman in 1960.[22]

Women in the Medical World

Relatively few women have had a place in the upper echelons of the Otago Medical School staff or on lists of highly achieving graduates. That women doctors have faced special problems in building careers in academic or research medicine is generally acknowledged. This raises the question of whether their achievements should be judged by criteria different from those applied to their male colleagues, taking into account the special difficulties they faced. There are disadvantages in doing this and the need for such positive discrimination lessens steadily. Nevertheless, accounts of the experiences of women doctors, as indicated in several published collections, suggest that their undoubted success has not come easily.[23] Hercus and Bell devote a brief chapter to the 'Women of the Otago Medical School'. They claim to approach the topic with diffidence, but begin by expressing the view that women are 'natural instinctive doctors with a strong bias to the simpler remedies', a remark that comes perilously close to the patronising. As the 'greatest woman graduate the School [had] turned out', they selected the second, Margaret Cruickshank, describing her as one of those who 'found their inner reward in spending their lives in serving a small country community'. It was a safe choice, endorsed by Muriel Bell, who herself must have had a strong claim for the title, because Cruickshank, intellectually brilliant and personally admirable, had died almost half a century before, a victim of the 1918 influenza pandemic. Cruickshank was a fine doctor and a fine person, but it is hard to imagine the accolade of greatest male medical graduate going to a junior partner in a rural practice.[24] Hercus and Bell also mention the women who 'came to distinction in the Children's Health Service'. A few did so, notably Ada Paterson, a 1906 graduate who had done postgraduate work in Dublin and been in private practice in Picton, before joining the service as one of the four original members in 1912. From 1923 until her death in 1937, she was Director of the Health Department's Division of School Hygiene and thus the senior woman public servant of her day. More typically, though, the service was a refuge for women doctors who could not find suitable work elsewhere. It had small appeal to male graduates and historian Michael Belgrave calls it a 'professional backwater'. He also argues convincingly that women went into the service because they were virtually excluded from the financial rewards of private practice. 'It was one thing to emerge with a medical degree', he comments, 'and quite another to earn a living.'[25]

Hercus and Bell discuss Emily Siedeberg and Margaret Cruickshank, then list the women who graduated from the School prior to World War I, before singling out ten outstanding women graduates. Most completed their training in the early 1920s, when the proportion of women medical students graduating from wartime classes was high. As a group, they can be used to illustrate the career paths of high-achieving women in the early-to mid-century. Four were on the staff of the Medical School for longer or shorter periods and two more had a smaller role in teaching medical students. Doris Jolly (later Gordon), a 1916 graduate, was the first woman from Australasia to gain a Fellowship of the Royal College of Surgeons of Edinburgh and lectured for a time in public health. She is best remembered as an obstetrician and fundraiser for the University's Chair in Obstetrics. Marion Whyte (later Cameron), a 1918 graduate, became the first lecturer in anaesthetics at the Medical School in 1928, where she served for twenty years. Her appointment signalled that the specialty had received proper recognition. With experience in Britain and the United States, she was 'a pioneer in the use of endotracheal intubation, the use of the gas machine, intravenous fluids and spinals.' She won the respect, and also the affection, of generations of students in her fifth-year anaesthetic course and remained in private practice until 1957.[26] The work, and recognition, of her contemporary Muriel Bell, has been noted already. Marjorie Barclay, a 1923 graduate, who gained a diploma in radiology from Edinburgh and later travelled to both Vienna and Boston to further her expertise, was an outstanding diagnostic radiologist. She lectured in radiology at the Medical School for eleven years, from 1931. Helen Deem (née Easterfield, 1925) became

Medical Officer to the Plunket Society in 1939. Her revised infant milk formula won the support of paediatricians who had been alienated from Plunket methods and dietary advice in the 1930s. From 1946, she lectured to medical students in preventive paediatrics.[27] Cecily Pickerill (née Clarkson) is not on the list, but was also a 1925 graduate. She was trained by, and later married, Professor Percy Pickerill, surgeon in charge of the facial and jaw hospital of the Medical School and Dean of the Dental School. In 1939, they opened the Bassam Hospital in Lower Hutt for children needing plastic surgery, mainly for cleft palates and hare lips. It was the first New Zealand hospital to offer live-in accommodation for mothers. Sometimes, the fact that Cecily Pickerill had performed an operation was kept from the family until it was over. She continued the work for a decade after Pickerill's death in 1956.[28]

Two women on the list won the Travelling Scholarship. Alice Rose (1925) MRCP, married and remained in England, working in paediatrics and, during World War II, anaesthetics. Sir Charles Burns wrote of her that 'she could have gone far in the world of academic medicine, but there were few worth while posts in London in those days.' Jean Sandel (1939) FRCS (Eng) took up her scholarship after the war, and returned to spend her working life as a highly regarded surgeon at New Plymouth Hospital. [29] Marian Stewart and Zoe Cuff Robertson (later Mason) were classmates, graduating in 1933. In England to pursue her specialty of obstetrics and gynaecology when the war broke out, Stewart remained for the duration, working as a GP in the Lake District. She returned to a job at Ashburton Hospital, where Zoe Robertson was radiologist, until Professor Dawson invited Stewart to join his department in the Medical School. As well as setting up in private practice, she served for twenty-three years in the Department of Obstetrics and Gynaecology, where she rose to senior lecturer status.[30]

Expatriates do not feature on Hercus and Bell's list. One, Sylvia Chapman, appears on the list of distinguished medical expatriates compiled for the 1966 *Encyclopaedia.* Chapman's long life (she graduated in 1921 and died in 1995)

encompassed two careers, the first before World War II in New Zealand, the second in postwar Greece and England. They are linked by a focus on humanitarian work. In her first career, she undertook research in toxaemia of pregnancy, was involved with the beginnings of the Family Planning Association and served as a government nominee on the Senate of the University of New Zealand. During the war, she worked for refugees and was medical adviser to the Polish Children's Hospitality Committee. In 1944, the New Zealand Council of Organisations for Relief Service Overseas (CORSO) was founded in her rooms. The following year, when CORSO linked up with the new United Nations Relief and Rehabilitation Administration, she was selected for the gruelling task of leading a medical team to Greece. She settled in England from 1946, where she worked as an obstetrician and anaesthetist. The two women from Hercus and Bell's list who settled overseas did so for reasons other than career: Alice Rose married in England and Marion Radcliffe-Taylor moved to Perth for health reasons. She went on to make her name in Australia as an orthopaedic surgeon. One other graduate of the early 1920s, a surprising omission from the list, made a career in London as a child psychiatrist. In the 1930s, Kathleen Todd was Director of the London Child Guidance Clinic, co-authored a best-selling book on *Child Treatment and the Therapy of Play* and ran a practice in Harley Street. She later set up a fund to enable young psychiatrists to study in Europe.[31]

While classes at the Medical School grew during the depressed 1930s, the proportion of women studying medicine shrank. Alice Bush, who graduated in 1937, was one of just four women in a class of sixty-three. She acted as locum for Dr Edward Sayers in Auckland for four years during the war, while her husband was also overseas. After the war, Sayers invited her to join him in a professional partnership. She was the first New Zealand woman to become a member of the Australasian College of Physicians and her family went with her to England so that she could do her MRCP and Diploma in Child Health. In 1950, she began private practice in Auckland as a child health specialist. In the 1960s, she had a high profile as the President of the Family Planning Association.[32]

In the University, the Microbiology Department was the base for two notable women who taught in the medical course. Educated at Somerville College Oxford (BA, MA, Dip. Ed.) Mary (Molly) Marples came to New Zealand with her husband in the 1930s. She graduated MB ChB from Otago in 1944, following up with an MD and a postgraduate qualification from the School of Tropical Medicine, London. She specialised in cutaneous microbiology and related clinical conditions. Twenty years or so later, Margaret Loutit also accompanied her husband to Dunedin from Australia, when he took a position in the Microbiology Department. She too enrolled for another degree, in this case a PhD, and joined the staff of the Microbiology Department, becoming a full professor in 1981. In 1996, she was awarded the CBE for services to science.[33]

Three women, classmates at their Auckland high school, who graduated in the late 1940s, attained a high level of professional achievement. Barbara Heslop (née Cupitt) became the first medically qualified woman professor at the Otago Medical School, Beryl Howie a professor in the University of the Punjab and Margaret Guthrie (née Hoodless, later Wray) the first woman medical superintendent of a metropolitan hospital in New Zealand. Barbara Heslop's very long career in the Medical School was outstanding in both teaching and research. As a pathologist, she had joined the transplant immunology team and was a powerful influence for surgical research, with an international reputation. Heslop mentored hundreds of aspiring young surgeons through her Part I Surgical Fellowship course, for which she was made a Fellow of the Royal Australasian College of Surgeons.[34]

Throughout her time at the Medical School, Barbara Heslop kept an eye on medical women, their career prospects and the obstacles in their path. A survey she and three women members of her research team published in the *New Zealand Medical Journal* in 1973 provided the first comprehensive figures on the professional activity of New Zealand medical women and factors influencing this. The response rate to the survey was high, with 313 of the 374 New Zealand women medical graduates still living filling in the forms. At that time, none held positions that would commonly be regarded as being at the highest level in the profession (as specialists in the top grades, for example), none were among the fifty-two professors and associate professors at the two Medical Schools, and none worked as full-time medical superintendents of major hospitals or in positions of responsibility in the Medical Council or the Medical Research Council. Most expressed no interest in holding such positions. Some women had reduced, or ceased, their paid employment to look after children and they reported a loss of confidence in returning to work.[35] Heslop followed up the survey with further articles on women in the profession, which focused on the incompatibility of family life and advanced medical training. She recounts how Alice Bush had remarked to her in the early 1970s that, in the future, women doctors might have to choose between having children (both women had two) and training for clinical specialties. Sceptical at the time, she later came round to a similar view. In 1987 she compared the position of women doctors at the beginning and end of the United Nations Decade for Women (1976–85). Heslop noted that, while women by this time made up half of the second-year class at Otago, they accounted for only a small proportion of the teachers. She argued that, if they had children, the system of postgraduate training effectively culled many of the women doctors from acquiring postgraduate qualifications. In 1993, in an article she called 'Postgraduate Training for Women; the Eternal Tug of War for Women and how it has got Tougher', Heslop argued that the conflicting pressures of family and specialisation in medicine had become harder than in her own day. She pointed out that, in 1991–92, the list of newly registered specialists in the clinical specialties contained only 10 per cent women.[36]

One student of the 1950s, Associate Professor Dame Norma Restieaux, did not conform to this pattern. Dunedin-born and educated, she completed a BMedSc in Neurophysiology before graduating in medicine in 1960. She then began training in the emerging discipline of cardiology

under 'cardiac pioneers', John Hunter and John Borrie. She spent several years in London and Boston gaining advanced training and experience in both adult and paediatric cardiology before returning to Otago in 1970, as lecturer in the Medical School and Consultant Cardiologist at the Hospital. A superb teacher and gifted clinical cardiologist, she led the Department over a period of extraordinary growth and increasing specialisation. Restieaux was made a Dame Commander of the British Empire in 1992.[37]

By 2000, the University of Otago Calendar showed some change in the pattern Heslop described. Professor Linda Holloway had just moved from her position, as the first woman Dean in the Otago Medical School (Wellington), to become the first woman Assistant Vice-Chancellor Health Sciences. In the four schools that now made up the University of Otago Medical School, there were six women professors or professorial research fellows among the fifty-five medical staff at this level. In 2000, Barbara Heslop was professor emeritus (1990). The professors were Sarah Romans (Psychological Medicine, Dunedin, 1993), Diana Hill (Biochemistry, Dunedin, 1997), Christine Winterbourn (Pathology, Christchurch, 1996) and the professorial research fellows, Philippa Gander (Public Health, Wellington), Ailsa Goulding (Medicine, Dunedin) and Margaret McCredie (Preventive and Social Medicine, Dunedin). Within the next few years, Sarah Romans left, Professor Charlotte Paul was promoted to a Chair in the largest department in the University, Preventive and Social Medicine, and Helen Nicholson became Dean of the School of Medical Sciences. As the twenty-first century gets under way, the barriers that have kept medical women academics in a separate category are falling.[38]

• • • • •

What of our younger high-achieving graduates? Initially the intention had been to round off this celebratory chapter by looking at some of their careers, either heading to peak or at an early stage. However, there are too many candidates, the information is patchy and inequities and inaccuracies are more likely to occur than with the older, more established and better documented group (and even with that group the selection makes no claim to comprehensiveness). On balance, it has seemed preferable to confine the discussion to those who have completed, or nearly completed, their professional careers. The younger generation deserve a volume of their own.

There is one final point to be made, however, about the high achievers of the future. In 2006, the New Zealand Medical Students' Association organised a Medical Leadership Development Seminar. Seventy students from around the country were selected from more than two hundred applicants. A remarkable group of health administrators and leaders in health care converged on Wellington for the occasion. They ranged from the Minister of Health and politicians of both major parties with an interest in health (one of whom was a medical specialist), such leaders in the profession as the Chairs of the New Zealand College of General Practitioners and the New Zealand Medical Association, to the heads of the two Medical Schools and doctors working in such specialist areas as Maori, Pacific Island and rural health. That they had all thought it important enough to give up their time and, in some cases, travel long distances to speak to, and interact with, the student participants, seems immensely heartening. The mentoring by staff and more senior practitioners that throughout the history of the Otago Medical School has smoothed the path of ambitious young graduates was still evident in the year the School graduated its 10,000th student. The future leaders of the profession, in whatever area they choose to work, are ready.[39]

CHAPTER 28

Medical School at the Millennium

WHEN J.C. Beaglehole came to write the final chapter of his history of the University of New Zealand, he began with an admission of unease. 'History, or rather the historian', he remarked, 'faced with the necessity of exploratory observations on a living institution, is apt to feel some embarrassment. The post-mortem, with all its candid nakedness, yet remains more tactful than vivisection.'[1] The comment seems especially pertinent to the recent history of a medical school.

The entire history of the Otago Medical School could be defined as recent. The children and grandchildren of early students and staff still live among us. In some families, the School has trained three generations of doctors, and students of some of the earliest teachers remember them in sharp focus. In about 1950, Dr Mullin recalled in engagingly human detail his first meeting with the young Professor Scott, accompanied by his wife and small child, in 1884. His experience has its parallel today, in the many former students who can still describe with affectionate respect Scott's first professorial colleague, 'little' Johnny Malcolm, whose teaching in the School spanned the years from 1905 to the very different world of 1943. The oral traditions that have built up around characters on the staff and among the students are well established, their authenticity vouched for by many of the people who were there at the time.

The strength of the oral traditions is doubtless enhanced by the fact that a few individuals dominated the School's affairs for quite unusually long periods. In the case of the first three Deans, the duration of their association with the School and the relatively untrammelled authority they enjoyed (although none of them would have agreed with that description) enabled Professor John Halliday Scott, from 1877 to 1914, Sir Lindo Ferguson, on the staff from 1886 until 1937, and Sir Charles Hercus, who enrolled as a medical student in 1914 and retired as Dean in 1958, to mould the School in a very powerful way. It is a commonplace to say there are no longer such dominant individuals. This has some truth, because Medical School Deans now serve for finite terms and are more directly accountable to the Government and the University. Furthermore, many of the crucial decisions are taken by committees, rather than individuals. Professorial Heads of Departments traditionally served until they retired, and some still do, but generally the God-Professor has been replaced by the team leader.

How does the Medical School at the millennium differ from that of a hundred, or even fifty years ago? The sheer scale of its operation is the most obvious point of difference. In 1878, one professor taught a part-course to five students in a single room. In 1909, seven part-time lecturers, appointed to handle the full course in the 1880s, were promoted part-time professors, sharing cramped accommodation in the main University complex. There were still only seven professors in 1940, when Patrick Moore so tellingly captured their likenesses, but now they occupied two imposing buildings opposite the Dunedin Hospital and were assisted by an academic staff of twenty-seven, many of them part-time clinicians. They were barely coping with an annual student intake newly limited to one hundred and which would shortly rise by another twenty. The second half of the century saw rapid expansion, especially in the boom time of the 1970s, when the student intake was increased to two hundred, medical schools were opened in Christchurch and Wellington, new buildings sprang up like mushrooms and new staff were appointed to occupy them. The momentum was not maintained. Even so, if we fast-forward to the year 2000, we find fifty-five professors in a Medical School that operates on three extensive campuses and whose academic staff take up thirty-six of the fifty-two pages of staff names listed in the University of Otago Calendar. By any standard, it is a massive development, even without factoring in the change from Scott's small-scale operation with a single technical assistant, at first part-time, and no secretary, to the army of technical and administrative staff that service the modern school.[2]

Departments proliferated, and new areas of teaching emerged as the focus of medical education shifted. Anatomy, the mainstay of the first Edinburgh-style curriculum, was ousted from its prime position, in favour of the anchor Departments of Medicine and Surgery and these, in turn, were subdivided. Surgery became increasingly specialised, including Orthopaedic, Thoracic, Plastic (for a time), Urological and Neurosurgical. A whole range of specialties developed out of Medicine, including Pharmacology and Therapeutics, Therapeutics, Psychiatry and Paediatrics. Physiology gave birth to Neurophysiology, Biochemistry and, for a time, Clinical Biochemistry. The early combination of Bacteriology and Public Health led to strong Departments of Microbiology and Preventive and Social Medicine. Over the years, the emphasis in training doctors changed from the purely scientific to being more patient-focused. General Practice came into the curriculum and an emphasis on communication skills and medical ethics was introduced.

There has been a striking contrast in the growth patterns of the basic medical sciences and clinical subjects of the medical course. As well as medical students, the basic science departments in Dunedin taught first-year students for other health-related courses and degree students in science, where the numbers were not capped. In the 1990s, they became a separate School of Medical Sciences, with each of the large component departments remaining a cost centre. They continue to expand, to the equivalent of 1516 full-time students in 2001, and almost 1814 by 2004, when some 80 per cent of their work took place outside the Medical School.[3]

The teaching of clinical subjects to medical students presented quite different problems. The main difficulty was accessing an adequate number of patients in Dunedin hospitals and this led, first, to the sixth-year students being sent to Auckland, Wellington and Christchurch hospitals – a system that was increasingly formalised and worked very effectively for some fifty years, from the 1920s to the 1970s. Following this, the most exciting innovation of the last thirty years occurred when the University of Otago Schools of Medicine and Health Sciences in Christchurch and Wellington were developed, with their own particular strengths and characteristics, and playing distinctive roles in their own communities. In the mid-1990s, some of the clinical departments in Dunedin were clustered together as a Department of Medical and Surgical Sciences. Currently, this includes Anaesthesia and Intensive Care, the Bioethics Research Centre, the Edgar Centre for Diabetes Research, Medicine, Sports Medicine, Orthopaedic Surgery, Ophthalmology and Surgery.

Research has come to play an increasingly important role in the Medical School and in the lives of staff. Until the 1930s, it was small scale, individual and fitted around a full timetable (although not insignificant, as the work on goitre or hydatids demonstrates). When the Medical Research Council was established in 1937, funding became available for long-term projects, with full-time researchers, almost all located in the Medical School in Dunedin. At the same time, Hercus was making appointments to the staff based on research interests and capacity, and encouraging research in the Branch Faculties. There has been no looking back and, over time, certain trends have emerged. Individual research has largely given way to multidisciplinary team projects, with collaborators located in various New Zealand centres and overseas. Governments have encouraged medical researchers to align their work with health policy and there is an emphasis on health promotion.

The Medical School has always had certain memorable teachers who were recognised for their brilliance, discipline, or sheer eccentricity, although not everyone who sat in the same class cherished similar memories. One of the acknowledged characters was Gowland, whose hearty manner, outrageous stories and teaching skill seem to have been universally appreciated. Opinion on Eccles is sharply divided, while Adams' tight discipline inspired admiration and fear in roughly equal proportions. Over the last twenty years, the style of teaching has changed, from a heavy emphasis on formal lectures and end-of-year examinations towards small-group, self-directed learning, and frequent assessment through self-administered computer tests and formative assessments.

Student numbers have increased, but the growth has been controlled, capped by government at what was considered, at any given time, an appropriate number to provide the doctors New Zealand needed. Because not all applicants can be accepted to the School, the criteria for admission have been a contentious issue. In the earliest days, young men were largely self-selected, on the basis of their own intelligence and their family's ability to pay for the course to be completed in Britain. For most of the period since, selection has been based on examination achievement in the Intermediate course, taken at any university college in the country or, since 1998, the first-year health sciences course at Otago. The student intake has also changed in its gender and ethnic composition. For many years after the first woman was admitted, in 1891, the number of women students was low and unevenly spaced. Following this, it remained steadily at about 10 per cent of the intake for so

long that the myth developed that it represented a formal quota. Discussion bubbled on for a remarkably long time as to whether medicine was a suitable occupation for women. From the 1980s, the gender balance equalised, then settled with a slight female preponderance. The ethnic homogeneity of the School's early student population has also been overturned. There were not many Maori students after the first, Sir Peter Buck (Te Rangi Hiroa), graduated in 1904. For many years, the proportion stood at about 5 per cent but the new century has seen an increase. In 2004, the centenary of Buck's graduation, there were sixteen Maori graduates, the largest group to that time. The number of Pacific Island students has remained even lower. Since the 1980s, full fee-paying students have entered the medical course from countries with an agreement with the University, first from Malaysia and then from other countries in Asia and the Middle East. It is a very different student population from that of fifty years ago.

Medical students have enriched and enlivened the extracurricular life of Otago University. For decades, they dominated student politics, Capping, sport, college and social life in Dunedin. This changed in the 1970s, when they became submerged in the vastly expanded student population and two thirds of the fourth-year class, with its more senior potential leaders, left Dunedin. At first tentatively, then with increasing confidence, they have built up their own Students' Associations in Christchurch and Wellington as well as Dunedin. Medical students have established their own annual revue, developed their own support networks, social and sporting fixtures and produced their own publications. They have also sought connections with medical students at the Auckland Medical School, in Australia and recently, internationally, through the International Federation of Medical Students' Associations.

We may ask what events, over the century and a quarter of the Medical School's life, have had the greatest impact. As for the country as a whole, the reply must begin with the two world wars, because of the fine service of medical graduates, a number of whom gave their lives with the armed forces, and also because each war marked a clear stage in the development of the School. In each case, the Government's need for doctors gave the Deans of the day strong leverage to negotiate significant new buildings – the Lindo Ferguson and the Hercus, appropriately named after them. During both wars, new staff were also appointed to cope with the postwar bulge in student numbers and before and during World War II highly trained German Jewish researchers, fleeing Nazi Germany, stimulated research in the School.

The expansion of the School can be traced through its building programme, which is both an effect and a cause of growth, so that the two building booms in its history must be noted here. The first, in the Ferguson era, included the Scott and Lindo Ferguson Buildings, the Queen Mary Maternity Hospital, and lecture theatres in the Dunedin Hospital. The second, in the early 1970s, included the Sayers and Adams Buildings, and the Biochemistry and Microbiology Buildings in Dunedin and the new Clinical Schools in Christchurch and Wellington. The determination of the successive Deans to have the School closely linked to the Hospital is evidenced in the succession of buildings along Great King Street and the embedding of high-grade teaching facilities in the new Dunedin Hospital in 1980.

In the 1960s the dismantling of the federal structure of the University of New Zealand, and the subsequent under-funding of the Medical School within the newly autonomous University of Otago, led directly to an event which time has confirmed as a major turning point. The 1968 Christie Report was the stimulus for the building boom of the 1970s and the formation of the Christchurch and Wellington Schools of Medicine and Health Sciences.

The economic situation of New Zealand and the policies of different governments, at different times, have affected the School, but often less deeply than might have been expected. The 1930s Depression, for example, did not reduce the number of aspiring medical students, although it did reduce the proportion of women among them. The introduction of social security in 1938 was opposed by most of the medical profession, but did not affect teaching at the School. In the 1980s and 1990s, the School adjusted, repeatedly if often unhappily, to the ongoing government health reforms. A longer-term change has been social rather than political: the demands that society, and especially women, have put on doctors to become accountable and to communicate with their patients.

There is no end point to the story. The Otago Medical School has changed, through the influence of individuals within it, by the impact of external events, because of government or university policy, or the interaction of its schools. It will continue to change and adapt and survive, buoyed by its traditions, absorbed by its research and constantly rejuvenated by its students. And beyond these social and political pressures there is an immensely powerful force that drives medical education and practice: the nature, scope and speed of advances in medical knowledge and technology. With the pace of change itself the major challenge, the profession must adapt rapidly to advances, both technical and philosophical, in the delivery of health care to the individual and to the population as a whole, in order to fulfil public and therefore political expectations.

AFTERWORD

Looking Forward

THE ACHIEVEMENTS of the Medical School at the University of Otago during the more than 130 years since it was founded allow it to be very proud of its place in history. From small beginnings in New Zealand's first tertiary education institution, it has grown to become a medical school with an enviable international reputation. It has produced medical practitioners who have practised and influenced medicine widely throughout the world, and its graduates have contributed greatly to the medical workforce, the health research environment, and health policy development nationally and globally.

Consistently important themes for the Medical School and its continuing development at the University of Otago have been curriculum development and learning, the changing emphasis of health care, research, and the workforce of the future. How are these themes likely to develop as the Medical School moves towards the future?

Curriculum and learning

The practice of medicine has, as its basic tenet, the health and wellbeing of the individual. The medical practitioner uses his or her knowledge, skills, and understanding of the wide-ranging facilities of the health system to achieve the best possible outcomes for the patient at all times.

These requirements of the medical practitioner will remain constant in the future. In designing and implementing any future curriculum in medicine, there will always be a need to understand and have extensive knowledge of the scientific principles underpinning the practice of medicine. Achieving a wide range of basic practical skills will remain a consistently important priority, as will the need to understand the general and broad nature of medicine before focusing on specialty components of practice. Ethical practice, cultural awareness and competence, interprofessional interactions, communication skills, and decision-making abilities will all continue to be of primary importance.

In years gone by, the basis of medical knowledge and expertise often changed relatively slowly. However in the world of today and tomorrow, new information, new technologies, and new demands will arise ever more rapidly, and the medical practitioner is and will be required to learn and develop new abilities at an unprecedented pace.

Therefore the medical student and the medical practitioner have learning horizons which will expand ever more rapidly through their practising lives. The medical student has to become increasingly skilled in learning how to learn, and how to select what is important to learn. The information gained today in areas such as genetics, molecular biology, cancer diagnosis and therapy, therapeutics, and pharmacology may be redundant in a few years' time, with totally new concepts and capabilities being introduced and being adapted to the health environment.

Thus the real change in medical education for

the individual student and medical practitioner is in the pace of change of knowledge. The student and practitioner will be required to develop increasing skills in managing and adapting to the changed capabilities and information available, and to recognise that embarking on a career is a commitment to lifelong learning at an ever-increasing pace.

Medical educationalists now have to provide learning and teaching environments supportive of this approach to learning. It is as important for the student to learn how to gather and assimilate information as it is to learn content and facts. It is also now important for the practitioner to assure and demonstrate to others that he or she is up to date with knowledge and skills on a regular basis for continuing employment, and for professional registration purposes. This has led to continuing professional development programmes and monitoring by vocational training bodies and by medical registration authorities.

But do the above requirements change what a medical school provides in its teaching programmes as we look forward? The answer, definitely, is yes.

Our future in curriculum development and learning is in assisting the student to gain these abilities in a wide variety of different ways. This involves knowledgeable use of electronic media, particularly for access to current medical literature, research and opinion, and for rapid communication with health facilities and networks locally, nationally and internationally. Self evaluation of the integrity of information available, and the ability to collate and apply the information gained to the particular health need, is now an integral component of the skills of the practitioner. Learning to use these resources, and to apply them, has become a primary part of the curriculum of any medical school.

The changing emphasis of health care

With changes in our ability to recognise and treat disease have come changes in the primary emphasis of medical practice. Improvement in the treatment and prevention of, many infectious diseases has changed the landscape of human existence during the last century. There have been outstanding advances also, for example, in the treatment of cardiovascular disease and hypertension, cancer and leukaemia, acute trauma management and intensive care management. Immunisation programmes and public health initiatives have ensured the survival to healthy productive adult life of many who in previous centuries died in their early years. The prevention, or delay, of the morbidity of many adult diseases has changed the age profile of peak health care expenditure to later decades of life.

An emphasis which is important for the medical practitioner now, and in the future, is ensuring a long and healthy life, and the active prevention of disease and attendant morbidity. This includes good nutrition at all stages of life, strategies for accident avoidance and safety in the home, public and workplace environment, early detection of disease and risk factors for disease, and informed life and health choices by the public. The wider health aspects of behaviour and its modifications, risk awareness, screening programmes and early interventions to avoid and ameliorate disease are just as important to doctors of today and tomorrow as are the mandates to cure disease when it occurs. Care of the aged, prevention of obesity, avoidance of the complications of diabetes, and provision of support services for those who are isolated and alone geographically and in our social structures are now all increasingly important areas of need and demand for health professionals.

Health care systems also are changing worldwide. Episodes of hospital care are increasingly and appropriately brief, broader aspects of preventive health care are an increasing component of governmental policies, and the availability of health information to the population at large has expanded exponentially. A feature of countries with excellent health care outcomes is the provision of well-resourced and effective primary health care systems, with an emphasis on education, healthy lifestyles and disease prevention.

As part of these developments, medical schools are leading the changes, with changes in their curricula and structures, as they always have done. Although learning at the bedside in the teaching hospital will continue to be a necessary part of any medical student's education, the student's wider education will be in an ever-increasing range of environments. Medical students will spend more and more time away from their home medical school base as they undertake their learning programmes. They will more frequently be in dispersed environments, with a need for access to videoconferencing and electronic communication. Teachers and supervisors in these environments also will need increasingly sophisticated support from the Medical School.

Learning is and will be increasingly in health care networks. The emphasis on primary health care and community health will increase. Interprofessional and team-based care will assume even more importance in all health care.

The continuity of learning will be evident from medical school onwards, with medical schools and professional registration and monitoring authorities collaborating to provide support for self-directed and self-enabled learning, development and maintenance of practical clinical skills, and self-assessment activities throughout the practising life of every doctor.

The challenges in these dispersed and continuing learning environments will be to provide the infrastructure needed for the wide variety of placements, student and staff travel and accommodation, and physical facilities.

Research

Research at all levels will continue to be the hallmark of successful and world-leading medical schools. Research is fundamental to and essential in the development of new knowledge, improved outcomes of care, and the effective use of health care resources.

As a University with a medical school, Otago has every reason to be proud of the many world-leading contributions it has made to medical research throughout its history. Research-informed teaching and learning has been and will continue to be the lifeblood of the Medical School at Otago. Medical research associated with the Faculty and its Schools will continue to grow and to make further contributions globally in future years.

Many of the successful research outcomes in health result from national and international research collaborations: major scientific advances come from shared information and complementary research themes. The evidence base for good medical care comes from carefully conducted and analysed clinical trials, often on a global basis. Medical research at Otago can be expected increasingly to be part of international collaborations, and with international funding sources.

An important component of future development and success in research within the Faculty and the University will be the leadership, funding and resources provided by government, funding agencies and the University as a whole to support large, multidisciplinary and world-leading research groups.

The workforce of the future

A medical school must be able to plan towards and assist with the provision of a suitable medical workforce for the future. The planning of undergraduate curriculum development, postgraduate training, and research development all must be in the context of national and international health needs. Medical schools must also be advocates for the health care of those who are disadvantaged, and those who have specific developmental and health needs.

Planning the numbers and characteristics of the workforce of the future needs to take account of rapidly developing new knowledge and technology, changes in the characteristics and welfare of the population, and changing work patterns of the health workforce. These characteristics will determine selection policies for training in medicine, government funding for training places, and the nature of the training programmes.

Such planning needs to be undertaken cooperatively in conjunction with those responsible for postgraduate vocational training programmes, government agencies including funding bodies, medical registration authorities, professional associations and policy-makers. An important aspect of future planning for the medical workforce is to ensure a collaborative and cooperative approach to such planning, with careful longitudinal data collection and analysis of changes introduced and their outcomes.

The future as a reflection of the past

The University of Otago's Medical School has achieved outstanding successes during its first 130 years. Its place in history is assured: its legacy of educators, clinicians, scientists and leaders is outstanding. Its contributions have been medical education, research and health care: its future, as for its past, will see these themes continued to the highest standards with enthusiasm, energy, and great pride in its achievements.

D.M. ROBERTON
Pro-Vice-Chancellor, Division of Health Sciences
Dean, Faculty of Medicine
University of Otago
2008

APPENDICES

Deans of Faculty and of the Otago, Christchurch and Wellington Schools, Assistant Vice-Chancellors (AVCs), later Pro-Vice-Chancellors (PVCs), Health Sciences, and Professors of the School 1874–2000

Faculty Deans

1891–1913	John Halliday Scott (Professor since 1877)
1914–1936	Henry Lindo Ferguson (Professor since 1909)
1937–1958	Charles Ernest Hercus (Professor since 1922)
1959–1967	Edward George Sayers (Professor since 1959)
1968–1973	William Edgar Adams (Professor since 1944)
1974–1977	John Desmond Hunter (Professor since1962)
1978–1983	Geoffrey Leonard Brinkman (Professor since 1976)
1986–1990	John Desmond Hunter (Professor since 1962) Inaugural AVC Health Sciences 1989–90
1991–1995	Ralph David Huston Stewart (Professor since 1974) AVC Health Sciences 1991–1998
1995–2004	Archibald John Campbell (Professor since 1984)
2005	Linda Jane Holloway (Professor since 1994) AVC (then PVC) Health Sciences 1999–2005
2006–Present	Donal Muir Roberton Also PVC Health Sciences, 2006–Present

The Otago Medical School: Deans

Until 1986 Deans of Faculty were also Otago Medical School (OMS) Deans.

1986–1990	Ralph David Huston Stewart (Professor since 1974) Dean of Faculty 1991-1995, AVC Health Sciences, 1991–1998.
1991–1996	John Graham Mortimer (Professor since 1977)

In 1996 the Otago School was divided into the Dunedin School of Medicine and the Otago School of Medical Sciences.

Dunedin School of Medicine (DSM)

1996–1997	John Graham Mortimer (Professor since 1974)
1998–2002	William John Gillespie (Professor since 1981)
2003–Present	Dr John Burman Adams

Otago School of Medical Sciences (OSMS)

1996–2006	David Todman Jones (Professor since 1989)
2007–Present	Helen Diana Nicholson (Professor since 2000)

The Northern Centres
Christchurch, Wellington and Auckland Branch Faculties 1938–c.1972: Sub-Deans

From the mid 1920s sixth year students were sent to Christchurch, Wellington and Auckland Hospitals for their clinical year. Between 1938 and about 1972 each centre was recognised as a Branch Faculty, under a Sub-Dean.

Christchurch		Wellington		Auckland	
1938–1952	Arthur Nelson	1938–1962	John Mercer	1938–1956	Walter Gilmour
1953–1957	Malcolm Gray	1963–1965	John Keeling	1956–1957	Edward Sayers
1958–1962	John Landreth	1966–1972	Guy Hallwright	1958–1961	Walter Henley
1963–1970	George Rolleston			1962–1972	Michael Gilmour

The Christchurch School: Deans

1970–80	George Lancelot Rolleston (Professor since 1970)
1982–1985	John Desmond Hunter (Professor since 1962)
1986–1993	Alan Maxwell Clarke (Professor since 1970)
1994–2001	Andrew Reed Hornblow (Professor since 1988)
2002–2005	George Ian Town (Professor since 2000.
2006–Present	Peter Richard Joyce (Professor since 1986)

The Wellington School: Deans

1972–1975	Graham Francis Hall (Professor since 1972)
1977–1985	Ralph Hudson Johnson (Professor since 1977)
1986–1991	Thomas Vianney O'Donnell (Professor since 1970)
1992–1994	Eru Woodbine Pomare (Professor since 1986)
1996–1998	Linda Jane Holloway (Professor since 1994)
	Dean of Faculty 1999; AVC, then PVC, Health Sciences 1999–2005
1998–2007	John Norman Nacey (Professor since 1998)
2008–Present	Peter Roy Crampton (Professor since 2004)

Professors of the Otago Medical Faculty 1874-2000

Included in this list are professors appointed before 2000, whose primary employment has been with the Otago Medical School. No distinction has been made between professors appointed to established chairs and personal professors. Since 1996, professors in Dunedin have been appointed to either the Dunedin School of Medicine (DSM) or the Otago School of Medical Sciences (OSMS).

Otago Medical School: Dunedin

M. Coughtrey	Anatomy and Physiology	1874–1876
J.H. Scott	Anatomy and Physiology	1877–1905
	Anatomy until 1914; Dean, 1891–1914	
J. Malcolm	Physiology	1905–1943
F. Ogston	Medical Jurisprudence and Public Health	1909–1911
	Medical Jurisprudence until 1916	
W.S. Roberts	Pathology	1909–1915
D. Colquhoun	Medicine	1909–1918
H. Lindo Ferguson	Ophthalmology	1909–1936
	Dean, 1914–1936	
F.C. Batchelor	Midwifery and Diseases of Women	1909–1910
L.E. Barnett	Surgery	1909–1915
S.T. Champtaloup	Bacteriology and Public Health	1911–1921
W.P. Gowland	Anatomy	1914–1940
A.M. Drennan	Clinical Pathology	1916–1928
D.W. Carmalt Jones	Systematic Medicine (Mary Glendining Chair)	1919–1939
F.W. Fitchett	Clinical Medicine and Therapeutics	1919–1939
F.G. Bell	Surgery (Ralph Barnett Chair)	1925–1952
F.R. Riley	Midwifery and Gynaecology	1929–1931
E.F. D'Ath	Pathology	1929–1962
J.B. Dawson	Obstetrics and Gynaecology	1931–1950
C.E. Hercus	Bacteriology and Public Health	1922–1958
	Preventive and Social Medicine from 1955;	
	Dean, 1937–1958	
F.H. Smirk	Medicine (Mary Glendining Chair)	1940–1962
	Research Medicine, Director of Wellcome Institute	1962–1968
J.C. Eccles	Physiology	1944–1950
W. E. Adams	Anatomy, Dean, 1968–1973	1944–1973
N.L. Edson	Biochemistry	1949–1966
A.K. McIntyre	Physiology	1951–1961
J.L. Wright	Obstetrics and Gynaecology	1951–1980
M.F.A. Woodruff	Surgery (Ralph Barnett Chair)	1953–1956
J.A.R. Miles	Microbiology	1955–1978
G.J. Fraenkel	Surgery (Ralph Barnett Chair)	1958–1969
C.W. Dixon	Preventive and Social Medicine	1959–1979
E.G. Sayers	Therapeutics, Dean	1959–1967
J.R. Robinson	Physiology (Wolff Harris Chair)	1961–1979
A. Wynn-Williams	Pathology	1963–1970
W. Ironside	Psychological Medicine	1962–1969
J.D. Hunter	Medicine (Mary Glendining Chair, 1962–1973)	1962–1990
	Dean, 1974–1977; 1986–1990; Christchurch,	
	1982–1985; AVC, 1989–1990	
J.M. Watt	Paediatrics and Child Health	1967–1976
J.G.T. Sneyd	Clinical Biochemistry	1967–1990
G.B. Petersen	Biochemistry	1968–1998
D.W. Taylor	Physiology	1968–1987

A.M.O. Veale	Human Genetics (MRC)	1968–1972
R.O.H. Irvine	Medicine	1969–1973
	Clinical Dean, 1969–1972; VC, 1973–1993	
B. James	Psychological Medicine	1969–1981
W.R. Trotter	Anatomy	1969–1982
F.N. Fastier	Pharmacology	1969–1980
J.B. Howie	Pathology	1969–1987
R.W. Medlicott	Psychological Medicine	1969–1978
A.M. Clarke	Surgery	1970–1993
	Ralph Barnett Chair 1970–1984;	
	Dean, Christchurch, 1986–1993	
J.S. Loutit	Microbiology	1970–1988
A.J. Alldred	Orthopaedic Surgery	1971–1981
J.B. Blennerhassett	Pathology	1971–1996
E.G. McQueen	Clinical Pharmacology	1971–1981
J.R. Hubbard	Physiology	1972–1995
F.O. Simpson	Medicine	1972–1989
P.J. Molloy	Cardiac Surgery	1973–1993
R.D.H. Stewart	Medicine (Mary Glendining Chair)	1974–1982
	Dean, OMS, 1986–1990; Dean of Faculty,	
	1991–1995; AVC, 1991–1998	
A.B. Baker	Anaesthesia	1975–1992
R.J. Seddon	Obstetrics and Gynaecology	1975–1991
	Wellington, 1975–1980	
G.L. Brinkman	Medicine, Dean, 1978–1985	1976–1985
T.C. Highton	Medicine	1976–1977
J.G. Mortimer	Paediatrics and Child Health	1977–1990
	Dean, OMS, 1991–1996; DSM, 1996–1997	
R.G. Robinson	Neurosurgery	1977–1980
J.C. Parr	Ophthalmology	1977–1986
S.W. Heap	Radiology	1978–1985
D.C.G. Skegg	Preventive and Social Medicine	1980–2004
	Vice-Chancellor, 2004–Present	
A.D.C. Macknight	Physiology (Wolff Harris Chair)	1980–2001
R. Laverty	Pharmacology	1980–1997
Margaret W. Loutit	Microbiology	1981–1990
P.E. Mullen	Psychological Medicine	1982–1992
A.K. Jeffery	Orthopaedic Surgery	1982–2000
D.G. Palmer	Medicine	1982–1992
G.O. Barbezat	Medicine (Mary Glendining Chair)	1983–2003
J.C. Murdoch	General Practice (Elaine Gurr Chair)	1983–1992
D.G. Jones	Anatomy	1983–2004
	Deputy-Vice-Chancellor, 2005–Present	
V.S. Chadwick	Experimental Medicine	1983–1994
Barbara F. Heslop	Surgery	1984–1989
A.J. Campbell	Medicine	1984–Present
	Dean of Faculty, 1995–2004	
A.M. van Rij	Surgery (Ralph Barnett Chair)	1985–Present
T.C.A. Doyle	Radiology	1988–Present
P.A. Sullivan	Biochemistry	1988–1995
W.P. Tate	Biochemistry	1989–Present
J.M. Elwood	Preventive and Social Medicine	1989–1999
	(Hugh Adam Cancer Epidemiology Unit)	
D.T. Jones	Microbiology; Dean, OSMS, 1996–2006	1989–2006
A.V. Campbell	Biomedical Ethics	1990–1996

M.W. Tilyard	General Practice (Elaine Gurr Chair)	1993–Present
Sarah E. Romans	Psychological Medicine	1993–2001
R.J. Olds	Pathology	1994–2007
J. Mann	Human Nutrition, 1988–Present; Joint with Medicine, 1995–Present	1995–Present
P.D. Wilson	Obstetrics and Gynaecology	1995–Present
G.R. Gillett	Biomedical Ethics Neurosurgery, 1995–2006	1995–Present
A.E. Braithwaite	Pathology	1995–Present
G.W. Tannock	Microbiology	1996–Present
D.M. Evans	Director, Bioethics Centre	1997–Present
J.F.T. Griffin	Microbiology	1997–Present
A.M. Wheatley	Physiology	1997–Present
A.E. Reeve	Biochemistry	1997–Present
Diana F. Hill	Biochemistry	1997–Present
B.J. Taylor	Paediatrics and Child Health	1998–Present
D.M. Jackson	Pharmacology	1999–2004
P.F. Smith	Pharmacology	1999–Present
J.D. Langley	Preventive and Social Medicine (HRC, ACC)	2000–Present
Helen D. Nicholson	Anatomy Dean, OSMS, 2007–Present	2000–2006

Christchurch

G.L. Rolleston	Radiology, Dean	1970–1980
D.W. Beaven	Medicine	1972–1989
W.A.A.G. Macbeth	Surgery	1972–1992
A.R. McGiven	Pathology	1972–1986
F.T. Shannon	Paediatrics and Child Health	1972–1990
D.R. Aickin	Obstetrics and Gynaecology	1972–1999
K. Schwarz	Preventive and Social Medicine	1973–1979
K.S. Adam	Psychological Medicine	1974–1978
R.W. Carrell	Pathology	1978–1986
E.A. Espiner	Medicine	1978–2000
J.M. Gibbs	Anaesthesia	1980–1995
W.J. Gillespie	Orthopaedic Surgery Dean, Dunedin School of Medicine, 1998–2002	1981–2002
P.C. Ney	Psychological Medicine	1980–1984
R.A. Donald	Medicine	1982–1997
P.R. Joyce	Psychological Medicine Dean, 2006–Present	1986–Present
A.R. Hornblow	Community Health, then Dean	1988–1993
D.R. Boswell	Pathology	1988–1996
A.G. Rothwell	Orthopaedic Surgery	1990–2005
M.G. Nicholls	Medicine	1991–2002
D.W. Teele	Paediatrics	1992–1999
R. Sainsbury	Medicine	1992–2005
S. Jane Chetwynd	Public Health	1994–1998
Rita L. Teele	Radiology	1994–1999
D.N.J. Hart	Pathology	1995–Present
T. Gin	Anaesthesia	1996–1999
Christine C. Winterbourn	Pathology (HRC)	1996–Present

A.M. Richards	Medicine (NHF)	1996–Present
S.W. Beasley	Paediatrics, Clinical Professor	1997–Present
R. Fraser	Pathology	1997–1998
L. Toop	General Practice (Pegasus Chair)	1997–Present
J.A. Roake	Surgery	1997–Present
H. Ikram	Medicine, Clinical Professor	1999–2002
P.B. Davis	Public Health	1999–2004
D.M. Fergusson	Psychological Medicine	1999–Present
B.A. Darlow	Paediatrics	2000–Present
	Cure Kids Chair in Paediatric Research from 2007	
F.A. Frizelle	Colorectal Surgery (Canterbury Health Chair)	2000–Present

Wellington

G.F. Hall	Medicine, Dean	1972–1975
T.V. O'Donnell	Medicine	1972–1991
	Chair, OMS, 1970–1972; Dean, 1986–1991	
W.E. Stehbens	Pathology	1974–1991
W.H. Isbister	Surgery	1975–1989
H.J. Weston	Paediatrics and Child Health	1975–1991
F.J. Roberts	Psychological Medicine	1975–1979
R.J. Seddon	Obstetrics and Gynaecology	1975–1980
R.H. Johnson	Medicine, Dean, 1977–1985	1977–1987
K.W. Newell	Community Health	1977–1982
G.W. Mellsop	Psychological Medicine	1982–1994
J.D. Hutton	Obstetrics and Gynaecology	1983–1994
L.A. Malcolm	Community Health	1984–1994
E.W. Pomare	Medicine, Dean, 1992–1994	1986–1994
J.G. Horne	Surgery	1990–2004
C.R.W. Beasley	Medicine	1993–2001
P.R. Stone	Obstetrics and Gynaecology	1994–1998
Linda J. Holloway	Pathology	1994–2005
	Dean, 1996–1998; AVC/PVC Health Sciences, OU, 1999–2005	
	Dean, Faculty of Medicine, 2005	
P.M. Ellis	Psychological Medicine	1994–Present
A.J. Woodward	Public Health	1995–2003
A.C. Dowell	General Practice (ACC Chair)	1997–Present
K. Grimwood	Paediatrics and Child Health	1997–2007
B. Delahunt	Pathology	1996–Present
N.E. Pearce	Medicine (HRC)	1998–2000
J.N. Nacey	?Medicine, Dean, 1998–2007	1998–Present
G.S. Le Gros	Medicine	2000–2004

Graduates of the Otago Medical School, 1887–2006

Graduates are listed by the year they qualified, with any scholarships or higher degrees in brackets after their names; MDs who did not have an Otago MB ChB are listed at the end of the relevant year. The surnames given for women graduates are those of their qualifying year; where known, their maiden or married names are given in brackets.

To compile this list, the Alumni Office's list of MB ChB graduates was checked against the Medical Faculty's loose-leaf typescript, and latterly database printout list of graduates and the bound volumes of the Faculty's *Register of Graduates*.

Up to 1924, the list of graduates was compiled from the list published in the Otago University Calendar for 1921, supplemented by the additional names in the 1925 calendar.

MD graduates' names were taken from the Faculty's list and also compared with the loose-leaf files listing all graduates.

Graduates whose names do not appear in the Medical Faculty's records have been checked in the *Roll of Graduates of the University of Otago* [to May 1988] ([Dunedin]: University of Otago, 1989); *University of New Zealand: Roll of Graduates* [1870–1961] (Christchurch: Whitcombe & Tombs for the University, [c. 1963]); and the relevant annual graduation booklets. From 2001, the Faculty's electronic records were used.

The list of scholarship holders was compiled from John Hunter, *Compendium of Historical Data 1873 to 1992*, Otago Medical School Alumnus Association, Dunedin, 1993, supplemented in the case of the Travelling Scholarship by the graduation booklets, and for the Rhodes Scholarships, the web-site of the Rhodes Trust.

1887
William Ledingham Christie (MD 1890)

1889
Herbert Clifford Barclay (MD 1895), George Anderson Copland (MD 1891), William Thomas Dermer, Walter Kerr Hislop, William John Mullin

1890
William Butement, William Allan Chapple (MD 1899), Percival Robert Cook, Ernest Edward Fooks, James Harper Reid

1891
William Watson Griffin, Alexander Hendry, Robert Henry Hogg, John Forbes Menzies, John Alexander Newall, Edward John Roberts

1892
Robert Church

1893
Charles Thomas Little, Kenneth McAdam, Murdoch William Ross, James Torrance

1894
Matthew Campbell, John Lovell Gregg

1896
John Morton Matthews, Emily Hancock Siedeberg, Andrew Stenhouse

1897
Margaret Barnett Cruickshank (MD 1903), Arthur Edward Albert Palmer

1898
George Patrick Brown, Alexander Robertson Falconer, William Archibald Logan, James Hardie Neil, Charles North, William Sutherland

1899
Eugene Joseph O'Neill, Ernest Harry Williams

1900
Douglas Home Blackader Bett, Francis Arnot Blackader Bett, William James Cran, Constance Helen Frost, William Edmund Gibson, Arthur James Hall, Jane Kinder, Daisy Elizabeth Platts (Platts-Mills), Carl Hermann Schumacher (Seaforth), Thomas Arthur Will, Alice Woodward (Horsley)

1901
Robert Noble Adams, Sydney John Cook, Walter William Moore (MD 1907), Michael Charles Frederick Morkane, John Bonwell Sale, Walter Moray Shand, Frank Ferdinand Aplin Ulrich

1902
Sydney Chalmers Allen (MD 1905), James Hamilton Hall Baillie, James Brugh, Andrew John Crawford, Colin Huntly Gordon, William McAra, Jessie Clarkson Maddison, Wilfred Thomas Simmons

1903
Eleanor Southey Baker (Baker-McLaglan), William Frederick Browne, Francis Rudolph Hotop, Charles Ogilvie Lillie, Ernest Millington Livesey, John Davis Marks, William Fergus Paterson, Russell Ian Ritchie, Leonard Smith Talbot, Isaac Thompson

1904
Agatha Helen Jane Adams (Monfries), Winifrede Ismay Bathgate, Peter Henry Buck (Te Rangi Hiroa) (MD 1909), Alexander Kinder, Thomas McKibbin, Gilbert Haywood Mirams, Emily Helen Violetta Nees (Ridley), James Herbert Graham Robertson, John Frew Robertson

1905
Casement Gordon Aickin, Robert Stephen Briffault, Alexander Francis Ritchie Crawford, William Aitken Fairclough, Thomas Fergus, Henry Ernest Howard, William Malcolm Thomson

1906
Archibald Turner McLeod Blair, William Elliot Carswell, Gabriel Michael Joseph East, Thomas Gilray, Harold Edward Jeffreys, Eric Lachlan Marchant, William Fulton Neil, Ada Gertrude Paterson, Thomas Charles Patterson, Hugh Edward Webb, James Thomas Wellington Wilkin

1907
Richard Amor Bagley, Robert Walter Baron, James Robert Closs, Alan Renata Green, John Patrick Hastings (MD 1910), William Hugh Clifford Patrick (MD 1908), Ivan Stuart Wilson (MD 1910), John McKeown Withers

1908
Stanley Eric Vincent Brown, James Garfield Crawford, Thomas Harrison, Eugene Trevelyan Rogers (MD 1912), Francis Arthur Scannell, Robert Alexander Shore, Sydney James Simpson, Arthur Charles Thompson, Tutere Wi-Repa

1909
James John Eade, Philip Stanley Foster, Sydney Hartley Hay, Arthur Noel Houghton, Thomas William James Johnson (Travelling Scholar 1909) (MD 1911), Leonard Arthur Line, William Huston Dodd McKee, William Haddow Pettit, David Steven (MD 1917)

1910
Edmund Ewart Brown, James Collins, Ina Burnham Dugleby (Moody), George William Gower (MD 1918), John Mickle Hyde, Leonard Hugh McBride (MD 1912), Arthur Dysart Nelson, Thomas Gordon Short, John Edward Llewellyn Simcox, Henry Caldwell Tait, Michael Herbert Watt (Travelling Scholar 1910) (MD 1912), Hatton Leslie Whetter, Philip Randall Woodhouse

1911
Patrick Augustine Ardagh, William Gillies Borrie, Robert Walker Edgar, David Eardley Fenwick (MD 1917), William Philip Johnston (Travelling Scholar 1911) (MD 1915), Robert Bernard Pearson Monson (MD 1916), Herbert O'Callaghan, Herbert Donald Robertson, Hugh Lawrence Widdowson, Catherie Louisa Will (Brookfield), William Balfour Wishart; MD: James Andrew Nixon Mulholland

1912
Athol William Purchas Brookfield, John Ebenezer Kelly Brown, Arthur Owen Evans, William Farquhar Findlay, Thomas Campbell Fraser, Thaddeus Julian (Travelling Scholar 1912), William Cuthbert McCaw, Arthur Stanley Moody (MD 1917), Walter Sneddon Robertson, Percy Peter James Stewart, William Howard Thomas, Leslie Joseph Thompson, Thomas Trench Thompson, James Renfrew White (Ch.M. 1923), David Whyte, Eric Arthur Widdowson, George Wishart Will

1913
Cyril Victor Atmore Baigent, Roger Buddle, Dugald George Matheson, James Garfield Mitchell, Thomas Harold Pettit, David Livingstone Sinclair, William Sowerby (Travelling Scholar 1913) (MD 1916), Leslie Alan Spedding, Alexander Meiklejohn Trotter, Kenneth Isaac Woodward

1914
Frederick Cameron, John Connor, Edward Kerr Edie, Erwin Eric Faris, Roland Arthur Hertslet Fulton (Travelling Scholar 1914), Bertram Hazelwood Gilmour, Charles Ernest Hercus (MD 1921), Philip John Jory, Gordon Napier MacDiarmid (MD 1923), Douglas Gordon MacPherson (MB 1914; ChB 1920), James Ayson Marshall, Donald Stuart Milne (Travelling Scholar 1915), Daniel Frank Myers, Thomas Russell Ritchie, Samuel Llewellyn Serpell, George Stanley Sharp, Hugh Short, Kenneth Edwin Tapper, Wilfred Stanley Wallis (MD 1922), William Watt

1915
William Aitken, Bertram Frederick Aldred, William Amos-Johnston, Robert Hector Baxter, Philip Blaxland Benham, Ivan Blaubaum, Norman Harrison Dempster, Henry Bayldon Ewen, Herbert Leslie Gould, John Graham Gow, Selwyn Langstaff Haslett, Herbert Miller Hay, Ronald George Keith Hodgson, Doris Clifton Jolly (Gordon), Kenneth MacCormick, Donald Mackay, Angus McPhee Marshall, David Douglas Wallace Martin, Francis Dewsbury Pinfold, George Redpath, Oswald James Reid, William Jamieson Reid, George Harold Robertson (MD 1921), Aubrey Vincent Short, Arthur Harry Aylmer Vivian, Ernest John Herbert Webb, Noel Stewart Whitton, Alexander Duncan Shanks Whyte, Warren Hastings Young

1916
William Fleming Currie, Mary Francesca Compere Dowling (Travelling Scholar 1916), Harold Ray Gibson (MD 1920), George Brownlee Isdale, Arthur Kidd, Stuart Scoular (MD 1918), Gladys Margaret Wilkes Shaw, William Henry Simpson, William Hunter Will, Irene Woodhouse, Eric Melvyn Wyllie

1917
Leonard Hugh Booth, Robert Lyall Christie, Donald Eric Currie, Christopher ap Rhys Davies, William Henry Davy, James Noel Edgar, Gerald Patrick Fitzgerald, William Douglas Fitzgerald, William Patteson Pollock Gordon, Mabel Aileen Hanron (Christie), Roy Harris, Ashley Aston Haworth, James Alfred Jenkins (Travelling Scholar 1917) (ChM 1924), Archibald Joseph, Iain Cameron Macintyre (MD 1920), Robert Roy Douglas Milligan, Frederick James Mulholland, Duncan Robertson Niven, Aeneas William Tolster O'Sullivan, Spencer Tauria Parker, Alexander Martin Ross, Everard Oswald Rowley, William Gladstone Scannell, Frederick Montgomery Spencer, Theodore Thomas Thomas, Dallas Bradlaugh Walker, John Russell Wells, James Leslie Allan Will, Robert Milne Wishart

1918
Frederick John Appleby, Humphrey James Barnicoat, Leslie George Bell, Francis Clough Blundell, William Makuri Cotter, Arthur John Cottrell (Travelling Scholar 1918), John Raymond Cuthbert, Geoffrey Jasper St. Clair Fisher, Robert Stephenson Jordan Fitzgerald, Wilfrid Thompson Glasgow, Charles Mills Greenslade, Richard John Burnside Hall, William David Hart, David Collingwood Low (MD 1921), Lawrence Carrington Mail, Alexander Smith Morton, Charles Stewart Murray, Victor Rylands Nicholson, Douglas McKnight Paterson, Grace Stevenson (MD 1922), Robert Burns Watson, Marion King Bennie Whyte (Cameron), Mary Phoebe Wilson

1919
Ivan McDonald Allen (MD 1920), Colin Campbell Anderson, Emma Gertrude Applegate (Atmore), David Alfred Bathgate, Louis Amos Bennett (Travelling Scholar 1919) (MD 1921), William Stephen Vincent Bransgrove, Howard Francis Buckley, Henry Mayall Budd, Sydney Rivers Cattell, Edward John Cronin, Edward Pohou Ellison, Charles Stanley Frederick Fraser, Arnold Gilray, Vincent Denis Griffen, John William Hall (MD 1921), Oswald Fyfe Lamb, James Tait Laurenson, Walter Watson Little, Samuel Lawrence Ludbrook, David Matthew

Mitchell, James Francis Cleveland Moore, Douglas Leonard Muir, Samuel Bertram Wanless Strain, Henry Howard Eric Vivian, George Edwin Waterworth, Robert Lanktree Withers, Robert Henry Wylie

1920
Percy Errol Allison, William Arthur Anderson, Beatrix Helen Bakewell, Geoffrey Michael Fulton Barnett, Andrew Muir Begg, Arama Thomas Begg, Harold Shaw Billcliff, Norman Francis Boag, Elspeth Mary Cameron (Fitzgerald), Colin James Campbell, Harry Kenrick Christie (ChM 1928), John Maxwell Clarke (ChM 1931), Herbert John Colvin, Joseph Roger de Witte Connolly, Arthur Herbert Driver, Rupert Selwyn Australia Graham, Alfred Smith Gray, Frank Copland Hutchison, Alfred Barrett Jameson, Cyril Arnold King (Travelling Scholar 1920), Lawrence Manning King, William Richard Lawrence, Graham Douglas Lindsay, Eric Howard Manley Luke, Albert George McClymont, John Campbell McKenzie, Hector Macdonald Monro, Alan Edwin Park, William Barnett Reekie, Alan Bruce Roy, Kenneth Guthrie Salmond, George Herbert Thomson, Henry Charles Tod, James Noble Waddell

1921
Moana Maru Anderson (Gow), Maurice Bevan Brown (Travelling Scholar 1921), Alexander Lionel Caselberg, Sylvia Gytha de Lancy Champman (MD 1934), Cecil Roy Childs, Rosina Dorothy Crawley (Richards), Eva Esther Day (Hill), John Dreadon, Walter Syme Eudey, Willliam Beaumont Fisher, Rita Ethel Osborne Gillies, Malcolm Kennedy Gray, Harold Edgar Harris, William Jack Pearson Hutchison, Ashley Selwyn McInnes, Morgan Patrick McSweeney (MB 1921; ChB 1923), Peter Milne, Arthur Alexander Reid, Charles Richard Stewart Roberts, Douglas Hutchinson Saunders, Hugh Roland Segar, James Jefcoate Valentine, Cecil Govett Romaine Wright

1922
Robert Stevenson Aitken (Travelling Scholar 1923) (Rhodes Scholar 1924) (MD 1939), Robert Findlay Allan, Harold Angell, James Bruce Baird, Robert Frescheville Bakewell, Muriel Emma Bell (MD 1926), Charles Ritchie Burns (Travelling Scholar 1922) (MD 1926), John Cairney, Roland Cashmore, Leopold Ransford de Castro, James Stuart Church, Robert Alan Harry Church, Ernest Young Comrie, John Winterton Costello, Thomas Beveridge Davis, Reginald George Dudding, Gerald Jacob Frengley, James Ian Roberts Gray, Eily Elaine Gurr, Phyllis Haddow, Cedric Stanton Hicks, Walter James Hope-Robertson, William Archibald Johnston, Ranfurly Percival Stanley Kelman, Grace Helena Kine (Proude), Russell David King, George Richard Kingston (MD 1933), Alexander Henderson Kirker, Cecil Edgar de Latour, Philip Patrick Lynch (MD 1925), Frances Isabella McAllister (Preston), Duncan Campbell MacDiarmid, Colin Campbell Maclaurin, Gilbert Maclean, David McMillan, Eric Snow McPhail, Augusta Manoy (Klippel), Norman Manson, Zealanda Marshall (Aitken), Phyllis Mather, Hessie Morton (McDermid), Henry Martin O'Connor, Lindsy Morgan Park, Hazel Rebecca Bryan Patterson (Allison), Arnold Perry, Marion Aroha Radcliffe-Taylor, Eric Jesse Rawnsley, Edgar Robert Reay, Mortimer Philip Reddington, Hubert George Rix, George Douglas Robb, Malcolm Robertson, Kenneth James Langlands Scott (MD 1923), David Neil McCulloch Scrymgeour, Ronald George Shackleton, William Francis Shirer, Susannah Catherine Campbell Sinclair, Ronald Douglas Stronach, Harold Bertram Turbott, John Maurice Watters, Charles Skinner Williams, John Harold Herbert Wood

1923
Duncan Roy Abernethy, Robert Findlay Aitken, Leslie Gordon Austin, Robert Leslie Grosvenor Barclay, Ruth Marjorie Cruickshank Barclay, William Alan Blomfield, Alister James

Brass, Walton Howarth Bremner, Eric Hattaway Bridgman, Kenneth Rex Brokenshire, William Henry Blinman Bull, Harold Douglas Cameron, Mary Anderson Champtaloup, Stewart White Crawford, Eric Frederick D'Ath, James Keith Davidson, Eric Tewson Dawson, Derek Ernest Denny-Brown (MD 1946), William Julius Dickel, John Paterson Donald, Mollie Fisher (Christie), Noel Edward Hertslet Fulton, Isabella Gault (Wise), Maurice Greville, Allan Hopkins, Edwin Warwick Hunt, James Dewar Hunter, John Alexander Douglas Iverach (Travelling Scholar 1924), Elizabeth Kate Jary (Hughes), David Richmond Jennings, John Faulks Landreth, Eric Roy Lange, Elizabeth Pretoria Lumsden (Hall), Dennis Douglas McCarthy (MD 1942), Eric Ian Alan Macdonald, Archibald Hector McIndoe, Allan Francis Mackay, Norman Reay MacKay (MD 1926), Donald Dixon McKenzie, James Gilbert MacKereth, Hector James Mail, Charles McIntosh Marshall, Aubrey James Mason (ChM 1933), Norman Murdoch Matheson, Edith Annie Mayo, George Inglis Miller, Horace Webster Nash, Claude Vincent Page, John Leonard Plimmer, Norman Rawstron, Henry Salisbury Ray, John Herbert Rule, Robert Gemmel Burnett Sinclair, Alfred Norman Slater, Marjorie Smith-Wilson, Norman Charles Speight, Caroline Morrow Stenhouse, Ralph Grainger Stokes, Angus Leslie Sutherland, Claude Alexander Taylor, Alan Arnold Tennent, Samuel James Thompson, Samuel Joseph Thomson, Kathleen Mary Todd, John Martin Twhigg, Francis Gerald Ward, Cyril Henry Williams, John Upham Williams (MD 1929), Jack MacKay Young

1924
Robert Erwin Austin, Morris Axford, Harold Havelock Barnett, Francis Eastham Bolt, Reynold Harold Boyd, Craig Edward Brown, Edward Brown, Edward Coventry Bydder, Winifred Ethel Cox (Morton), Alexander Cumming, Ronald Otway Davidson, Lyell Stanley Davis, Kenrick Holt Dean, Muriel Helen Easterfield (MD 1927), William Rognvald Fea, James Fitzsimons (Travelling Scholar 1925), Robert Searson Rodney Francis, Sylvester Lot Geerin, Robinson Early Hall, William Keith Renwick Hamilton, Benjamin David Hart, Eric Robin Harty, Adam Hamilton Harvie, Keith Hoani Holdgate, Roy Humphrey Howells, Clifford Samuel James, Brian Maruice Johns, Harry Selwyn Kenrick, Frederick Alexander Lamb, Robert Gordon Butler Lusk, Eugene Gribben Lynch, Gladys Muirson MacAlister (Bremner), Allan Augustus MacDonald, Lawrence Cradock McNickle, John Mark, Richard Bowden Martin, Robert James Maunsell, Margaret Joan Mayfield (Williams), Kenneth William Miller, Oscar Carl Moller, Arthur Rainsford Mowlem, Charles Everard North, Roland Glyndwr Phillips-Turner, Charles David Read, Reginald Francombe Roberts, Alice Campbell Rose (Tallerman) (Travelling Scholar 1925), Carl Xavier Ruhen, Wilfred Robert Ryburn, Edward George Sayers (MD 1959), Frederick Rich Smale, Kingsley Rupert Steenson, William Raymond Courtney Stowe, Dorothy Sweeney (McKeefrey), Edward Harold Harvey Taylor, Patrick Arthur Treahy, Norman Waddle, Edward Baden Powell Watson, Frederick Edward Webster (ChM 1938), Roy Samuel Whiteside, James Lewis Wicken, David Arthur Callender Will, Basil Laun Wilson, Jeanie Gardner Wood (Fougere); MD: Munro May Hockin

1925
Catherine Ellen Weppener Anderson, James Henry Beaumont, Francis Oswald Bennett (MD 1946), Hugh Barton Berney, Robert Eldred Beven Brown, William Anderson Bird, Keith Buchanan Bridge, Percy Charles Edward Brunette, Eardley Lorimer Button, Gordon Bertram Campbell, Eric Candy, Cecily Mary Aroha Wise Clarkson (Pickerill), Trevor Grahame De Clive-Lowe, James Jackson Crawshaw, Leonard Kerr Crow, John Alexander Dale, David McKee Dickson, Mary Douglas, Archibald Durward (Travelling Scholar 1926), Theodora Clemens Easterfield (Hall), William James Edginton, David Nathan Eppstein, Henry Walden Fitzgerald, Robert Louttit

Flett, William Swan Fogg, John Cennick Forsyth, Ernest Sydney Fossey, Ian Comyn Fraser, Desmond Makgill Frengley, Carlyle Bond Gilberd, Philip Vernon Graves, Henry Percival Gray, Frederick William Helmore, Owen Stanmore Hetherington, Nina Catharine Howard (Muir), Adam Irvine Hunter, Stewart Hunter, Cedric Walter Isaac, Hoani Turner Jennings, Alvert Edward King, Charles Herbert King, Moe Kronfeld, Harold Braithwaite Lang, Ella Langley (Connolly), Francis Reginald Leonard, Chisholm McDowell, John Bell McMiken (MD 1943), Joseph Patrick McQuilkin, Samuel Thomas Martin, Cecil David Meadowcroft, William Eric Minty, Effie Muriel Morgan, Frank Adrian Morton, James Aitkenhead Paterson, Charles Edward Reid, Bruce Clarkson Rennie, Gordon Francis Rich (ChM 1933), William Gordon Rich, Leith Alexander Riddell, Roy Vernon Shaw, Frederick Charles Merritt Shortt, Edward Battersby William Smyth, Philip Edwin Starr, James Garfield Stewart, Uriti May Strack, Sydney Herbert Swift, Graeme Gibson Talbot, Edgar Frederick Thomson, Thomas Howard Thorp, John Fortescue Zohrab

1926

Eleanor Kathleen Abbott, Rodger Anker Bakewell, Frederick G. Barrowclough, Raymond Edward Bridge, William George Bridgman, Douglas James Brown, Joseph John Brownlee, Corban Assid Corban, Newell Raine Cotton, Fawcitt Miller Dodds, George Morton Evans, James Herbert Fahey, Margaret Marion Grater (Lemon), Janette Muir Grave (King), Melville Simpson Harris, Robert Turnbull Hay, Keith Norris Hiskins, Henry Nicholas Johnson, Ronald George T. Lewis, Helen Edith Lochhead (Dougall), Joseph Cecil Douglas Macky, Bertram George Mitford, Phyllis Maude Moir (Babington), Walter Gordon Paterson (MD 1931), Basil Ainslie Porritt, Newton Quilliam, Lindsay Sangster Rogers (Travelling Scholar 1927), Thomas William Stoddart, Arthur Beresford Sturtevant, Felicia Walmsley, Archibald Wallace Wilkinson, George Wood

1927

Melville Huia Aiken, Jessie Alexander (Burnett), Henry Campbell Barrett, Horace Laurenson Bowell, Leslie Melville Burnett, Ernest Edward Butler, Alfred Bramwell Cook (Travelling Scholar 1927) (MD 1944), Charles Desmond Costello, Edgar Francis Fowler, Donald Joseph Goodwin, Thomas Bennett Hamilton, Alfred Josiah Clark Hanan, John Telford Harding, Cyril Michael Thomas Hastings, Barbara Hay Henry (Roche), Lewis Edmund Jordan, Beryl Jessie Lawrence, Selwyn Graham de Clive Lowe, Stuart Bain MacKay, Leonard George McQueen, Alexandra Carson Mathieson, Trevlyn Ernest Miller, Alexander George Minn, Noel Thorpe Mirams, D'Arcy Harper Moir, James Duncan Murdoch, Alfred Lionel de Berri Noakes, John Havelock North, John Arthur Rolland O'Regan, Rahiri Hildyard Pitcaithly, Leonard Randell, Mary Jane Hulse Russell, William George Eric Shand, Edwin Patrick Spencer, Charles Keith Vautier, Morris Netterville Watt, Pauline Catherine Witherow (Simcock)

1928

William Bale Andrew, Dudley Walker Ashcroft, Raymond Ward Bellringer, Reginald Charles Bonnington, Alan Murison Bowie, Cedric John Charles Britton (MD 1937), Henry Burrell, Frederick Russell Chisholm, Ronald Frederick Clare, Leslie Gordon Cook, Lionel Hildreth Cordery, James Joseph Dee Foley, John Richard Hertslet Fulton, Frederick Plimmer Furkert, Ellensleigh Denny Gordon Gillies, Erin Michael Griffin, Eustatius Wm. Barton Griffiths, Jack Carl Rudolph Hindenach (Travelling Scholar 1928) (MD 1931), Horace Emerton Hodge, Helen Isabel Houghton, George William Lock, David Gervan McMillan, Richard William David Maxwell, John Cubridge Mercer, Edward Thomas Gordon Miller, Kenneth Frederick Mulcock, David Oswald Paterson, Alan Alexander Pullar, Russell Vernon Ritchie, Archibald

Murray Scott, Walter Netley Searle, Douglas Thomas Swift, Stanley Livingstone Wilson

1929

Denis Frank Armstrong, George Percy Bardsley, Raeburn Neil Campbell, John Egerton Caughey (MD 1939), Bettina Matraves Collier (Hamilton), Gordon Owen Lindsay Dempster, Joseph Leonard Dimond, Brian John David Dunn, Grahame Stoddart Erwin (MD 1942), Hugh Stuart Fleming, Murray Hamilton Heycock, Bernard Trevor Hooper, Nola Mary Ivory, Douglas Waddell Jolly, Claud Wilfred Alfred Kimbell, Rosalind Brackenbury Latter, Ian James Hamersley Logan, Edward Kenmure McLean, William Wallace Main, Eric Vener Maxwell (Travelling Scholar 1929), Selwyn Bentham Morris, Russell Redvere Murray, David Elmore Orchard, Herbert Kenneth Pacey, Trevor Edward Palmer, Bernard William Pearcy, Kathleen Anuei Pih (Chang), Norman Nathanael Porterfield, Louis Hauiti Potaka, Dorothy Smith, Thomas Malcolm Smith, Donald Robert Louis Stevenson, William James Crosbie Wells, Roland Francis Wilson

1930

Patrick Clarence Anderson (MD 1939), William Brown, Stuart Cordingley Colbeck, Hugh Stewart Douglas, Lennox Douglas, Norman Lowther Edson (Travelling Scholar 1930), Paul Joseph Fogarty, Howard James Gaudin, Ellen Gough Heycock (Boddy), Fred Hodgkiss, John Woodward Horsley, Alfred Tennyson Howie, Brian Tyrwhitt Wyn Irwin, Clive Reginald Lambert, Douglas Masson Logan, Elfie McCaskill (Needham; Connall), Alexander McIlroy, Herbert Frank McNickle, Archibald Robert Alex. Marshall, Thomas Seton Norris, Desmond Patrick O'Brien, Adah Hamilton Evelyn Platts-Mills (Blomfield), Ian Marshall Rutherford, Arthur Leslie Sheild, John Arthur Stallworthy, Anne Margaret Thomson, William Goddard Volckman, Donald George Wallace, Maurice Sinclair Wells, Charles Debden Wilkins

1931

Donald Young Allan (MD 1936), George Richard Butterfield, Thomas Enright Caffell, Archibald Murdoch Douglas, Thomas Michael Francis Fitzgerald, Thomas Russell Cumming Fraser (Travelling Scholar 1931) (MD 1946), Eric Worton Gibbs, Theodor Anton Green, Robert Burns Grey, Anna Lydia Hansen (Nannestad), Katherine Milner Hastie, James Paul Kennedy, George Raymond Kirk, Leonard Hugh Marshall, Norman William Martin, Karl Iversen Nissen, Alfred Cecil Wallace Oakey, Adam Russell Ross, Frank Finley Sligo, Garth Rivers Stoneham, Arthur Wemyss Gordon Sutherland, Joseph Robert Gibson Thompson, William Guildford Todd, Eben Lambert Wilson

1932

Arthur George Bell, Hedley Ernest Bellringer, Rex Blunden, James Verney Cable (Travelling Scholar 1932) (MD 1937), Arthur Wilfred Fletcher Cole, Florence Aileen Craig, Teresa Imelda Craig (Thompson), John Rawson Elder, Gordon Neville Findlay, William Alfred Fitzherbert, Ian Donald Gebbie, Edward Harold Walter Gifford, Martha Kirkland Grigor (Gregory), Sydney Wallace Jefcoate Harbutt, Thomas Henry Jagusch, Charles Wynn Squire Jerram, Golan Haberfield Maaka, Graham Campbell MacDiarmid, Albert Matthews McGavin, Murray McGeorge (MD 1939), Neil Hugh Allan MacKinnon, Neil Gordon McLean, Gordon Logie McLeod, Meredith Conley Moore, Edward Keith Mulinder, Geoffrey Alexander Myers, James Keith O'Dea, Leslie Ian Parton, William Rowland Phillipps, Thomas Robert Plunket, Basil Oswald Quin, William Henry Rothwell, Hugh Alan Small, Eric Newman Smith, Sidney S. Smith, Margaret Ruth Sneddon, Robert Francis Stenhouse, Ronald Swanson Stewart, Marie Payne Stringer (Buchler), Raeburn Rodd Talbot, William Fitzgerald Watters, Hilton Leonard Willcox

1933

Vivian D'Arcy Blackburn, Beryl Eveline G. Bowden (Douglas), John Frederick Bradbury, Winston Stephen Charters, Leslie Peter Clark, Edgar Herman Clarke, Allan Gordon Cumming, John Keith Cunninghame, Joseph Richard Dawson, William Lillico Dodds, Alan Wilson Douglas, Owen Lamont Eaton, Murray Alexander Falconer, Norman Frank Greenslade, Murray Thomson Greig, Albert Moor Hartnell, William Bremner Highet, Arthur Hallam Howie, Gordon Alexander Irwin, Edward Speid Jamieson, Trevor Harold Knights, Robert John McGill (Travelling Scholar 1933), Malcolm Lionel Robert Morley, Noel Hunter North, Richard Orgias, William Murray Porteous (MD 1946), William Alec Priest, Norman William Pryde, Peter William Stewart Riley, John Russell Ritchie, Zoe Cuff Rutherford (Mason), Colin Ross Stevenson, Dorothy Marian Stewart, Thomas Campbell Sutherland, Russell Felstead Thomas, Alan Lambert Wilson, Robert Alan Wilson

1934

Edmund Peter Allen, David Athol Arnott, Beauchamp d'Epinsy Barclay, Arthur Charles Belfield, Ruth Margaret Boyd-Wilson (Hill), Evelyn Joyce Burley (Lester), David Craig Lloyd Clay, Graham Bruce Alastair Cowie, Jione Antonio Dovi, John Boyd Wallace Dunlop, Bruce Walton Grieve (Travelling Scholar 1935), Douglas William Guthrie, William Hawksworth, Noel Frederick Charles Hill, Charles Barclay Innes, Rupert Desmond Keenan, James McHaffie, David Gilmour McLachlan (MD 1941), William Macky MacLaurin, Vine Carey Martin, Benno Mongeimer, Robert David Morrow, Elizabeth Vivien Newlands, Geoffrey Buckland Orbell, Thomas Max Pemberton, Douglas George Phillips, Kenneth Rees-Thomas, Allenson Gordon Rutter (Travelling Scholar 1934), Cleveland Latimer Edward Lilly Sheppard, Irwin Bruce Speight, Marion Kerr Steven, Kenneth Rees Thomas, Ian Douglas Thomson, Alan Keith Tulloch, Mary Watson, William James Watt, Gertrude Aphra Willis (Morley)

1935

George Potter Adams, William Edgar Adams, Clive Murray Arthur, Alexander Charles Begg (MD 1947), Margaret Annie Birks (Begg), William Lindsay Barron Burns, Wallace Neil Campbell, Fred Lawrence Clark, Arthur Percival Cotter, George Mudie Foote, Richard John Gillett, Neil Thomas Philip Hardie, Frank Leo Hutter, Norman Kenneth Bernard Kimbell, Richard Arthur Lucas, Thomas Alastair MacFarlane, Harvard Northcroft Merrington, George Edward Moloney (Travelling Scholar 1935), Gordon William Moore, Charles Marwood Mules, Francis Arthur Hatherall Neate, Thomas Phillips Neil (Hardie), Philip John Orton, Ralph George Park (MD 1945), William Mummery Platts, Donald Finlay Price, Charles Graham Riley, Gavin Lindsey Miles Scholefield, Benjamin Gibson Spiers, Kenneth James Talbot, John Dalrymple Willis, Mabel Collis Wood (Laing)

1936

Leicester Hammond Aitken, Harold Basil Alexander (Travelling Scholar 1936), William Somerville Baber, Diamond Allan Ballantyne, John Netterville Barron, Robert Douglas Neil Bissett, Margaret Elizabeth Wilson Christie (MacDonald), Robert Lawrence Mowbray Christie, William Hector Davis, Alexander MacKay Trotter Dickie, Geoffrey Thornton Dudley, Eric William Duncan, Francis Barette Edmundson, Eric Mitchell Elder, Gertrude Louisa Galliers (Brosnahan), Charles George Dines Halstead, Leo Gordon Hannah, Thomas Wishart Harrison, Colin Graeme Hunter (MD 1958), John Colin Lopdell, Bernard Edward Paul McCullough, Alexander Ironside Littlejohn MacDiarmid, Joseph Neil MacFarlane, Terence Arthur Mears Maunsell, Francis Russell Miller, Reginald Moore, Hubert Morrison, George Rowan Nicks, Harry Leslie Palmer, Claude Percival S. Riddell, Margaret Stuart Riddell (Smith), Leslie John Roy, Francis Norman

Sharpe, Alice Grace Stanley (Armour), Dora Mary Stevenson-Wright (Young), Denis Tiffin Stewart (MD 1950), Myrtle Inez Thew (Hill), Claudia Lilian Weston(Cottrell), Edmund Gillow Young

1937

John Wynyard Bartrum, Annie Hayes Berry, William Melville Will Brookfield, Graeme Campbell Taylor Burns, Walter Irving (Tony) Cawkwell, Oliver Westby Chapman, Hono Evan Horrell Denham, Ernest Hugh Densem, Eugen Jeno Fischmann, Marcus Rattray Fitchett, Harold Mason Foreman, Walter Lewis MacLeod Gilmour, Robert Renton Grigor, Alan MacKenzie Gunn, Joseph George Harkness, Reginald George Harper, John Robert Hinds (MD 1955), Howard Hunter, Margaret Robina Jackson (Chieffi), George Clifford Jennings, Lannes Fullarton Johnson, Alexander Stuart King, Harvey Tuarangi Knight, Frederick Boyes Korkis, George Lemchen, Ernest Going Loten, Thomas John MacCormac, William James Buchanan McFarland, Vincent John McGovern (MD 1954), William Richard McKechnie, Colvin Hugh McKenzie, Iain Lumsden MacKinnon (MD 1961), Kevin Nicholas McNamara, William Maxwell Manchester (Travelling Scholar 1937), Alan Francis Marshall, Roger Thornton Marshall, Reginald Warren Medlicott, Patrick Alexander Harding Moore, Beatrice Esther Nelson (Schuchard), Charles Plummer Powles, Chris Stains Preston, Walter James Ramsay, Charles Calvin Ring, Derek Raymond Ryder, Peter Reid Skinner, Jack Ajzyk Slucki, Alice Mary Stanton (Bush), Earl Stevenson-Wright, Alexander Cuthbertson Stewart, David Uttley Strang, Frederick Alexander Sundstrum, Alistair James Thomson, John Douglas Thomson, Hector Charles Tremewan, James Ronald Turner, James MacKenzie Tyler, Ronald Wagstaff, Colin Edward Watson, Thomas Alastair Watson, James Michael Watt, David Renfrew White, Stephen Empson Williams, James Lawrence Wright

1938

Sydney Graham Aitken, Ivan Allan Alexander, Leo Solomon Antonoff Lewis (MD 1951), Kenneth Richard Archer, John Borrie (MD 1954), William Roy Carswell, Claude Lewis Carter Cook, Mitford William Alfred Cowles, David Leonides Cropp, Douglas Gordon Cumming, Campbell Newman Smith D'Arcy, James Dempsey, Aland Richmond Ellis, Gavin Hannay Forrest, Thomas Oswald Gilbert, Alastair Gordon Gilchrist, William Gelston Gray, Bruce MacFarlane Hay, Charles Peter Howden, Cuthbert Hatherly Hughes-Johnson, Margaret Fraser Hunter (Gatman), Douglas McKelvie Jack, Hal Jacobs, Alan Rutherford Johnson, Robert Middleton De Lambert, Harold Dixon Law, John Alistair Loan, Alan Lionel Lomas, William Brian de Laval Lusk, Thomas Macallan, Norman Dryburgh McCreath, Ronald Alexander MacDonald, Lindsay MacDougall, Kenneth Penn Leslie MacGregor, John Lewis McIver, James Samuel McVeigh, John Laurence Malcolm, John Anthony Meade, Donald James Hildreth Meredith, Robert Frederick Moody, Charles Stuart Moore, John Robert Jellicoe Moore, Gilbert Murray, Hamish Coates Neale, Allan North, John Penman, Hugh Coleman Petherick, James Ramsay, Judah Laurence Reynolds, Anthony Trevelyan Rogers, Mutyala Satyanand, Joseph Lindsell Simcock, Dorothy Spence-Sales, Kenneth Robert Stallworthy (Travelling Scholar 1938), John Malfroy Staveley, Murray Alexander Stewart, Lester Wycherley Suckling, Alan William Sutherland, Colin Kemp Swallow, Derek Henry Symes, Peter Christopher Stanley Unwin, Kenneth Frank McNeill Uttley, Molly Wagstaff (Smith), Richard Joseph Walton, John Kinder Ferrier Watson, Cornelius William Whetter, Ernest Edwyn Willoughby, Charles Frederick Wilson

1939

Albert Burman Adams, John Raymond Addison, Dennis Newton Allen, John Norman Armour, Robert Buchanan Beattie, Alexander William Huntly Borrie, John Joseph

Bourke, Warren John Boyd, Percy James Brown, Eric Dawson Burnard, Cyril Thomas Collins, Wyvern Grey Cook, Denholm Carncross Cuddie, Richard Henry Dawson, Desmond John Andrew Doyle, Walter Ronald Easton, Allen Edward Erenstrom, Charles Patrick Marshall Feltham, Richard John Lillico Feltham, George de Lacy Fenwick, Roderick Graeme Stewart Ferguson, Harold Faber Fookes, Thomas Grahame Fox, Harold Henry Gilbert, Hilgrove John Gosset, Albert James Henderson, Patrick Fraser Howden, John Arthur Keeling, Douglas Peter Kennedy, William Ross Lane, Garsie Aris De Latour, George Hector Levien, John Douglas Lough, George Ian Louisson, Leo Charles McCarthy, Robert Gair MacDonald, Donald Stewart Malcolm (MD 1948), Anthony Howard Marsh, Alison Jean Marshall, Hagbarth Ernest Moller, Norma May Morey (Witters), Eric Musard Nanson, John Warrington Newlands, John Robert Mills Nicholson, Brian Wotherspoon Nixon, William Irvine Paterson, Frederick Charles Platts, Eric Solomon Raudnic, Louis Robinson, Noel William Robson, Dennis Rogers, George Lancelot Rolleston, Alexander Mathieson Rutherford, Bruce Wyville Rutherfurd, Jean Mary Sandel (Travelling Scholar 1939), John Thomas Shearer, Lawrence George Stephenson, Sydney Allan Struthers, Edward Sydney Thodey, Samuel Bruce Thompson, Alan Samuel Turner, Harry Jenner Wales, Adrian Herbert Webb, John Hallam Webber, Vivian Ian Edgar Whitehead (MD 1950), Henry Edward Martyn Williams, Walter Williams, Noel Henry Wilson

1940
John Lewis Adams (MD 1959), Alexander Godfrey Armitage, John William Avery, Vance Leonard Barber, Neil Colquhoun Begg, Norma Beatrice Benson, Lindsay John McFarlane Black, Albert Damer Gibson Blanc, Stanley Burnham Lake Bowker, Allen Lindsay Bryant, Selwyn Kerry Burcher, Francis John Cairns (MD 1948), Graham Lelliott Clark (MD 1948), Balfour William Clouston, James Lewis Colgrave, George Burall Courtis, John Andrew Kirby Cuningham, William Gordon Davidson, Edward Owen Dawson, John Dickie, John Ross Duff Eaton, Robert Stewart Edward, Keith Munroe Emanuel, Kurt Erber, Thomas Hill Fisher, Colin Clifton Foote, Donald Bartlett Gash, Douglas Alexander Gordon, Graham Francis Hall, William Wybrow Hallwright (Travelling Scholar 1940), Charles Warrington Howden, William Lumley Hughes-Jackson, Barry Hamilton Irvine, Richard Myles Irwin, Walter Ruthven Lang, James Joseph McDonald, Victor Bauchop McGeorge, Neil Joseph McIlroy, Eunice Janet McLean (Loan), Athol Ewan McMillan, Jack Dilworth Haslett Matthews, John Forbes Menzies, John Keith Michelle, Thomas Finlayson Miller, Anne Helen Morgan-Coakle, Michael Noel Oliver, Thomas Milne Ongley, Keith Leslie Park, Victor Tomlinson Pearse, Colin Thomas Bushby Pearson, Herbert Dudley Purves, William Hanson Reid, John Rich, Anthony William Stuart Ritchie, Percival Curwen Service, Louis Percy Simmons, Derek Grey Simpson, Gordon Allan Smith, Harman Gilbert Smith, William Joseph Smith, Christabel Mary Spence-Sales (Wallace), Hugh Allen Alexander Stevely, Allan Henderson Stewart, Lindsay Rutherford Stewart, John Charles Davis Sutherland, Charles Herbert Thomson, Peter Mowbray Tripp, Harold Charles Tuck, Donald William Urquhart, Malcolm Watt, Gordon Henry Beckett Whitta, Thomas Kenneth Williams, Francis Jamieson Wilson, Paul Wynne Wishart, William Sealy Wood

1941
Richard Nichols Akel, Thomas Ritchie Anderson, Clifford Henderson Baird, Stephen de Carteret Barclay, Meynell Francis Henry Blain, John Peter Broad, Irene Glenwynne Burford (Rhodes), David Charles Campbell, Tom Dick Collingwood Childs, Redmond Brett Gould Cook, Ellis Thacker Dick, Ross Graham Dreadon, Hugh Patrick Dunn, John Alex Duthie, Irwin Bruce Faris, John Farquhar Findlay, Iain Henry Fletcher,

Alan Harvey Foate, Clive Houghton Garlick, Mervyn William Arthur Gatman (Travelling Scholar 1941), Elsie Craig Gibbons, Humphrey Walter Gowland, Christopher Gresson, Guy Pieremont Hallwright, Reginald Henry Hamlin (Travelling Scholar 1941), Cecilia Ellen Hands, Arthur Gordon Harper, Newenham Deane Maurice Harvey, Alfred Heppner, H.L. Hersch, Gordon George Jenner, David Dagobert Kallman, Kurt Kent-Koplowitz, Franz Kral, Victor Shirle Land, David Levinsohn, Maris Laline McClymont (MacDougall), William Frederick McConnell, Robert Alexander McDowell, Peter George McLeod, Richard Maunsell Martin, Stanley William Paterson Mirams, Charles Joseph James Morkane, Trevor Adolphus Morris, William Arthur Dysart Nelson, Catherine Newman, William Dorrien Nichol, James Raymond Norris, William Charles Raymond North, Paul Oestreicher, Geoffrey Orchard, Oswald Richard Brooks Pringle, Morris John Purdy, John Wellesley Evan Raine, Richard Ewart Rawstron (MD 1973), Heinrich Schmidt, Robert Duncan Scott, Lionel Arthur Scrivin, Olga Wilhelmina Lina Semon, Francis Harding Sims (MD 1991), Richard Ivan Rapley Skelley, John Steven, James Marshall Stewart, Hugh Cyril William Stringer, Robert Thomson Sutherland, Franklyn Hugh Swan, Charles Swanston, Arthur Newton Talbot, Mary Lorraine Talbot, Robert Lawson Thompson, Graham Morris Thomson, Geoffrey Townsend, Thomas Charles Trott, Richard Peter Tuckey, Ernest John Velvin, Allan Edwin Walton, Stewart Kennerley Watson, Jakob Weiser, Jack Mackay Wogan

1942
William Ross Aitchison, William Stewart Alexander (MD 1950), Alan Joseph Alldred, Ian Douglas Auld, John Colin Baird, Margaret McBeth Beedie (Buxton), Murray Lionel Benson, Lewis (Ludwig) Bieder, Leslie Winston Blain, Cyril Lindsay Breeze, Hamish Grant Bremner, Elizabeth Rae Brown, Gerald Morgan Brown, Joseph Burstein, Ronald Hugh Caughey (MD 1957), Roma Holbrook Chatfield (Roberts), Lloyd Woodrow Cox, Marjorie Elizabeth Cuttle (Macready), Margaret Isabel Elliott (Giles), Hilda Fleischl, Thomas Campbell Fraser, Noel Russell Freeman, Iris Mabel Emily Hamlin, Solomon Hass, Alan Colin Hayton, John Cowley Hazledine, Cyril Ashley Heaphy, Michael James Hewitt, Nancy Jocelyn Hunter (Gruar), Lionel Allenby Jacobs, Ian Reuben Bailie Jacobson, Norris Roy Jefferson, John Alexander Kilpatrick (MD 1947), Basil Marmaduke De Lambert, Keith Remington Lothian (Travelling Scholar 1942), John Bennett MacKay, Edwin Keith MacLeod, John Clarke McNeur, Thomas John Miles, Henry Britton Coates Milsom, Patrick William Eisdell Moore, Edgar Atheling Morris, Colin Samuel Morrison, Robert Flaxley Mulligan, Peter Desmond Nathan, Kenneth Hardie Patterson, Stewart Cunningham Peddie, Marcel Reichmann, Albert Glynn Roberts, Thomas Arvon Roberts, Roland Arnold Rodda (MD 1951), Marjorie Dorothea Rohan, Patrick Philip Eric Savage, Ewing Kirkland Scorgie, Bernard Shieff, Laurence Herbert Simpson, Alan Smith, Mark Graham Somerville, David Upham Steven, Geoffrey James Taine, Owen Lewis Thomas (MD 1947), Robert Bayne Topping, Henry Earl Windle, Margaret Isabel Wishart, Frederick Brian Masgrave Woodhouse

1943
Colin James Alexander (MD 1964), William Birch Allen, Robert Edmund Ballantyne, Jack Ballin, Peter Franklin Bartley, Douglas Trevor Beetham, Rowland Bramwell Bell, Henry Rongomau Bennett, John Daniel Bergin, Keith Hilliard Black, Molly Joan Boyes (Woodroffe), Leonard William Broughton, Melville Bryan Bruce, Douglas John Clifford, Arthur Charles Atkin Coombes, Thomas Henry Cornish, Patrick William Cotter, John Robert Earle Dobson, Robert Charles Doherty, Robert Bruce Duncan, John Edwin Raymond Edgar, Thomas Oliver Enticott, Sholto Grant Faris, Arthur Macky Fisher, Patricia Rae Ford (McDonald), Patrick Burnham Fox, Harold

Hugh Francis, Edward Lear Gillies, Arthur Oswald Gilmour, Martin Girling-Butcher, Gerald Lynch Gleeson, Earle William Glenn, Godfrey Matthew Goodson, Frederick John Gruar, Denis McRae Hanna, John Martin Hansen, Victor Harris, Sidney Caslake Hawes, Brian Henry Rowland Hill, Kenneth Morton Hole, Alfred Hoppner, Alison Hunter, Jean Dudley Margaret Jerram (Savage), William Halley Johnston, Ross Lyle Jones, James Ralston Kirker, John Martin Langham, John Spencer Bonar Lindsay (MD 1953), Jeffery Melville Louisson, Douglas David Lyness, Joan Katherine McDougall (Griggs), John Woodward Mandeno, Rachel Mark, Edward John Marshall, Norman Graeme Marshall, Reginald Tice Martin, Aileen Nada Maxwell, Curt Sally Meyer, David John Miller, Graham Anderson Milne, Stephen Moor (MD 1956), Graeme Murray Morice, William Murphy (MD 1955), Margaret Isobel Erskine Neave, Ian Lawrie Oliver, Monica Annie Ongley (Neville), Desmond Ernest Quick, Whitworth Atholstone Russell, Anthony Crowley Sandston, John Hutchison Saunders, Patrick Carroll Skinner, Charles Naughton Taylor, Lionel F. John Taylor, Heath Thurlow Thompson, Duncan Munro Todd, Wilmot John Trezise, Caleb Lewis Tucker, Robert Algar Warren, Robert Tannahill Watson, Windsor John Weston (Travelling Scholar 1943) (MD 1979), Allan Neil White, Ian Kennedy Wilson

1944
Chalmers Allen, Shirley Juliette Appleton (Dowding), James Warne Ardagh, Cecil Douglas Banks, John Stott Beedie, Lenn Gifford Bell, Lynton McHardie Berry, Hamilton Donald Walter Black, Harry Black, Eric Robert Blakely, John Alexander Macdonald Boyd, Kelson Brasted, Geoffrey Leonard Brinkman (MD 1952), William Henry Brockett, John Kirk Brown, George Nevil Brownlee, Robert George Bruce, Alastair Gordon Buist, Thomas George MacDonald Burnett, Jack French Burton (MD 1951), Clive Bremner Cameron (MD 1960), Douglas Ian Chisholm, Keith Wallace Cochrane, Allan Richmond Cockerell, Patrick William Conlon, Glyndwr Thorsby Davies, Patrick John Dowling, Robert Walter Evan Edgar, Max Farb, Keith Mickle France, Karl Gerstl, Ada Maisie Gilling, Laurie Kalman Gluckman (MD 1963), David John Gudex, Robert Henry Trevor Holmden, Ian Leslie Graham Hutchison, Thomas Jenkins, Daniel Grant Johnston, Joyce May Emery Jones (Merriman), Brian Joseph Kelly, Robert Fyffe Lamb, Peter Joseph Edward Lewis, William Allan Liddell, John Wilfred Logan, Patrick Corbett Loudon, Donald McAllister, Walter Victor Macfarlane (Travelling Scholar 1944), Colin Fulton McKee, Archibald Bruce Mackenzie, Neil Perry Markham (MD 1964), Mary Joyce Marples (MD 1951), Wilfrid Christie Mills, Margaret Isabel Moore (Wishart), Daphne Phyllis Morrison (Adams), Bernard William Murphy, Murray John Murray (MD 1954), Neil Gray Murray, Terence Michael O'Brien, Patrick Augustine Ongley, Maurice John Otley, Andrew John Paterson, Athol James Patterson, Alan William Pearson, Eric Harold Peat, June Esther Reid (Kriechbaum), Rex William David Renton, Alexander Charles Ritchie, Donald Walton Rowntree, Bruce Osborne Ryburn, Jakob Segal, Alfred Farquhar Shaw, Warwick Mayne Smeeton (MD 1957), Flora Smith, Ross Smith, Robert Russell Spencer, Kenneth Ernest Stone, Theodore Felstead Thomas, Alfred Lawrence Thompson, Warren Leishman Thompson, Derrick Tomlinson, William Reisiswyl Trotter, John Moore Tweed, Alexander Durell Warren, William John Watt, Graham Kemble Welch, James Stewart Wilson, Keith Barrington Forbes Witcombe

1945
David Hartley Abbott, Ashley Morton Aitken (MD 1968), James Aitken Baird, Ronald Albert Barker, Harry Andrew Beagley, Frederick Guy Trevor Beetham, Robert Bradley, Maureen Bridgman (Dingwall), Ian Sinclair de B. Broadfoot, Ross Fordyce Burton, David Graeme Campbell, David

Bernard Caro, Leslie Charles Carter, Noel Chambers, Robert James Maunsell Coates, Charles Maxwell Collins, Brian Morrison Corkill, Shirley Lyford Curtis (Tonkin), Thomas Robert Alexander Harries Davis, Noel Percival Dowsett, Leo Charles Dunn, Clifton Elliot, Leonard Gordon Ellis, Warren Jack Enticott, Alan Derek Fair, James Hilliard Gane, Theodore MacKay Gray, George Herbert Green, Bevan Bentley Hall, James Henry Douglas Hall, Rodney Chisenhall Hamerton, Nigel Bendyshe Hannay, Bruce Robertson Hay, Jack Mitchell Hay, John Samuel Hopkirk, Gerald Ernest Hoult, John Bruce Howie (MD 1968), Stanley Regnault Hunt, Jean Winsome Isdale (McLean), Victor David Morrow Jacobson, Helen Maxwell Jeans, Peter Vaughan Jenkins, Barry Kahlenberg, Desmond Anderson Kernahan, Paul Kunguviel, Alan Stoddart Lambert, Richard Brooke Langley, Ian James Leitch, Lindsay Robert Lidd, Henry David Livingstone, Jack Marshall MacDonald (MD 1968), Edward Morris McLachlan (MD 1970), Bertrand Anthony McLaughlin, Donald Houston McLean, Cecil William Malthus, Robert George Mathieson, Allan Douglas Muir, Dennis Michael O'Donoghue, Manahi Nitama Paewai, John Cuthbert Parr (Travelling Scholar 1945), John Shirley Phillips, Alfred Philip Poole, Ian Ambury Miller Prior (MD 1954), John David Reid (MD 1951), Francis Knox Rennie, Joan Eleanor Robertson (Walton), William Norrie Rogers, Richard Desmond Rowe (MD 1968), Abdul Habib Sahu Khan, Timothy Savage, Diana Manby Shaw (Mason), Norma Claire Campbell Sheperd, Norma Claire Shepherd (Kent), Douglas Paviour Short, Graeme Purves Gilbert Sim, John Hamlyn Stewart, Phyllis Mary Stockdill, Graham Alexander Tait, Kenneth Ross Tyler, William Leslie Francis Utley, Geoffrey Llewellyn Walton, Patricia Hunter Will (Cook), Juliet Carleton Williams (Harrison), AlistairMacdonald Wilson, Mollie Marmion Wood (Pryor)

1946
John Douglas Allen, Richard John Bogle Anderson, Dengate Robert Armstrong, Archie Stapylton Badger, Brian Gerald Barratt-Boyes (ChM 1962), Donald Maurice Geddes Beasley, James Ainslie Begg, Henry Robert Clifford Benny, Eric Paul Brasted, James Deen Brosnan, Stuart Hawksworth Brown, Alexander George Lyell Bruce, Nancy Serena Geddes Butt, Vincent Bernard Barnabas Conaglen, Oswin John Connor, Charles Bruce Cornish, Richard Lindsay Cotton, Jack Thompson Doyle, Stuart Given Elder, Randal Forbes Elliott, George McKenzie Emery (MD 1960), Maurice White Falloon, Richard Henry Lindo Ferguson, Hugh Alexander Fleming (Travelling Scholar 1946) (MD 1952), Duncan Mowat Forrest, Noel Upton Colston Godfrey, Ross Clifton Gordon, Joseph Francis Hare, Gilbert Charles Robertson Hay, John Charles Hayes, Patrick Terence Llewlyn Hitchings, Campbell Munro Hockin, Anthony Frederick Hunter, Thomas Albert Henry Hurrell, Margaret Mary Isdale (Clayton), John Bruce Jameson, Barrie Russell Jones, Paul Danby Kempthorne, James Kenneth Laing, Derek Alexander Larnder, Ronald Knox McFarlane, Donald Wallace McGregor, Maurice Dominic Match, Reginald Conrad Melsom, Brian Oliver Mulvihill, Oliver Ross Nicholson, Patrick Desmond O'Donoghue, William John Oram, Kenneth Reid Orr, Colin Benjamin Oxner, Derek James Patterson, Gordon Schofield Pettit, Leo Issie Phillips, Brian Errol Pierard, Neil Gorman Prentice, William James Pryor, David Henry Hamilton Pullon, Desmond Alexander Purdie, Peter Allan Restall, Keith Langdon Robertson, David Brockway Rogers, Laurence Hawford Scott, Ralph William Harvey Simmons, Michael Fryer Soper, William Ross Stewart, William Howard Conway Teppett, Robert Francis Thorburn, William Dalrymple Trotter, Norman Derek Walker, Ian Burns Watson, Malcolm Hames Watson, John Bruce Russell Wells, Sheila Frances Wilding, Andrew Cameron Howitt Wilkinson, James Milroy Wilson, Raymond James Wilson, Derek Ernest Nelson Wood, Ngaire Alexander Woods, Rex Earl Wright-St Clair (MD 1971), Stephanie Joy Wylie (Ellis)

1947

Warwick Norman Andrews, Lancelot McCready Armstrong, Alfred Maxwell Bradfield, Lawrence Henry Brett, Timothy John Buckley, Harry Anderson Budd, Gilbert Gillies Burness, Brian Lindsay Campbell, Gordon Melville Campbell, Leslie Raymond Chapman, Jeremiah Alfred Chunn, James Escott Church, Colin Richmond Climie, Graham Lawson Cochrane, Judy Anne David Collins (Wilson), Jack Atkin Coombes, Alister Winston Cooper, Irvine Crawford Cowie, William Bruce Craig, Miroslav Crkbenac, Winifred Mary Croke (Staple), Anthony Morgan Dignan, Neville Walter Dorrington, Philip Gladstone Downey, Ian Gordon Drury, Henry Richard England, Judith Moyra de Vernot Faris (McCann), Herbert George (Barney) Feltham, Geoffrey Noel Ferner, Prudence Anne Fitzgerald (Abrahams), Joseph Maxwell Foreman, Stanley Gibson Fraser, William Alexander Fraser, Joseph Victor Goodman, Geoffrey Donald Gordon, Barbara McLeod Graham (Allen), Peter Court Grayson, Francis Joseph Hall, David Stanley Hanna, Edward Francis Cule Hefford, Denys Heginbotham, Alexander David Hodge, Jack William Hoe, Irwin Colin Isdale, Malcolm Hindmarsh Jameson, Bernard Vance Kyle, Roy Ting Law, Neil Campbell Little, David Wilson Low, Edith Jean Lyness, John Donal McCreanor, Donald Michael Fraser McDonald, Jean Macdonald (Boyd), Colin Hill Macgibbon, John Butler Macgibbon, Evan Robert McKenzie, John Alexander McQueen, Peter Somerville Malthus, Diana Marcia Morton, Keith Gordon Neill, Peter Wynn Nicholson, John Henry Nind, Kevin John O'Connor, John Kenneth Paterson, James Duncan Paton, Max Pearl, Edmund Justin Peterson, Garth George Powell, Herbert Dick Rawson, David Lloyd Rees-Jones, Nancy Margaret Salmond (Saunders), Graeme Calderwood Schofield (MD 1954), Graham Alexander Shanks, Harry Ansell Shaw, Rex Livingston Sinclair, William Wallace Stevens, Henry Stone (MD 1961), Maire Jean Tait (Smith), Robert Browne Tennent, Mary Alice Theodore Tolley, Roy Taylor Wade, Gerard Aloysius Wall, Raymond Arthur Wanty, Clement Arthur Cornelius Wiggins, David Whatton Wilkie, Kenneth James Wilson, Helen Rarity Young (McCreanor) (Travelling Scholar 1947) (MD 1972), Laurence Gowan Young, Sydney Ronald Young

1948

Anthony James Allison, Alan Frank Gordon Anderson, Colin Graeme Anderson, Peter Apthorp, Murray Richard Ashbridge, Donald Ward Beaven, Keith Ellis Berendsen, William Faithfull Bindon, Fay Booth (Young), Helen Kathleen Borg, John Stuart Boyd-Wilson, Lawrence Gordon Brock, Benjamin Buckley, Andrew Kennedy Burt, Thomas Patrick Cannon, Bryan William Christmas (MD 1971), David Simpson Cole, James Douglas Colonna, Vernon Bruce Cook, Roslyn Woodrow Cox (MD 1955), Arthur Robinson Craig, James Gordon Craig, Robert John Croke, John Alexander Cunninghame, Barbara Farnsworth Cupit (Heslop) (MD 1954), Joseph William Davies, Donald Joseph Dobson, Ronald Basil Dorofaeff, Keith Douglas Drayton, Frank Roderick Duncanson, Robert Gordon Dykes, Ronald Rutherford Elvidge, William Avison Evans, Keith McDowell Ewen, Alexander Fergus Ferguson, Marianne Fillenz, Peter Fleischl, Kenneth Hugo Friedlander, John Campbell Gillman, Gavin Lawrence Glasgow, John Edwin Goodyear, Maxine Winslow Gray (Wanty), Robert Graham Gudex, Mary Hanafin (Coldham), Harold McLean Harding, Robert Boyd Hardy, Denis Brian Hewat, Herbert John Hall Hiddlestone (MD 1954), Geoffrey Warren Holland, Keith Edward Holmes, Selwyn Howard Hope, Alan Bernard Howard Howes, Elaine Valerie Hulse (Osmond), John Desmond Hunter (Travelling Scholar 1948) (MD 1962), Leonard Stanley James, Eadmund Bede Jenner, Bryan George Jew, Tame Ngahiwi Kawe, William Lempfert Kenealy (MD 1962), Alexander Vincent Kurta, Paul Kurzweil, Charles Edward Laverty, Owen Lawrence, Graham Collingwood Liggins, David Alexander John Luke, Henry Robert McCoy,

Ellison James McInnes, Millen Gordon MacKay, Malcolm Robert McLean (MD 1957), John Alexander McLeod, Thomas Ernest George Mark, Andrew Richmond Martin, William Dickson Meldrum, Murray Neale Menzies, Thomas William Milliken, Rachel Monk, Diana Montgomery (Edwards), Rina Winifred Moore (nee Ropiha), Alan Grenfell Morgan, Arthur Jefferson Moss, Paul Frederick Mountfort, Kenneth Wyatt Newell, Robert Anthony Sinclair Ongley, David Duncan Pottinger, John Richard Presland, Frank Mitchell Ramsay, John Archdall Raymond, Peter William Richmond, Donald Malcolm Rickard, Shirley Blyth Robertson, Leonard Richard Robinson (MD 1960), Ian Douglas Ronayne, Noel Roydhouse (Ch.M. 1970), Ian Schneideman, Brian Walter Scott, Alan Ashley Skinner, Olga Dorothea Skousgaard (Batt), David Ross Smith, Zoe Petronella Smuts-Kennedy (During), Peter Cameron Stichbury, Arthur Richard Stone, Peter Desmond Swinburn (MD 1957), Robert Charles Taylor, Ronald Ernest Tingey, Linnie Bryant Tombleson (Calvert), Dorothy Field Usher (Potter), Geoffrey Charles White Maclaren Wallis, Sydney Rae West, Richard Anthony Drumond Wigley, Carl Shiley Willis, George John Alexander Wilson, Patricia Wilson (MacKay), Bruce Armstrong Worley, Noel Raymond Young

1949

Duncan Dartrey Adams (MD 1962), Ruth Evelyn Adams (Mitchell) (MD 1968), William Ward Akroyd, Margaret Shirley Andrews (Tennent), John Apthorp, John Desmond Baeyertz, Stuart Alexander Ballantyne, June Barclay, Thelma Constance Becroft, Charles Humphrey Belton, Stephen George Bishop, Jack Boston, Nevill Hamilton Brooke, Beverley Jean Brown (Luke), David Byron Brown, John Joseph Brunt, Ransford George Kerr de Castro, David Barry Chrisp, Noeline Clemens (Burn), Rosemary Agatha Clendon (Faull), Peter Stowell Cook, David John Cross, Barry Mitchell Dallas, Noel Thomas Dalton (MD 1968), Desmond Stewart Peter Dickson, Peter James Dowsett, Hubert Francis Drake, Keith Edward Debney Eyre (MD 1957), Solomon Faine (MD 1959), Geoffrey Elliot Fairbrother, James Patrick Beaumont Fitzgerald (ChM 1966), Michael James Foley, Deryck Joseph Austin Gallagher, Kenneth Miller Galloway, John William Gerald Gibb, Earle Craig Neil Gray, Malcolm Bryce Gunn, Peter Hall, Ivan Harper, Thomas Guy Hawley, John Herbert Heslop (ChM 1959), John Joseph Horan, Richard William Hornabrook, Stella Lindsay Horwell (Johnstone), Beresford Wallace Houghton-Allen, Milton Frank Howes, Beryl Overton Howie, Yue Leonard Jackson, Ivan John Jeffery, Graeme Vaughan Jenkins, Oliver Alexander Johnstone, Owen John Lewis (MD 1959), Charles Marshall Luke, Ronald Diarmid MacDiarmid, Campbell Heywood MacLaurin, Denis Thorpe Mathews, Robert Mervyn Mitchell (Travelling Scholar 1949) (ChM 1957), Kenneth Noel Nicholas, John Terence O'Brien (MD 1959), William Grattan O'Connell, Thomas Vianney O'Donnell (MD 1959), Charles Eric Parr, Elman William Poole, Donald David Porter, Noel Travers Potter, George Stuart Purvis, Humphrey Barton Rainey, Jason Charles Prier Reade, Jack Reuben Salas, James Miller Saunders, Edwin Sayes, Alwyn James Seeley, Leon Isaac Shenken, Frederick Bernard Sill, Dudley Ian Moffett Sinclair, Ian Henry Westbrooke Squires, David Sturman (MD 1976), Roderick Duncan Suckling, Kenneth Edgeworth Ussher, George Alexander Waddell, Dion Wilson Warren, Henry Keith Watt, John Brian Wells, Henry Jeffray Weston, Norman Graham Wimsett, David Govett Romaine Wright, Geoffrey Wynne-Jones, Gordon Hastings Young

1950

Philip Maxwell Allingham, Bernard William Andrews, Sydney Ronald Arthur Ayling, Jane Aylward (Munro), William Burleigh Barlow, Brian Jonathan Barrett, Arthur Wynyard Beasley, Donald Henry Ashdown Blackley, Kathleen Elsie Brown (Wake), Mary Litster Burnet (O'Halloran), Craig Donald Burrell, Cyril Gavin Burt, Thomas Patrick Casey (MD 1965),

William Edward Chisholm, Derek Erle Hislop Clarke, Harold Collinson, Keitha Corlett (Farmer), Stephen John Hindmarsh Cox, Henry George Crofts, Kenneth Richard Dalley, Frank Harman Davie, Frederick Bernard Desmond, Brian Harrison Doherty, Fritz Emmanuel Dreifuss, Malcolm Noel Ellis, Shirley Elizabeth Entrican, Rolfe Baxter Finn, Henry William Joseph Fox, John David Frankish, Robert Donald Fraser, Rainsford Rhodes Freeman, James Francis Gwynne (MD 1958), David Russell Hay (MD 1960), Thomas Lonnen Hayes, William Roy Holmes, Noel Keith Honey, Michael Fitzherbert Horrocks, Ronald Gordon Howes, John Leslie Hunt, Robert Hunt, Miles Wilson Hursthouse, Henry Kaye Ibbertson, Griffith Jones, Susi Ruth Levinsohn (Levene), Thomas Christie Macbeth Lonie, Allan William McArthur, Selwyn Roy McCabe, James Edmond McCoy, William Arthur McIndoe, Malcolm McKellar (MD 1964), Desmond Alexander McQuillan, Hugh Marwick, William Rex Morris (MD 1959), Terence Victor Nelson, John Derek Kingsley North (Rhodes Scholar 1950), Walter John O'Halloran, Ian Raymond Alvon Overton, Derek John Perry (MD 1960), Edward George Perry, William Owen Sawtell Phillipps, Lindsay William Poole, Owen Fordham Prior, Howard Desmond Prisk, Alan William Roberts, David William Acton Rodwell, Margaret Elizabeth Rudd (Coop), James Fraser Ryan, Helen Florence Salkeld (Wood), John William Saunders (Travelling Scholar 1950), Keith Richards Simcock, John Desmond Sinclair (MD 1955), Charles Notley Sorrell, Gerald Cedric Staniland, Harold Trevor Staub, David Johnston Stephen, John Joseph Sullivan, Nicholas Theodore Taptiklis, Nils Carl Theilman, Ernest James Thompson, John Joseph Valentine, Arthur Milton Oliver Veale, Ernst Karl Willi Wilzek, Charles Wong, John Wilkinson Wray

1951

Ronald Thomas Hardy Adlam, Deirdre Morag Airey, John Finlay Aitken, Alfred Robert Anderson, Charles Peter Anyon, Alan George Austin, Lancelot Frederick Austin, Robert Donald Barclay, Ian William Barrowclough, Douglas Barrie Berryman, Henry Charles Bethune (MD 1961), Trevor Harold Bierre, Stanley De Bonnaire, John Brian Booth, Norman Lewis Sidney Bourchier, William Alston Bovaird Brabazon, Herbert Arnold Brant, Richard Henry Burrell, Alastair Fleet Burry (MD 1956), Leonard Raymond Butterfield, Peter Frederick Caldwell, Peter Frederick Calvert, Stuart Maxwell Cameron, Vincent Ward Davidson Campbell, Ronald John Cantwell, Ivan Cher, William Norman Clay, Reginald Bruce Conyngham, Roger Hector Culpan, Douglas Herbert Cummack, Richard Dyer von Dadelszen, Roy Edward William Darby, John Michael Davis, Athol James Duke, Bernard Leslie Dunn, Peter William Dykes, Hugh Alexander Eaton, JohnJoseph Enwright, Denis Wordsworth Feeney, Colin Robert Fenton, Ashton John Fitchett, Sydney Allen Fitzgerald, Patricia Elizabeth Gardner, Arthur David Gillman, James Ritchie Gilmour, Maxwell George Goodey, Graham Rothwell Gordon, Charlton Morpeth Greig, Crellin Balfour Grieve-Dingwall, Meredyth Colston Gunn (Wilson), John Douglas Guy, Brian George Hay, James Rudd Hay, Ronald Hamilton Hayward, Douglas Jonathan Hibbs, George Condor Hitchcock (MD 1968), Neville William Hogg, Roy Frederick Hough, Tremayne Everard Hardy Hunt, Bruce Irving Hunter, Gordon Clifford Jacobsen, Ann Priscilla Jarvis (McKinnon), Walter James Jarvis, Lloyd Henry Johns, Anthony Lloyd Johnston, Graham Frank Joplin, Marjorie Joyce King (Seymour), Brian William Alfred Leeming, Cyril Levene (MD 1961), Arthur William Lewis, Hubert Douglas John Lovell-Smith, John Bird Lovell-Smith, Hamish Heathcote McCrostie, David Malcolm McIlroy, Ian Noble Radcliffe McKay, David Scott McKenzie, Kenneth Christopher Bruce MacKenzie, Shona McLeod (Hodgson), Ernest David Lindsay Marsden, Isidore Adair Marsden, Alan Henderson Meikleham, Wilbur Harry Mercer, Colin Marcus Miln, James Frederick Moodie, Jane Munro (Harrison), Thomas William Murray, Max Dickson Nash, Eric

Russell Overton, Alan Howard Paul, Douglas Gordon Potts (MD 1960), James Graham Power, Norman Jack Prichard, Desmond Maurice Vincent Rea, Laurence Ian Rhodes, William Worsley Richardson, Teras Patricia Riordan, Geoffrey Lawson Rollo, Augustin Anton Schiessel, Brian Alexander Scobie (MD 1972), Frederick Thomas Shannon, Marie Margaret Simpson, Ralph Stephen Wallis Skinner, Allan Gibson Smith, Lawrence James Smith, William James Smith, Brian Douglas Stringer, Christopher Morgan Stubbs (Travelling Scholar 1951), Stephen Watson Taylor, Eric Edgar Tilson, John Douglas Todd, Leonard Lawrence Treadgold, Arthur Neil Turnbull, Leo James Walker, James Graeme Walkinshaw, Milton Walters, William Edward Walton, William Maxwell Wearne, William Kerr Webster, Graham Arnold West, John Hunter Williams, Douglas Leonard Williamson, Ian Irvine Wilson, Raymond Victor James Windsor, Margaret Winn Wray (Hoodless; Guthrie), Bertram Herries Young, Marjorie Rose Young

1952

Ian Aarons (MD 1968), Alan Robert Anderson, Alan Gibson Baird, Ronald Thomas Ewen Baker, David Maxwell O'Neill Becroft (MD 1962), Edith Ruth Blumenthal (Black), Kelvin Reid Bremner, Robert John Wilson Buick, David Cranleigh Thomson Bush, Richard Thomson Bush, Graeme Dickinson Desmond Cable, Brian James Caldwell, Alan Donaldson Cameron, Ian Kenneth Campbell, Joan Dorothy Anne Casserley, Douglas Harold Coop, Lionel Lingwood David Cordery, Derek James Crawford, John Daniel Crowley, Robert Morrison Davie, Michael de la Cour Davies, Alan Arthur Dawson, John Douglas Denford, Tenick Carr Dennison, Ernest Raymond Dowden, Peter Calder Durward, Athol John Erenstrom, Donald Wakefield Eyre-Walker, Muriel Blanche Elizabeth Berney Falcon (Mason), Edwin Robert Fawcett, Peter Hugo Friedlander, Bruce Robert Noel Golden, Georg Graetzer, Charles Desmond Hall, Errol Everard Hannah, James Vincent Hodge (MD 1959), Arthur Welton Hogg, William Barrie Jackson (MD 1958), Graham Harry Jeffries (Rhodes Scholar 1952), Gavin Stewart McLaren Kellaway (MD 1960), Patrick Robert Kelleher, Edward Hibell Kerkin, Keith Edward Kibblewhite, Peter Graham Lindsay, Murray Joseph Angland McDonald, Ray McKenzie, Brian Philip MacLaurin (MD 1971), Peter Elder McNab, Gilpin Marryatt, John Graham Masterson, Patrick John Molloy, William Denis Moloney, Graham John Tarr Moore, Rodney Robert Winston Morrison, Whitley Francis Otway, Renzi George Palmer, Roderick Sheppard Rowe, George Herbert Sanders, John Heriot Seddon, Edward Petrie Shilton, William Copland Shirer, Thomas Alexander Bain Sinclair, Mary Lillian David Skinner, William Sprott, Leslie Credis Stewart (Travelling Scholar 1952), Thomas Bertram Humphrey Strain, James Calvert Uren Tait, Robert Cecil Tait, Graham Denis Tills, Kenneth John Urwin, Roger Neale Wallis, Edward Cameron Watson, Harry George Watts, Selwyn James Smith Webb, Leon Trevor Williams,Montague Edward Williams, Wilfred Travis Wilson, Leopold Otto Winter, Desmond John Woods, Margaret Woods, William Robert Young

1953

Richard Thomas Aldridge, Roger Clement Bartley, Edward Bassett, Oliver Bowes Bond, Bernard James Bowden, Alister George Douglas Bowron, Phyllis Muriel Brass, James MacAlister Bremner, John Ernest Butt, Neil Callahan, Alan Herbert Caselberg, Philip Louis Cassin, David Thomas Clouston, Gregory Bede Conlon, Colleen Anne Conyngham (Hall), Brian Winfield Cook, Leo Joseph Cooney, Michael Henderson Cooper, Dawson Albert Cotton, James Blackett Cotton, John Piercy Coutts, Margot Ronson Craw (Gardner), Adrienne Lorraine Croucher (Gibson), Peter Miller Dennis, Alistair David Dick, Geoffrey William Dodd, Alan Ellis Dugdale (MD 1962), Graeme Ross Duncan, Jack William Edgar Eton, Daniel William Fairclough, Joan Jessep Fitchett

(Kay; Presland), William George Flux, Anthony Francis Foley, Rex Thomas Garlick, Peter Leon Gibson, David Henry Ewart Gillingham, Bryce Donald Glennie, Harold Haydon Gray, Bruce William Griffith, George Grundy, John Hall, John Hall-Jones, Barry Robin Hardwick-Smith, Bernard Edmund Heine, Graeme David Henderson, Eva Ruth Hersch (Seelye), Klaus Guenter Heymann, David Andrew Hogg, Garth Grierson Holdaway, Helen Margaret Irwin Hunt (Liley), Robert Russell Hunter, Beverley John Herbert Insull, Robin Orlando Hamilton Irvine (MD 1958), Clara Elizabeth Jackson (Rawley), Graham Lincoln Jackson, James Lewis Jardine, Ronald Geoffrey Kay, Geoffrey Bruce Kiddle, Marcus Louis Langley, Richard George Lawrence, Ernest Peter Lippa, Ronald Derry Lockhart, John Ludbrook (Travelling Scholar 1953) (ChM 1961) (MD 1973), Alistair Macaskill MacLeod, Cathel Alexander MacLeod, Laurence Allan Malcolm (MD 1969), Robert Ross Manning, Rodger Heath Maxwell, Kendall Maurice Mayo, George Peter Mellor, Ramon Richard Menendez, Gordon Walter Mills, Clive Robert Moody, Ross Osborne Moore, David Hope Mowbray, Victor Blythe Newman, William Henry Olds, Graeme Henley Overton, William Bruce Paton, Mary Max Patrick, Neil Andrew Philip, Hugh Bradbury Pratt, John Sinclair Rea, Keith Woodham Ridings, Thomas John Bruce Ritchie, Brian Robertson, Selma Roniger-Hahn, Richard Peter Gorton Rothwell, Dorian Michael Saker, Lawrence Sanson, Graeme Ralph Sharp, Dharam Singh, Leslie Errol Spencer, Raymond Harry Spitz, Kathleen Rose Standage, Russel Ivan Steel, Leslie Herbert Stevens, Sione Tapa, John Heywood Taylor, Harold Thomas, James Duncan Forrester Thomson, Brian Ernest Tomlinson, Bruce Carncross Turnbull, Douglas Peter Wallace, Reginald Terence Ward, Archibald Westgate, Thomas Shailer Weston, Senga Florence Whittingham, Henry James G. Whyte, John Cyprian Phipps Williams, Woodrow Gilbert Wilson, Liam Hugh Wright

1954

Irene Abrahamson (Valentine), Neil Albert Algar, Philip Middleton Barham, Elizabeth Beauchamp (Naylor), John Morrison Bird, Peter Walter Theodore Brandt, John Philip Broad, William David Bruce, Hugh Cameron Burry, Hugh Cameron Butel, Robert Reid Cameron, Selwyn James Carson, Richard Edward Carter, Alan Maxwell Chirnside, Robin Macfarlane Chrisp, Robert Harry Kenrick Christie, Patricia Ann Coates (Weston), Jack Murray Costello, James Robin Musgrave Davidson, Peter George Reed Dawe, William Edward Dervan, James Anthony Dick, Lloyd Allister Drake, Hamish Robert Earl, John David Earwaker, Ian Harold Ellerm, Leo Asher Faigan, Ross Alexander Fairgray, Ian Calderwood Fleming, George Douglas Smith Forster, Warren Neil Cranston Fraser, Trevor Gebbie, Robin Danby Gibson, Patrick Francis Hunter Giles, Geoffrey Maitland Gray, Arthur Henry Hackett, Victor Desmond Hadlow, Ronald James Hamer, Philip David Harkness, Margaret Mirriam Hart (Belton), Donald Urquhart Hay, George Stanley Derek Heather, Colin Holloway Hooker, Cedric Howard Hoskins, Kathleen Audrey Johnstone (Bradford), Denis Miles King, Frank William Kwok, Murray Alexander Lamb, Peter Richard Lamb, George Richard Laurenson, Gavin Grant Liddell, Albert William Liley (Travelling Scholar 1954), Evelyn Belle Lind, Peter John Little, John Edward Ross Lorimer, Murray James Loughlin, Ray Richard Otto Lycette (MD 1962), Alan Robert McKenzie, James Richard Colin MacLaurin, Peter Mann Meffan, James Armour Monro, Gerald Louis Morris, Donald James Mulheron, Brian Robertson Neill, William Ngan Kee, Malcolm John Nicolson, Kenneth Alfred Kingsley North (Rhodes Scholar 1954), Gerald Jack Ogg, Natalia Pachomov (Venetz), Peter Douglas Pedlow, Wayne Valentine Petch, James Lanyon Poor, John Leslie Derwentwater Radcliffe, Frank Purvis Rawley, Murray Spencer Robertson, Robin Anthony Roche, John McKenzie Ross, Kevin Fitzmaurice Ross, Robin Stuart Charters Scoular, Richard John Seddon, Michael Elliott Shackleton,

Robert Leslie Shannon, Peter Floyd Sheppard, Duncan Harry James Shine, Margaret Clare Sidey (Gibberd), Allan James Kings Simmance, Graeme Ballantyne Smaill, Dennis Bernard Spackman, Trevor Charles Svensen, Peter Wilfred Tapsell, Katharine Helen Campbell Thomson (Bowden), Blair Lawrence Jervis Treadwell, John Lewis Veale, Alfred James Vincent, John Evens Weblin, Robert Cecil Bruce Webster, Bernard Welford, Charles Francis Whittington, Howie Keith Forbes Wilson, Clarence Mong Wong, Mohammed Yusuff; MD: Joy Krishna Mohanty

1955

John Philip Andrew, Thomas Leslie Francis Averill, Heather Baillie (Thomson), Mercia Annette Barnes, Brian Maurice Barrett, Patricia Bassett, Edward Fletcher Battersby, Warwick Francis Bennett, Michael Nathaniel Berry (MD 1961), William Henley Bird, Bronwen Eileen Broomfield (Robinson), Joseph John Brownlee, John Cairney, Ronald Douglas Cameron, Graeme Douglas Campbell, Richard Arthur Cartwright, John Atherton Cashmore, Jack Chuen Chin, Charlotte Lilian Christie (Robertson), Richard Campbell Clark, Basil Frank Clarke, Barry Malcolm Colls, John Axford Kenneth Commons, Robert Bruce Cook, Lawrence Alan Day, Constance Marguerita Dennehy, Graeme Pat Duffy, Leslie Morgan Dugdale (MD 1966), Nigel Onslow Eastgate, Henry John Espiner, Thomas Farrar, Anthony James Francis, Denis Hugo Friedlander, Gerrit Carel Geel, Robert James Golding, Robert George Batthews Graham, Albert Green, Roger Gardner Greenhough, Kenneth Newman Haldane, Ian Sinclair Hamilton, Lawrence Herbert Hansen, Murray Selwyn Haslett, Gwenyth Marie Hookings (Allison), Robert Hughes, Sidney John Ivil, Ivor Francis Joseph, John Patrick Kelly, Margaret Iris King (Meffan), Derek Heathcote Livingston, Arthur Irwin Logan, James Duncan Campbell Macdiarmid, Cathryn Anne McIver (Christie), Keith Grace McKenzie, William Dacre McKenzie, Brian Thomas McMahon, John Edward Keith McNaughton, Marc Albert Matsas, Patricia Claire Meikle (Cairney), Kenneth Norman Paul Mickleson, Clarice Lora Moore (Main), Roderick Bruce Ian Morrison (MD 1960), Roderick Thomas Muirhead, Stanislaw Jozef Muller, John Panton Musgrove, Ram Narayan, Donald Craig Neilson, Jules Joseph Armand Nihotte, Robin MacKenzie Norris, John Joseph O'Hagan, Brian Eden Oldham, Desmond Oswald Oliver, David George Palmer (Travelling Scholar 1955) (MD 1961), William Frederick Parkes, Stanley William Parkinson, Margaret Dawn Parsonage (Maxwell), Chunilal Madhiv Patel, John Gwyther Richards, Hamish MacLeod Roake, Anthony St John, Philip John Scott, Ernest Lloyd Sear, Bryan Lee William Seymour, Gordon Raymond Joseph Sheehan, Cleveland Ross Sheppard, Earle James Cecil Shine, Donald Carrick Simpson, Harold Lawrence McIntyre Smith, Douglas William Stewart, Alison Myra Tarrant (Gaitonde), Tania Roberta Tarulevicz (Gunn), Allan John Taylor (Travelling Scholar 1955), David Emil Mynott Taylor, Richard James Graham Thomson, William James Treadwell, William Nichol Tucker, Kenneth Robert Ullrich, Peter van Praagh, David Russell Wallace, John Scott Werry (MD 1975), Charles Miles Williamson, David Gordon Wilson

1956

John Duncan Abernethy, Athol Maurice Abrahams, Brian Fitzgerald Allen, John Gavin Andrews (MD 1965), Noel Richard Godfrey Badham, John Campbell Barrett, Graham Beale, Francis Rayner Bernard, Alistair Duncan Bird, John Bartlett Blennerhassett, Elizabeth Anne Bowie, Carleton Murray Bullivant, Alan Riddle Burnet, David Egerton Caughey, David Crosby Chatterton, Alan Maxwell Clarke (ChM 1969), James Ivor Clayton, Elizabeth Mary Corbett (Irvine), Pamela Mary Dawe (McGruer), Owen William Lee Dine, Arthur Wong Doo, Trevor Watson Doouss (ChM 1970), Ronald William Ensor, Brian George Henley Enticott, Royce Ormond Farrelly,

Norman Walden Fitzgerald (MD 1961), Thomas Richardson Fogg, Bruce Arthur Ford, Desmond Wilson Frengley, Robin George Gee, William Ivan Glass, Norman Garrick Graham, David Templeton Gray, Kenneth Allen Handcock, Brian Robert James Harris, Thomas Connell Henshall, Brian Francis Heyward, Frederick Cossom Hollows, Ross Nisbet Howie, Donald Robert Ingram, Clifford Tasman Jones, Judith Karaitiana (Hall), Bruce Albert Kaye, James Thomas Kearney, Peter Knowles-Smith, Geoffrey Fyffe Lamb, Phillip William Bruce Lane, On Kit Law, Stanley Peter Lay, Peter Noel Leslie, John Garland Lester, Kendal Graeme Lewis, Annie Low (Moy), David Whibley Ludbrook, Ian William McDougall, John McKay, Ian Sword MacKenzie, John Kirk McKenzie (MD 1963), Munro Bruce MacKereth (MD 1973), Ngaire Margaret McKerrow (Walsh) (MD 1963), Thomas Francis Mackie, Neil Francis McLeod, Ian Alan McPhail, Raymond John Patrick Meehan, James Webster Mewett, Michael Robert Miles, Robert Frank Moginie, John Bentham Morris, John Graham Mortimer, Ian Stuart O'Connor, Eugene Stern Paykel (MD 1970), Graham Albert Pope, Heemi Parore Te Awha Rankin, Hendry Robertson, Philip Waldo Robinson, David William Sabiston, Arthur Kelvin Saxton, David John Scott, Thomas Derisley Stuart Seddon, Colin Stanley Smith, John Huston Stewart, Ralph David Huston Stewart (Travelling Scholar 1956) (MD 1968), Jerzy Surynt, William Ashley Symmans, Anthony Robert Taylor, Alfred Campbell Trousdale, Henry Lum King Wah, Paul Bernard Walmsley, Michael Anthony Valintine Watson, Henry Selwyn Wilcox

1957
Ian Alan George Abernethy, William Nelson Adams Smith (MD 1970), Robert William Reid Archibald, Warren Iver Austad, Peter Dean Bamford, Brian Manson Barraclough (MD 1986), John Trevor Barrett, Lewis Rene Beale, Allan Roy Bean, Jocelyn Valerie Bell (Hay), Felix Alexander Biland, David Andrew Bremner, John Gordon Buchanan, John Burd Carman, James Francis Carter, Richard Terry Maidstone Caseley, Maurice Kiran Chandulal, Joan Shirley Chapple, Sydney Tasman Choy, Lyndon Van Christie, Patricia Mary Clarkson, Simme Coggin, Colin Leithead Crawford, Allan Roy Deed, Peter St John Dignan, Peter Brian Doak, Malcolm Gordon Dunshea, Ellis Ross Earnshaw, Eric Arnold Espiner (MD 1964), Peter Jones Eynon, Donald Wallace Farquhar, Robert Murray Fergusson, Cressy William Free, Ian Sills Everard Gibbons, Irwin Hunter Hanan, Edward Litton Telford Harding, Lesley Kathleen Harries (Doak), George Hing, Michael David Henry Holdaway, Paul Brendan Jenner, Graeme Roland Jensen, Brian Lexington Jones, Alan Ronald Kerr, Graeme Douglas Kerr, Trevor Richard King, Gordon Murray Kirk, David Robert Laing, Murray Railley Laird, Susanna Renate Lemchen (Williams), Brian John McConville, John Charles MacCormick, William Ian McDonald, John McIlwaine, John Scott MacLaurin, Hubert Edward McMillan, Leonard Mark Ante Marinovich, John Nicholas Mein, Christopher John Mercer, Ronald James Methven, Peter James Middleton (MD 1963), David Fairfax Minnitt, Paul Alexander Monro, Raymond George Ross Moon, Gordon Ian Nicholson, Roger Valentine Nicoll, Kevin Patrick O'Brien, Desmond Edward Parfoot, Richard Keith Pears, Neil Richard Perrett, Elizabeth Margaret Rich, Kevin Patrick Sanders, Edwin Fong Sang, John Armstrong Searle, James Henry Weir Short, Judith Cherry Smith (Wardill) (MD 1967), Clive Bryan Stanley Stephenson, Michael John Tait, John David de Villiers Taylor, Leonard James Thompson, Ernest Hugh Thomson, David James Vey, Hendrika Jacoba Waal-Manning (MD 1982), Roger Archibald Wilkinson, William Patrick Williams, Jennifer Colston Wilson, Gerald Wong, Paul Bowah Wong

1958
Donald Russell Aickin, Douglas Graham Allan, Donald Edward Allen, Helen Beaumont Angus, Athol Bruce Arthur,

John Richard Barnett, Arthur Leslie Batt, Arthur David Beck (ChM 1970), Murray John Bishop, Pamela Brown (Jones), Patricia Marie Buckfield (MD 1979), James Burkinshaw, David Gordon Campbell, George Shannon Chisholm, Hugh James Clarkson, James Ambrose Collins, Harold Valentine Coop, Richard Anthony Cox, John Howard Exton (MD 1984), Ian David Fleming, Peter Ronald Garrod (Travelling Scholar 1958), John Michael Gibbs (MD 1978), Annetta Elsie Alexandra Gillies, Gerard John Green, Ian Strachan Greig, Cameron Ross Gribben, Herbert Graham Hall, Jack Wilfred Hamer, James Clarke Hanan, Gordon James Harris, Robert Graham Hay, John Hayward Henderson, Charles McKinnon Holmes, Cornelis Hoogland, John Edwin Horton, Peter Geoffrey Hurst, Ailao Imo, John Rex Inder, Alexander Keith Jeffery (ChM 1975), Frederick Owen Jensen, John Peter Kania, Neil Hylton Le Grice, Norman Harrison Leslie, Donald Wallace Liddell, John Francis McCafferty, Donald MacCulloch, John Bruce McCully, Donald MacDonald, Alexander Roy McGiven (MD 1963), Henry Ralph McKinlay, Bruce McLean, Graham Michael McLeod, Ian Gordon McPherson, Kenneth Eric Webley Melvin, Laughton Eric Martyn Miles (MD 1966), John Zinzan Montgomerie, Allen Martin Moore, John Dermot Mora, Grenville Ross Mosley, Maurice Cyril Nathan, John Murray Neutze (MD 1968), Anthony John Newson, William Fredrick Oakley, Philip Harry Palmer, Vallabh Unka Patel, Alan Thomas Perry Patterson, William John Pattison, Anthony David Perrett (MD 1968), James Graham Perry, John Desmond Pollard, Martin Pollock, Peter Ian Clarkson Rennie (MD 1970), Maxwell Duers James Robertson, Ross Saunders, Andrew Sharard (MD 1969), Kum Cheung Shum, Helen Maud Simpson (Bichan), Alec Jardine Sinclair, Vivian Francis Sorrell, Patrick Hugh Spencer, Bede Harold Squire, John Steiner, Hugh Edward George Stevens, Geoffrey James Stokes, Johannes Swier, Gabriel David Tetro, David Erskine Tolhurst, David Wilson Virtue, David Charles Warnock, Gerrit Jan Michel Westerink, Tristram Peter Dennitts Willcox, Leslie Wong Shee, Allen Edward Madfield Zohrab, George Zwonnikoff

1959
Trevor Malvin Agnew, Elizabeth Aitken (Ramage), Donald Melville Angus, Gerald Lane Batchelor, Melvin Athol Brieseman, Barry Jeffery Bruns, Francis Fabian Bryant, David Stanley Campion (MD 1966), Barry Ronald Cant, Robin Wayne Carrell, John Page Chambers, Kathleen Mary Christian (Lawther), Russell Evan Heath Comber, Herbert Bramwell Cook, Ashwin Alexander Corbett, Raymond Bodley Cossham, David Morris Coulter, Lindsay Howard Couper, Robert Stanley Craven, Rosalie Davida-Horvath, Lanktree John Humphrey Davies, Edwin Francis Dempsey, Ernest George Dominikovich, Brian Stewart Douglas, Michael Nansen Eade, Morgan Francis Fahey, Brian James Francis, James Dermot Frengley, Ian Bruce Fulton, Neville Henry Fursdon, Jean Fyfe (Bryant), Charles Murray Goodall (MD 1964), Bryan George Hardie Boys, Denis Astley Harding, Roy Douglas Harris, John Goldie Hawkes, Viola Cornelia Heine (Palmer), Peter Barrie Herdson (Travelling Scholar 1959), Rodger William Hilliker, Jeremy Dashwood Phelps Hopkins, Braida Merle Hopper, Csaba Imre Gyorgy Horvath, Rexley Blake Hunton, Basil Rockliff Hutchinson, Trevor Stephen Jaquiery, William Angus Johnston, David Thomas Kelly, Leonard Robert Kitson, Andrew David Eric Knight, Brian Murray Laugesen, Gam Poi Lee, John Reginald Little (MD 1994), David Alistair Lonie, William Luey, Brian Charles McCluskey, Janice Marion McKay (McConville), Bruce Stuart McMillan, Rosalie Helen McPherson (Sneyd), Richard Freeman Mark, Frederick Samuel Martin, Peter Walton Martin, Malcolm Ross Mowat, Kenneth John Newton, James Ng, Edwin Dominick O'Donnell, Maurice Jack Orpin, Robert Douglas Peter, Michael Ambrose Martin Rea, Linsell Donald Richards, Ralph Charles Riseley, John Richard Roberts, George Barrie Scholes, George Ansley Schuster, David Gordon Seay, Colin Arthur Shanks (MD 1975),

Michael Joseph Simcock, Duncan Jules Simon, Colin Charles Skelton, Roger Morton Ridley Smith, John Graham Trevellyan Sneyd, John Harrison Spencer, Andrew Carlyle Stenhouse (MD 1968), Ronald Graham Stephens, Gilbert Barrie Tait, John Chalmers Thomson, Paul Donald GriffithsWilson, Michael Wise, Thomas Richard Young

1960

Edwin Paterson Arnold, Glenys Patricia Arthur (nee Smart), John Arthur Avery, John Ronald Ayers, Peter Harold Bannister, David Townson Bathgate, Graham Berman, Barrie Graeme Bird, David Andrew Blaiklock, Alastair Roland Brown, George Earle Dunlop Brown, Elizabeth Waugh Burns (Berry) (MD 1972), Bernard Ruane Casey, Roger McKenzie Chambers, Sun Onn Chin, Jonathan Cohen, Richard Selwyn Croxson, Marcus Oliver Dill-Macky, Richard Allen Donald (MD 1966), Paul Lydon Dowd, Desmond Dowse, Ronald Newman Easthope, Michael John Paul Fogarty, Raymond Fong, Eric Raymond Foster, Clive Lindsay Francis, Miriam Frank, Jack Fraser, David Fung, Peter William Gage, Michele Delahaye Goddard, Peter James Gormly, Peter Wynne Grant, Bruce Peter Milburn Hamilton, James Edmund Herrick Hefford, Elizabeth Ann Hodge (Hewitt), William Peter Holloway, David A'Court Horton, Patricia Houghton (Wood), Philip Houghton, John Campbell Kennedy, Michael McKenzie Kerr, Anthony Raymond Kirk, Julian Alastair Kirk, Alison Jean Knox (Sommerville), Ian Edward Langbein, Selwyn Robert Leeks, Isla Ellen Lonie (Frew), John Milne Loughlin, Heather Macallan (Leslie), Peter John McCleave, Kenneth Blair McCredie, Graeme Marlow MacDonald, Kantha Madhavji (Soni), John Trevor Matthews, Thomas Duthie Mills, James Cleveland Moore, Roger James Morrison, Leon Raymond Mortensen, Brian James Muir, Warren John Richard Muirhead, Michael James Murdoch, Grenfell Bertram Louis Parker, Kanoo Dayal Nana Patel, Raman Unka Patel, Peter Samuel Perry, Hew Crichton Prain, Thomas Desmond Prendergast, Robert Greig Pringle, Judith Anne Radcliffe (Barfoot), Colin Peter Reece, Richard Greig Reed (MD 1978), Norma Jean Restieaux (MD 1973), Guy David Sarfati, John Licco Sarfati, Alister James Scott (Travelling Scholar 1960), Rachel Emily Senn (Maule), Peter Mills Shaw, David Colquhoun Shove, Jonathan Peter Simcock, Bhawar Singh, Ailsa Mary Smith (Morrison-Galt), John Graeme Speirs, Donald James du Temple, Brian Curtis Thomson, Bernard Treister, Bryan John Trenwith, William David Troughton, Graham Stanley Tucker, Edgar Dunstan Turner, Elaine Mary Tutchen, Noeline Lillian Beatrice Walker (Carrington), Martin Russell Wallace, Joseph Williams, Earle William Wilson, Roma Agnes Wilson, Po Hing Wong, David Graeme Woodfield, Murray Edward Wyatt, Ronald George Young

1961

Trevor Charles Adams, John Sutcliffe Allan, John Verrall Allison (Travelling Scholar 1961), Edward David Anderson, Michael Richard Andress, Patrick Jerome Beehan, Boyd Lovell Blake, Ross Wilson Blue, Ian Douglas Brown, Thomas Pendreigh Brown, Louis John Harrison Butterfield, Sun Sung Chau, Wei Nien Cheng, Vallabh Chunilal, Geoffrey Bolton Clarke, James Farquhar Cleland, Ian McMillan Connor, John Wilson Crawford, John Cameron Cullen, Ian Wallace Davidson, Ram Dayal, Pauline Anne Ellis (Blue), Peter Gaetano Fama, John Gerard Flannery, Barry Betham Grimmond, William Peter Harper, Henry James Heron, Rodney Fergus Jardine Hickey, Tatyana Hillerby (Godyaew), Norman Robert Honey, Peter Richard Norie Horne, Michael Lesslie Hucks, Keith Raymond Humphries, Mark William Irwin, Barrie Montague Jackson, Graham George Jackson, Murray Patrick Kelly, John Fullwood Kent, Andrew Leslie Kepes, Barry George Lavery, Jack Graham Learmonth, Brian Charles Leary, Brian Joseph Linehan, Robert James McAllister, Gary James McBrearty, Joseph Anthony William McCoy, Graham Herbert McLellan,

Lindsay Gerald Moffatt, John Bower Morton, Gerald Anthony Moss, Roy Charles Muir, Walter Balfour Peter Murray, Laurence Ross Neill, Harry Kay Morrell Nicholls, Dennis Richard Osborne, Barry William Oliver Partridge, Maganbhai Chhibubhai Patel, Ian Charles Prangnell, Reginald Satyaprakash Prasad, Thomas Rankin Pryde, Lindsay Bruce Quennell, Parshu Ram, Peter Graeme Alexander Reid, Paul Graham Ricketts, Graeme Allan Robbie, Graeme James Roberts, Mirdza Robins (Palmer), Antony Henry Roche, John Roberts Roke, John David Frederick Roy-Smith, George Cockburn Salmond, Robert Bernard William Smith, Charles Steiner, EricJohn Wayne Stephens, Adrian David Stewart, Frederick Edward Strange, Janis Lorin Sutherland (Oliver), Phyllis Margaret Taylor (Charlton), William Taylor, Nicholas Peter Thomson, Ronald Valentine Trubuhovich, Ernest Twose, Brian Hazelton Walsh (MD 1987), Ralph Marcus Lawson Whitlock, Hugh Patrick Williams, William Williamson, Herbert Bruce Wilson, John Douglas Wilson, James Bing Wong

1962

Allan Carson Adair, Clive Owen Bell, Dorothy Haydn Bell (Cameron), Ashleigh Alick Bishop, Charles Angelos Blades, Graeme Bertram Blake, Graeme Rutherford Blyth, Robert Albert Boas, Hugh Russell Bodle, David Bruton, Keith Robert John Cameron, Graeme Melrose Campbell, Wei Chhi Cheng, Matthew Stephen Shearburn Clark, Richard Sneyd Clemett, Richard Harding Coates, Paul Gillespie Cooke, George Martin Cornish, Gale Mervyn Curtis, Michael Francis Cussen, Donal Dalziell, David Hugh Coverdale Davidson, Lance James Day, Trevor Lancelot Dobbinson, Hugh Douglas, Barnett Rae Eades, Dean Patrick Eyre, Richard Hartley Ferrar, Roger Geoffrey Foote, Richard Charles Fowler, Efstathios George Gallate, Michael Bedford Gill, Howard Christie Gorton, Kenneth John Graham, Ronald Graham Grant, Ronald James Kay Grieve, Laurence Grundy, Nigel Neill Hamilton-Gibbs, John Hanley, Roger William Hay, Helen Robyn Hewland, Edgar Hans Josef Hift, Roger Stockwell Hill, Peter Eugene Holst, Francis Turner Logan Hull, Peter John Hurley (MD 1969), Edward George Jones (MD 1970), Barry Caine Knight, Dorothy Jean Kral, David Walling Leslie, Maureen Joan Lester (Peskett) (Travelling Scholar 1962), Alexander Richard Lo Su Fook, Maxwell John Lovie, John Farnie Butler Lusk, Niall Caville MacKenzie, William James Mackey, Cecily Anne McNulty (Cowie), Papali'i Semisi Ma'ia'i, Mary Victoria Miller (Cameron), Barry James Mills, Peter William Moller, Ronald John Molony, Robert Bruce Morrison, Tadeusz Andrzej Musialkowski, Brian Kingsford Otto, Jagdish Chandra Parmeshwar, Garry James Prockter, Robert Bohdan Mikolaj Ravich, David Eric Richmond (MD 1977), Stewart Maitland Robinson, John Ellis Rouse, Mark Aldred Sapsford, Peter de Schweitzer, Murray Selig, Peter Roderick Seville, Meon Carolyn Shand, John Harold Sheat, Brian John Shivnan, Thomas Kay Sidey, Malcolm James Simons (MD 1976), Avtar Ganga Singh, Lorraine Elsa Smith, Howard George Stephens, Michael Goldring Stephens, Walter Stewart James Tongue, John Kingsley Walsh, James William Beresford Walshe, Nigel James Warden, William John Wattie, Dean Carey Williams, John Gardner Williams, James Cornfoot Jarvis Willis, Stanley Peter Woodhouse; MD: George Gustav Somjen

1963

Stephen Percy Balme, David Prescott Baron, David Michael Joseph Barry, Robert Bruce Bell, Richard Mason Bernau, Martin George Betro, John Derek Billings, Christopher John Bossley, Frank Peter Botica, Philip Edward Boulton, Stafford Daniel Bourke, John Audley Bowbyes, George Robert Boyd, William Baring Brabant, Bevan Edgar Wilson Brownlie (MD 1970), Daumants David Bucens, Andrew Frank Cameron, Andrew Huang Chong, Rodger Frederick Colbert, John Innes Colegrove, Boris Matthew Corbett, Sydney Douglas Cox,

Donald Richard Dalley, Philip John Dee, Leslie Ding, Stephen Richard Dixon, Victor Dolby, John Charles Doran, James Innis Doull, Peter Cuthbert Dukes, Mason Harold Durie, Gavin Francis Farr, Russell Stuart Ferguson, Helen Brading Foreman (MacNeill), John Alan Ross Fountain, Florence Anne Fraser, Alan Gillard Frazer, Anthony Michael Bowker Gebbie, Peter Gianoutsos, Ronald John Goodey, Alistair McLean Gordon, Alan John Gray, Murray Hickson Greig, John McLeod Gordon Grigor, Hester Nina Grudnoff (Squire), Harold John Beecher Guy, Peter Neill Hamilton-Gibbs, Ronald Kenneth Haydon, Mary Robertson Heyhoe, David Graham Hill, Graham Lancelot Hill, Saba La Hood, Anthony Peter Hura, Janet Rickord McCall Irwin (Smith), John Alexander Ives, Robin Valentine Jackson, David Laurence Jamison, Gary Roy Johnstone, Donald John Jones, Per Brandt Jorgensen, Errol Valeno Kelly, Ian McConachie Kendall-Smith, Owen Berkeley King, John Campbell Larking, Robert Archibald Leathem, Ronald Alexander Leng, John Howard Lidgard, Peter McCormick, Iain James Alister MacFarlane, Barry Scott McGuinness, Russell Frederick McIlroy, Peter Alexander McKinnon, Anthony Dunstan Crawford Macknight (MD 1969), Jocelyn Mabel MacKnight, Noel Keith MacLaren, Mark Haswell McMillan, Peter David Martin, David Charles Mauger, Frederick Edward Mayell, Marcus Webley Melvin, Chee Yu Mok, Richard Tanner Moloney, Clifford Raymond Munro, Jack David Murdoch, Maureen Anne O'Brien (Bassili), Lesley Anne Palmer (Smith), Bruce James Pardy (ChM 1980), Paul Thomas Patten, Roger Worsley Peak, Graham Harrison Perry, John Ewart Pettit (MD 1974), Jean Dominique Peyroux, Kow Weng Phang, Richard George Pirrit, Billie Rosemary Jane Porter (Campbell), Colin Neil Pullar, Ian Read, Brian John Robb, Raymond Reeves Robinson, Barry Douglas Rutherford, Katherine Jean Scott (Lennane), Ian Robert Sewell, Bramah Nand Singh (Travelling Scholar 1963) (MD 1975), Evan Ross Smith, Margaret June Sparrow (Muir), Peter Charles Methven Sparrow, Alexander Waddell Squire, Donald Charles Stewart, Austin John Sumner, Bruce Barry Taylor, Broughton Beauchamp Thomas, John Beveridge Truman, Ngaire Jean Twose (Jeffreys), Malcolm Norman Waddle, Edward Peter Ward, Graham Wardrope, David Ashton Warner, Peter Caradus Wellings, Harvey Edward Williams, Michael Joseph Basil Wilson, Graham John Woods, Wilson Godfrey James Wylie; MD: J.B. MacKereth, Kailash Chandra Nathsarma

1964

George David Abbott (MD 1971), Viopapa Edwina Annandale (Atherton), Ross Raymond Bailey (MD 1970), Frederick William Banks, Donald William Bardin, Anthony Terrence Batistich, Paul Randolph Berry, John Edward Blackburn, Douglas John Bolitho, Francis Tudor Bostock, Thomas Raymond Bracken, Murray Frederick Brennan (ChM 1983) (MD 1983), David Anthony Brodie, Andrew Sutherland Brook, Marion Ruth Bucens (Fromm), Edmund Samuel Cadogan, Lucy Fong King Chung (Chan), Kerry Edgar Clark, Lowrie Arthur Cotterell, Brian Richard Cross, Judith Anne Daniels (Driscoll), William Lawrence Daniels, Marion Joy Dewar (Carey-Smith), Victor Howard Wong Doo, James Robert Elder, Ian Desmond Elliott, Thomas Nigel Ellison, Jon Evans, Rex David Fairbairn, Winifred Anne Fisher (Kennedy), Colin Barrett Fitzpatrick, Karen Thelma France (Palmer), Ian Ross Gardner, Jacob Johannes de Geus, Richard Lewis Graham, Alastair William Grant, Donald Harley Gray (ChM 1974), William Payne Greenslade, David Ross Hamilton, Brian Eric Hardy, Guy David James Harper, Nicholas Walter Harry, Barry von Hartitzsch, Anthea Helen Hatfield (Wheeler), Peter John Hatfield, Anthony Maurice Hewlett, Grahame William Davison Hinkley, Edison Rae Hobson, Helen Ann James, Evan Wilson Jamieson, Peter Nicol Jennings, Ronald William Jones, Marion Joan Kral (Boock), John Jamieson Landreth, Peter Wade Law, Joseph George Anthony Lee, Anthony Bruce

McCallum, David James McCleave, Robert Duncan McFarlane, Marion Joy McInnes (Hamilton), Donald Angus Ross McKay, Winston Irving McKean, Neil Gordon MacKenzie, Margaret Alison McLagan (Rainer), Barrie Craig McLeay, Duncan Joseph McVey, Ian Grant Malcolm, Stuart Bruce Malcolm, Thomas Michael James Maling (MD 1977), Michael John Mant, Colin David Mantell, Thomas Harry Marshall, Roderick George Martin, Evelyn Jean Martindale (Mander), Peter John Mayerhofler, Aeneas David Mee, Michael Aloysius Menzies, Harvey MacDonald Morgan, Eric Ronald Muncaster, Denis Gerard O'Connor, Neil MacDonald Fraser Officer, Thomas Anthony Ord, Ian Robertson Phillips, Ian Graham Renner, Brian Max Robertson, Ian Alasdair Robertson, Jeffrey Bartlett Stevens, Ruth Harriett Stevenson (Schell), Graeme McNee Stone, Graeme John Taylor (Travelling Scholar 1964) (MD 1990), Maurice Campbell Tennent, David McAuley Thomson, Ngaamo Russell Thomson, Matthew Holder Tizard, Guildford Bruce Todd, Colin Arthur Tourelle, James Bellord Waldron, William Thomas Raeburn Ward, Kingsley William Warden, Evan Charles Watts, Howard Keith Way, Boyd Hustler Webster, Desmond Frank Wilson, James Young Yee, Karen Deborah Zelas (Williams)

1965

Anthony Joseph Ansford, Edric Sargisson Baker, Graeme Laurence Barnes (MD 1974), Julian Peter Bell, Peter Robert Bell, Anthony Marcus Benjamin, Bryan Barrie Berkeley, Ross Douglas Blair, David William Boldt, John Dudley Bonifant, Robin Helen Briant (MD 1973), Gerald William Kershaw Bridge, Nicholas Roger Guy Broadbent, Gael Brook (McLean), Leo Francis John Buchanan, Richard Bruce Burnet, Graham Dene Burrows, Percy Vaughn Bydder, Douglas Friars Carnachan, Richard Harold Claridge, Edward Desmond Clarke, David Barry Crabb, Michael Sutherland Croxson, Margaret Christine Cunningham (Croxson), John Campbell Cunninghame, Edward Bolton Dakin, William Anthony Davies, Dorothy Edith Dowd (Stevens), Roderick Boyd Ellis-Pegler, Christopher John Evans, Richard Evans, Murray Leonard Farrant, Christopher John Rowland Feltham, Graeme Holt Fenton, Roderick Stuart Ferguson, George Allan Foote, Alastair John Forrest, Rex Noel Frye, Duncan Stuart Gibbs, Lindsay Franklin Haas, Thiers John Halliwell, John Hancock, Ian Bruce Hassall, Christopher John Heath, Patrick David Hertnon, Anthony Mark Hoby, Ian MacMurray Holdaway (Travelling Scholar 1965) (MD 1973), Anthony John House, Maxwell Kenneth Johnson, Rees Hollier John Jones, David Herbert Kitchen, David Rogan MacDuff Latham, Humphry Ian de Lautour, Peter Leathem, Brian James Leitch, James John MacDonald, Beth Janice Leslie MacGregor (Synek), John Robert McKinnon, Ian Grant McNickle, Colin Ulric McRae, Kevin Vincent Marriott, David Frederick Marris, Raymond John Marsh, Timothy Dennison Medlicott, John Hollingsworth Moore, Murray Neil Muir, Peter Ian Parkinson, Yogesh Chandra Patel, Richard Milgrew Power, Anthony Geoffrey Poynter, Peter Charles Rea, Alister Heaton Rhodes, Stuart Allan Ross, Alastair Gardner Rothwell (MD 1987), Ian Michael St George (MD 1991), Merrick Clifford Sanderson, David John Scott, Malcolm Raymond Sears, Enn Sepp, Kenneth Lincoln Settle, Edward Gordon Simpson, Clive Anthony Smith, Graham Peter Snodgrass, Peter Grahame Snow, Murray John Stanton, Ann Elizabeth Minnie Steele, Richard John Stewart (ChM 1978), Peter Lincoln Stokes (MD 1974), Peter James Harvey Strang, Denys Shane Sumner, John Raeburn Talbot, Richard George Talbot, Hugh Barclay Tapper, Kenneth James Thompson, Garnet Donald Tregonning, James Victor Vaughan, Christopher Joseph Wakem, Brian Robert Weston, Alan Grant Williams, Terence Glynn Wilson, John Martin Wishart, Sun Wong, Russell John Worth, Peter Yee, Trevor Cedric Young, William John Zohrab; MD: Stanley Hickling

1966

Philip Francis Waren Airey, Bruce Donald Alexander, Malcom Lawrence Baigent, Michael Anthony Hugh Baird, Winton John Sugden Barnes, John Eldon Barry, Donald Harry Bashford, Lawrence Arnould Bates, Allan Clifford Binnie, John Lind Bradley, Peter John Buckley, William James Burton, Murray John Bycroft, George Dennis Calvert (MD 1974), Malcolm Maben Cameron, Keith Alexander Carey-Smith, Alexander Russell Chang (MD 1988), David Graeme Edgar Clarke, Gabrielle Brett Collison (Doyle), Brian John Crichton, Anthony Bernard Cull, Peter Robert Cunningham, John Wayne Delahunt, Alexander George Dempster, Ivan MacGregor Donaldson (MD 1976), Stewart Grant Drysdale, Mark Bevan Duffill, Russell James Falconer, Joan Lorraine Faoagali (Wilson), Thomas Mackenzie Fiddes, Graeme Reynold Ford, Patrick Andrew Frengley, Bryan Richard Melville Frost, Stephen Thomas James Gilbert, David James Stuart Gray, Bruce Craig Robertson Gregory, Anthony Arthur Griffin, Suzanne Helen Hatch (East), Jack Hilton Havill, Patrick Grahame Henley, Anna Astrid Holst (Orgill), Ivan Philip Howie, Martin James Hudson, David Barclay Innes, Mark Francis Jagusch, Ripley Donald Newton Jones, Andrew Kaegi, Jill Juanita Kelly (Calveley), Alan Archibald Kerr, Lynsie Ruth Kerr (Kitchen), Michael John Knapton, Graham Francis Kyd, Peter Lee (MD 1975), Richard John Lennane, Antony Peter Rex Ludbrook, John McGarvin McIlwraith, Murray Osborne McLachlan, Colin Gordon MacLeod, Warren Maxwell McNaughton, James Orton Maguire, John Richard Delahunt Matthews, Ronald Gordon Meikle, Graham Wilfred Mellsop, John Glanville Miller,Malcolm Kenneth Milmine, Robin Noel Moir, Donald Hugh Montgomery, Antony Trevor Morris, John Humphrey Morris, John Irwin Newstead, Stephen George Kitch Packer, Grahame James Pohlen, Neil Ashley Pollock, Eru Woodbine Pomare, Zbigniew Jan Poplawski, Alexander Charles Peter Powles, Anthony John Rockel (MD 1978), Barbara Jean Rusbatch (Hooker), Robert Francis Salamonsen (MD 1977), Christopher Terence Savill, Paul John Sheehan, Paul Stewart Simcock, Ian James Simpson, Walter Gordon Harris Smithson, Allan James Smyth, Gregory Norman Steele, Robert Maxwell Stevenson, John Marshall Stewart, Allan Frederick Neil Sutherland, Kenneth William Talbot, Brent William Taylor, Clinton Adam Teague, Marise Anne Thacker, Lindsay Graham Thomas, Winston Tong, Stuart West Twemlow, Graham Oliver Ward, Karen Margaret Leslie Ward, David Anthony Wilde, Brian James Williams, John Lindsay Wilson, Anthony David Wong, Douglas Wong, Leslie Wong, Maurice Edward Robert Wood, James Joseph Wright (MD 1973), Mary Anthea Wright (Ellis) (Travelling Scholar 1966)

1967

John William Luther Ainsworth, Patrick Geoffrey Alley, Anthony Eric Armstrong, Ailsa Clyne Heath Barker, Jonathan James Baskett, John Philip Ronald Bell, Dennis Gordon Bentley, Lance David Blumhardt (MD 1980), Doreen Constance Bolton, Stephen Layton Rumbold Bowker, Michael Russell Mark Broadbent, John Melville Broadfoot, Brian Campbell Broom, John Edward Brunton, Noeline Margaret Butcher, Colin John Calcinai, Stephen Blake Calveley, Leigh Robert Campbell, William Deryck Charters, John Ewen Clarkson, John Gerard Clarkson, Patricia Dorothy Cruickshank (Hill), Bernard Joseph Cummings, Paul James Dempsey, James Donald Devane, Bruce Anthony James Dewe, Ynys Tamazin Douglas, Douglas Bruce Drysdale, Gerald Barrington Duff (MD 1984), David James Dunlop, Thomas Richard Ellingham, David Robert Ellis, Patrick Joseph Farry, Peter Macalister Feltham, Russell Charles Franklin, John Geoffrey Gilbert, Neil McNaughton Gilchrist, Henry Ronald Ross Glennie, Stuart Peter Gowland, Peter Michael Graham, Robert Renton Grigor, Michael Reid Grimstone, Osmond Bruce Hadden, Fredrick Arthur Hamilton, Norman Montague Hartwell,

Paul Christopher Herrick, George Alistair Holmes, Gerald Stephen Irwin, Robin James Irwin, Geoffrey Peter Keller, Ann Lang (Philipp), Selwyn Douglas Ruthven Lang, Beryl Monica Lewis (Moody), Gerald Richard Lewis (MD 1977), Janet Antonoff Lewis (Dunlop), Ernest Going Loten, Christopher John Lovell-Smith, Kenneth Henry Low, David Lawrence McAuley, Patrick Francis McEvedy, Vianney George McGirr, Ian Leslie MacGregor (MD 1978), John William McLeod, Anthony Brian Marks, Graham Hawe Mason, Murray Hugh Matthewson, Peter Britton Milsom, Dermot Dubrelle Morrah, Christopher John Lester Newth, Jonathan Guy Pascoe, Anthony William Pierre, Ewan Alistair Porter, Elizabeth Celia Purves (Travelling Scholar 1967), Basil Paul Quin, David Eric Rawlings, Russell Warwick Stedman Reid, Leonardus Johannes Roborgh, Roger Bernard Scown, Kevin Patrick Shannon, Robert Stuart Simons, Graeme Rex Simpson, Bruce Arthur Skinner, Kevin Paul Smidt, Howard John Smith (MD 1977), Norman John Stokes, Robert Ian Symes, David Leonard Talbot, Brian Meredith Teviotdale, Harilal Thakorlal, Ronald Thomas Bruce Thompson, Kenneth John Thomson, Paul Derek Trolove, Garth John Turbott, Malcolm Ernest Turner, Kenneth Bedford Vallance, Hendrik De Vetter, John Stuart Wakeman, Paul Fred Walker, Jeremy Kenneth Walton, Euan Warnock Watson, Graham Donald Watson, Robert Peter Welsh, Paul Robert White, Jocelyn Mary Williams, Laurence Anthony Wilson, Miles Roger Wislang, William Leonard Wright, Arthur Albert Young

1968

John Dickson Adams, Robert Elliott Aitken, Stuart Allan, Kenneth Ritchie Anderson, Geoffrey Carter Archibald, Norman Montyque Arnott, William John Baber, Robert Beaglehole (Travelling Scholar 1968) (MD 1977), Margaret Helen Bell (Chacko), Forbes Eadie Bennett, James Alan Boyne, Geoffrey Errol Bradley, Robert William Bramley, Peter Shackleton Brooke, Alan Claude Brookes, Michael James Butler, Graeme Robert Carlaw, David Graham Carroll, David George Chaplow, Luk Sun Chin, Christine Mary Conolly (Roke), Kenneth Gordon Couper, Gaia Erika Cox, Paul Grave Crozier, Clyde Gordon Cumming, John Graham Davison, Evan William Dry (Dryson), Christine Lillian Dunbar (Jaworski), Toomas Eisler, Elizabeth Ellen Eliot, Graham Walter Erceg, Ian Robert Holms Falloon, John Cornelius Finlay, Stuart David Foote, Beris Ford, David Cornelius Freeman, Donald Bruce Fulton, Robert James McKinlay Gardner, Leo Garmonsway, Alastair Hugh Bruce Gillies, Wendy Elizabeth Hadden (Fitzwilliam), Warwick Rhys Harding, Anthony Eric Hardy, Raymond Reginald Harvey, John Wilton Henley, Thomas Michael Hewitt, Peter Reginald Honeyfield, Grahame Arthur Hookway, Michael Noel Hosking, Alan Wilfred Hull, Robert Lewis Hungerford, John David Hutton, Rodger Jackson, Edward Denis Janus (MD 1976), James Arthur Judson, Richard George Keightley, Douglas Herbert Knight, Robert John Kyd, Russell Theodore Lienert, Margaret Florence Lovell-Smith (Carter), Jeffery Luey, David Wayne McGregor, Andrew Ronald MacKintosh, David John McNicoll, Allen William Marx, Graeme Sidney Mawson, Roger Beach Balfour Mee, Peter Ronald Meech, John Eisdell Moodie, Mischel Elden Neill, George Ngaei, Michael Gary Nicholls (MD 1976), Noel Winston Nicholson, Eoin Dodds MacGregor Park, David Luke Pascoe, Mahendrakumar Chhaganlal Patel, Warren Max Paykel, Jill Peckham (Brady), Joseph Edmund Petoe, Dennis Louis Pezaro, Robin Philipp, Antony Martin Felton Reeve, James Henry Alexander Robertson, Derek Leslie Rothwell, Glenis Elizabeth Ruge (Tiller), Ian Henry Sampson, Roger Millan Scott, David Norman Sharpe (MD 1982), Helen Kelsey Sill (Tasker), Warren Morrison Smith, Brian Grove Spackman, Lindsay John William Strang, Murray John Summerfield, Royden George Tallon, Ian Murray Mynott Taylor, Kenneth Robert Thomson, John Walter Gill Tiller, Russell John Tregonning, Marion Anne Upsdell, Alison Rae Varcoe, Ronald

Edward Vlietstra, Leigh Ashton Warner, William Graham Alexander Watkins, Michael William Watt, Henry James Wernham, Michael Andrew Wilson, David Erami Tohengaroa Yates, Alan Yee; MD: Francis Alexander de Hamel

1969

Adarine Mary Anderson, Jessie Christine Anderson, Ross Charles Anderton, Julia Anne Aranui-Faed (Baird), Eric Verdun Arbuthnot, Timothy Malcolm Astley, George Peter John Atlas, Rosemary Jane Hazel Avery, Diane Margaret Baguley, John Hamilton Betteridge, Jonathan Glover Bibby (MD 1981), Calder Howard Botting, Patrick Joseph Bradley, Judith Bruton (Baranyai), Graeme Mervyn Bydder, Archibald John Campbell (MD 1983), John Seymour Chapman-Smith, Charles Bevan Chilcott, Mary Margaret Gillian Clover, Francis Allan Cockburn, Raymond William Cook, Michael David Cresswell, Ross George Davidson, Teresa Catherine Dawe (Turnbull), Ian Dean, Gavin Scott Douglas, Peter John Dunn (MD 1978), Robert John Eastwood, Graeme Robert Edgeley, James David Ross Elliott, James Matheson Faed, Michael William Fancourt, Robin Frances Fancourt (Allen), Malcolm McDougal Fisher (MD 1987), Allen Rex Fraser, Gary Ernest Fraser, Roger Henry Gilbert, Allan Anthony Colston Godfrey, Myles John Grant, Allen James Gray, Bruce Stephen Greenfield, Richard Stanley Grenfell, Richard Haskell, Ian Hass, Angela Dale Hawes (Deacon), John Lyndon McLeod Hawk (MD 1992), Gerald John Lachlan Hewitt, John Robert George Hilton, John Leicester Reed Hodge, Michael Geoffrey Holmes, Hamish McKinlay Horton, Graeme Henry Johnson, Lannes Fullarton Johnson, Dale Laura Johnston, Ian Stuart Crawford Jones (ChM 1977), Elizabeth Ann Rhodes Kaegi (Ritchie), Alan Robert King, Darion Mary Letford (Rowan), John Cameron Lindsay, Graeme Ronald Linfoot, Hugh William Baird Litchfield, Kevin Luey, Donald Evan Murray MacCormick, Garth Raymond McDonald, John Richard MacDonald, David James McHaffie, Andrew John McKenzie, Fiona Margaret McKinnon, Norman Edgar MacLean, Ramanlal Madhav, Aidene Rosalind Mason (Urquhart), Jann Medlicott, Richard James Meech, Peter Russell Miller, David Selwyn Morris, Maxwell Clarke Morris, Keith Mervyn Muir, Warren David George Nicholls, Campbell Gerald Odlin, Penelope Grace Palmer (Cook), Stephen John Palmer, Richard Lionel Pardy, Rasik Patel, David John Peddie, Robert William Percival, Christine Ann Quin, Christopher George Randell, Errol Thomas Raumati, James John Reid, Annabel Frances Ross, Cynthia Jean Rutherford (Kerr), John Douglas Rutherford, John Alexander Ryder, Graeme Gordon St John, Ian Kevin Scott, Andrew Lindsay Sew Hoy, Judith Elizabeth Sill (Cogan), Ross William Sinclair, Robin Fred Smart, Ngaire Adrienne Smidt (Carter), Hugh Timothy Spencer, Bruce James Spittle (Travelling Scholar 1969), William Joseph Sugrue, James Leonard Talbot, Suzanna Taryan (Svirskis), Robert Gibson Tiller, Ross Clifton Tovey, Anthony Haydon Townsend, John Gregory Turner (MD 1977), Peter Sinclair Warren, Peter James Watt, Brian Mostyn Williams, Ernest Walter Willoughby, Douglas William Wilson

1970

Gary Edward Aitcheson, Timothy Allen Alexander, Simon Bruce Colfox Baker, Antony Nigel Barker, Alastair Charles Begg, Peter Alexander Borrie, Graeme Henry Brown, Stuart Whitaker Brown, Kenneth Leslie Buck, Robert Loudon Cable, John Arthur Calder, Robert William Cameron, Cyril James Chapman, Barry Ronald Claridge, Anthony Ridgway Coates (Travelling Scholar 1970), Kenneth Raymond Cooke, Howard Arthur Coverdale, John Richard Davis, Christopher Richard Donald, John Dale Drummond, Richard Michael Edmond, David Eric Elder, John Cecil Munroe Emanuel, Richard Lewis Maxwell Faull, Anthony Everard James Fitchett, Joseph Fliegner, Kenneth Charles Fox, Jeffrey Brendan Friis, William Terry Gavin, John David Gillies, Peter William Gould, Peter

James Gow, Lindsay Atholstan Green, David Verran Greer, Alastair James Haslam, Robert Steuart Henderson, James Geoffrey Horne, Noemi Horvath, Roger William House, Charles Paul Telford Hutchison, Gordon Elliott Jackson, Murray Grenfell Jamieson (Rhodes Scholar 1970), Peter James Keary, Thomas Desmond Keenan, James Clark Kerr, Lewis Edward James King, Bruce McNeill Kinloch, Frederick David Lane, Martin Rodger Laurent (MD 1983), Allan John Lester, Wendy Rose Isbell Low (Bartley), Michael Brian Lusk, John Ewing McArthur, Ian James Macbeth, Noel Robert McCleave, Alistair Peter McGeorge, Barbara McKean (Westra), John Dugald Stewart McKean, William Gordon McNickle, Timothy James Bromley Maling (MD 1993), Robin Macdonald Marchant, Alistair Graeme Marshall, Ross Howard Martin, Ata Matatumua, Campbell John Miller, Ian Keith Milne, Peter James Stewart Moodie, John Drakely Moore, Paratene (Pat) Ngata, John Charles Opie, William Leslie Page, Allan Leslie Panting, Philip John Parkin, Bryan Ronald Parry (MD 1988), Gareth John Glyn Parry, Graham Keith Parry, Linda Margaret Parry (Bealing), John Greig Pearce, Edward Arthur Pearson, Susan Mary Perry (Wily), Kevin Craig Pringle, Stephen Harry Raymond, William James Reeder, Roger George Price Rees, John Kingston Reeve, Ralph Andrew Reeves, Charles Peter Ring, Malcolm Clive Robinson, David Graeme Ross, Karla Maxine Ross (Rix-Trott), Anthony Ansley Ruakere, Michael Geoffrey Sargent, Norman Shum, Barbara Mary Simons (Bull), Rene Smit, Allan Herries Smith, Bruce Linton Smith, Robert Kennedy Smith, Judith Claire Somerfield (Herd), Stanley David Somerfield, Judith Margaret Stewart (Wright), Clive Warwick Stone, David Charles Sutherland, Paul Dennis Sutherland, Gillian Stephanie Tregenza (Bourne), Adrianus Marie Van Rij (MD 1986), Lyall Hopkirk Varlow, David Anthony Waite, Edmond Freeland Walford, David Ivon Walton, Rodney Falcon Waterworth, Garry Robert Werner, Alison Winifred Wesley, Edwin Andrew Whiteside; MD: Edward Morris McLachlan, Tapendra Mohan Mukherjee

1971

Robert John Anderson, John Halsey Andrew, Anthony Arnold Atkinson, Stuart Francis Avery, Robert John Barton, Lorraine Joyce Beard (Travelling Scholar 1971), Winfield Malloch Bennett, Hilary Ann Blacklock, John Baker Boulton, David George Brabyn, David Leslie Bratt, Rex Leslie Browne, William John Loudon Cable, John Scott Carnachan, Maxwell Roy Chalmers, Christina Zenobia Clee (Clarkson), David Glyndwr Clee, Peter John Conolly, Pamela Margaret Cooper (Elder), Diana Ruth Dent (Plummer), Peter Dodwell, Alan Malcolm Donoghue, George Downward, Lesley Margaret Drummond-Borg (MD 1983), Gary Malcolm Duncan, John Charles Eliott, Peter Richard Fisher, Richard Mottram Forster, Kevin John Gaskin, Derek Clifton Gibbons, Alan John David Gillies, Peter David Gluckman, Kenneth John Greer, John Nevinson Harrison, Rosemary Eraine Hawkins (Parkin), Anthony Pierce Hay, Ross Gordon Gilbert Hayton, Mila Hill, Elizabeth Mary Hudson (Speer), Warwick Stanley Hunter, Brian Frederick Issell, Pauline Judith Johannesson (Murdoch), John Samuel Huston Jones, John Lawrence Karalus, Peter Edwin Keeley, Andrew Graeme Stuart King, Douglas Allister Lingard, Alan Reed List, David Kingsley Lascelles Lyall, Kelvin Lewis Lynn, Owen Roy McAuley, William James McBeath, Marie Elizabeth McCarthy, Donald Ian McDonald, William George McFarland, Donald George McInnes, Michael John Mackay, Raymond Douglas McKenzie, Allan Bruce MacLean (MD 1984), Logan James McLennan, Patrick John McNaught, Patricia McVeagh, Anthony Ross Marshall, Patrick Arnold Warren Medlicott, Timothy Eisdell Moore, Leo Kelvin Morresey, David John Murchison, Thomas James Neale (MD 1986), Herewini Muturangi Ngata, Paul Fred Nicholson, Alan Miller Nicoll, Colleen Donna Patterson, Charlotte Entrican Paul, Ronald Arthur Peach, James Huia Penniket, Allan David Pettigrew, Murray Vincent Pfeifer, Robert Dudley Purves,

Ian Lester Rafter, Dinah Susan Reddihough, Donal Muir Roberton (MD 1979), Trevor John Roberts, John Robert Matheson Rogers, Sarah Elizabeth Romans-Clarkson (MD 1989), Philip Charles Ruge, David Andrew Scollay, Keith Richard Searle, Anna Lise Seifert (Koefoed), Peter Hugh Sharr, Nigel Edmund Sharrock, John Edward Shevland, Bernard John Sill, Paul Francis Silvester, Calvin Wilfred Royce Simons, Wayne Richard Frederick Smallman, Warwick Macdonald Ian Smeeton, Martyn Wade Smith, Anthony Peter John Snell, Mark Graham Somerville, Geoffrey Paul Stephens, John Martin Patrick Sullivan, David Alfred Thompson, Barry Ross Tietjens, Hugh Edward Townend, George Christopher Tripe, Paul Ronald Trotman, Peter Gunther Turner, Wilfred (Bill) Edward Dampney Turner, James Rowland Tyler, John Edgar Upsdell, Raman Lakha Vasan, Elwyn Peter Walker, Philip Nelham Watson, Robert Graham Weatherhead, Denis Edward Whittle, Owen Ralph Wiles, Laurie Colin Williams, Gavin Neil Wilton, Alastair Graeme Yule

1972
Barbara Jean Adkins, Terence Russell Aitken, Clive Carlisle Allcock, Paul Christopher Armour, Mark Llewellyn Bassett, John Neville Baxter, Gregory Marc Beacham, Jennifer May Berryman, Glenys Fay Blackburn, Robert John Blackmore, Karin Leonie Blaymires, John Douglas Bourke, Leonard William Brake, Roland Spencer Broadbent, Jessica Mary Brown (Kirker), Terence Vicary Kerry Burcher, Charles William Cameron, Craig Henry Campbell, Sylvia Anne Carlisle, Elizabeth Mary Chalmers (Doherty), Christopher John Wesley Chambers, Bruce Andrew Chapman, Brian Lewis Clarke, Daphne Lesley Climie (Kay), Karen Ann Colgan (de Luen), Maurice James Colgan, Denys John Court, Michael John Crooke, Kevin John Davey, Duncan Andrew Doig, Terence Charles Anthony Doyle, Charles Geoffrey Dunckley, Gavin Kenneth Earles, Roger William Farrow, Bernard Michael Fitzharris (MD 1983), Penelope Frances Fitzharris (Gibson) (MD 1983), David Seymour Francis, Robert-Jan Fris, Douglas John Gillanders, Phillip James Godfrey, Cary Victor Griffiths, David William Gudex, John Gilbert Harris, Peter Geoffrey Harty, Nicholas Gerard Hassan, Colin Angus Heinz, Christopher John Heron, John Highton (MD 1983), Murray Alfred Hodder, Christopher Francis Hoskins, Errol Lloyd Hudson, Stephen James Hyde, Maurice Stuart Carson Jolly, Christopher John Kempthorne, John Brian Kenny, David Kilpatrick (MD 1981), James Alexander Kirker, Geoffrey James Kivell, Robert Ross Kydd, Michael Guy Laney, Ian Robert Lange, David John Alfred Langford, Vaughan Gilbert Laurenson, Diana Rosemary Lennon, Juliet Alice Liddell (Broadmore), Robert MacLean Loan, Charlie Luen, John Francis McGettigan, Malcolm Bruce McKerchar, TimothyWilson McKergow, Anthony Richard Marsland, Donald Paul Martin, Sylvester Wayne Miles (MD 1982), Fiona Bayard Millard (Stewart), John Wilfrid Mills, Janet Theo Milne (Scott), Peter Ian Moody, Anthony William Eisdell Moore, Christopher Owen Morgan, Robert Marwood Mules, John Edmund Newman, John Andrew Ormiston, Robin John Palmer, Trevor John Parry, Graham Malcolm Patrick, Christine Joan Perkins (Arnold), John Stanley Francis Pollock, James Hubert Primrose, Mason Philip Ramsay, Martin James Wheatcroft Rees, Peter John Rich, Allan John Robert, Geoffrey Maxwell Robinson, Peter Huntly Robinson, Robert Simon Hearn Rowley, Iain Allan Russell, Richard Sainsbury, Neil John William Scholes, Peter John Schwarz, Russell Sinclair Scott, Peter James Sears, Michael Anthony Sexton, Jillian Ruth Shanks, Neil William Grahame Shaw, David John Shipp, Robert Graeme Sim, Stewart William Sinclair, David Christopher Graham Skegg (Travelling Scholar 1972) (Rhodes Scholar 1972), Richard James Somerville, Ralph William Souter, Ian David Stephens, Michael John Stephenson, Kenneth Hamilton Tarr, Nicholas Peter Terpstra, William John Thompson, Alan James Thurston, Peter Valentine Twigg, Paul Davidson Veitch,

David Stanley Velvin, Clyde Mervyn Wade, Colin Frederick Wakefield, Graeme Frederic Washer, Anthony John Wilson, Roland John Wilson, Suzanne Lee Wilson (Davis), Ho Leng Young; MD: E.W. Berry, Jeffrey Samuel Dodge

1973
Kenneth William Adams, Rodney Kenneth Allen, Graham Symon Armstrong, Patrick Robert Bary, Richard Michael Dorrington Batt, Peter Scott Benny, Ross Lewis Bohm, Ian Lindsay Breeze, Peter James Cairney, Peter Marsden Cardon, Timothy Kenred Carey-Smith, James William Frederick Cashman, Mervyn Joseph Ah Chan, John Douglas Clark, Stuart James Cleland, Howard Murray Clentworth, Lyall Graham Clyne, Alastair John Corbett (Travelling Scholar 1973) (MD 1987), Christopher Douglas Cotter, Geoffrey Ronald Cutfield, Christopher John Dawe, Noel Kenelm Digby, John Roger Doig, Alan Doube, Alan Farnell, Richard Lillico Feltham, Alan Bryden Foote, Murray Raymond Fosbender, Conan Fowler, Darryl Lindsay Fry, Wayne Richard Gillett (MD 1991), Peter Lear Gillies, Ian James Griffiths, Anthony Micheal Guy, Barend Ter Haar, David Charles Hall, Roger Gaythorne Harris, John Murray Hedley, Kevin William Hill, Michael Cadness Hobbs, Henry Alfred Holmes, Peter James Horsfall, Lewis John Hudson, Gregor James Hunter, Neil Alexander Hutchison, David Arthur Jacks, Simon L'Moine James, Stephen Leonard Johns, Eric Mervyn Jones, Stephen Nicholas Kardos, Philip Kelly, David William Kerr, Graeme Warren Kidd, Peter Thomas Kyne, Anthony Roy Law, Richard Alistair Loan, Iain MacDonald, Donald John Lewis McIver, Janice Marilyn McKenzie, Ian Bruce McPherson, Richard Stanley Marks, Laraine Ruth Martin (Ruthborn), Timothy John Mason, John Dunstan Mercer, Wallace Howard Metcalfe, David Jeffery Meuli, Francine Aleida Meuli (Hupkens Van Der Elst), Thomas Michael Miller, Michael Peter Moore, Neil David Morrison, Richard Calvert Muir, Ronald George Neal, John Dannefaerd Nealie, Charles James Newhook, John Patrick O'Connor, Eric Frank Orgias, Ashton John Parker, Trevor Murray Parr, Brian John Percival, Ross Alan Pettigrew, Jordan Pishief, Stamatis Pishief, Karen Olive Poutasi (Davidson), Philip Anthony Reid Railton, Anthony Evan Gerald Raine (Rhodes Scholar 1973), James Patrick Raleigh, Judith Anne Reeve (Scott; Gough), Bruce Edwin Rhind, Terry George Richardson, Charles Robert Riley, Patricia Mary Robertson, Peter John Lindsey Rodwell, Alexander John Fergus Ross, Garythe Mary Samuda-Evans, Graeme Brian Scrivener, Branko Sijnja, Christopher Simpson, Terence John Sinton, Keren Mary Skegg (Cargo), John Wright Skelley, Ralph Brock Smith, David Thomas Somerton, Richard Allan Speed, Nigel Henry Stace, Andrew Philip Stewart, Aage Heert Terpstra, Donald Mackie Thomson, Michael John Thorpy, Stuart Henry Tiller, Leslie John Tonkin, Julia Helen Tyler (Jorgensen), Richard James Tyler, Harvey Douglas White, Janette Frances White (Venus), Janice Linda Whyte, John Gordon Wilson, Stuart Elwyn Wilson, Keith Stuart Christopher Wong, Michael Colin Wong, Kathleen Patricia Wood (Bode), Antony Ivan Yelavich; MD: Reynold Francis Xavier Noronha

1974
Victor John Allcock, Michael Harding Anderson, Aloiamoa Rainsford Anesi, David Alan Ansell, Ava Ruth Baker, Judith Mary Bent, Stephen Charles Bentley, John Berry, Lesley Ann Bond, Peter Robert Bradley, Ralph Thomas Bright, Samuel James Broome, Graeme Edward Browne, Guy Philip Bryant, Colin Chin, Richard James Coleman, John Francis Collins, Anthony Michael Cook, Susan Margaret Craw, Francis Donald Cullen, Kevin John Dallimore, Geoffrey Michael Davis, John Charles Christopher Davison, John Alastair Didsbury, Andrew Graeme Divett, Stephanie DuFresne, Howard Robin Eastcott, Rex Douglas Faulknor, Robert John Fearon, Philippa Constance Flavell (Wylde), Helen May Gardyne, Stephen Stewart Gibbons, Lesley Claire Gilbertson (Rothwell), Nigel

Leslie Gilchrist, Matea William Gillies, Allan Craig Grant, Samuel John Greaves, John James Guthrie, Noeline Anne Hammond (Tanner), Simon Edward Hammond, Timothy Michael Healy, Robert Weston Hill, Hamish MacGregor Holland, Clive Douglas Hunter, Peter Grant Johnston, Robert McLaren Jones, Tessa Elizabeth Jones, Richard John Kyngdon, Alistair George Leggat, Christopher Vaughan Leigh, Priscilla Leone, Coleen Jonanne Lewis (McKeay), David Sterland Loeber, Timothy Graham Lynskey, Ian Francis McCullough, John Melville McDougall, Robert Malcolm McIlroy, Richard John Mackay (Travelling Scholar 1974), Heather Thomasina Mackintosh, Alastair Donald Macleod, Peter Boyce John McLeod, Ian William McQuillan, John Brian Malcolm, Lorna Ageatha Martin, John Alexander Matheson (Rhodes Scholar 1975), Robert Douglas Maunsell, Michael John Robert Milburn, Rodger William Mills, Herbert James Montague-Brown, Anthony James Morkane, Marilyn Rae Mortimore (Mackinder), Marten Muis, Edmund Frith Newman, Susan Joyce Newton, Robert James Marshall Norman, Paul Gerard O'Brien, Russell William O'Neil, Victoria Ann Tomlinson Pearse, Thomas Matthew Peyton, Anne Maude Phillips (Heays), Lloyd Martin Phillips, Afzal Mohammed Rehman, Gayle Lynley Roberton (Holdaway), Kenneth Robert Romeril, Brian Colin Ross, Elizabeth Jane Round (Chapman), John Melville Wellsted Russell, David John Sage, Mark Neville Sanford, Peter Richard Imlay Saunders, Martyn Robert Seay, James Henry Farquhar Shaw (MD 1986), Marc Timothy Malcolm Shaw, Douglas Hilton Sherwin, Murray William Smith, Victoria Jane Smith (Smeeton), Denis Walter Steeper, Paul Haydn Stephens, Gregory Dawson Taylor, Robert John Utley, Graeme Douglas Wards, Alastair William James Watt, Michael John Whitwell, Anthony Russell Wiles, Brian Norman Wills, Patricia Margaret Yelavich (Gallagher)

1975

Richard Hugh Acland, Christopher Howard Alldred, John Douglas Armstrong, Christopher Hugh Atkinson, James MacKenzie Aubrey, John Richard Baker, Philip James Barnes, David Michael Benson-Cooper, David Lloyd Bird, Barnett Roy Bond, Anthony John Bouckoms, Andrew Charles Rumbold Bowker, Lynley Margaret Brown, Heather Lesley Calder (Burnett), Clive David Bremner Cameron, Robert Geoffrey David Campbell, Malcolm Ronald Curtis Capon, Simon James Carson, Deborah Leigh Carter (Antcliff), John Manley Carter, Melton Gordon Clark, John Samuel Cook, Gregor David Coster, Anthony Kevin Daynes, John Leonard Dewsbury, Christopher Mark Dominick, Edwin Brennian Dorman, David John Downey, Desmond Mark Epp, Karen Christina Evans (Moyle; Linde-Thomsen), Lindsay Ross Fieldes, Mark Robert Fraundorfer, Cherrie Ann Galletly (Smith), Duncan Charles Galletly (MD 2004), Brian Jonathan Gibson, William Gin (MD 1988), Louise Isabel Goldwater (Stockley), Adrian John Gray, Lorraine Hamilton Griffin (Smith), Derek Nigel John Hart (Travelling Scholar 1975) (Rhodes Scholar 1975), Fiona Ellen Hawker (Caldwell), Marie Madeleine Henderson (Geelen De Kabath), Simon John Hooton, Jeremy Hornibrook, Adrian Regnault Hunt, James William Jerram, Geoffrey Verne Johnson, Diane Valerie Jones, Annabelle Joy Kaspar (Babbage), John Hendy Kay, Peter Maurice Kempthorne, Peter King, Christopher Reuben Knight, Ramesh Lala, Elizabeth Jane Lange (Taylor), Helena Geraldine Lash (Wynniatt), Stephen Lillioja, Stephen Paul McCormack, Paul Lawrence McNamara, Alan John Mangan, Peter Manson, Murray Frank Matangi, Donald Maxwell Melville, Keith Edwin Menzies, John Charles Mercer, Nigel David Miller, Alistair Joseph Moffitt, Raymond Moore, Erin Juanita Moran, Kevin Alec Morris, Sandra Lee Morris (Swallow), Stuart Scott Mossman (MD 1989), Anne Florence Murphy (Hodgson), Vincent John Murphy, Philip Leigh Nairn, Guillaume Michael Newburn, Richard Oliver Nicol, Paul Stanley Noonan, Stephen James O'Flaherty, Neville Richard Palmer, Caroline Jane Parker, Vivienne Joan

Peterson (Carlton), Kathryn Mary Powell (Reynolds), Richard Desmond Price, Peter John Pryor, Deborah de Berri Quilter (Broadfoot), Margaret Anne Rawnsley (Burtenshaw), Richard Ronald Rax, Paul Raymond Revell, Roger Michael Reynolds, Vaughan Francis Richardson, Robert William Robertson, Peter Neville Robinson, Henk Roozendaal, Alexander Douglas Rutherford, Michael George Sargent, Michael Duff Short, Michael James Short, Donald George Simmers, Anthony Carl Smith, Gordon Stephen Smith, Grant Farrar Smith, Andrew Duncan Spiers, Robin Stephen, Donald Edward Stewart, John Peter Sumich, Janice Clare Swindells (Hay), Barry James Taylor, John Stanley Vercoe, Albert Willem Vorstman (Ch.M. 1988), Lester Alan Walton, Ross Wilfred Warring, Martin Lyth Watt, Richard Kenneth Watt, John McKenzie Weir, Albert Edward White, William Peter Widdowson, Colin John Wilson, Leona Fay Wilson, John Derek Wood, Antony Todd Young, David William Young, Douglas Kum Young, Rennie James Young

1976

John Burman Adams, Eileen Mary Allan, Peter Francis Allen, Robert Seymour Allison, John Royden Almond, Jennifer Lesley Andrewes (Percival), David Drummond Archibald, David John Arcus, Denis Raymond Atkinson, Grant Roger Ayling, William Gordon Babe, Tony Ramon Bai (MD 1987), Roger Alexander Baillie, David Rhys Bassett, Spencer Wynyard Beasley, Graeme Paul Bennetts, Timothy Robert Bevin, Roderick Lloyd Bird, Michael John Borrie, David Bourchier, Noel Sydney Bourke, Eileen Anne Brosnan, Evan Christopher Brown, Richard Waldron Bunton, Stephen Thomas Chambers (MD 1990), Peter Chapman-Smith, Hamish Alister Charleson, Richard James Chisholm, John Vincent Conaglen (MD 1985), Gillian Mary Corbett, Andrew Cressett Corser, Ian Allan Cowan, Jonathan Mark D'Arcy, Mark Davis, Colin Ding, Peter Richard Downey, Quentin John Durward (MD 1984), Charles Frank Farthing, Anthony John Ferris, Kelvin Robert Finlay, John Sixten Fisher, Vincent Allan Friend, Stephen Alexander Gardner, Jeffrey Ernest Garrett, Alison Heather Gaston (Bown), William Thomson Cramond Gilkison, Anthony Neil Graham, Lewis Stephen Gray, John Dean Greenwood, John Edgar Harman, Anthony John Haycock, Jacqueline Judith Ho (East), David Wallace Hope, Phillip Francis Hughes, Carl Theo Jacobsen, Krystyn Dayll Jensen, Kenneth McCrae Johnson, Graeme Kenneth Johnstone, Larry Alexander Jordan, Stuart Kennedy, Peter John Kershaw, Mark Odtarm Lee, Ann Maree Leonard (Holland), Trevor Ian Lloyd, Iain Stuart Loan, Andrew John Logan, Brigid Mary Loughnan, David Scott Low, John Rarity McCreanor, Donald Mark MacKenzie, Michael David McKenzie, Bruce John McLeod, Helen Jean Mansfield (Moriarty), Keith Frederick Maslin, Neil Bernard John Matson, Grant Royden Maxted, Suzanne Valerie Mazey (McDiarmid), Edward William Mee, Julie Patricia Mellor, Jeffrey Thomas Miller, Trevor James Mitchell, Alexander Moreland, Roger Morgan, Christopher John Moughan, Robert John Moyle, Jan Catherine O'Brien (Reeves), Geoffrey Edward Olsen, Steven John Reuben Patchett, Ian Malcolm Petersen, Jennifer Pauline Pilgrim (Travelling Scholar 1976), Felicity Anne Plunkett, Robert John Reekie, Mark Langdon Robertson, David John Rowe, John Roy, Robert Andrew Sapsford, Dianne Margaret Sharp, Eugene Sherry (Hartley), Jillian Mary Sherwood, Graeme Bruce Skeggs, John Lawrence Smale, Ian Charles Smith, Derek Frank Snelling, Gillian Anne Spark (Stonelake), Gregory Durham Spark, Elizabeth Moira Stella Stein (Iost Alcalde), Richard Strawson Stubbs (MD 1985), Ian Douglas Sullivan, John Tangney Sullivan, Christopher Howard Thomas, Bryan John Thorn, Antje Johanna van der Linden, Geoffrey Henry James Vause, John Geoffrey Walker, John Charles Welch, Philip White, Jonathan Andrew Dowling Whitty, Charles Frances Williams, David Scott Williams, Alastair Kennedy Wilson, Janice Marjorie Wilson, Martin Alexander Wilson, Dennis Wong, Michael Ivan Yee, Stephen Kum Young, Rex Maurice Yule

1977

Michael William Thomas Alexander, Simon John Alexander, David Stanley Allen, Nigel Graeme Anderson, Anthony John Appleyard, Randal Garth Bailey, Denise Anne Baker, Thomas John Baster, Graeme Winston Bishop, Neil Buddicom, Sandra Janette Byers (Dinihan), Andrew Colin Lindsay Campbell, Peter Laurence Catt, Roderick Hanbury Chisholm, John Montague Chrisp, Richard John Christie, Malcolm John Clark, Colin James Conaghan, Graham Petersen Cooke, David John Cox, Lyndall Jean Crampton, Paul William Crone, Ross Gerard Denton, Anne Elizabeth Dick (Walsham), Alan Alexander Drage, Harry Kingsley Dye, Colin Harold Dykes, Paul Frederick Freeman Egden, Ross Malcolm English, Eoin David Fehsenfeld, Albert John Feisst, Prudence Linley Field, Hilda Marie Firth, Simon John Fleming (MD 1988), Jeremy Michael Foley, Garry Vernon Forgeson, Kevin Douglas Forsyth (MD 1990), Elizabetha Westerbeek Galloway (Van Eerten), Paul Donald Galloway, Neil Denis Garbett, David John Geard, Peter William Gendall, David Francis Gerrard, Francis Dominic Gilchrist, Robert Farrer Gilmour, Richard Warwick Gorringe, Robyn Mary Goss (Hunt), Frances Margaret Greaves (McDowell), Ronald Lindsay Griffiths, Keith Grimwood, Christopher Alan Gross, John Zsolt Gyenge, Peter Mark Hanan, Brian William Thomas Hanning, Suzanne Margaret Hayde (Senior), Roy Haywood, Sandra Jill Hicks (Meldrum), Mark Kirby Holland, Lauree Arlene Hunter, Philip Rowan Hyde, John Chirnside Hyndman, Grahame Sanderson Inglis, Rosemary Ann Johnston, Janice Mary Frances Jolly (Elliott), Murray John Judge, Christian Kalderimis, Michael Leslie Huriwai Karetai, Gabrielle Mary Keating, John David Kennelly, Myrto Tattaraki Kenny, Russell Edwin Kiddle, Brett Lee Krause, Petronella (Elly) Maria Kroef, Karin Elizabeth Lamb, Richard Oliver Lander, Kevin Ross Lee, David Ronald Alexander Leonard, Stephen Laurence Lewis, David Gordon Lichter, Jonathan Lloyd Lichter, Pamela Heather Lyttle (Broadbent), Christopher Neill McEwan, Simon Patrick McGuire, Kevin John McKerrow, Anthony Stuart McLean, Helene Margaret MacNab, Clifford Paul Mason, Maurice Dominic Matich, Stephanie Mary Matich, Margaret Moira Metherell, Roy Warwick Morris, Brian Patrick Mullan, Neil Douglas Munro, Colin Trevor Myers, John Norman Nacey (MD 1987), Ernest Narodetsky, David Stewart Howard Nicholls, Sandra Elizabeth Oates (Webb), Roger Simon Strachan Parr, Rosemary Anne Pedley (Bunn), Henry John Poczwa, Simon David Prior, Brian Robert Quick, Lewis John Randal, Shirley Margaret Rawstron (Hayward), David Alexander Ritchie, Bridget Anne Robinson (Travelling Scholar 1977) (MD 1987), Richard Garth Robinson, Richard Austin Robson, Bevan Lloyd Rogers, Brett Lachlan Rogers, Dawn Lesley Ross (Miller), David Peter Sampson, Brent Stephen Savage, Alison Margaret Scandrett (Forbes), Gary Raymond Seifert-Jones, James Stanley Shanks, Harvey Dickwin Wai Shing, Murray John Sinclair, Pauline Therese Smale (Daly), John James Smalley, Colin Leonard Smith, Peter Roland Francis Sparks, Graeme Paul Spry, Hans Robert Stegehuis, Anne Elizabeth Stephenson (Reynolds), Ian David Stewart, William Hedley Taine, Murray Donald Taylor, Donald Henry Theobald, Jane Laura Thomson (Batchelor), Murray Bruce Thorn, Robin Deborah Suzanne Treadwell, Richard Neil Tremewan, Beatrix Christina Treuren, Ian Murray Turfus, Geoffrey Alan Lindsay Turner, John William De Vries, Christopher Hereward Wake, Paul Richard Wanty, Maxine Judith Watson (Inglis), Stewart John Wells, John Robert Whittaker, Peter Wilkinson, Gail Williams (Phillips), Helen Patricia Williams (Loan), Roger Denis Wilson, Roger Lennox Kirkland Wilson, Timothy James Wilson, Poleon Yee, David Kenneth Young, David William Young

1978

Melanie Susan Mary Abernethy, John Leonard Ayers, Jill Elizabeth Baird (Sheaks), Graeme William Balch, Colin Stuart Barber, Kathryn Elizabeth Barber (Barnett; Crosier), Barry John Barnes, William Henry Barnes, John Theodorus Louis Beaumont, Alison Frances Begg, Sheril-Ann Bendall (Wilson), Paul Charles Bennett, Philip George Bobby, Philip Merrifield Borrie, Russell Grant Bourchier, David Ralph Bowie, Lorraine Agnes Broad (Welch), Raewyn Alice Brockway, Bronislawa Maria Brooks (Zazulak), David Ian Brougham, Henare Renata Broughton, Sally Lenise Buchan, Geoffrey Robert Buckett, Gerald Burgess, Geoffrey Charles Bye, Christopher Stewart Calder, Michael Andrew Caughey, Craig Gavin Cherry, Simon Ernest Chin, Vivienne Anne Clark (Aarons), Michael Hugh Cleary, David James Colquhoun, Jennifer Jocelyn Cook (Couper), Trevor Graham Cook, Richard Thomas Lee Couper, Fay Janet Craig (Woolfield), John Adrian Crawshaw, Jacqueline Anne Cripps, Alison Jane Crisford (MacDonald), Ian George Crozier (MD 1988), Brett Delahunt (MD 1995), Joanna Delahunt (Dabbs; MacDonald), Andrew Sutherland Dickie, John Doran, Crawford James Hood Duncan, Robert John Ebert, Andrew James Edwards, John Randal Elliott, Gerard Charles Fairhall, Stephen Matthew Fallow, Stephen James Faulkner, Kevin Barry Fitzsimons, Jeremy Aylwin Foate, David William Glasson, Nina Catherine Gresson, John Stanley Groom, Anne Denise Guy, Christopher Hartley, Glenn Arthur Hayward, Diane Christine Hodges (Jones), Bernard Keith Holmes, Gary John Hooper, Alison Jean Jenkin (Moore), Thomas Michael Jenkin, Peter Stuart Johnston, Peter Richard Joyce (MD 2005), Marjan Kljakovic, Mohan Parbhu Lala, Gail Houng Lee (Wong), Diane Marie Leighton, Jennifer Susan Lewis (Wren), Hugh David Lovell-Smith, Richard Andrew Luke, David William Lyon, Graham Macdonald, Neil John McHugh (MD 1989), David Wilson Mann, David Frank Cadman Mason, Rua Roxane Mercier, Alister Hugh Miller, David Hugh Miller (MD 1988), Stella Ruth Milsom (Monk), John Martin Monash, Stephen Richard Munn (Travelling Scholar 1978), Elizabeth Eli Nannestad, Phillip John Noble, David Joseph O'Connor, Kaye Dallas Ottaway, Mary Carmel Owens, Richard Hamilton Washbourne Parker, Lynette Ann Pascoe, Richard Edward Perry, Mary Kathryn Pinfold (McLean), Enid Pugmire, Susan Ruth Hamilton Pullon, Roselyn Winifred Quick (Parker), Michael Andrew Raynes, Darag Stuart Rennie, Arthur Mark Rennie (MD 1986), Simon Glenn Riddell, Susan Beatrice Roberts, Ian Graham Robinson, Jeffrey Mark Robinson, Timothy Sean Kirshaw Rooke, Philippa Margaret Rumble (MacKay), Christopher Gerard Ryan, Peter Lindsay Sandin, Murray Sheriff Shaw, Helen Elizabeth Shiach, Fiona Mary Smaill, Jillian Margaret Smith (Warlow), John Pattison Smyth, Nicholas Adrian Staats, Andrew Benjamin Stewart, Glenn John Sutcliffe, John Campbell Sutherland, Boyd Anthony Swinburn (MD 1994), Huta Tangaroa, Janice Mae Tate (Sargent), Neil John Thomson, Robert Raymond Van Rij, Alan Ronald Walker, Susan Elizabeth Walthert-Divett, Alistair Burns Watson, Geoffrey James Welsh, Gerard Thomas Wilkins, Hamish John Wilson, Nigel John Wilson, Sonny Jen Hong Wong, Nicholas Fawcett Woolfield, Peter Raymond Woolford, David John Wylie; MD: Norman McIlrath James

1979

David Alexander Abernethy, Peter Adam, Vasanthi Selvarani Arulambalam (Bradley), Charles Richard William Beasley, Alison Joy Belton (King), Catherine Joan Belton (McArthur), Gillian Frances Bishop, Janet Mary Blackman, Glenn Clifford Blanchette, Bruce Blyth (MD 1989), Joanne Marie Bowler (Thornton), John William MacDonald Boyd, Garry Robert Brian, David Michael Broad, Roger James Franklin Brown, Mark Anthony Oakley Browne, Diana Kim Hill Burgess, Wayne Elliot Butt, Peter Richard Cameron, Eleanor Margaret Carmichael (Lamb), Malcolm John Carmichael, Grant Thomas Carr, Mark Henry Chapman, Timothy Irving Christmas (MD 1993), Anne Melton Clark, Michael John Cleary, Lee Torine Coleman, Hugh Shackleton Cooke, Shane Patrick Cross,

Martin Campbell Davis, Denis Charles Delany, Ian James Dinihan, Joanne Wendy Dixon, Ian Alfred Duncan, Angela Joan Dunlop (Towler), Robert John Dunlop, John Michael Elliott, David Michael Ewen, Margaret Jane Fairhurst, Keith Charles Fay, Peter Finlayson, Sydney Ross Fitzsimons, John Murray Fleischl, Peter Charles Fleischl, Brigid Anne Forrest (Moriarty), Alastair William Fraser, John Kerswell French, Richard Anthony Galea, Guy William Forbes Gardiner, Helen Elizabeth Gilson (Carter) (MD 1995), Ian Amos Glass (MD 1991), Rodney Graeme Gordon, Susan Mary Gordon, Helen Frances Grace (Crampton), Joan Selina Green (Buckingham), Jo-Anne Guy (Reynolds), Martin Frederick Harris, Leon George Heron, Jean Lesley Herron, Hamish Renwick Hilson, Christopher Michael Holdaway, Mary Majella Holden (McSherry), York Nien-Hsiung Hsiang, Richard John Hursthouse, Geoffrey Mark Insull, Timothy John Insull, Franklyn Jay Ives, Christine Mary Jackson, Kathryn Elizabeth James, Richard Gerard Janus, Lewis Main Johnson, Sharleen Kay Johnston, Kenneth David Jolly, Ronda Verina Jolly, Colin Edmund Jones, Lissa Elaine Judd, Louise Ann Kane, Matthew Gerald Kenealy, Brian Donald King, Bruce Willfred Kirkham (MD 1991), Anthony James Reid Kriechbaum, Robert Ernst Guenther Kusel, Santi Parbhu Lala, John Alan Lambe, Bruce Malcolm Lintern, Gillian Elspeth Logan (Morris), Anthony Brears Lynch, Lindsay John McBride, Alison Jane McFarlane (Slattery), Kenneth Robert McFarlane, Frances Margaret McGrath, Peter Francis McKernan, Mark James McLaughlin, Gerald Jonathan Maclaurin, Jioji Tuwai Yacomaikilakeba Malani, Russell George Meads, Tracey David Meech, Carole Anne Millichip, Carol Anne Mitchell (Veale), Alexandra Deborah Moore, Aynsley David Adair Moore, Mark Ronald Jenkins Morris, Wayne D'Arcy Morris, Jann Isabel Muggeridge (Singer), Russell Alec Eric Muirhead, Geoffrey Martin Nichol, Robert Marama Teika-Moeaua Nicholas, Patricia Mary O'Brien, John Liston O'Donnell, William Dalton Olds, Robert Benjamin Greenslade Oxner, David Victor Le Page, Philip John Polkinghorne, Marion Rosalind Poore, Robin Pratt, Brendon Geoffrey Rae, Sudhindra Narayana Rao, John Dereck Antony Richmond, Duncan William Roberts, Patricia Leigh Robertson, Glenys Norma Round (Bennett), Grant Leonard Russell, David Schroeder (Travelling Scholar 1979), John Paul Scott (MD 1991), Francesca Sewell (Kelly), Debra Leone Sharp, Graham James Sharpe, Michael John Dennistoun Shaw, Philip John Shoemack, Michael John Sim, Paul Quirinus Smeele, Sara Mayne Smeeton, Sandra Elizabeth Staples (Rattenbury), Paul Wesley Stenberg, James Tear Stewart (MD 1991), Catherine Beryl Stone, Katherine Dana Stone, Jan Swinnen, Gillian Henton Tate (McCalman), Murray Campbell Thorburn, Deborah Jane Thornton, Joanna Mary Thwaites, Michael Robin Tills, Elizabeth Ann Tobin (Millow), Gillian Mary Trebilco (Brown), Patrick Gerald Tuohy, Brenda Mary Turner (Carlisle), Kevin Edward Tyree, Sally Elizabeth Anne Urry (Higgs), Andrew George Veale, Peter Tony Vujcich, Murray Edward Wackrow, Robert James Walker (MD 1990), Mark Bradford Watts, Mark Wilson Ian Webster, Athol Umfrey Wells (MD 1998), Davinia Marion White, Jonathan Beauchamp Wilcox, Christine Margaret Williams, Christine Wendy Williamson (Budd), Michael Francis Willis, Margaret Lesley Wilsher (MD 1989), Glenys Margaret Wilson (Weir), Rachael Joan Wilson, Janice Helen Windsor, Helene Margaret Winter (Pearson), Derek Wong, Marisa Moana Wong (Stevenson), William Wong, Elizabeth Anne Worsnop, Christopher Carlisle Wright, Mark Stephen Wright, Brendan Davidson Yates, Stephen Paul Young

1980

Timothy Robert Akroyd, Bruce Cashmore Allen, Janet Margaret Allwood (O'Reilly), Brent William James Anderson, Brian Joseph Anderson, Geoffrey John Anderson, Neil Bryce Averis, Susan Joan Ballantyne (Fancourt), Alison Margaret Barthow (Vogel), David Charles Bawden, Simon James Baxter, Tammy Elizabeth Haynes Beadel (Eaton), Sue Lorraine Belgrave, Clive John Bensemann, Mark Edward Bevin, Dennis Boon von Ochssee, Elizabeth Mary Bostock (Narbey; née Ross), Catherine Zoe Bourke, Michael Frank Bradley, Susan Kiddle Brann (Bennett), Debra Jan Bromiley, Peter John Browett (Travelling Scholar 1980), Jane Bridget Buckley, Thomas Anthony Buckley, Peter James Burn, Nicola Frances Carey, Julia Merle Carr, Ian Warwick Chambers, Jonathon Hinton Peter Chambers, Sulochana Anjali Chand, Sydney Bernard Choy, David Michael Coleman, Peter Richard Coleman, Christopher Charles Collins, Timothy John Cookson, Michael Martin Corkill, John Peter Coughlan, Grant Nigel Coulter, John Howard Coverdale (MD 2004), Robyn Dorothy Crighton, Anne-Marie D'Arcy Cullen (Williamson), Ian William Dallison, Richard Norman Davis, Peter Bernard Didsbury, Leone Esther Dillon (Rankin), Keith Michael Downer, Mavis Joy Duncanson, Ross Henderson Dysart, Gordon Arthur Eckert, Antony Spencer Edwards, Shan Edwards, Dawn Elizabeth Elder, Bruce William Eyers, Richard Robert Faris, Michael James Fisk, Timothy George Fletcher, Christine Margaret Foley, Christopher Henry Fox, Alan Gordon Fraser (MD 1994), Barbara Mary Fraser (Lane), Geoffrey Graham Fraser, Graeme Thomas French, Mark Gary Gazley, Michael Haigh Glen, Paul William Glue, Linda Margaret Graham (Wixon), Patrick Bernard Grant, Benjamin Vincent Gray, James Philip Gray, Stewart James Hastie, Philip Louis Hazell, Helen Elisabeth Heslop (MD 1990), Michael Hodges, Leigh Ann Hooper (Nightingale), Allan Neil Hopkins, Linda Ann Howell (McHugh), John David Hudson, Michael Howard Hunter, John Lewis Hutchison, Jennifer Jean Johnson-Barrett, Rodney Bert Keillor, Timothy William Kenealy, Richard James Kenner, Julie Edith Kidd (Collins), Julie Kimber, Joseph Michael Kirk, Michael Frederick Klaassen, Christine Lacy, Christine Lynette Lambie, Sally Jane Langley, Anne Brigid Lavin (Simpson), Christine Alison Laws, Alison Elizabeth McAlwee, Gillian Mary McBreen (Churchman), Alan Ross McCormack, Stephen Allan McGregor, Nicholas Paul McIvor, Nicola Anne McKay (Hendtlass), Donald George McKirdy, Robert Malcolm Stuart McLean, Quentin Charles MacMurray, Andrew Graham McNab, Fiona Marion McQueen, Lyndell Anne Maher (Gibson), Wendy Anne Maidment, Donald Paschal Matheson, Alan Crawford Meads, Prudence Anne Miller (Murdoch), Thomas David Milliken, Frederick Paget Milsom, Mark Harold Moore, Ishavar Morar, Christine Maree Morgan, Christine Elizabeth Moss, Roger Tony Mulder, Henry George Murray, Hamish John Cunningham Neill, Turi Mark Osborne, Terissa Anne Page, Thomas George Palfi, Martin Clive Palmer, David Charles Parker, Rhonda Wendy Patterson (Holmes Turner), Brendon Edward Pauley, Helen Marie Phillips (Richardson), Prudence Mary Pullar, Glenn Norman Richards, Christopher Horace Ridings, John Philip Riordan, John Malcolm Riseborough, Helen Wilhelmina Rodenburg, Christina Margaret Rogers, Gordon Alistair Royle, Margaret Joy Sage, John Douglas Sellman, Ian King Shaw, Paul Jonathan Simmons, Jean Starling, Stephen, Rowan Elizabeth Stephens, Christopher Mawson Stewart, Nigel Lawrence Stewart, Graeme Edward Stokes, Richard John Street, Antony Graeme Svensen, Bruce John Taylor, Glynmor Trevor Thomas, Thomas James Thompson, Rosemary Jane Thomson (Fenwicke), Murray William Tilyard (MD 1995), Graeme Ronald Tingey, Jacqueline Louise Virtue, Lesley Marian Voss, Leonard Gordon Bruce Wakefield, Jayne Louise Ward (Leaper), Andrew Worrall Webster, Philip Alan Weeks, Jeremy Robert West, Philip John Weston, Lynette Elizabeth White (Hearn), Murray George Wiggins, Ross Gregory Wilson, Susan Prudence Wilson (Campion), Christopher John Wynne

1981

Margaret Clare Adams, Graham Adler, Ronald James Alcorn, Richard Spence Alexander, Matthew Newton Allen, Jean

Avery (Bowie), Kathryn Ann Elené Baddock (Lipscombe), Jeremy James Squires Baker, Katherine Frances Bayston, Richard John Beedie, James Edward Trevor Beetham, Peter Stephen Bergin (MD 1995), Peter Bruce Bethwaite (Travelling Scholar 1981), Dianne Grace Bluett (Hollis), Brent Patrick Boon, Gabrielle Mary Brown (Ruben), Stephen David Brown, Joseph John Brownlee, Cheryl Ruth Brunton, Grant Noel Buxton, Ruth Ngaire Carter, Linda Mary Chaffey (McKillop), John Lloyd Chapman, Sally May Chartres, John William Arnold Cheesman, Kenneth Fredrick Clark, Hugh Oswald Clarkson, David Peter Clews, Ivan Frank Connell, Catherine Helen Cooper, Denise Cooper (Symonds; Dalziel), Judith Alice Corkill (Stone), Edward Paul Coughlan, Brian Cox, Joseph Gerard Craig, Tony Norman Crutchley, Peter James Trolove Davidson, Gavin Michael Davis, Anthony James Doyle, Raymond Deane Drew, Christopher Graeme Duffy, Margaret Fisher, Karen Patricia Flamank (Wood), Julie Margaret Fletcher, Peter James Foley, Andrea Margaret Forde, Richard Anthony Franklin, Sirovai Fuatai, David Alan Galler, Alastair James Gibson, Tony Gin (MD 1992), Philip Michael Gluckman, John Charles Goldsmith, Catherine Mary Hadley, Nicholas David Hanna, Mark Philip Hawken, Lesley May Hawkins, Spencer Charles Heald, Seton John Henderson, Mark Scott Henley, Jane Christine Henrys, Henry Andrew Herbert, Peter Allenby Herbert, Christopher Denis Hill, Timothy Richard Hitchings, Richard Derek Hudson, Gregory Brian Hunt, Brian Ian Hyland, Mark Andrew Irwin, Amanda Helen Isdale, Philip Mark Jacobs, Jonathan Nicholas Jarman, Grahame Mark Jeffery, Michael Lloyd Jenkinson, Mark Alistair Johnston, Jennifer Anne Jones, Ian James Kelso, Mark Patrick Kennedy, Robert Ross Kennedy, Gavin John King, Lise Mary Stewart Kljakovic (Scott), Marko Kljakovic, Antony Robert Koerbin, Donald Corrie Lake, Bruce Stuart Lambie, Heather Lawson, Denis Kai Fong Lee, Barry Denison Lewis, Anne Marguerite Liddell (MacVicar), Patricia Margaret Alison Liddell (Ritchie), Andrew Long, Jeffery Stuart Louitt, Graham Spencer Loveridge, Glenys Kay Lowe, Stuart Grant Lydiard, Lesley Jane McDougall, Alistair Roy McGregor, Murray Fraser MacKay, Alan James McKenzie, Peter John McKenzie, James Gerard McKevitt, Don Graeme McLeod, Reta Mary McLeod, Simon Francis McMahon, Brett Stuart Mann, Maureen-Anne Meates (Meates-Dennis), Ernestine Margaret Chryshanthie de Mel (Cabraal), David Richard Mercier, Lars Jorgen Koefoed Molving, Peter James Moore, Suzanne Patricia Morris, Jayanti Mudaliar (Teh), Blair John Munford, Kerry Elizabeth Neilson, Sally Jane Newell, Emiel Christopher Neynens, Helen Denise Nicholson, Eleni Nikolau (Clews), Alan Edward Norrish, Fiona Mary North, Patrick Myles O'Connor, Lynne Maree Anne O'Donnell (Tonks), Therese Siobhan O'Donnell, Paul Lawrence O'Gorman, Robin John Olds, Malathi Pasupati, Nalini Patel (Hira), Murray David Patton, Ruth Anne Pearson (Brown), Ian David Penny, Mark Kingston Peterson, Christopher James Pottinger, Lynn Margaret Price, Catherina Elisabeth Maria Pronk (Karen), Ruth Annette Quinney, Wendy Jane Rae (Busby), Deborah Anne Read, Barry Gordon Reeve, Sandra Meryl Rhind, Brent Vincent Richards, Margaret Elinor Rind (Robinson), Justin Alan Roake, Christopher Ian Robinson, David George Robson, Murray Robert Robson, Toby Francis Rose, Janet Simpson Saunders, Paul William Schimmel, Belinda Mary Denise Scott, Paul Arthur Searle, Christopher Jon Seeley, Maithili Sellathurai (Pasupati), David William Shaw, Timothy Gordon Short (MD 1993), Allan James Simpson, Elizabeth Ruth Simpson (Ridgen), Jennifer Anne Simpson, Lorraine Clare Smith (Bright), Rebecca Morton Smith (Henderson), Hans Theodoor Eduard Snoek, Veronica Anne Spencer, Gordon Robin Spooner, Odette Wilhelmina Spruyt, Diana Staniforth, Julie Dawn Steele, Maryanne Robina Stemmer, Ralph Alan Huston Stewart (MD 1993), Caroline Marjorie Stone (Corkill), Lydia Sulima-Rogaczewskia, Nigel Purcell Tapper, Lochie Rodrick Teague, Ian Armstrong Thomson,

George Ian Town, Janet Catherine Turnbull, John van Dalen, Anthony Clifton Van Der Oest, Deborah Jean Verran, Peter Robert Wall, Anne Elizabeth Sumner Walsh (MD 1995), Margaret Anne Wanty, Jonathan Hugh Warren, Stephanie Elise Weinrauch, Elizabeth Marion Whitcombe, Andrew MacLachlan Wilson, Philip John Wiren, Bruce Jen On Wong, Colin Stephen Wong, Lincoln William Wong, Victor Wong, Philip Clive Wood, Graeme Clifford Wright; ChM:, William John Gillespie; MD: David Kirkpatrick

1982

Richard Mark Adcroft, Kathryn Jane Aitken, Jacqueline Sherburd Te Makahi Allan, Derek Norman Allen, Timothy John Anderson (MD 2002), Nicola Cecile Austin, Angus Talbot Baird, Wame Raratabu Baravilala, Antoinette Alma Bearman, Sean Jeremy Beehan, Christopher Dennis Stanley Boberg, Michael William Carston Booth, James Howard Borthwick, Sharon Elizabeth Brinsdon, Keith Frederick Brockway, Raymond McWilliam Bruce, Timothy Michael Buckenham, Alastair Gordon Buckman, John Francis Cameron, Quentin Robert Stuart Cameron, Derek Colin Campbell, Robert David Carpenter, Annie Chen-Green, Harsed Hiralal Chhima, Susan Marion Clark, Jonathan Bernard Cleary, Jennifer Helen Clifton (Nicholson), Christopher Paul Cochrane, Nicholas William Louis Cochrane, Gary Collinson, Paul Alfred Corwin, John Patrick Cosgriff, Marjory Jean Craig, Dwayne Edward Nicol Crombie, Sally Anne Davidson, Helen Anna Davies, Jonathan Charles Davies, Mary Phillipa Davison, Brian John Deavoll, Simon Mark Dempsey, Catherine Rose Dobbie, Alexander Steven Donn, John Ranald Elliot, Andrew Donald Fairgray, Shanthi Neranjana Fernando (Ameratunga), Deborah Mary Kaye Gilbert (Proverbs), Peter John Gilling, Paul William Glover, Benjamin Joseph Goddard, Nell Belinda De Graaf, Mark Hilary Gray, Normal McLeod Gray, Wendy Ann Gray, Alistair Jan Gunn, Pamela Alison Hale, Roger Michael Owen Hall, Susan Hallwright, Margaret Shiell Hamilton, Ross Alistair Henderson, Kerry Denis Hennessy, Robert Stanley Hepburn, Judith Ann O'Brien Heyworth (O'Brien), Ruth Margaret Highet, Christopher Healy Hobson, Barbara Eva Hochstein, Charles John Perry Hollings, Andrew Cedric Holmes, Beverly Dawn Hopkins (Smith), Stephen John Houston, David Ormond Hutchinson, Peter Martin Jansen, David Lewis Jardine (MD. 2004), David Alan Jenkins, Guy Philip Jenner, Peter Arthur Benjamin Johnson, Peter Ormond Johnstone, Richard Geoffrey Keddell, John Myles Kenealy, Paul Kerdemelidis, Ziyad Khouri, Denis Robert King, Stephen Maxwell Kyle, Euan Ronald Laird, Neil Keith Lambie, Geoffrey Euan Laney, Gareth John Laws, David Alexander Lawson, Mark Robert Leadbitter, Bruce Kenneth Lockett, Julian Argus Lofts, Ian Robert Lord, Stephen Wilson Low, Anne Catherine Lowe (Campbell), John Lindsay McCall (MD 1993), Hylton Greig McCormick, Mark James McKeage, William Alexander MacLaurin, Andrew Ian McLeod, Anne Elaine McNamara (Lord), Peter Anthony McSweeney, William Paul McSweeney, Raewyn Julie Mair, Brigette Mary Meehan, Patrick James Meffan, Philippa Mary Mercer, Andrew Peter Miller, Ross Irwin Mills, Mary Leigh Moore, Robert Mackay Morton, Vivienne Mary Mountier, Marea Wyn Murray (Fortune), Nigel John Murray, Charlie Ng, Kingsley Ng-Waishing, William Ross Nicholson, Susan Kay Nightingale, Lesley Unity Nutt (Joblin), Dermot Roderick Michael O'Connor, Mark Harold George Overton, Paul Hartley Owen, Philip Ralph Palmer, Stephen Geoffrey Palmer, Paresh Patel, Gordon Livingstone Patrick (Travelling Scholar 1982), Lynne Marie Penman (Lane), Paul David Peterson, Adrienne Jill Prestidge (Mills), Rodney Gerard Radich, David Bruce Rankin, Barbara Jean Richards (Hart), Sally Louise Rishworth (Hadfield), Peter Alexander Robertson (MD 1997), Sally Rosa Robilliard, John Leonard Rowland, Duncan Malcolm Roy, Vicki Louise Royfee (Robertson), Allison Bernice Ryan (Reuben), Susan Isobel Savage (O'Malley), Robert Scott Schmidli, Elizabeth Margaret

Scott, Helen Scott, Richard Seeman, Peter Herbert Christopher Sew Hoy, Jill Margaret Shepherd, John Peter Eugene Shepherd, Derek Robert Sherwood, Alexander Ian Frederic Simpson, Russell Bruce Smart, Brenda Elizabeth Smith, Penny Elizabeth Speary, Grant Matthew Spence, Timothy William Sprott, Dougal John Steel, Duncan Scott Stevenson, James Frederick Garaeld Stewart, Barbara Ann Stockdill (O'Connell), Dianne Stokes, Christopher Noel Strack, Nancy Jennifer Sturman (Rhodes Scholar 1983), Alexandra Elizabeth Styche, Valerie Anne Takas (Sharp; Howells), Laurence Sinclair Thomson, Christopher Kenneth Thorn, Spencer Ting, Peter Alistair Tomkins, Robyn Jennifer Toomath, Robert William Ure, Christina Hendrika van der Oest, Melissa Anne Wake, Madeleine Frances Wall, Karen Jennifer Wardill, Linda Susan Mary Wells, Allan James Wellwood, Andrea Claire Wheeler, Paul Stephen White, Jeffery Russell Wickens, Miles Grant Williams, Murray Lesley Williams, Kerry Robin Willoughby, Deborah Ann Wilson, Ian Robert Wilson, Ross Malcolm Wilson, Christopher Michael Wong, Frank Jen Toon Wong, James David Woodfine, Susan Margaret Young

1983

Rosemary Anderson, Mark Boyd Austin, Kim Katherine Badham (Pasley), Bartrum William Baker, Patricia Anne Bassett, John Samuel Beca, Mary-Anne Bellamy (Dunlop), Colin David Craig Bennett, Stephen James Best, Wilhelm Andreas von Biel, Michael Robert Brewer, Michael David Buist, John Gorrie Burton, John Patrick Richard Cantillon, Barbara Carran (Seeley), Judith Anne Chappell (Anson), Janine Hilda Close (Crofts), Jennie Lynne Connor, James Walter Corbett, Spencer John Craft, Ashok Dahya, Michael John Dally, Kathleen Mary Davey (Young), Christopher Robin Denz, Peter Andrew Devane, Rosemary Claire Dodd, Glenys Marie Dore, Carol Mary Elizabeth Douglas (Waugh), Nicholas Patrick Duffy, Paul Michael Duggan, John Douglas Dunbar, Hamish Carson Dunn, Richard Shane Dunphy, Anne Elizabeth Edwards (Brown), Mark John Elder (MD 1995), Richard Willis Everett, John Charles Fanning, Christopher Alan Fawcett, Catherine Ann Ferguson, Catherine Mary Ferguson, Michael Peter Neville Findlay (MD 1994), Martyn Donald Fisher, Paul Alexander French, Philip Martin Frost, James Douglas Fulton, Michael Robert Futter, Edward John Gane (MD 1998), Timothy Lindsay Gardner, Kevin John Giles, David Spencer Gilgen, Robyn Lynette Gough (Crow), Christopher Michael Graham, David Alexander Graham, Kerry Nevyne Gunn, Hugh Carl Hanger, Michael John Hardie Boys, Sophia Harris, Phillipa Jane Hay (Pile) (MD 1993), Lesley Anne Hoy, Alan Grant Huber, Christopher John Hughes, Dermot Sherbrooke Fitzmaurice Hurly, Bruce Valintine Jack, Catherine Gillian Jackson, Leslie Ian Johansen, Paul Laurence Johnston, Gerald Scott Johnstone, Christopher John Joyce, David Lempfert Kenealy, Ian Colin Stuart Kennedy (Travelling Scholar 1983) (MD 1993), Sharon Yiu-Lan King (Law), Suzanne Barbara Knapp, Ruth Lindsay Knowles, Erich Joseph Kusel, Rosemary Joan Laing, Paul Christopher Lane, David Ralph Leadbetter, Daniel James Lee, Amanda Tessa Lennon (Harlow), Ruth Yvonne Lennox, Philippa Hilary Leys, Shelley Lichter, John Duncan Little, Philippa Anne Loan, Peter Anthony Louisson, Clive John Scrimgeour Low, Kerryn Lesley Lum (Estall), Martin Elvis Lum, Hugh Donell McCabe, Bronwyn Joy McFarlane (Daniels), David Whitehead MacFarlane, Jennifer Ann McGechie, Neil Lyle Macindoe, David John Barron McKenzie-Pollock, Susan Mackersey, Simon Campbell Maclaurin, Neil Fraser Maclennan, Helen Margaret McMaster, Paul Murdo Macpherson, Selaima Likuvutia Malani, Lynda Ruth Malin, Stephen Dwight Mark, David Martin Markie, Wendy Nicola Marshall, Lasantha Martinus, John Francis Mathews, Richard Peter Mercer, Ashley Clinton Milne, Arthur James Morris, Graham Peter Morrissey, Dilip Kumar Naik, Jonathan Charles Nelson, Roy Nicholson, Liam Quinlan O'Connor, Ann Greenslade Oxner (Woods), David Anthony

Palmer, Gail Christine Pearson, Johan Peters, Ruth Pettengell, Kevin David Pile (MD 1994), Athula Keminda Polonowita, Satya Prakash, Stephen Harper Purchas, Arvind Ranchhod, Philippa Dianne Reeve, Andrew John Cheyne Reid, Ann Kathleen Richardson, David Leslie Robinson, Matthew John Robinson, James MacLean Ross, John Victor Russell, Sarah Anne Sawrey (McDonald), Helen Kathleen Sayer, Marina Dawn Sew Hoy, Susan Kathleen Shand, Robyn Anne-Marie Shaw (MD 1995), Trevor Ian Shum, Peter Graeme Barclay Sim, Beverley-Anne Singe (Lawton), Mark Stephen Slater, Alison Mary Smith, Catherine Louise Spencer (Spencer-Taylor), Bruce Dougal Stewart, Neal Robert Stewart, Marcus Kopell Stone, Colleen Elizabeth Surridge, Tala Taavao, Maelen Stanford Tongia Tagelagi, Robyn Matira Taikato, Peter David Tobin, Matthew Peter William Tomlinson, Frances Margaret Townsend, Jeremy Francis Tuohy, Susan Elizabeth Tutty (Tait), Lynn Usmar (Samuels), Kristine Ann van der Beek, Hendrik Eduward van Roekel, Stewart John Walsh, Joanne Mary Ward, Christine Alicia Ware, Donald Robertson Menzies Watson, Sarah Katherine Waymouth, Elizabeth Diane Couper Whyte, Timothy Rex Wilkinson, Brett Nicholas Wilson, Richard Scott Wilson, Terence David Wong, Duncan Alan Wood, Marianne Margaret Wood, Michael James Woodbridge, Russell Alan Wright (MD 1993), John William Wyeth (MD 1995), Kris Pik Yet Yee, David Riyyad Zarifeh, Peter Zink

1984

Malcolm James Abernethy, Richard Paul Aickin, Dallas Ann Alexander (Andrews), Michael Warne Ardagh, Susan Cresswell Ashe (Millard), David Lancelot Austin, David Edward Baldwin, Steven Marshall Bannister, Murray Lindsay Barclay (MD 1997), Janice Marie Barrett, David George Bathgate, Blair Douglas Bermingham, Timothy Killoch Blackmore, Alastair George Wattie Borwick, Peter Mark Boyd-Wilson, Peter Reid Bremner (MD 1996), Simon Paul Brokenshire, Nigel Ross Brown, Megan Beverley Bryan, Margaret Marie Phillips Bryant, William James Buchanan, Sarah Jane Buckley, John Robert Burnett (MD 2004), Michael John Burt (Travelling Scholar 1984), Andrew Arthur Burton, Alain Guillaume Carbonatto, Graeme George Carpenter, Simon Richard Edward Carter, Rosemary Nicola Chambers, Peter Timothy Chapman (MD 1997), Alan Chin, Kenneth Chin, Bruce Duncan Chisholm, Elizabeth Ann Christie, Simon Peter Clark, Michael John Clarke, Catherine Diane Collings, Gavin Maxwell Colthart, Bernard Douglas Coombs, Gordon Dean Coote (Millar-Coote), Richard John Coutts, Trudy Anne Cowley (Honore), Helena Louise Cox, Timothy Cummack, Eva Frances Currie, Ian James Currie, Peter von Dadelszen, Judith Ann Davis, Stephen Gerard Delany, Kalawati Magan Deva, Stephen Grant Duffy, Peter Roderick Dunbar, David Stewart Duncan, Gerard Martin Eagar, Jonathan David Eames, Thomas Bartlett Elliott, Evan Richard Everest, Simon Pascoe Ewen, Peretiso Faletoese, David Fearnley, Roderick Peter Ferguson, Peter Norman Gerald Fitzgerald, Elizabeth Jean Fitzmaurice (Tennent), Andrew Paul Forrest, Jocelyn Doreen Fougère (Heard), Russell Malcolm Fowler, Stephan Garry Foy (MD 1996), Susan O'Neill French, Philip Ivor Bruce Garden, Marianne Patricia Gardenier (O'Connell), Jane Gabrielle Gardner (O'Brien), Brenda Valerie Gibson, Kevin William Gilbert, Marc Louis Gimblett, Deborah Joy Goodall, Peter Robert Findlay Gootjes, Malcolm Keith Gordon, Cameron Charles Grant, Iain Lachlan Grant, Lynda Maree Gray (Stack), Allan Mark Griffiths, Peter Harvey Griffiths, Susan Lyndall Hamer, Paul Michael Hantz, Stephen Beaumont Harris, Graeme John Hart, Nicola Mary Hay, Tracey Claire Heads (MD 1992), Peter James Henderson, David John Hepburn, Andrew John Herbert, Andrew Alexander Hill, Christopher William Hoffman, Andrew Hugh Holden, Bruce George Honore, David Maitland Hough, Sandra Jan Ibbetson, David Arthur Sinclair Jackson, Grant Dale Jackson, Suzanne Alison Jackson, Alastair Blair Johnston, Ross John Keenan, David

McKenzie Kerr, Ngaire Margaret Kerse, Michael Richard King, David Edward Kirk (Rhodes Scholar 1985), John Michael de Langen, Andrew Stansfield Lawson, Malcolm Paul Lay, Christopher John Leaper, Timothy Joseph Linton, Anne Elizabeth Loughlin, Jeffrey Andrew Lowe, Alan Peter Luchie, John David McCartie, Dynes Tracey McConnell, Kirsten Kathleen McDonald (Gendall), John Mackenzie, Mark Donald McKenzie, Timothy Paul McKenzie, Mary Heather McPherson (MD 1995), Christopher James Mansell, Caroline Helen Maskill, Alistair Rodney Maxwell, Ursula Mayr, Russell Frederick Metcalfe, Jeremy Laurence Millar, Ian Malcolm Morison, Peter Graeme Morrison, John William Arnold Mulder, Lynette Mary Murdoch, Patricia Frances Neal, Ross Neville-Lamb, Richard Anthony Victor Newman, Luke Langston Newnham, Christopher Morris Nunn, David John Ross Napier Orsbourn, Michael James Partington, Ashwinkumar Kanji Patel, Graham Douglas Paterson, Beth Hamilton Pearson, Paul Baden Phibbs, Gregory Thomas Musgrove Phillipson, Narella Elizabeth Plant (George), Jocelyn Anne Poland (Murphy), Christopher William Prowse, Anthony Gerard Quinn, Nigel John Raymond, Donald James Riseborough, Gregory McBey Robertson, David Richard Rogers, William Blair Rhodes Rolleston, David Hugh Rollinson, William Rex Rowe, Christine Joy Rushton (Jackson), Rodney John Sayer, Christopher Edward Dennistoun Shaw (MD 1997), David Peter Shaw, Victoria Shirley Shaw, Lily Shue, Mark Bernard Simmonds, David Alan Sinclair, Harrinder Singh, John Faulkner Sligo, Bruce Andrew Small, Don Edward Smith (MD 1993), Timothy Stapleton Smith, Brian Andrew Soundy, Stephen, Timothy Charles Tasman-Jones, Colin Fraser Thompson, Stuart David Thomson, Paul Leonard Timmings, Alistair James Tulett, Annette Mary Turley (Collins), Christiaan Pieter van Oeveren, Paschasius Mathys Sier Vermunt, David Murray Voss, Colin Paul Wackrow, Mark Andrew Ward, Peter David Watson, Mark Weatherall, Teresa Marie West (Hunt; Kelly), Michael Vance Whiley, James Edward Thomas White, Martin Ross Whitehead, Mark Anthony Whittington, Timothy James Wilkinson, Christopher Prior Williams, Deborah Isobel Williams (Gibson), Forbes John Williams, Jerome Wladyslaw Wisniewski, Helen Margaret Wood, Leon Russell Wright, Michael Koi Young; MD: Lybus Chester Manning (Hillman)

1985
Margot Allen, Chanaka Amarasinghe, John Colin Rowland Arnold, Daphne Isabelle Austin, Emma Catherine Baird, Peter John Bannister, Miriam Ruth Barnett, Rosemary Anne Barnett, Anthony John Beaven, Stephen James Bentall, Valerie Clare Black (Woodfield), John Philip Joseph Bourke, John Campbell Brebner, William Lee Brown, Cameron Craig Rutherford Buchanan, David Howard Francis Buckley, Raffaela Angela Buonocore, David Patrick Burke, Robert Victor Carlson, Nicholas John Chamberlain, Michael John Chin, Sandhya Chunilal, Kevin Joseph Cleary, Penelope Gail Clifford, Anne Bernadette Condon, Lynley Ann Cook, Alison Margaret Craig, Peter Roy Crampton, David Matthew Dalziel, Gregory John Denny, Anne Maree Dibley, Leigh Shenton Duncan, Andrew Carson Dunn, Karleen Michelle Edwards, Matthew James Frazer Eggleston, Jeremy Charles Evison, John Clayton Fenwick, Francis Antony Frizelle, Linda Marie Garrett, Michael David Grubb, Peter Douglas Guy, Martin Antony Hadler, Andrew Warwick Hamer, Rachel Maryann Hardie Boys (Watters), Stewart Lowry Hardy, Murray Lennard Harty, Katherine Ann Hayes (Shaw), Matthew John Hills, David Lewis Hingston, Robin Leigh Holland, Charles William Hornabrook, Jennifer Ruth Hosking, Timothy Hou, Hamish Stevenson Howie, Martin Kent Hunn, Mary Louise Hutchinson, Karl Louis Rewi Jansen, Anne Louise Jaquiery, Kathryn Jane Jeffery, Simon Francis Charteris Jordan, Ichiro Kawachi, Gregory George King, Janet Elizabeth Kirby, Jennifer Lea, Joan Deborah Leighton (Moody), Robyn Jean McArthur, David Craig McCormick, Deborah Frances

MacFarlane, Anne-Thea McGill, Richard Graham McGrath, Iain Lachlan McLean, Stuart Bruce McNicoll, Derelie Ann Mangin (Richards), Kerry Jane Mannis (Skidmore), Colin Peter Marsland, Rhett Bennett Mason, Richard John Massey, Elizabeth Ann Middleton, Graham David Mills (MD 2006), Helen Joy Mills (Tricker; Tobin), Stephen Mathew Mills, Khalid David Mohammed, Stuart John Monk, Vinu Morar, Philip Neil Morreau, Bernadette Therese Mullin, David Roger Murdoch (MD 2002), Alister McKenzie Neill (MD 2005), Timothy Frank Ngan Kee, Rhoderick Gordon Nicholson, Christopher Jules Nihotte, Anthony Phillip Nixon, Diana Alison North, Batsile Maitshupo Nyoni (Matlhaga), Jason Charles O'Connell, Lianne Ruth Parkin, Naresh Parsotam, Neeraja Pasupati (Surendran), Sallyanne Tonya Patchett, Donald Colin Patterson, Alexander Stephen Philip, Garth Harcourt Poole, David James Porter, Barbara Louise Poskitt (Reiche) (MD 2002), Jane Sinclair Renwick, Anthony Peter Richards, Deborah Jane Robinson, Carole Anne Ross (Tancredi), Nicola Margaret Scott (Matthews), Jane Elizabeth Seeley, Geoffrey Mark Shaw, Nigel Ralph Skjellerup, Mark Patrick Smith, Verne Gullen Smith, Bruce Lou Solomon, Dereck James Souter, Paul Jeffrey Carlyle Stoddart, Michael Dashwood James Strettell, Michael James Sullivan, Christopher Sutcliffe, Beverley Anne Taylor (Mounsey), Colin Robert Thomas, John Hugh Joseph Thwaites, Fraser Caird Todd, Anthony Mark Tonks, Peter John Trye, Roelof (Ralph) Meindert van Dalen, Peter John Van Dyk, Phil Mary Elizabeth Waite, Christopher Morice Ward (Travelling Scholar 1985), Malcolm Robert Ward, Mark Jeremy Wardill, Scott William Wells, Erica Jayne White, Michael John Anderson Williams (MD 1999), Anne Catherine Wilson (Young), Christopher David Bruce Wisely, Conroy Allan Wong, Rodney James Wynne-Jones, Penelope Ann Wytenburg (Holmes), Alistair Arthur Young, Anis Yusuf; MD: Adrian Donald Hibberd

1986
Semisi Larkin le Tagaloa Aiono, Robert Paul Anderson, Susan Jane Argent, Jan Elizabeth Arnold, David Asboe, Garry James Barron, Justin Brian Barry-Walsh, Mary Philomena Basire, Leanne Carol Berkahn, Neville Patrick Andrew Berry, Robert Hank Beulink, Pradip Bhula, Thomas Arnim von Biel, Maria Johanna Anna Boers, Michael Robert Boland, Malcolm John Bollen, Brendon Douglas Bowkett, Louise Grace Boyd, Glenn Andrew Brennan, Colin Robert Scott Brown, Timothy Graham Buckleton, Neil James Bungard, Genevieve Marie Marguerite Carbonatto, Annabel Mary Carter, Michael Glenn Catton, Fiona Margaret Clendon, Kirsten Jane Coppell, Jonathan Charles Craig, Susan Veronica Crombie, Brendan James Daly, Dhammika Pradeepa Dassanayake, Michael John Davison, Andrew Stewart Day (MD 2002), Penelope Anne Day, Mark Christopher Devcich, Ann Marie Diggins, Ian David Dittmer, John David Dockerty, Michael Seymour Dray, Paul Anthony Ellis (MD 1997), Erica Jane Fairbairn, Sharron Ruth Flahive, Colin Fong, Richard James Fong, Nicholas Kinnear Foster, Grant James Freear, Stuart David Gardiner, Nicholas John Giblin, Ian John Goodwin, John William Goulden, David James Greening, Francis Thomas Hall, Anthony Hannah, Ruth Margaret Harkett, Andrew Alan Harrison, Peter Frank Noel Harrop, Murray John Hay, Anita Hegde, Allan Edward Herbison, Phillip Nicholas Hider, Catherine Grace Hill, Joanna Mary Phelps Hopkins, Mary Jane Houliston, Deborah Jane Ingham, Maki Ruston Mary Jagose, Malcolm John Armstrong Joblin, Kevin Young Kan, Brent Andrew Krivan, John Francis Kusel, Dean Matea Larkin, Jan Denise Lavery, Lance James Lawler, Philip Leadbitter, Malcolm Erskine Legget, Clement John Le Lievre, Timothy William Love, Janet Rose McDonald, Patrick James David McHugh, Kay Elizabeth McIntyre, Blair Richard McLaren, Andrew John McNeill, Dean Lawrence Mannis, Tearikivao Maoate, Jacques Renard Marchand, Craig Scott Marshall, Donna Maree Marshall, Ate Folole Moala, Peter Robert Montgomery, Justin

Stewart Mora, Alexander Keith Wright Morgan, Robert Ian Murphy, Garry Harold Nixon, Paul Stephen Norton, Timothy John O'Meeghan, Christina Clare Page, Jacqueline Therese Papesch (Jansen), Michael Eric Papesch, Kiran Patel, Adrian Leslie Pepperell, Tania Ann Phillips, Grant Bruce Pidgeon (MD 1996), Patricia Caroline Priest, Christopher John Read, Iain Charles Reid, Dominic Sean Riminton, Alison Gardner Ross, Grant Ryan, Mary Agnes Scanlon (English), Philip Peter Schroeder, Douglas Stanley Scott, Martin Robert Seers, Mary Jane Sneyd, Anthony James Stoop, Matthew Francis Strack, Jacqueline Maria Elizabeth Stumpel, Anna Joy Sullivan, Rohan Senaka Swaris, Apisalome Talemaitoga, Nevin William Taylor, Rajivini Mohana Thiruchelvam, Barry Ian Turner, Patricia Eleanor Van Kralingen, Jennifer Theresa Visser, Richard James Walsh, Duncan Wright Watts, Margaret Ann Weston, Anthony Campbell White (Travelling Scholar 1986), Philippa Lynne White (De Hamel), Agadha Crisantha Wickremesekera, Anthony Brendan Williams, Bridget Frances Williams, Hammond Gwyn Williamson, Philip Paul Wong, Andrew Francis Woodhouse, Robert Peter Young

1987

Gillian Mary Aburn, Stephen Andrew Aitken, Douglas John Annan, Michael Antoniadis, Susan Maree Bain, Giles Timothy Harding Bates, Murray John Beagley, Bryan William Robert Betty, Kelvin Wilson Gwynne Billinghurst, Philip Antony Bird, Robyn Joy Sawatski Blackhall (Webber), Jan Elizabeth Bone, Andrew John Bowers, Jan David Breward, Andrew John Broad, Cynthia Irene Buchanan (McQuillan), Noelyn Ann Buisman (Hung), Isabelle Catherine Jacqueline Carbonatto (Bowkett), Angus Martin Chambers, Margaret Helen Chavasse (Mollison), David Robert Harry Christie, Desmond Edward Chung, Andrew Charles Clark, Hilary Janet Cleland, Judith Ann Clemett, Judith Anne Collett, Jennifer Anne Cooke, Charlotte Maryann Cox, Susan Jane Creighton, Thomas Edward Currie, Fenella Jane Devereux (Duncan), Marshall Francis Antony Donnelly, Alan Michael Donoghue, Ngaire June Ellis, Gregory Miles Emerson, Geoffrey Michael Esterman, Ceri Lee Evans (Rhodes Scholar 1988), Susan Lesley Evans, Helen Jacqueline Fahey, Bernard Murdoch Fanning, Mark Andrew Featherston, David Wayne Ferrar, David Finlay, Rodger John Fitzgerald, Carolyn Gaye Fowler, Caroline Ann Gibb, Gillian Ruth Gibson, David Robert James Gill, Andrew Gin, Anne Marie Greening, Rowena Maria Gregoire (Poole), Diane Catherine Hampton (Young), Drusilla Susmita Harichandran, Christopher Richard Harman, Timothy Lee Hawkins, Beena Hegde, Andrew Millar Henderson, Joanne Claire Holdaway (McMaster), Penelope Anne Holdaway, Helen Patricia Holden, Richard Sidney Lewis Hornabrook, Graham William Johnston, Christopher Robert Johnstone, Nicholas Francis Jones, Nicola Alison Jordan, Christopher Peter Henry Kalinowski, Kaye Joanne Kehely, Sophia Kwan Mei Kennelly (Chan), Grant John Kiddle, Marie Samantha King, Arthur Richard Kitching (Travelling Scholar 1987), Jane Caroline Knowles (Couch), Nicholas David Lawn, Richard Michael Lloydd, Steven Raymond Low, Christopher David Lynch (MD 2004), Kirsty Dorothea McKellar, Wayne James McKenzie, Michael James MacKey, David Hector McLean, Seamus Vincent McNulty, Maletino Mafi, Andrew Mark Manning, Alana Marie Marshall (Wilson), Vicki Anne Martin, David Robert Matthews, Rina Mehrotra, Shawn Patrick John Millin, Janet Marie Moloney, Wendy Kay Morgan, Andrew Julius Chan Mow, Michelle Frances Mullin, Donald Alexander Munro, Sally Elizabeth Murdoch, Christopher John Murphy, Martha Payom Na Nagara, Gopinath Nayar, Ramesh Nayar, Stephen Genn Jueng Ng, Wayne Douglas Nicholls, Bart Nuijsink, Paul Andrew Ogilvie-Lee, Jennie Mary Oliver, Annabelle Jean Olliver (Claridge), David Colin Anthony Oxner, Jo-Ann Elizabeth Pahl, Amanda Carolyn Parkin, Gail Antonia Roshan Perera, Nicolette Lachlan Perkins, Susan Rachael Peters (Sutherland), Robert Grant Phibbs, Warren

Paul Pickering, David Robert Pickett, Dianne Heather Poad, Mythi Ponnapa, James Alexander Stuart Reid, Bastiankoralage Belinda Valerie Jayamaha Rodrigo, Graham Marshall Roper, Greig Kelman Gray Russell, Nicole Maya Sauerland (Anderson), Adrian Hamilton Secker, Mary Elizabeth Seddon, Margaret Susan Senvicky, Philippa Jane Michelle Shine, Glen Smith, Paul Laurence Snelling, John Gardner Speirs, Graham Sue, Sally Elizabeth Talbot, Paul David Taylor, Beven Telfer, Shane Martin Tibby, Paul John Albert Trott, Leanne Kaye Tyrie, Meiapo Tiui Uili (Schmidt-Uili), Christine Janice van Dalen, Gregory Paul Van Schie, Jan Marie Webber (Craik), Helen Margaret Weir, Robert Peter Weir, Robert David Wilks, Alexander Philip Williams, Brent Alan Williams, Nigel John Willis, Russell Peter Wills, Callum John Wilson, Rosalind Margaret Wilson, Stephen George Withington, Jeffrey Kwok Wah Wong; MD: Robin Fraser

1988

Louise Elizabeth Aldridge, Michael Liong Tiong Ang, Kerri May Angell, Richard Malcolm Byres Annand, Helen Maree Austin, Peter Mark Ayson, Peter Alan Barber, Sheryl Anne Barnes, Nicholas Soheil Bashir-Elahi, Kaye Jeannette Basire, Dominic Joseph Gerard Bell, Mark Andrew Beniston, Hugh Robert Loreburn Blackley, Gareth Lee Blackshaw, Douglas John Braithwaite, William Mark Bridgman, Mary Elizabeth Brooker, Stephen Grant Brown, Sarah Anne Bullen (Moss), Linda Catherine Burgess, Martyn Buyck, Robert Maxwell Campbell, Mark Geoffrey Clatworthy, Mark Robert Cohen, Birgit Dijkstra, Sandra Carol Dinsdale, Teresa Donnelly, Clare Mary Doocey, Ross Drake, Wendyl Jude D'Souza, Clare Marie Dudding, Gregory Lawrence Dunn, Mary Anne Faigan, Anthony John Farrell, Penaia Albert Faumui, Martyn Edwin Flahive, Lois Fong, John Stevens Fountain, Stephen John French, Tracey Jan Giddings, Gwyneth Elaine Graham, Howard Granger, Garry Richard Grubb, Thomas Khee Kian Ha (MD 1999), Caroline Jane Hampton, Nora Elizabeth Hanke, Mark Robert Haywood, Michael Patrick Hewson, Michael Alan Holmes, Richard John Holmes, Kirsten Margaret Holst, Catherine Jin-Young Hong, James Daniel Houghton, Franz John Hubmann, Penelope Jane Hunt (Burn) (MD 1997), Tania Jane Hunter, Terrie Eleanor Inder (Foster) (Travelling Scholar 1988) (MD 1997), Warrick John Inder (MD 1997), Albertine Adriana Ireland (Bielski), Neil David Jamieson, Mary Elizabeth Jones (Holden), Nigel Alistair Kim, Colin Paul King, Antony Richard Aylmer Lafferty, John George Lainchbury (MD 1998), Andrew David Philip Laing, Patrick Eugene Leary, Nigel Adrian Lever, Karen Gaye McCartney, Jennifer Anne McDonald, David Owen Ross McGregor, Gerard James McHugh, David Peter Robert McKay, Duncan Joseph McKay, Suzanne Elizabeth McKeage, Alastair William McLean, Stuart McMaster, Andrew Ronald Malcolm, Ben Matalavea, Anthony John Matthews, Shreeram Sudhakar Mayadeo, Gary Stuart Mitchell, Nina May Molteno (Taylor), Anna Margit Ledgard Moor, Patricia Moira Moore, Wayne William Morriss, Samantha Anne Murton, Raewyn Cheryll Mutch, Grant McKay Neumegen, Peter David Norrie, Gabrielle Anne Nuthall, Anne Evelyn O'Donnell, Lucy Clare O'Hagan, Christopher John O'Meeghan, Trevor John Palairet, Nicholas Bruce Palmer, Scott John Pearson, Jane Margaret Pepper, Krishnan Ramanathan, Mark Campbell Reddy, Bryan Reginald Russ, Kevin William Russell, Philippa Mary Ryan, Joanne Sayers (Macgregor), Lauren Patricia Seel (McGifford), Clair Louise Shadbolt, Jane Shapleske, Harpal Singh-Sandhu, Fuia'Ava Pokotoa Sipeli, Keith McEwen Small, Murray Russell Smith, Simon Robert Stables, Phillipa Alice Story, Mark James Sycamore, Rees Tohiteuru Rangi Tapsell, Jane Margaret Tarbotton, Susan Maree Taylor, Christopher James Roland Thomson, Malcolm Ewen Thomson, Penelope Susan Alexandra Thomson, Michael Francis Joseph Thwaites, Paul Jeremy Clive Trotman, Julie Hong Tsung, John Andrew Tuckey, Christine Leigh Walker (Taylor), Muir Livingstone

Wallace, Elizabeth Catherine Weston, Jeffrey Stuart Wong, Janette Merlene Woolerton, Paul Abraham Wotherspoon; MD: Francis Michael Davis

1989
Kay Doris Abraham, Judith Frances Adams (Matheson), Lee Rachel Allen, Jason McGregor Armstrong, Carol Margaret Atmore, Lynette Myrelle Austen (Yates), Janine Maria Bailey (Travelling Scholar 1989), David Leslie Bain, Andrew Charles Robert Baldey, Karen Andrea Baynon, Bhamidimarri Theresa Jean Lacava, Robyn Joy Blake, Martinus Hubertus Bonne, Teresa Michelle Booth, Susan Rita Boswell, Timothy John Bradley, Simon Roger Brebner, Paul Gavin Bridgman (MD 2003), Amanda Pauline Brown, Helen Moyra Brown, Adrienne Yee-Bo Sun Chin, John Hugh Clarkson, Mark Harding Coates, Julia Leigh Collett, David Graeme Cooksley, Marjolein Jannette Copland (Van De Kuilen), Michael Corbett, Lynda Bellamy Croft, Bernard Denis Cummings, Alastair Wilson Edward Currie, Alison Jane Daniell, Glen Adam Davies, Veena Farah Deobhakta, Edward Ward TeKanawa Douglas, Sarah Jane Mary Eglinton (Hartshorn), Richard John Evans, Stuart D'Arcy Farmer, Cameron Stuart Feint, Leeanne Frances Fisher, Susan Lianne Foot, Sarah Marion Seabourne Ford, Kim Belle Glass, Fiona Leigh Gordon, Alistair John Gray, Anna Hillary Bolman Gray, David Graham Grayson, Leye Mary Greenslade, Nicola Jane Gwatkin (Hartland), Timothy Scott Hampton, David John Hartshorn, Joseph Gerard Hassan, Emma Jane Henderson, Rosemary Jane Henderson, Terry Beaumont Hercock, Jack Simon Hill, Guy Richard Hingston, Helen Margaret Hingston (Malcolm), Julie Anne Holden, Lisa Jayne Horrell, Nicholas Peter Samuel Humphries, Kathryn Barbara Hunt, Nirmala Jeevaratnam, Julie-Anne Frances Jones, Vicki Lee Jones, Andrea Mary Judd, Patrick Ian Kay, Andrew Francis Kelly, Kenneth Donald Kuen, Thomas Kuruvilla, Andrew Jeffrey Joseph Law, Jeffrey Yen Law (Yen), Martyn William Lemberg, Denise Helena Limby, Christine Lipyeat, Conrad Ernest Loten, Bevan Michael Lowe, Theresa Jane Lum, Margaret Josephine Lusk, Sally Josephine Lyttleton, Deidre Anne McAlpine, Shona Ann McDowell, James Roy McGiven, Peter James McIlroy, Clare Kathleen McKay, Craig Andrew MacKinnon, Karin Vendela Victoria McNamara, Claire Richardyne McNee (West), Murray Stuart Malcolm, Gregory Michael Malham, Lea-Anne May, Iain Craig Melton, Andrew Martin Miller, Florina Chan Mow, Roderick David Mulgan, Thomas Allan Mulholland, Roland Ng, Susan Rosemary Nicoll, Jennifer Maree O'Donnell, Hock Lai Ooi, Jodie Jane O'Sullivan, Leaanne Elizabeth O'Sullivan, Karen Nina Parkes, Denesh Chhotu Patel, John Eric Peebles, William Suttle Peters, Andre Christopher Peyroux, Timothy Lionel Phillips, Helen Linda Pilmore (Jones) (MD 2000), Leon Shane Prendergast, Vijay Ranchhod, Susan Jean Read (Pearce), David Stuart Ritchie, Anne Frances Roche, Richard Hugh Stephen Roxburgh, Helen Brackenbury Sadler, Prudence Anna Elizabeth Scott (Rhodes Scholar 1990), Elizabeth Sewell (Crooks), David Andrew Sidebotham, Milne James Simpson, Komudi Pulsara Siriwardena, Murray John Smith, Maria Stavrinos, Richard Henderson Steele, Antony Clyde Wilson Taylor, James William Taylor, Malcolm Roslyn Thompson, Anna Nicole Twhigg, Hilary Mary Tyler, Indrani Vetharaniam, Andrew Brian Vincent, Graham Paul Viney, Stephen Paul Voss, Iain Gordon Ward, Edward William Watson, Helen Lucy Wemyss, Jan Elizabeth Widdowson, Michelle Irene Wilde, Daniel John Williams, Adrienne Alison Williamson, Esko James Wiltshire (MD 2002), Sharon Rose-Anne Winters, Selwyn Patrick Wong, John Campbell Woodfield, Rodney Ewen Wu, Angie Young, Stanley Arthur Zambazos, Adam Leonard Zyskowski; MD: Edmund Anthony Severn Nelson

1990
Christopher Donald Adams, Caroline Aiau, William Scott Babington, Geraldine Rosa Baker (Hill), Susan Jane Bargh, Gordon Pitt Beadel, Iain James Alexander Bell, Joanne Marie Berkahn, Jacqueline Frances Blunt, Andrea Jane Boon, Charles Eric Noel Bradfield, Katherine Ann Bristow, Raewyn Carol Broady, Kathryn Beatrice Burnell, Allister John Bush, John Lancelot Bush, Angus Donald Byars, Janine Jane Bycroft, John Robert Cameron, John Christopher Canton, Diane Margaret Carter (Gee), Tina Marie Cartmell, Chun Sing Chan, Colin Yee Ying Kit Chin, Jane Elizabeth Christiansen, Brett Francis Christmas, William Andrew Clement, Glenn Hamilton Coltman, Sara Lyla Cooksley (Gilkison), Christine Marie Coulter, Ian Robert Coutts, Andrea Kay Crichton, Timothy Scott Cunningham, Sarah Mary Elaine Cutts, Elizabeth Rose Dennett, Harsha Rohan Dias, Claire Patricia Dillon, Steven Leslie Ding, David Glyn Eastgate, Christine Frances Elder, Kerry Lee English, Cecile Therese Evans (Jansen), Andrew Thomas Stanley Falloon, Sandra Joy Flooks, Matthew Scott Gentry, Catherine Elizabeth Gibbs (Swan), David Douglas Gibbs, Andrew Bruce Glenny, David Stephen Goh, Stephen John Graham, Kirstie Sue Harris, Miranda Christina Harvie, James Richard Hattaway, Christopher Kerry Hawke, Landon Robert Katene Hepi, Donna Louise Holdgate, Simon David Jensen, Keith Joe, Charlotte Sarah Hope Johnstone, Peter Graham Jones, Warrick Brian Jones, Anne Maree Judkins, Simon Michael Kelly, Nicola Jane Kennedy, Andrew John Kerr, Paul Frederic Keys, Jeffrey George Kirwan, Jeannie Margaret Knapp, James Christopher Knight, Rebecca Doak Langley, Kathryn May Leslie, Michelle Robyn Le Lievre, David Kenneth Linscott, Vivienne Elizabeth Linscott (Anderson), Helen Marie Long, Michael Peter Loten, Francesca Therese McCaul (Walkey), Dougal Russell McClean (MD 2001), Jane Theresa MacDonald, Paul Desmond McGeown, Cameron Sinclair McKay, Frances Janet McKellar, Martin Stephen McKendry, Caroline Mary MacKenzie, Steven Neil Mackey, Elizabeth Helen McLeay (Hayes), Wendy Marie McRae, Kim Tautai Ma'ia'i, Christine Ann March, Nicola Dawn Marris, David Michael Mason, Jeremy Bernard Alan Meates, Hamish Meldrum, Mark Andrew Milner, Anthea Maree Murray (Prentice), Stephen John Neas, Clare Patricia O'Donnell, Robin Athol Ojala, Jeannie Susan Oliphant, Stephen Charles Parkinson, Christopher Sushil Parshuram, Giresh Kanji Patel, Paul Cameron Phillips, Prudence Mary Poole, Keri Huia Ratima, William Glenn Reeve, Fiona Margaret Rennie, Katherine Anne Richards, Jonathan Paul Richardson, Philip Grant Richardson, John Adrian Rietveld, Susan Janice Rive, Michael John Roberts, Stephen Peter Robertson (Travelling Scholar 1990), Helen Elizabeth Russell, Deborah Suitafa Ryan, Paul Francis Sabonadiere, Lynette Grant Sadleir (MD 2004), Louise Maree Sang, Dean Richard Schluter, Lisa Michelle Searle, Stephen John Searle, Ramon Edward Sheehan, Grant Russell Shrimpton, Dimitria Simatos, Ellis Leva Situe, Hannah Marion Small (Bates), Cecilia Casware Smith, Kathryn Laura Smith, Diane Elizabeth Sommerville, Viliame Trusttum Karayame Sotutu, Katherine Anne Sowden, Ivan Ivitza Srzich, Hilary Jane Stevenson, Kathryn Barbara Stewart, Geoffrey Maurice Street, Dean John Stubbs, Daniel Svoboda, Elsa Medland Taylor, Justine Elizabeth Taylor (Lancaster), Paul Michael Templer, Aravinda Thiagalingam, Jane Mary Thomas, Thomas Douglas Thomson, Jonathan Gerald Tisch, Michelle Marie Todd, Adam Paul Tucker, Belinda Jane Turnbull, Geoffrey Martin Tvrdeich, Janet Audrey Vaughan, Louisa Eugenia Voight, David Mark Wallace, Tania Wallace (Lewis), Katharine Ann Wallis, Michael William Watson, Janet Patricia Whineray, Elizabeth Margaret White (Adkin), Lucille Marie Wilkinson, Graham Ashley Wilson, Duane Mathew Winter, Malcolm Gavin Wong, Peter Martyn Wright, Heather Mary Young, Sonia Jean Young (Wong), Stavro Zambazos

1991
Marguerite Annan (Kuipers), David William Ardern, Catherine Barrow, Suhanthini Baskaranathan, Katherine Louise Bate (Travelling Scholar 1991), Kristin Delia Bell,

Michelle Lara Bennett, Neil James Beumelburg, Maria Louisa Bews-Hair, Antony Arthur Blakely, Catherine Mary Bollard (MD 2005), Susannah Ruth Bone, Pauline Anne Booth, Cushla Sue Borthwick, Helen Dian Brasch, Fraser Martin McKirdie Brown, Paul Brydon, Peter George Burt, Stephen John Busby, Stephen Robert Campbell, Anna Margaret Catherwood, Bridget Mary Chang, Pauline Yee Po Lan Chin, Ronald Blair Christian, Jasmine Mei Chua, Dara Chung, Amanda Mary Clarke, Nigel Forsyth Clarke, Louise Ann Cole, Shelley Erin Collings, Justine Cooper, Paul David Cooper, Paul Geoffrey Cosgrove, Michael David Cox, Arran John Culver, Helen Victoria Danesh-Meyer, Lesli Sharon Davies, Simon Lee Edwin Dodge, Peter Seamus Doran, Paul Francis Edgar, Rosalie Elizabeth Elder, Helen Anne Fieldes, Gavin Fraser Fincher, John Newton Fink, Mark David Floyd, Mark Gerard Foley, Sai Yan Fong, Sharyn Lee Fryett, Kathryn Nola Gadd, Martin Richard Gardner, Rosemary Ann Brander Gittos, Catherine Joy Goold (Ripley), Noelyn Gordon-Glassford, Steven William Alexander Grant, Karen Elizabeth Gray (Edgar; Skinner), Marilyn Gay Griffiths (Coventry), Robin Glyn Griffiths, Janine Catherine Hancock (Rasmussen), James Derenzy Harman, Elizabeth Lynn Harris (Eccles), Leslie Jane Havard, Wendy Jane Hawke, David Kevin Hayes, Pauline Joan Horrill, Maureen Houstoun, Mary Louise Hull, Anne Margaret Hunter, Rosemary Gwyneth Irwin (Edwards), Pamela Margaret Jackson, Karen Finlay Jensen, Richard William Kain, Harpreet Kaur (Aulakh), Joanne Maree Keaney, Malcolm Kendall-Smith, Michael George Kerr, Philip Graeme Knight, Jeremy David Krebs (MD 2003), Richard Thomas Laing, Ruth Alexa Laird (Lucey), Carlene Meryl Margaret Lawes, Kim Maree Lawson, Brigid Mary Lee, Yun Chor Lee, Leinani Salamasinia Aiono Le-Tagaloa, Maree Catherine Lindsay, Agnes Cynthia Lin-Mey Liong (Ngan Kee), Andrew Craig Lynch, Rachel Nola McCoy, Timothy James McCullough, Simone Lynley McLeavey, Fiona Jane McPherson, Andrew Gregory Marshall, Joanna Francesca Martino, Christopher William Masters, Philip James Matheson, Paula Susan Mathieson (Jones), Kirsty Rachel Maule (Jordan), Richard Hugo Medlicott, Maria Jane Middlemiss (Au Young), Kevin James Moginie, Susan Clare Moller, Thomas Ramsay Morton, Phillipa Jane Murray, Kim Marie Nester, Patricia Anne Newell, Gillian Michelle Nixon, Derek Ross Parkes, Lloyd Wentworth Peterson, Anthony Ronald John Phillips, Rebecca Margaret Pope, Nicola Kazia Poplawski (MD 2001), Ivan Nelson Popoff, Andrew Bryon Porteous, Paul James Quigley, Sarah Anne Rathie Redfern, Amanda Jane Renfree, David Marc Rentoul, Harvey Jason Rigby, Dominic James Rillstone, Elizabeth Caroline Roberts, David Rillstone Robertson, Simon Rae Robinson, Lauren Kim Roche, Susan Helen Rouse, Dean Robert Ruske, Leonie Kay Russell, Caroline Anne Ryan, Karen Ann Ryan, Tessa Joyce Ryder, David Robert Sandford, Diana Sarfati, Andrew Robert Scott, Christopher Mark Sealey, Robert Paul Sew Hoy, Mark John Sherwood, Philippa Margaret Shirtcliffe, Andrew Campbell Smillie, Dianne Marie Smith (Davis), Robyn Lee Smith, David Luton Sturge, Lisa Ann Sweetman (Boston), Jacqueline Karen Tam, Ramani Shobana Thiruchelvam, Louise Elizabeth Jane Thomson, Gillian Therase Todd (Penno), Philippa Mary Tremewan, Lynn Maree Twigley, Vicki Janette Tyrrell (Cunningham), George Varsanyi, Maraia Korina Marama Waibuta, Stephen Craig Walsh, Leanna Gaye Ward (Dodge), Adam Stewart John Watson, Anthony Philip Wells, Yvonne Isobel Olive Wharerimu, Annabel Margret White (Collecutt), Julian Blair White, Katherine Prudence White, Susrutha Kusal Wickremesekera, Angela Jane Williams, Sharyn Elizabeth Willis (Johnston), Brent Anderson Wishart, Rosamond Robertson Withers (Bridgman), Roland Wong, Jason Peter Woodrow, Angela Joan Worsley (Dowie), Anthony Yung

1992

Christopher George Abbott, Clare Johanna Ainsworth, Paul James Ainsworth, Nicola Mary Alsop (McKendrey), Ruth Margaret Angell, Lynda Ashton (Vis), Wayne John Bailey, Diana Elizabeth Ballantyne (Maxwell), Julie Elizabeth Barber, John Mark Barnett, Sriskanthan Baskaranathan, Anne Elizabeth Baxter, Chantal Yvonne Best (Taylor), Karen Lee Bisley, Damon Andrew Blair, Katherine Anne Bourke (Ferrier), Marise Ailsa Brice, Andrew Mark Broadbent, Jennifer Susan Brown (Clayton; Grew), Jan Louise Bryham, Fiona Margaret Burns, Nicholas Ellis Carney, Margaret Ruth Caughley (Walker), Trevor Andrew Chan, Amanda Charlton, Nelson Chen, Helen Andrea Chidgey (Mayall), Christopher Wayne Chin, Grant Robert Christey, Malcolm Alexander Christie, Robert Francis Coup, Murray Alan Cox, Sandra Margaret Crofts, Daelyn Margretta Cullen, Robyn Frances Dalziel (Chirnside), John David Danesh (Travelling Scholar 1992) (Rhodes Scholar 1992), Aaron Blair Penfold Donaldson, Annette Rosemary Downey, Paul David Dukes, Gaye Andrea Eden, Anna Kate Eglinton, Campbell Bryan Emmerton, Brett Ferguson, Siale Alokihakau Foliaki, Lisa Marie Fox, Robert Wilson Frengley, Bharathy Ganeshanathan (Bahirathan), Flora Helen Gastrell (Ward), Alanagh Elizabeth Gilbert-Jacobs, Kathleen Joy Gillies (Read), Anthony Douglas Goh, Alison Jane Goodwin, Hamish David Gray, Katherine Mary Hall, Derek John Hann, Scott Andrew Harding, Jason Paul Harper, Simone Patrice Hart, Caroline Ellen Hastrop, Ian Murray Hayes, Janet Emily Hayward, Paul James Healy, Katrina Marie Heer, Tiwini Hemi, Richard James Hillock, Leanne Susan Hulbert, Timothy Llewellyn Jackson, Mohan Vasantha Jayasundera, Samuel Havelock Knox Jerram, Alison May Kirkman, Lee-Ann Margaret Kitto, George Robert Laking, Sally Joy Lane (Wootton), Jo-Dee Leanne Lattimore, Michael Buong Ying Lau, Warren Kenneth Lee, Alina Janet Leigh, Hamish Donald Hunter Leslie, Patrick William Lascell Lyall, Brett David Lyons, Kirsten Anne McAuley, Sharon Jean McHardy, Anne Lorraine MacKay-Bell, Bruce Cameron McKenzie, Virginia Anne McLaughlin, Bryan Frederick MacLeod, Ross Ian MacLeod, Darren Mark Malone, Nicola Fleur Manttan, Deborah Fleur Mason, Evan Graham Mason, Richard Antony Matsas, Kim Suzanne Mawson, Catherine Ann Mills, Joanne Louise Mitchell (Dockerty), Marcos Erik Monasterio, Helen Margaret Moore, Louise Ann Moore, Joseph Robert Morahan, Andrew Ronald Gordon Muncaster, Glen Phillip Murphy, Annette Deborah Nesdale, Garry Richard Nind, David Bruce Nixon, Michelle Kathrine Nottage, Anne Bernadette O'Connor, Karaponi Okesene-Gafa, Robyn Louise Oldfield, Hamish Robert Osborne, Keryn Lee Painter (Powell), Merryl Eileen Park, Sanjiv Ramanlal Patel, David William Peacock, Toni Elizabeth Petterson, Krishna Charles Pillai, Sarita Rosheen Pillai, Kevin Robert Plumpton, David Robert Porter, Justin Gregory Pratt, Mark John Pratt (Courtney), Joanna Louise Alexandra Prendergast, Jenepher Anne Press, Anne Preston-Thomas, Michael Vijay Reddy, Shirin Lisa Robinson, Graham Philip Sceats, Donna Miranda Schakelaar, Carole Ann Searle (Reeve), Paul Hilton Sherwin, Anna Mary Sinclair, Manvir Singh, Carolyn Marlene Smale, Brendan Paul Smith, Richard Lloyd Somerville, Faafetai Sopoaga, Rowena Marie Sosich, Joanna Phyllis Standage, Catherine Ann Stedman, Julian Reiss Stoddart, Jonathan William Leslie Sturm, Deborah Ann Sum, Michael Leonard Talbot, Anthony Tam, Graeme Bevan Taylor, Frank Neville Thomas, Merlin Christopher Thomas, Sean Douglas Thomson, Craig Norman Thornley, Penelope Jane Thornton (Mitchell), Fiona Jane Timms, Fiona Mary Turnbull, Bridget Margaret Turner (Kelly), Nilesh Raman Vasan, Sarah Jane Wadsworth, Craig Innes Wallace, Tony Martin Walls, Carleen Mary Ward, Stuart John Watchman, Jonathan William Webster, Andre Marcel Westenberg, Gerard Peter Willemsen, Benjamin Kenneth Joseph Wilson, Andrea Stephanie Wong, Vanessa Jeanne Wood (Ellison),

Gillian Elizabeth Yardley, Brendon John Yee, Edward Shouen Yee, Stephanie Kim Young, Anna Marie Zender, Andrew Paul Zimmerman

1993

David Geoffrey Allen, Michael John Anscombe, Cheryl Ruth Archer, Rachel Ellenore M. Atkinson, Sukhdeep Singh Aulakh, Philip Edwin Baigent, Jeremy Baily-Gibson, Glenda Margaret Barber, Katya Rosaline Bazley, Grant Rocco Beban, Aaron James Bell, Adam Bialostocki, Carolyn May Bilbrough, Susan Billington (Reynolds), Campbell Raymond Boswell, Meryl Anne Bramley (Nicol), Lisa Judith Bron, Hubertus Carolus E. Buyck, Karen Elizabeth Cairns, Alastair John Cameron, Helen Claire Campbell (Taylor), Priscilla Louise Campbell-Stokes, Miriam Canham, Cherie Katherine Castaing, Victoria Louise Chadwick, Lisa Jane Chapman, Stephanie Jane Charteris, Lynette Marie Cherry, Kheang Chheng Heang, Shane Edward Christensen, Caroline Margaret Christie, Matthew Edward P. Claridge, Paul William Clarkson, Saxon John Connor, Catherine Louise Conway, Louise Frances Couch, Bronwyn Anne Cowley, Chris Cresswell, John Andrew Crump, Geoffrey Todd Cunningham, Shona Dawn Dalzell, Anna Helen Davison, Thomas Andrew Dawson, Charlotte Mary Dempster, Glen Anthony Devcich, Michael Francis Devlin, Richard Thomas Doocey, Paul Edward Downing, Alwyn Bernard d'Souza, Niels Robert Dugan, Peter Bruno Egli, Joanna Carmel Emanuel, Peter Thomas Enright, Siavash Es'Haghi, Glenn James Farrant, Michael Francis Fay, Carissa Yuen Kim Fong, Kolin Stanley Foo, Alan Thomas Forrester, Sandra Marie Fountain, Lisa Christine Fuller (Eskildsen), Mark Robert Gardener, Murray Donald Govan, Andrew Stuart Granger, Brendon Mark Gray, Andrew Lloyd Greensmith, Katyleen (Katya) Annetta Gunn (Woods), Kirsten Louise Haggitt (Cunningham), David Neil Hailes (Travelling Scholar 1993), Bruce Harvey Hamilton, Phillip Craig Hamilton, Rupert Lauriston Handy, Christopher Michael Hanna, Lynne Marie Harris (Birnie), Fleur Cecilia Hart, Timothy Michael Harvey, Andrea Lesley Hedgland, Katherine Mary Henry (Swanson), Benita Leigh Higgins (Douglas), Michael Charles Hlavac, Brendon James Hock, Celine Ann Holland, Sheryl Dawn Howarth, Stephanie Jane Inder, Clare Rachel Jansen (Anderson), Penelope Anne Jeffery, Amanda Jane Johnston (D'Souza), Philippa Johnstone, Brendan Patrick Kane, Stephanie Louise Keel, Kristin Mary Kenrick, Sylvia Rae Kupenga, Prudence Rosalind Lamb, Michael David Lattimore, Gabriel Buong Hung Lau, Peter Anthony Laws, James Andrew Letts, Andrea Evelyn McBride, Sharyn Leigh Shirley MacDonald, Tinika Louise MacDonald, Rachael Leigh McEwing, James Andrew McGuire, Ross Peter Vernon McKellar, Jillian Kaye McKenzie, Maria Mackey, Jonathan Charles McKinnon, Emily Jane W. McLauchlan, Rachael Mira McLean, Ramila Magan, Anthony Selwyn March, Jennifer Helen Martin (Rhodes Scholar 1993), Stefan Mark Mazur, Luci Monette Mellsop (Montgomerie), Naresh Kumar Mondraty, Robyn Margaret Moss, Dawson Charles W. Muir, Paula Munro, Paul Alexander Murphy, Sarah Amanda Nicolson, Andrew Reinholds Palmer, Manish Thakorbhai Patel, Sandra Kaye Paterson, Joanne Elizabeth Paver, Rebecca Dilrukshidevi Perinpanayagam (Rasiah), Stephen Timothy Pitman, David John Priest, Lynda Jane Priest (Moore), Dean Richard Quinn, Kim Margaret Rapson, Richard Ian Reid, Neil MacDonald Renwick, Brandon Geoffrey Rickards, James Jude Riddell, Joanna Margaret Rose, John Christian Rouse, Matthew John Rowbotham, Bevan Wayne Roy, Andrew Stuart Russell, Katrina Louise Sandford (Allen), Antonia Weston Shand, Helen Kathleen Sharp, Isabel Sarah Sharpe, Andrew Ian Sidwell, Jeremy William Simcock, Jeremy John William Smillie, Janine Margot Smith, Kerry Anne Smith (MacAskill-Smith), Louise Helen L. Spellman, Jeanette Ann Spencer, Jennifer Mary Spring, Alexander Joseph Srzich, Lisa Katrina Stamp, Paul Alastair Stevens, Anna Elizabeth Stevenson (Bashford), Robert Alexander Story, Thomas James Studholme, Antony James Suter, Penelope Jane Symes, Tevita Taka, Teresa Mary Thompson, Jacqueline Maree Z. Thomson, Rachel Moana Thomson, Vi Hien Thi Tran, Michael John Tustin, Andrew Graham Usher, Lilian Geraldine Van Alphen, Shirani Vetharaniam, Kuinileti Tamato Chang Wai, Gerrard Matthew Walker, Janaka Kesara Wickremesekera, Andrew James Wilde, David Christopher Williams, Mark James Wilsher, Kay Anne Wilson, Michelle Louise Wilson, Deanne Lyndsey Wong, Katrina Wong, James Peter Worthington

1994

Keri Aile Alexander, Jason Bernard Alexandre, Kate Elizabeth Allan, Anna-Karenia Patricia Anderson, Rosalind Frances Anderson (Raine), Craig Robert Andrews, Michelle Ruth Andrews, Andrew Audeau, Duncan Alan John Baird, Rosemary Ruth Baker, Mark Jason Barlow, Joanna Mary Barron, Geoffrey Robert Barton, Anna Jacqueline Bashford (Christie), Rachel Helen Beard, Iliesa Sasala Beci, Andrew James Bell, David John Como Bettany, Matthew William Bevin, Brendon John Bigwood, Vivien Michelle Binney, Angus Bruce Binnie, Jane Lesley Birss, Catherine Caroline Blackie, Kathleen Margaret Blacktop, John Stephen Britten, Campbell Kenneth Brodie Brown, Rosemary Maxina Bruce (Stoddart), Simon Lloyd Mortlock Burrows, Paul Andrew Butel, Rachael Annette Byars, Andrew Melville Carll, Jennifer Barbara Chadderton (Woods), Neroli Anne Chadderton, Winston Kuen Cheung, Grant Irwin Gordon Christie, Siew-Siew Chua, Trevor Michael Claridge, Lloyd Taylor Clarke, Gina De Cleene, Karen Maree Cleveland, Antony Keith Clough, Shelley Janice Coldham (Reilly), John William Corboy, Jan Elizabeth Cottle (Hurring), Edward Erle Coxon, Roy Andrew Craig, Melinie Jane Culverhouse (Hansen), Paromita Dasgupta, Rosemary Kay Davey (Neild), David Llywelyn Davies-Payne, Mark Edward Davis, Philippa Jane Depree,(Travelling Scholar) Bronwyn Christine Dingle (Graham), Will Jonathan Dransfield, Thomas Eade, Kathryn Jane Edwards, Mark Lewis Edwards, Bryan Craig Ellis, Rachel May Evans, Carolyn Clare Falkner, Jonathan Patrick Feltham, Joanne Therese Finlay, Marcus Anthony Reginald Fitchett, Victoria Paula Flight, Anthony Joseph Freeman, Brett Matthew Gerrard, Jill Lynette Gibson, Ainsley Kate Goodman, Michael Gerald Goodwin, Peter William Hadden, Vivienne Ann Hancock, Sarah Linden Alethea Hart, Elaine Ruth Harvey, Glen Campbell Hawkins, Robyn Ann Hay, Erfan Hedayati, Sonya Louise Hockey (Bennett), Erika Anne Hollow (Klier), Deanne Marion Horton (Bedggood), Rachel June Hoyle, Rodney Jason Hughes, Christopher Denis Hutchinson, Benedict Olisaemeka Isichei, Tony William Jackson, Paul Andrew James, Terence Mark James, Dilan Sudarsh Jayawardena, Elaine Mary Jeffrey, Stuart Ian Johnson, Peter Kannu, Allan Trotter Keast, Jane Margaret Kennedy, Kerrie Sarah Morgan Knapp, Caroline Helen Lara (Fraser), Blair Peter Duncan Leslie, Thomas Mark Levien, Antonia Janet Lile, Huei-Fu Jack Lin, Janene Margaret Lindsay, Michael Charles McCabe, Andrew Kenneth MacCormick, Fiona Margaret Victoria McCrimmon, Beth Mary McDonald, Paul Dickson McMurray, Theo Leonard De Malmanche, Anne Teresa Maloney, Jacqueline Rachael Maplesden, Alastair John Mark, Timothy Joseph Adrian Marr, Ana-Louise Elaine Martin, Miriam Lynley Martin, Richard Charles Wilson Martin, Napolione Masirewa, Caroline Mary Meade, Grant Robert Meikle, Rosalind Frances Elizabeth Menzies, Janeen Elizabeth Milner, Terry Andrew Mitchell, Coral Jeannie Morris (Battensby), Peter Philip Morrison, Andrew Scott Murray, Raymond Chee Hui Ng, Sarah Ly Nguyen, Sean Jason Nicholson, Jeanine Patricia Nunn, Andrew Peter Oakley, David William Orr, Margot Winifred Parkes, Margaret Parle, Maria-Lee Pearse, Colin Mark Peebles, Deirdre Chiara Percy, Linda Margaret Pirrit, David James Poff, Christopher John Wheelans Porter, Helen Judith Pratt, Natasha Jane Rafter, Mark John Ralfe, Rebecca Anne Randerson, Maya Natu Ravaji, John Noble James Reynolds, Andrew Francis Cameron Riley,

Miranda Elise Robinson, Timothy Richard Sheat Rumball, Matthew Kevin Russell, Jamie Christopher Ryan, Simon Norman Ryder-Lewis, Rahul Sant-Ram, Elizabeth Anne Schroder, Michael William Scott, Sarah Ann Seay (Wakeman), Jeremy Alistair Sheard, Barbara Lea Sinclair (Wensley), Sara Jane Souter, Denise Alice Stapleton, David William Steven, Jane Louise Strang, Richard Nigel Sullivan, Simon Peter Talbot, Bernard Tamba-Lebbie, Andrew Huck Hoe Tan, Iona Patricia Thomas, Gerard Martin Thyne, Andrew Edwin Tse, Alainuanua Diana Tupai, Andrew John Turbott, Justine Claire Turnbull, Arlo Jane Upton, Richard Milne Ussher, Garry Gerrit Van Der Veen, Michael Gerard Francis Van Gulik, Mark Stuart Waddington, Rokoveivuke Lalakonadokoulu Waqanisau, Rachael Elizabeth Waters, Mark David Wilkinson, Stephen John Williams, David Jeremy Williamson, Esther Elizabeth Willis, John Murray Wilson, Astrid Ursula Windfuhr, Lisa Cherie Wynne, Michael Robert Wynn-Williams, Roslyn Ann Yeoman, Calum McDonald Young, Peter Wilson Young; MD: Helen Elizabeth Carter, Gary Allen Wittert

1995

Barbara Mavis Adams, Bronwyn Jane Armstrong, Fareed Bahrami, Adrian Gallus Balasingam, Taraneh Bashir-Elahi, Angela Claire Beard, Tina Yvonne Bergen, Ivan James Bergman, Latham John Berry, Felicity Anne Elizabeth Bettle (Smith), Margaret Jean Bickerstaff, Christopher Lawrence Birks, Nicola Justine Blair, James William Heyward Blake, Andrew Arnold Blunt, Owen David Boswell, Andrew McDonald Botting, Scott Faulkner Boyes, Susan Jane Bray, Janene Rochelle Brown, Peter John Campbell, Kerryn Jennifer Carter, Nancy Johanna Carter, Paula Jane Carter, Michael Bruce Causer, Vicki Marie Cavanagh (Vertongen), Victor Hsi Tai Chen, Gary Cheung (Chi-Wah), Antonia Cole, Karl Geoffrey Cole, Terrence Anthony Creagh, Nicola Jane Dalbeth (Moore) (Travelling Scholar 1995) (MD 2005), Shelley Jane Dalzell (Robinson), Shailesh Chand Dass, James Carline Davidson, Adam John Wallace Davies, Gareth John Reynolds Davies, Stephen Nicholas Dee, Gaurav Atma Deva, Karen Jean Dickinson, Tony Ian Diprose, Owen Doran, Jeremy Mark Dryden, Sarah Louise Dunlop, Philip Martin Eames, Marianne Susan Elston, Kate Elizabeth France, Jolene Mary Fraser, Greg Arana Frazer, Richard Blair Gearry, Debra Jane Gibb, Andrew James Gillespie, Prakriti Gopinathan, Suetonia Cressida Green, Edwina Valmai Guard, Rosemary Megan Hall, Ricci Bernette Harris, Penelope Angelique Harvey, Jeremy Elliott Hay, Philip Haywood, Meredith Johanne Hicks, Susan Michelle Hing, Brett Manarangi Tauu Isaja Hoggard, Matthew Justin Holton, Maraekura Horsfall, Carl Augustus Edward Horsley, Jane Howe, Wendy Anne Hunter, Rachel Elizabeth Inder, Anna Mary St Clair Inglis, Stephen James Inns, Nabura Ioteb'a, Andrew Donald Jackson, Mary Anne Jamison (Abrahams), Timothy Scott Jefferies, Wikitoria Ella Jenkins (Lins), Helen Ruth Johnston, Stuart Lawrence Jones, Ciandra Jane Keenan, Alexander Basil King, Nicholas Chee Kong Lam, David Peter Langston, Ywain Thomas Lawrey, Susannah Kate Lewis (Cunningham), Cynthia Yeng Lim, Danny Boyd de Lore, Caroline Elizabeth Lovelock, Samantha Lowndes (Bendall), Graham Ralph Lowry, Rachelle Fay Lumsden, Sarah Juliet Lynn, Geoffrey Robert McGrath, Glenn Stuart McKay, David Garth McKenzie, Alison Margaret MacLean, Anthony Duncan William McNaughton, Rupa Natasha Maitra, Grace Riria Malcolm, Salina Lo Pui Man (Lupati), Rebecca Frances Marson, Richard Jordan Frank Martin, Sarah Catherine Lena Metcalf, Andrew Murray Mitchell, Andrew Robert Moot, Andrew Russell Munro, Simon Philip Murphy, Gwynifer Ruth Napier, Kimberley Rae Naylor (Alexander), Lisa Ng, Michael Glenn Nightingale, Clare Patricia O'Brien, Tracey Anne O'Brien, Rebecca Mary O'Connell, Nigel Colin Parr, Sanjeevan Pasupati, David Apollo Paul-Jama, Diana Jane Purvis, Yasantha Ranjeeva Rajapakse, Damayanthi Sulochana Rasanathan, Michael Ratna, Sureka Ratnavadivel,

Helen Jane Rawlinson, Sally Rentoul, Ian Alasdair Revfeim, Vernon Leslie Reynolds, Graeme John Roadley, Imogen Anne Robertson, Barbara Joy Robinson, Peter James Ryan, Rachel Elizabeth Sawyer, John Benedict William Schollum, Katrina Louise Scott, Meredith Louise Simcock, Warren John Simpson, Garth Reginald Smith, Jeffrey Bruce Smith, Gregory Matthew Spencer, Claire Giselle Spooner, Martin Kingsland Stiles, Andrew Peter Stokes, Victoria Louise Stott, Tralee May Sugrue, Qalo Sukabula, Malama Laura Tafuna'i, Kim Christina Tanner, Lynda Jane Thwaites, Frans Robert Jan Visser, Brent Randolph Daley Waldron, Catherine Anne Walker (Becker), Joanne Amanda Wall, Dean Patrick Walsh, Matthew Thomas Walsh, Patrick Ryan Walsh, Rachel Jo-Anne Wensley, Erica Louise Whineray (Kelly-Whineray), Jeremy Grant Whiting, Michael Patrick Wilson, Sarah Joanne Wilson (Painter), Mark Andrew Winstanley, Andrew Ching Wong, Nicholas John Woods, Anna Jane Wyeth, Henry Yau-Ching Yong

1996

John Joseph Ah-Chan, Jennifer Maree Aitken (Butler), Lee Anne Anderson, Russell William Anscombe, Christopher Ross Bain, Kim Charlene Baker, Janet Alison Ballantyne, Karen Louise Barclay, Peter John Barwell, Celia Abigail Mary Baskett, Anthony Maxwell Becker, Antony Edward Bedggood, Annabel Jane Begg, Christopher Graeme Bell, Kirsty Grace Bennett, Sandra Catherine Bennett, Juliet Elizabeth Berkeley, Stuart Randolph Berry, James Peter Berryman, Barbara Helen Blok, Sarah Jane Bowie (Carr), Jill Christian Buchan, Simon Andrew Bugden, Nicola Anne Butler, Jane Frances Calder, Zoey Ann Calman (Irvine), Robyn Denise Carey, Harriette Jane Carr, Derek James Chan, Lau Hui Chiong, Deborah Anne Chitty, Neil John Cochrane, Bridget Mary Collins (Louie), Brigid Nancy Connor, Stuart Ryan Dalziel, Cameron Grant Dickson, Maureen Joan Dingwall, Stephen Paul Dinniss, Bronwyn Eleanor Dixon, Jonathan David Lewin Dryburgh, Emma Bernice Dunning, Timothy Wilfred Eglinton, Gordon Calum Faulds, Janet Helen Ferguson, Antony John Finch Field, Aaron Dominic Fleischer, Lindy Grace Fookes, James Addison Foulds, Sarah Anne Fountain, Deborah Marianne Gardiner, Katherine Rachel Gardner, Marysha Jane Gardner, Craig Alastair Gedye, Janet Patricia Gentry (Robinson), Andrew Timothy Paul Gibson, Kim Annette Margaret Gidall, Julia Ruth Given (Crook), Andrew John Gooding, Anganette Betty-May Hall, Reece Craig Hall, Bruce Richard John Hammonds, Paula Maree Hanley, Azani Hasan, Jason Leonard Henwood, Sarah Elizabeth Hill, Louise Maria Hitchings, Grant Lindsay Hounsell, Miriam Louise Hurst, John Richard Jarvis, Stephanie Lisa Jones, Michael John Charles Kennedy, Maree Jacqueline Kerr (Spencer), Beheshteh Khoshaeen, Robert Peter Kieboom, Tee Ban Kiem, Jorian Russell Kippax, Joseph Kimmanje Kizito, Bridget Alexandria Kuzma, Phoebe Kar Wai Lam, Mark Graham Lawrence, Matthew Richard Leaper, Julie Anne Lincoln, Paul Francis Lockington, Eunice Aunette Low, Carmen Ruth Lowe, Penelope Chantelle Lowe, Dennis Jonathan Kar Que Lum, Adrienne Mary Lynn, Samuel Vincent McBride, Lauren Jane McCormack, Mary-Elizabeth McDevitt, Winston Andrew McEwan, Kim Margrethe McFadden (Travelling Scholar 1996), Ian Duncan Henare McKay, Adam Mark McLeay, Catherine Jane McMurray, Hayden James McRobbie, Laurens Aarnoud Manning, Kerryn Margaret Martin, Laura Mary Martin, Zara Susan Kathleen Mason, Andrew Graham Meads, Luke Ian Merriman, Goswin Yason Meyer-Rochow, Andrew Livingstone Miller, Joanna Mary Mills (Blakey), Joellene Rae Mitchell, Zachary Moaveni, Lada Moeung, Katherine Sarah Stewart Moodie, Anna Mary Murphy, Alastair Burgoyne Murray, Rozeena Musa, Katherine Ruth Neas, Jason Martin Nebbs, Bridget Marie Neveldsen, Anna Marie Nicholson, Lance Arthur Nicholson, Sarah Louise Olson, Brendan Charles O'Neill, Abdul Karim Othman, Robyn Suzanne Parker, Kathryn Lorraine Patchett, Jodie Maree Paterson, Kirsten Jane Pearce, Robyn Peters,

Richard Charles Peterson, Julian Alexander McCoy Pettit, Stuart Alexander Philip, Fredrick Thomas Stephen Phillips, David Llewellyn Pilbrow, Margaret Joan Pohl (Meads), Raoul Edward Pope, Ioselani Pouesi, John Albert Rawstron, Matthew Charles Reid, Kent Thomas Robinson, Philip Aaron Robinson, Grant Richard Rogers, Rebecca Jane Rowe, Anikha Lee Sanders, Gabrielle Satterthwaite, Sarah Jane Scott, Sharifah Hildah Shahab, Jeremy Russell Peter Sharr, Leanne Shaw, Anne Sheehan (Lear), Dilprasan De Silva, Maithri Jill Siriwardena, Rebecca Louise De Souza, Justine Speedy, Jonathon Lindsay Spencer, Camilla Holly Stevens, Phillipa Helen Tanner, Kim Oraline Taylor, Hua Sieng Ting, Justin Travers, Perry Charles Turner, Ann Van Der Veen, Devonie Sylviane Waaka, Christopher John Wakeman, Miranda Jean Walkinton, Jane Helen Walton, Daniel Roland Watson, Gretchen Ann Willis, Liam Clifford Wilson, Tanya Louise Wilton, Andrew Charles Woollons, Timothy David Wright, Loong Aun Terence Yang; MD: Naga Mani Pavuluri

1997

Sarah Jane Abrahamson, Michael John Aitkenhead, Zairani Alias, Caroline Rose Allum, Riki Bridget Anderson, Nathaniel James Anglem, Dion Raymond Astwood, Amanda Joy Aveling-Rowe (Thompson), Michelle Amanda Bailey, Michelle Nicole Diana Balm, Stephanie Louise Bardsley, Scott Ian Barker, Sally Liza Barlow, Thomas John Scott Barry, Michelle Kim Bawden, Ben Beaglehole, Catherine Jean Lesley Bell, Alexandra Catherine Anne Bennett (Taylor), Stephen Marc Berrill, Tabwe Bio, Pita Birch, Paul Martin Blundell, Christian Nicolas Honor Brett, Shona Mary Bright, Jennifer Kyra Broom, Roger Malcolm Browning, Christopher James Callaghan, Scott Robert Cameron, Andrew Neil Causer, Rebecca Jane Chalmers, Colin Gemin Chan, Shirley Chan, Timothy Chi Chan, Bernard Teck Luk Cheu, Chhay Jason Ly Ching Chhay, Allen Norman Cockfield, Carin Jeanette Conaghan, Angela Bridget Craig, Nicholas Bruce Cross, Judith Lynn Cubitt, Paula Maree Cummings, Philip John Davis, Christopher John Daynes, David John Doig, Annabelle Denise Donaldson, Matthew Philip Doogue, Kathryn Sarah Edward, James Edward Edwards, Kumudith Chameekara Ekanayake, Nicola Ann Elliot, James Michael Evans, Vanessa Anne Farr, Tracey Diane Fay, Caroline Fenton, Ross Howell Fountain, Dale Deirdre Fox, Dean Allan James Frear, Anusha Ganeshalingham, David Robert Gilbert, Adrian Howard Beaumont Gilliland, Anne Katherine Graham, Rebecca Grainger (Travelling Scholar 1997), Hadrian Alexander Luscombe Green, Joegelia Careso Green (Bacolcol), Nicholas Mathew Roberts Griffin, Jacquelin Lee Hall, Christopher Russell Harrington, Justine Leigh Harris, Michael Anthony Haymes, Karl James Hellyer, Simon David Hendl, Nicola Maret Hill, Jenny Ho, Selena Ann Hunter, Jennifer Etienne Hutton, Izan Ibrahim, Tristram Richard Ingham, Nicholas Dean Jacob, Anthony John Jacobson, Deborah Jane Jessup (Mitchell), Lisa Jane Johansson, Ingrid Jane Jolley, Nathan Reece Joseph, Shalini Devi Karan, Nor Afidah Karim, Steven John Kelly, Jonathan Donald Kennedy, Nee Chen Khoo, Cem Rahim Kibar, James Nicholas King, George Peter Kini, Oleg Kiriaev, Vincent Yan Lau Kai Kit, Michelle Elinor Lavill, Adeline Chern Yee Lee, Shuh Fen Lee (Moy), Kuok Aun Leow, Peter John Llewellin, Paul Martin Lodge, Hamish John Ernest Love, James Andrew MacDonald, Anne Louise McGregor, Michelle Kaye Dorman Mckinlay (McKinlay), Maria Mackintosh, Andrew James McLachlan, William Mitchell McMillan, Masliza Mahmod, Hasmannizar Abdul Manap, Fazal Karim Mann, Jarad Marcus Martin, Andrew Philip Matthews, Muhamad Khairudin Menon, Martin Alan Minehan, Alvin Denver Lagaluga Mitikulena, Todd Christopher Moesbergen, Norazhana Mohamad, Susannah May Mourton (Beehan), Jonathan Terence Moy, Achdiat Mahpha Fansuri Mustapa, Lawrence Ng, Jarrod Robert Ngan, Christopher James Nicholson, Brigid Maree O'Brien, Heidi Elizabeth Oettli (Conway),Gerardine

Mary O'Kelly, Dick Montague Ongley, Byron John Oram, Hairol Azrin Othman, Robert Eoin Park, Matthew Alan Paul, Judith Paull (Pain), Kyle Gareth Perrin, Rochelle Marie Phipps, Andrew John Pitcher, Kathleen Potter, Godfrey Jason Quin, Norhaslira Abdul Rahim, Eta Tavakuru Raicebe, Bishan Nishantha Rajapakse, Arun Ratnavadivel, Claire Aileen Reilly, Heidi Rentoul (McMillan), Megan Jayne Reynolds, Bronwen Jane Rhodes, Dean Stuart Robertson, Martin John Robinson, John David Robson, Amira Roessler (McMurray), Justine Elizabeth Candida Roots (Gearry), Rachael Kathleen Rowley, Mohd Fahmey Sabudin, Mohd Salleh Abdul Samad, Rohit Santram, Malcolm Richard Ian Scott, Sharyn-Jayne Seaboryne (Hayes), Richard Bryan Shepherd, Sharon Leighann Sime, Louise Margaret Sivertsen, Andrew William Smith, Kylie Jayne Smith, Nicole Robyn Smith, Mohd Ali Hanafiah Mat Soad, Chao Yang Soon, Amy Donna Stanway, Janet Sara Stedman (Geddes), Catherine Isobel Stewart, Nina Mary Stupples, Viktoria M. Sundakov, Hayley Joy Sweatman, Sanjeevana Roshan de Sylva, Kang Wei Tan, Eng Wei Tang, Dit Khiong Tee, Jeanne Tie, Stuart Lok Jiu Tie, Liam Kevin Tranter, Amanda Jane Turnbull, Margrietha Magdaleen van Wyk (Bismark), Nicholas George Waldron, Richard Thomas Wall, Eldon William Ward, Rachel Helena Webb, Sharmila Dharshini Weerasinghe (Bernau), Penelope Jayne Weir, Sarah Helen Welch, Heidi Leigh Werder (Waldron), Graham Clifford Wesley, David John Whitley, Dyanne Alison Wilson, Iain Malcolm Stewart Wilson, Anna Christine Winter (Bruce), Keith Neville Winters, Chi Wing Wong, Sue Chin Jennifer Wong, Khairulamir Zainuddin, Muhd Zanapiah Zakaria

1998

Zulkernain Ahmad, Sue Young Ahn, Lance David Anderson, Noraliza Bt Mohd Ariffin, Katherine Sarah Armour, Rachel Margaret Arms, Rosemary Helen Ayers, Sharul Abdul Aziz, Adam Alexander Bailey, Andrew Edward Baker, Christina Jane Baker (Lind), Mohammed Faizal Bakhtiar, Katherine Louise Bannehr (Speedy), Helen Louise Bird, Emma Jane Blair, Samuel Geoffrey Bloore, Christopher Peter Bowen, Sarah Penelope Bradford, Nicola Anne Broadbent, Robert John Bryant, Daren Carl Buhrkuhl, Terasa Frances Bulger, Arif Anuar Burhan, Anthony Philip Butler, Leanne Cameron (Travelling Scholar 1998), Matthew David Chacko, Mui Khoon Chang, Ramandeish Megen Chatha (Wood), Chien-fang Megan Chiu, Pai-yi Chou, Jacqueline Ann Claridge, Rachel Hong Clarke, Paul Lloyd Coceancig, Rosalind Marcella Crawford, Hamish Graeme Curry, Azlan Darus, Ilse Dirkzwager, Tania Claire Dryburgh (Stokes), Adam Walter Durrant, Rowan Louise Durward-Saunders, Tony John Falkiner, Adrian Lachlan Feint, Joanna Louise Fenwick, Bridget Ann Fogarty, Tailulu Luisa Fonua, Nicola Jane Ford, Annette Elizabeth Forrest, Claire Louise Frampton, Claire Kirsten Frizzell, John Marshall Garrett, Brent James Gaskin, John Andrew Alfred Geddes, Kelly Louise Gibbs, Iain Charles Gilmore, Heather Joy Guy, Hazlee Abdul Hadi, Gregory James Harkness, Azlina Binti Ali Abul Hassan, Joelon Martin Hays, Jeremy Michael Hickling, Lu Wei Hii, Richard Lu Hii, Kate Barbara Hill, Adrian George Hindes, Timothy Peter Hodgson, Ann Barbara Horner, Mark Edmund Houghton, Todd Geoffrey Hulbert, Gavin Charles Hutana, John Hamilton Irvine, Graham Joseph Jeffs, Ben Joss Johnston, Shamsul Anuar Kamarudin, Cameron James Lacey, Heather Patricia Lane, Wai John Lee, David Murray John Lienert, Ee Wei Lim, Karen Sok-Hian Lim, Christopher Raymond Peter Lind, Yow Oh (Simon) Ling, Kaye Elizabeth Logan, Brendan Charles Luey, Michael John McArtney, Anna Frances McConnell, Samuel Ross McCormack, Geoffrey Boyce McCracken, Tristan McGeorge, Joanne Helen McGregor, Matthew Ian MacKay, Bruce Norman McKinnon, Geraldine Anne Mackle, Peter Ian McQuillan, Giritharan Mahadevan, Vance Neville Manins, Paul Raymond Manley, Janine Maree Rashid Mardani, Benjamin Charles Margetts, Alan John Mawhinney, Kenneth Paul Melvin, Stephen Christopher

Merrilees, Christopher Millar, Helen Elizabeth Miller, Jan Vladimir Miller, Allen Mervin Saifoloi Mitikulena, Michael Charles Morrison, Geoffrey Kafutee Mudu (Muduioa), Zulkeflee Muhammad,Katherine Pamela Muir, Peter Andrew Newton-Howes, Simon Paul Nicholas, Mark Arthur Nixon, Nicholas Grant Norman, Katherine Margaret Norton, Bradley David O'Connor, Tracey Maree O'Flynn, Shen Tat Ooi, Robert Joseph Orec, Genevieve Tyra Ostring, Homizarina Bte Othman, Nik Adilah Nik Othman, Maree Louise Owen, David Lachlan Palmer, Leanne Carol Parker, Bhaveshkumar Patel, Hussain Yusuf Patel, Richard James Pendleton, Rachel Marama Potae, Marianne Power, Syed Fairuzelnajeeb Syed Abdul Rahman, Muhammad Ramnizar Ramli, Anil Manu Ranchord, Azlinazura Abd Rasid, Richard Andrew Rawstron, Graham Matthew Balfour Reeves, Gareth John Richards, Christopher William Rumball, Shamnika Deepal Rupasinghe, Soheila Rashid Safari, Nor Azimah Salleh, Marina Abdullah Sani, Vanessa Selak, Kerry Anne Sexton, Mohna Sudha Sharma, Caroline Victoria Shaw, Robert Alistair Shaw, Hamish Gregor Simmers, Rachael Amy Smith, Andrew John Snell, Rebecca Ruth Stack, Catherine Elizabeth Stone, Olivia Ann Stuart, Richard Paul Sullivan, Elaine Ik Ling Tan, Song Liang Tan, Deborah Sandra Mary Taylor (Smith), Belinda Jan Thompson, Isileli Ma'Afu Tonga, Benedict Ka-Wai Tseung, Katherine Tuck, Maartje Johanna Tulp, Peni Vaha, Brigitte Eve Waibel, John Su-Wun Wang, Andrew James Warnock, Helen Weston, Stephen Keith Whiting, Justin Robert Wilde, David Iain Wilson, Aroha Murchie Winsome (Dacker), Siaw Jin Wong, Duncan Morris Wood, Gemma Wood, Michael John Woodfield, Sally Ann Wright, Kah Mun Yee, Chong-Meng Yeo, Cheryl Lok See Yeung, Zamsyari Zakaria; MD; Sharifah Noor Akmal

1999

Kara Riria Ackerman, Scott Gordon Adams, Robyn Louise Aldridge, Stewart Alexander Allan, Jeremy Bernard Allen, Stephen Timothy Andrews, Yama Atal, Kelly Jean Austin, Rebecca Selina Ayers, Kelvin John Badham, Mark James Bailey, Alexander Robert Baker, Sharmila Balanathan, Sandra Helen Barr, Alan David Barton, Jason Murray Barton, Sarah Rachel Barton, Nicholas Dodgshun Bedford, Karel Beeby (Voice), Ian Reginald Best, Karena Jan Binnie, Timothy Leonard William Blackstock, Lauren Jaqueline Brenner, John Barry Bridgman, Danielle Louise Brown, Nicholas Charles Buchan, Allannah Maree Burke, Wayne Carstens, Reuben James Casey, Poh Juan Chai, Vimal Girdhari Chand, Ya-Shu Chang, Mee-Yew Chen, Hui Kiun Chin, Andrew Cho, Kok Foong Choo, Alexandra Cole, Joanne Elizabeth Cole, Naomi Elizabeth Collins (Dunwoodie), Gareth William Coulter, Timothy James Currie, Nicholas John Cutfield, Joanna Louise Davis, Matthew James Debenham, John Raymond Denton, Glenn Doherty, Jason Terry Donovan, Andrew Jeremy Dunkley, Josephine Anne Easton, Kathleen Maire Fay, Jane Nicola Fielder, Fiona Joy Findlay, Jennifer Margaret Francis, Joshua Troy Freeman, Mark Geoffrey Gilbert, Jacqui Lee Gore (Young), Timothy Christian Gavin Grice, Jennifer Mary Griffin, Haron Rahmat bin Harun, Christopher David Haslett, Robert John Hensen, Michael John Herd, Jennifer Anne Hill (Davies), Timothy Matthew Hill, Brad Michael Hockey, Joanne Carol Holden, David Hou, James Philip Houghton, Pei-Chin Hsieh, Steven Marshall Hudson, Melissa June Hull (Audeau), Mohd Nor Akmal Husin, Nicholas James Hutton, Iliza Idris, James Anthony Innes, Nahla Irtiza Ismail, Donald James Jap, Dumindu Sanjeewa Jayasinghe, Sarah Elizabeth Jenkins, Sarah Robyn Jordan, Nurul Aida Binti Selamat Keliwon, Paul Antony Kelly, Sarah Megan Kennedy, Lift Hiong Khoo, Shih-Wei Kuo, Joanna Elizabeth Lambert, Geoffrey Lee, Tom Chao-Nan Lee, Marianka Sophie Leenheer-Langemeijer, Bernard Joseph Leuthart, Ana Licina, Chong Wan Lim, Kirstin Lindberg, Karen Pui Wee Ling, Kenneth Lee Maan Liong, Edward Joseph Livshin, Irene Ching Low, Mathew William Ludgate,

Derek Jah-Yuen Luo, Geoffrey Dougal McAlpine, James Israel McCormick, Vini Teresa MacDonald, Kylie Jayne McGregor, Hamish Douglas Robertson McKee, Barry Douglas McKenzie, Michael William McKewen, Nicola Jane Maddren, Alicia Celeste Massarotto, Wan Rahiza Wan Mat, Oliver John Watson Matthewson, Sameer Memon, Suzanne Edith Miles, Rosemary Jane Miller, Mazlina Mohamed, Catherine Tanya Moor, Fiona Jane Morris, Michael Neville Morrison, Christopher George Munns, Ingrid Ann Naden, Fatmawati Noseri Nazri, Jessica May Yoke Ng, Richard Mark Ng, Wai Leap Ng, Jing Hieng Ngu, Martha de Launey Nicholson, Fariz Safhan Mohamad Nor, Syafinaz Amin Nordin, Azizan Omar, Suhaila Omar, Eu Geen Ong, Michael Peter O'Reilly, Mohd Rozaidil HJ Othman, Kathryn Ann Payne, Sandhya Balakrishna Pillai, Chen Hui Po, Jonathan Charles Potter, Vaughan Richard Poutawera, Megan Annette Pow, Heidi Marie Pridmore, Geetha Sujatha Rajan, Lorna Gail Rankin, Edrin Nazri Abdul Rasib, Michelle Angela Reeves, Brenda Sally Rimkeit, Struan Charles Robertson, Catherine Amelia Robinson, Karl Heinz Rodins, Penelope Joy Rowley, Cameron John Ryan, Paul Benjamin Samson, Rowan Schouten, Ralph Ewing Scorgie, Kylie Louise Sellwood, Claire Suzanne Shadwell, Salesh Sharma, Matthew Gordon Shaw, Jake Shortt (Travelling Scholar 1999), Craig Nicholas Temple Skidmore, Eileen Yin Yin Sung, Juliet Ee-May Tay, Jennifer Ann Taylor, Lai Peng Tham, Caroline Chia-Ling Tsai, Andrew Murray Ure, James Edgeworth Ussher, Eline van Empel (Thomson), Fipi Lagilagi Vatucicila, Nova Emily Waaka, Camie Wang, Gavin James Watson, Brenda Dianne Welsh (Poutawera), David Edwin Whybrew, William Matthew Widdowson, Gregory David Williams, Lisa Ann Williamson, Katherine Ann Wilson, Nicola Alice Wing, Catalina Sui-Kit Wong, Wen Giock Wong, Virginia Jane Wootton, Nik Ahmad Zahar Nik Yah, Maylin Anne Yap, Azlin Yusma MD Yusup, Azmil Farid Zabir, Shazharn Muhammad Zain, Khairul Anuar Zainun; MD: Robert John Hancox

2000

Nik Nairan Abdullah, Hamdi Najman Achok, Mohd Jamal Ahmad, Raja Elina Afzan Binti Raja Ahmad, Zaid Mahboob Ali, Yvonne Claire Anderson, Nicholas Anticich, Mohamed Ashraff Bin Mohd Ariff, Dianne Ruth Avery, Raflis Ruzairee Bin Awang, Damir Azhar, Graeme Michael Bain, Amil Suresh Balu, Narmali Kristina DeSaa Bandaranayake, Rachel Margaret Barber, Peter William Beggs, Damon Andrew Bell, Kristin Shirley Bell, Patrick John Beverley, Duncan James Oke Blaikie, Timothy James Bolter, Matthew James Boyd, James Harry Bradshaw, Arihia Maia Brewerton, Brent Ower Caldwell, Christina Rae Cameron, James Paul Cameron, Grant Haynes Cavit, Brendon Mathew Ah Chan, Damian Robert Clark, Craig Bryan Collie, Philip Daniel Conaglen, Fiona Lai Shan Connell, Sean Patrick Cope, Andrew James Coster, Veronica Bernadette Crawford, Ruth Cunningham, Lesley Adrienne Cupitt, Catherine Ann Davidson, Kimberley Joy Davies, Michaela Jayne Dawson, Liza Kathleen Edmonds, Patrick Oliver Munroe Emanuel, Ivana Erac, Ahmad Afkhar Fakhrizzaki, Andrew William Fenton, Margaret Woon Man Fok, Katherine Anna Foulds, Kim Lisa Fuller, Henry Matthew Gallagher, Denzil James Gill, Anna Isabelle Gilmour (Heenan), Huan-Tzin Goh, Lynn Heather Graham, Shaun Henri Grant, Hamish Steven Gray, Helwa Binti Abdul Hafidz, Stuart Barclay Hall, Julie Ann Hamilton, Stephen Benjamin Hamilton, James Rowan Harraway, Marie Renee Mane Hartley, Nigel Ian Hartnett, Thomas John Swanley Harwood, Anna Catherine Healy, Nigel James Henderson, Alastair James Hepburn, Wendy Tzu-Yun Huang, Zubin Othman Ibrahim, Alastair James Ineson, James Robert Irwin, Tineke Aleasha Iversen, Hayati Bte Jaafar, Christopher Glyn Charles Alexander Jackson, Hamish Arthur Jamieson, Matthew Alexander Jenks, Melanie Kay Johns, Christopher Simon Jones, Paul Anthony Jones, Vaughan Allan Jones, Annuar Deen Mohd Kamal, Rachel Petra Kan, Janet Fiona Kelly, Mulvey John Kelly, Nicholas

Acland Kenning, Kushlani Shiromala Kumarasinghe, Amanda Lorraine Landers, David Lindsay Lang, Rebecca Becca Chaw Lau, Tessa Faith Clare Lavaris, Anna Michele Lawrence, David Lap Yan Lee, Jun Lee, Kuo Luong Lee, Haida Leung, Glen Mark Alan Lightbody, Gary Joo-Meng Lim, Chin-Wei Lin, Wenyuan Liu, Andrew Roland Lucas, Christopher Edward Luey, Amiria Catherine Lynch, David Gordon McKenzie, James Mark McKevith, Aidalina Bt Mahmud, Chee Dick Mak, Gillian Claire Mann, Christopher Sylvan Manning, Nicholas Webster Marks, Nitin Mathur, Sachin Mathur, Nicholas Graham Mellsop, Oliver Hamish Menzies, Katherine Aleida Meuli, Christopher David Miller, Sarah Anne Mills, Juliana Jao-Eingld Lo Ming, Adrienne Melissa Mafaligi Mitikulena, Raimie Moljono, Mohale Phillip Mongalo, Matthew John Anthony Monk, Stewart Edward Montgomery, Ian Robert Lewis Munro, Los Vincent Newton, Siti Salmy Mat Nor, Brendon James O'Donoghue, Claire Tracey Olsson, Claire Louise Palmer, Craig Anthony Pelvin, Judith Anne Penney, Sarah Jane Perano, Sonya Jane Peters, Jody Anne Porter, Saurabh Prakash, Neil Robert Price, Victoria Louise Quin, Thuhairah Hasrah Abdul Rahman, Nicholas Jason Christopher Randall, Maivili Mathavi Raveenthiran, Victoria Jean Ring, Belinda Jane Robb, Adam Michael Roberts, Nicolas William Rogers, Juliet Mary Louise Rumball, David Matthew Rusk, Thomas Joseph Matiu Sanders, Inga Petrice Schader, Gabrielle Karen Scott (McDonald), Matthew Richard Scott, Brian John Scrimshaw, Elango Selvarajah, Sarah Lauren Sew Hoy, Sumitra Shankar, Peter Jonathan Hugh Sharr, Jamie Watson Shepherd, Adam James Harper Sims, Maria Sippen, Anna Catherine Skinner, Jonathan Alastair Smiles, Saxon Donald Smith, Anita Soma, Paul Miles Morell Stevenson, Peter Noel Stiven, Elke Patricia Strating, Sonali Disna De Sylva, Davina Lisa Tai, Kuan Shin Tan, Glenys Christine Tayles (Currie), Fraser James Taylor, Katriona Jane Thompson, Angela Ruth Thomson (Stephen), Hsien Kim Thoo, Kerry Jane Thornbury, Thomas Townend, Andrew Gordon Tucker, Clinton Paul Turner, Gianluca Valsenti, Catherine Sarah Vickers, Kirsten Anne Wadsworth, Anna Margaret Walker (Teata), Heidi Christian Walker (Travelling Scholar 2000), Laurence James Cedric Walker, Heather Jean Ward, Nicola Ward, Mary Rachel Warren, Gerald Philip Waters, Matthew Robert Webber, Sara Lilian Whimster (Baker), David John Whitehead, Fiona Kate Wilson, Heather Dawn Wishart, Gee Hing Wong, King Kiet Wong, Nur Yazmin Bte Yaacob, Handurugamage Manisha Namalee Yapa (Perera), Haur Sen Yew, Azny Syahirah Bt Mohamad Yusof, Rosmiyati Mohammed Zabidi

2001

Mahnaz Afsari, Steven Denis Alexander, Lakshman Thevakumar Anandanayagam, Khairullah Bin Anuar, Catherine Elizabeth Appleby, Astrid Elizabeth Anna Atlas, Noorul-Izzah Binte Mohd Azmi, Sonya Heidi Bader, Matthew Bailey, Tania Marie Bailey, Nor'Arifah Bt Abu Bakar, Jo-anne Dorothy Barclay, Adele Marie Barr, Emma Jane Beech, Sarah Jane Bellhouse, Dane Blackford, Thomas Boakye, Sonja Marie Bodley, Philippa Jane Bolton, Sharon Elizabeth Brandon, Louise Catherine Bremer (Donovan), Allan James Brown, Sarah Jane Buller, Nicholas Graeme Burgess, Michele Cameron (Causer), Benjamin Luke Hunter Campbell, Wan Yiu Wandy Chan, Timothy Mark Chapman, Isobella Cheung, Jenny Hui Chia Chieng, Ken Leong Chin, Tarragon MacLeod Chisholm, Wee Hin Chiu, Boon Ghee Chong, Chester Lun Yin Chong, Dyi-Jiunn Chuang, Shunn Miin Chuang, Deborah Ann Clarke, Sarah Jane Cooper, Karen Alice Court (Lewthwaite), Kendall Ann Crossen, Simon Charles Dalton, Kristian Garde Boyce Dalzell, Ohad Dar, Christopher William Davison, Saira Sonia Dayal, Patricia Ying Jia Ding, Magid Atif Fahim, Susan Leigh Fairbrother, Peter Maurer Ferguson, Evelyn Jayne Finlay (Gerrish), Julie Marie Fitzjohn (Travelling Scholar 2001), Angela Joy George, Derek William Goodisson, Nicola Helen Graham, Maryke

Griessel, Stephen Leonard Gunn, John Andrew Harrison, Michelle Heather Heaps (Cliffe), I-Li Ho, Samuel Hung Wai Ho, Sarah Ellen Howard, Adibah Bt Ibrahim, Antony James Inder, Mazuan Ismail, Carmel Maree Jacobs, Juliana Binti Jalil, James Paul Jarman, Oliver John Jeffery, Janice Margaret Jensen (Allfrey), Susan Caroline Johns, Kyra Louise Jones, Amir Reza Kalanie, Ami Kamdar, Joshua Timothy Kempthorne, Melissa Jenny Kerdemelidis, Ee Min Kho, Hae Won Kim, Stefan Dougal Kuiper, Julie Marie Lamont, Louis Meng-Yun Lao, Andrew Russell Lienert, Yu-Min Lin, Matthew Ka Wah Lo, Rachael Marion Loan, Conlin Wayne Locke, Jasmine Marie Chiou Iang Low, Jye Ru Lu, Abigail Jane Lynch, Bridgett Kay McDiarmid, Maya Macfarlane, Susan Heather Macleod (Grindlay), Rebecca Louise McNearnie, Jeremy Benjamin Madigan, Miswanudin Muizudin Mahyudin, Najwa Binti Mansor, Sherry Leigh Martin (Meek), Eileen Grace Merriman (Thompson), Krys Alistair Milburn, Natasha Jane Milestone, Logan Vaughan Mitchell, Ahmad Mahyuddin Bin Mohamed, Nik Rowina Binti Nik Mohammed, Chanel Moran, Siti Farah Alwani Bt Mohd Nawi, Nazatul Shahnaz Binti Mohd Nazri, Seamus John Newell, Sarah Louise Newton, Marie Neylon, Amane Nukada, Judy Frances Ormandy, Lauren Ovens, Clinton George Paine, Travis Niroshan Perera, Daniel John Pettigrew, Ruth Lim Shyh Ping, Clara Pishief, Jacqueline Marie Pitchforth (Chilcott), Ruhaila Binti Abdul Rahim, Marzilawati Binti Abd Rahman, Arvind Raju Ganga Raju, Kim Ann Ramjan, Suraya Binti Abdul Razak, Ahmad Riaz Fami bin Razali, Penelope Jane Rice-Wilson, Anjana Sonali De Rosairo (de Almeida), Paul Nicholas Rowan, Sharon Sagee (Leitch), Katherine Jessie Salmond, William Thomas Paul Simcock, Michelle Rose Simmons, Martyn Craig Sims, Rajdev Singh, Robert John Slade, Alistair James Smith, Natasha Maree Smith, Rebecca Mary Smith, Richard Donald Briton Smith, Richard Graeme Stubbs, Karl Peter Sturm, Aneta Krystyna Suder, Aqmar Suraya Binti Sulaiman, Su Yin Tang, Stephanie Louise Taylor (Jones), Michael Antonio Albert Thomson, Charles Lok Hui Tie, Sonya Nadine Towns, Charles Chao Chun Tsang, Kit Yung Karen Tsui, Christopher Ian Turnbull, Kate Cherie Ure (Eyre), Alexia Jane Urlwin, Paul Grant van Wijngaarden, Chi Hung Andy Watt, Heather Wehman, Kim Yuh-Kuan Weng, Miriam Elisabeth Wenzel, Benjamin John Wheeler, Miriam Louise Wheeler, Angus Munro Wickham, Angela Ruth Williams, Aron Hayden James Withers, Bronwyn Caryl Wong, Lai Yee Belinda Wong, Emma Elizabeth Yates, Po Yee Yip, King Wei Yong, Emma Mei-Leung Young, Simon William Young, Tony Jerng Che Young, Stanley L. Yu, Nurzeiti Yuslinda Bt Yusof, Afida Sohana Binti Awang Soh Yusoff

2002

Anis Ezdiana bt Abdul Aziz, Nor Azlina Binti Ahmad, Ali Omar Mustafa Al-Dameh, Farah bt Alwi, Amer Siddiq bin Amer Nordin, Ranil Dimanka Appuhamy, Azira bt Azmi, Simon Patrick Baker, David Robert Bartle, Darin Paul Bilish, Sainimere Lico Boladuadua, Sarah Emily Bowker, Shelley Anne Boyd, Lucinda Kathleen Boyer, Justine Louise Bradley, Emma Joan Britton, Michael Stewart Buckley, Cheryl Anne Lacson Buhay, Megan Tracey Calcott, Ruth Ann Cameron, Ian James Cathro, Joyce Chai, Huan Wee Chan, Chia-ti Cheng, Eddy Hiu Wa Cheng, James Philip Chisnall, Lisa Joy Claxton (Karl), Angus Norman Colquhoun, Marnie Robyn Cox, Rosalind Dana Crombie, Julie Marie Curry, Mark Leonard Dagger, Matthew George Daly, Chamila Shamala De Alwis, Joana De Sousa, Carol Marie Dean, Michael Jeremy Dick, Patricia Diotto, Richard James Downing, Samuel Ariki Dunn, Linieta Eades, Erica Epstein, Daniel Joseph Exeter, James Andrew Falconer, Sarah Anne Fargher, Hina Feki, Jeremy Ranil Fernando, 'Emeline Falengameesi Fonua, Monica Leeanne Ford, Mark Simon Fry, Kirsten Gaerty, Sean David Galvin, Sasi Rekha Ganga Raju, Veronica Christina Gin, Andrew James Greer, Susan Val Gunn (Plunkett), Hye Won Han, Stephen Walter Harris, Hafizah bt Hashim, David Joseph Hassan,

Rebecca Mary Hayman, Sam Bolton Hazledine, Bridget Fleur Healy, David Thomas Highton, Timothy Bih Kien Hii, Jennifer Claire Hill, Benjamin Russell Hindson, Steven Szu-wei Ho, Stephen Joseph Hoskin, Gerome Tze Wei Hsiung, Richard Tremain Hurley, Richard Stewart Jaine, Antony Phillips Jenks, Thomas James Jerram, Kent Rangitewhiria John Johnston, Jin Sung Joung, Luke Kain, Toral H Kamdar, Matthew Jacob Kelly, William George Kenyon, Alice Catherine Kevern, Jane Khaw Lih Jye, Cho Yee Kim, Tracey Lam, Damon Paul William Lane, Eva Leonora Lange, Nicholas John Lash, Mohammad Haroon Latif, Catherine Faleola Latu, Mon Hoo Lau, Joseph Lau Chung Heng, Vivienne Mary Law, Nicola Jayne Lawrey (van der Hulst), Quoa Young Lee, Lee Hui Yann, Lee Wai Gin, Arna Felicity Letica, Mou Kow Martin Leung, Martin Hsiu-Chu Lin, Emily Liu, Tin Heng Lock, Nicholas James Longley, Li Nyuk Loo, Ken Looi, Simon John McDowell, Glenn John McKay, Grace Elizabeth McPherson, Paula Jane MacRury, Daniel Charles Marshall, Vinita Mathew, Ruth Emily Mattingley (Wright), Michael James Maze, Robert Thomas Mitchell, Ahmad Farihan bin Mohd Don, Mohd Iskandar bin Mohd Ghazali, Barnaby Henare Montgomery, Conrad Jurek Morze, Jessica Caroline Mouat, Sharmini Muttaiyah, Seon Young Nam, Virginia Patricia Newman, Grabiel Kei Yiu Ng, Long Van Nguyen, Lesley Marie Nicol (Rumball), Khairun Nain bin Nor Aripin, Joanna Robyn O'Keefe, Penina Caroline Pereira, Jann Pickard, Justine Louise Pickett, Estelle Louise Pointon, James Richard Pole, Aleksandra Popadich, Sevvandi Premachandra, Patrick Julien Frederik Pritzwald-Stegmann, Evelyn Pui Wee Wee, Deborah Maree Rea (Barham), Penelope Jayne Rickman, Timothy David Deans Ritchie, Lucien Dominic Robie, Caroline Jane Robins, Philip Cameron Robinson, Emily Caroline Ross, Bryony Katharine Ryder, Andre Nicholas Schultz, Jeanette Mary Scott, Rebekah Ankusha Shaw, Halpewattege Isabelle Chrishendri Dilushini Silva, Hayley Anne Simpson, Elizabeth Jane Smaill, Richard Ian Smiley, Timothy Hugh Snook, Christopher Paul Spencer, Janine Toni Stevens, Henry Dominic Stracey Clitherow, Fairulliza bt Suha, Jaynaya Kathleen Thrush (Marlow), Christina Tuyet Ngoc Tieu, Courtenay James Tiffen, Clifton Edwin Timmins, Tam Hien Hien Trinh, David Graham Tripp, Stephen Charles Howard Tripp, James Jonathan Tuckett, Ritva Vyas, Christopher John Warren, Vanessa Joan Weenink, Asha Samantha Wettasinghe, Loretta Teresa Wigg, Andrew Keith Williams, Francessa Louise Wilson, Scott William Wilson, Aileen Li Ho Wong, James Pak-Wei Wong, Lee Hao Wong, Jordan Gardiner Wood, Hsin-Yu Sally Wu, Arthur Shang-Che Yang, Yu-ting Yeh, Deane Li-Shen Yim, Vincent Chung Ting Yiu, King Yee Yong, Jill Yu (Chi-Yuan Yu), Homayoun Zargar Shoshtari, Caroline Chunlei Zhou. MD: Evan James Begg

2003

Brandon Michael Adams, Hamish Stewart Alexander, Mohammed Imran Asaf Ali, Nagham A.H. Ali Al-Mozany, Daniel James Anderson, Joseph Frederick Baker, Colin Stewart Barnes, Irma Bilgrami, Michelle Anne Bloor, Kathryn Bray, Rebecca Louise Bond (Velluppillai), Helen Mary Bray, Robert Bruce Brown, Lauren Nadia Browne, Rebecca Jane Buchan, Nicholas Charles Butterfield, Sarah Catherine Callaghan, Laird Bruce Cameron, Joy Krishna Chakraborty, Mandira Chakraborty, Christina Wei-Hsin Chan, Huan Keat Chan, Hsien Cheng Chang, Winston Shyh Jye Chang, Hua Kiat Chen, Nicholas David Child, Tin Lok Chiu, Tin Lun Chiu, Julia Anne Cole, Jason Priestley Cook, Jacqueline Anne Copland (Shaw), Eloise Catrine Cottee, Kirsten Marie Crooke, Mya Cubitt, Neil Patrick Curran, Rachel Anne Davidson, Kathryn Frances Dawson, Ilaitia Tikotikovakadi Delasau, Emma Jordan Deverall, Catherine Margaret Dick, Thomas Marcel Douglas (Rhodes Scholar=2003), Rosemary Kaye Duckett, Robert Stuart James Elliott, Jason Yen Kang Feng, Sarah Joanne Fitzsimons, Miriam Karen Gavin-Franklin, Emily Anne Gill, Tiffany Sheryn Glass, Joanna Moira Glengarry,

Matthew Jay Goodyer, Bernadette Mary Laura Green, Alice Kathleen Guidera, Alana Jane Heath, Marissa Candace Henderson, Tanya Joan Henderson, Aidan Murray Hodges, Kieran Mark Holland, Todd Anton Hore, John Chen Hsiang, I-Pen Hsu, Hsuan-Ting Huang, Jannatul Ferdous Jaforullah, Ryan Jinu Jang (Jin Woo Jang), Suren Kaushal Jayaweera, Angus Cordner Jennings, Helen Jo, Sarah Annabella Johri, Alveera Raffiq Karim, Debbie Maree Keith-Dance (Higgins), Amirala Khalessi, Vivienne Kim, Katrina Kirikino, Andrew Simbwa Kibuka Kiyingi, Ilamaran Kumarasamy, Christiana Lisa-Rosa Lafferty, Tracey Kathryn Lang, Katrina Leah Langley, Dipti Lath, Rowena Anne Lawson, Grace Lee, Kyung Lee, Ming Lee, Yu Hang Leung, Guang Min Li, Yung Lung Liang, Nicholas James Lightfoot, David Tien Ang Lim, Tien Ming Lim, Chou Yen Lin, Frank Po-Yen Lin, Keng Hsin Lo, Frances Hui Leng Loo, Rebecca Sue-Ai Loo, Simon Ming-Yan Lou, Melissa Anne Low, Justine Sylvia McCallum, Christy Anna Macdonald, Michelle Kay MacDonald, Hamish Stuart Mace, Jeffrey Brian Macemon, Bjorn Dax Makein, Damian Kevin Marsh, Ineke Carmelita Clara Meredith, Reuben John Miller, Jonathan Douglas Minton, Thomas John Moodie, Koon Ling Mooi, Bronwyn Elizabeth Morris, Joanna Claire Muir, Nisha Nair, Sheetal Natha, Sharon Meei Ay Ngu, Huu Hoai Nam Nguyen, Jacob Yoong Leong Oh, Anselm Swee Kiet Ong, Nicholas James Oscroft, Catherine Leigh Parker, Rajeshbhai Kantibhai Patel, Vipul Patel, Sharon Tracy Pattison, Jake Nathaniel Pearson, Fiona Dorothy Perelini, Yih Jia Poh, Shalvin Rusheel Prasad, Julie Marie Price, Tracey Lee Putt (Coutts), Jessamine Reddy, Juliette Natalie Renaud, Jonathon Lee Richards, Frances Elizabeth Robbins, Logan Dudley Robinson, Lisa Helen Rofe (Mortimer), Anna Louise Scott, Ann Elizabeth Sears, Eugene Sien Deng Sia, Emerine Cherumi Dhanukshi Silva, Christina Yin Lei Sin, Adriane Jane Sinclair, Mark Alexander Smith, Troy Hampden Smithers, Sarah Victoria Sparks, Georgia Frances Stefanko, Gwendolyn-Mary Stewart, Michael Blair Stewart, Kate Strachan, Philip Alan Suisted, Raymond James Tai, Eugene Ewe Jin Tan, Olivia Lee Ting Tan, Rebecca Jody Tapp, Daryoush Tavanaiepour, Wei Han Tee, Angeline Teo Mei-Ping, Daniel Wen Chung Then, Kimberley Joanna Thomson, Ann Deborah Thornton (Guy), Katrina 'Oto'ota Tonga, Ailsa Claire Tuck, Sherry Tuiuli Mu Tagaloa, Sarah Jane Usmar, Marilize Ussher (de la Porte), Simon Henry Ussher, Silvia Judith Valsenti, Ansulette Van Splunder (Kay), Caleb Nathaniel Kai-Lik Vossen-Chong, Christopher David Walker, Jeremy George Webber, Melanie Dawn Webster, Yuranga Dilan Weerakkody, Travis Riley Westcott, Kenneth Barry White, April Zin Huey Wong, Sam Wong, Matthew John Wilson Wright, Ching Wan Wu, Kang-yu Wu, Michael Chi Wah Yip, Po Che Yip, Robin David Young, Kamran Zargar Shoshtari

2004

Jaslina Abdul Aziz, Sinan Albayati, Placide Vaune Elvis Alexis, Christy Ann Allan, Jessica Jane Allen, Marwan Momtaz Yousi Al-Zibari, Sahan Chathura Amarasena, Cameron Mahon Anderson, Kirsten Jessie Jane Anderson, Daniel Scott Andrews, Mary Wagih Fakhry Azer, Jean-Paul Marc Banane, Rita Banhalmi, Katherine Alice Bartlett, Jodie Emma Battley, Tristan Robert Bennett, Michael John Bergin, Nina Francis Bevin, Alicia Rose Blaikie, Kirsten Rosalie Lamont Bond, Sandra Elma Perdue Bourke, Angela Louise Butler, Geoffrey Paul Carden, Benjamin Hugh Carpenter, Natalie Jane Carter, Christopher Brian Cederwall, I-Ting Chan, Michael Chun Lap Chan, Chia-Fu Chen, Frank Cheng Fan Chen, Wai Li Chew, Yun Seo Choi, Yee Hui Chong, Annie I-Wen Chou, Chuan-tsung Chou, Tina Yu-Ting Chou, Anwar Shahzad Choudhary, Yuan Chu, Nola Adria Cobcroft, Adele Louise Colville, Shaun Jeremy Counsell, Ro Miriama Saunayalewa Delaibatiki, Raminder Singh Dhillon, Kandath Girijashankar Dhiraj, Michelle Louise Dickson, Hannah Joan Donaldson, Natalie Sylvia Marie Durup, James Beckham Duthie, Nicola

Jane Dykes, Nicola Anne Emslie, Peter Nabil Awadalla Fahmy, Jonathan Won-Hau Foo, Inga Jade Frederikson, David Ziggy Fyfe, Kelly Ann Gendall, Danielle Leigh Gerrard, Shiree Jasmine Gibbs, Wayne Kelson Gillingham, James Lawrence Glasgow, Ruchith Prasanna Gooneratne, Samuel Rollison Greig, Benjamin James Griffiths, Michael James Roy Halstead, Marissa Parrott Hampson, Harriet Eve Harper, Anna Louise Harris, Linda Talimoka Head, Andrew James Herd, David Hernandez, Rachel Clare Highton, Charlotte Jane Hill, Daniel Richard Hobbs, David Paul Hobbs, Richard John Holland, Claudia Daria Ursula Ho-Peng, Anthony Peter Houlding, Wayne Fang Wei Hsueh, William Hsin-Chieh Huang, Kate Louise James, Damian Hee-Sung Jiang, Joshua Matthew Pirini Johnstone, Evan Alan Jolliffe, Vincent Sze Sern King, Matthew Stephen Kirk-Jones, Lukasz Wojciech Klobukowski, Jonathan James Knight, Joseph Ming Kwan Koh, Rajiv Kumar, Andrew Vaughan Laurenson, Jethro Michael LeRoy, Daniel Mattathiah Levine, Anna Megan Levy, Kaylie Helen Lewell, Steven Tien Chai Lim, Vaughan Robert Lock, Bernard Christopher McCarthy, Kylee Hannah Maclachlan, Andrew Charles McLaughlin, Andrew John McNally, David Johnathan McQuade, Adrian Jules Macquet, Pralene Renu Maharaj, Rachelle Jenny Mason, Daniel Richard Mattingley, Felicity Claire Meikle, Sohrabh Memon, Stuart Michael Millar, WendyElizabeth Miller, Dominic Monaghan, Benjamin Gerald Moon, Samuel Thomas Moon, Louine Renee Bernadette Morel, Justin Bernard Morze, William Nepia Moss, Alison Rose Moulton, Benjamin James O'Leary, Anita Angela Page, Brooke Elizabeth Paisley, Timothy Maxwell Gray Panckhurst, Jung Moon Park, Sarah Catherine Parker, Christopher Tino Hamana Pene, Lisa Jane Percy, Samuel Stuart Phillips, Zelda Shanti Hattie Voigt Pick, Rupesh Kumar Puna, Gayathri Ramani, Thilini Ranasinghe, Tamsin Melanie Roberts, Joanne Clare Rogers, Aflah Roohullah, Naomi Amiria Schumacher, Allanah Catherine Scott, Kontoku Yoon Shimokawa, Ruoh Whay Sim, Kellie Lee Sizemore (Perrie), Lachlan Maurice Smith, Stephanie Jane Smith, Zafar Basil Viliamu Smith, Hee Jin Song, Maya Jane Steeper, Monique Francoise Stravens, Heidi Yi-han Su, Hugh Sung, Kirstine Jane Sutton, Sunaina Talwar, Aik Haw Tan, Michael Nader Zaki Tawadrous, Jonathan Colin Kersley Taylor, Claire Louise Thurlow, Chiew Ling Ting, Darryl Chan Tong, Sidharth Trivedi, Catherine Marie Truman, Han Tuan Truong, Vanessa Victoria Vallely, Gregory Adrian Van Der Hulst, Matthew Graham Van Rij, Ayesha Jennifer Verrall, Brooke Jean Vickerman, Hayden Francis Waghorn, David Richard Waterhouse, George William Waterworth, Wharemarama Marihi Wepa, Oonagh Ruth Margaret Wesley-Smith, Daniel Paul Weston, Jonathon Matthew White, Priscilla Jane Wildbore, Lauren Joy Williamson, Sarah Elvira Wilson, Prasangika Wimalasena, Martin John Wolley, Andrew Vincent Wong Ming, Daniel Brook Wood, Karen Robyn Hilary Wright, Scott Yu-Chun Wu, Catherine Guanlian Xu, Mrudula Yeletotadahalli Krishnaswamy, Pranavan Yoganathan, Mayada M. Yahya Zaki; MD: David Gareth Jones

2005
Damien Laurie Ah Yen, Erik William Andersen, Rebecca Margaret Ashman (Hughes), Jordan James Baker, Rachel Abigail Balfour (Caswell-Smith), Edward Douglas Graham Bebb, Sarah Louise Beck, Susan Rosemary Stella Bibby, Hermione Jane Binnie, Patricia Ann Boyd, Chelsea Brindle, Katrina Claire Brougham, Shelley May Bruce (Thomson), Richard James Burt, Victoria Louise Campion, Anthony James Carrie, Rebecca Jane Carroll, Peter Andrew Caswell-Smith, Anannya Chakrabarti, Jonathon David Chambers, Joe Harn Chang, Yuan-Hsuan Chang, Yi-Hsuan Chen, Yu-Shian Cheng, Kim Michelle Chilman-Blair (Glasgow), Hwee Sin Chong, Chih Ching Choong, Chi-Ying Chou, Kent Tsz Kit Chow, Fiona Amiria Christian, Jen Jie Chu, Aimee Marie Clark, James Stuart Clark, Richard Paul Collins, Tania Ellen Cooper, Lauren Alice Cross, Matthew James Herman Dalman,

Alexander Paul Benjamin Dalzell, Rachel Clair Dempsey, Kaveh Djamali, Roana Donohue, George Stanley Downward, Leanne Jennifer Drew (Garcia), Joseph Lawrence Earles, Alice Pamela Jane Edgar, Sarah Mary English, Gregory Ralph Evans, Katherine Fairbrother, Caroline Diana Fairhall, Sophie Jane Febery, Rebecca Anne Field, Yukio Conrad Flinte, Victoria Christina Francis, Bridget Lea Fry, Jesse Gale, Russell James Gear, Premjit Kaur Gill, Jonathan Wayne Graham, Christopher Mark Gray, Emma Louise Griffiths, Nourul Hayati Azrina Binti Haji Jaman, Haji Mohammad Khamirol Hidzan, Haji Satry Haji Sani, Carl Francis Harmer, Kelli Hart, Benjamin John Hayward, Sanjeeva Chandika Herath, Kushlin Rachel Higgie, Fiona Annette Hobbs, Nicola Jane Holdgate, Wei-Hsun Hsu, Kimberley Anne Hurlow (Shaw), Benjamin James Image, Andrew Kenneth Irving, Nicholas Robert Johnston, Nicholas John Kennedy, Christine Mei Chin Khoo, Hyun Ah Kim, Jae-Heon Kim, Lawrence Hyun Chul Kim, Woo Sung Kim, Michael James Kimber, San Shuen Ku, Sherman Shu Han Kueh, Nadine Frances Kuiper, Vivek Kumbhari, Fiona Lai Hui San, Karoline Esther Lalahi, Heath William Roy Lash, Ying Miin Law, Campbell John Le Heron, Sau Kai Lee, Yoo Young Lee, Cameron David Lewis, Marianne Margaret Lill, Heather Bronwen Little, Benjamin Hon Kuen Liu, Jui Liu, Chi Chun Adeline Lo, Giovanni Simon Losco, Amanda Jane McConnell, Caleb Errington McCullough, Jade McCurdie, Julie Clare McDonald, Mark William Macdonald, Md Ali Shabbana Bin Mohd Yassin, Richard David More, Frances Laura Morrison, Katherine Blair Mullin, Uma Muthu Naguleswaran, Timothy Kenneth Neve, Scott William Raymond Newburn, Rachael Marie Norman (Marks), Maartje Gertrudis Susanna O'Brien (Beckers), Beth O'Connor, Ken Okawa, Charlotte Jane Muriel Oyston, Hana Pak, Sze Yin Pan, Catherine Elizabeth Ann Parker, Emily Tine Perelini, Jyotika Devi Prasad, David Samuel Prior, Hannah Frances Ross, Andrew Grayson Rowan, Arapera Hapuku Salter, Rachel Ann Sara, John Paul Scarlett, Monique Kyle Scott, Angus Shao, Andrea Nicole Sievwright, Clare Louise Smith, Tara Mae Smith, Angela Mairi Spalding, Amy Victoria Spark, Suzanne Frances Stainer, Kate Stanbridge, George William Stephenson, Elizabeth Ann Stockman, Alannah Morag Stockwell, Kuei-Chun Su, Aik Lyn Tan, Eunice Chern Lin Tan, Helen Louise Tanner, Bogna Irena Targonska, Anna Michelle Taylor, Elisabeth Switzer Taylor, Keryn Louise Taylor, Lara Ann Temple-Doig, Thu Thi Thach, Lucinda Katherine Thatcher, Dougal Newstead Thorburn, Kung How Ting, Reuben James Tomlinson, Cindy Renee Towns, Simon Richard Townsend, Laura Vercoe, Nathan Thomas Watkins, Bridget Jane Watson, Dayna Louise Weake, Susan Enid Weggery, Catherine Anne Venus White, Shashi Wijesinghe, Samantha Annabel Hope Williamson, Kate Louise Willoughby-Martin, Duncan Richard Wilson, Meg Olivia Wilson, Olivia Wong Siaw Wui, Jennifer Anne Wright, Cheng-Ai Wu, Wan-Ling Miriam Wu, Sofie Ann Yelavich, Shin Jee Yi, Yeh Won Yoo, Ming-Chang Yu, Nusrat Zahan, Jie Zhang

2006
Sarah Catherine Abbott, Placide Vaune Elvis Alexis, Bassal A. Al-Nasrallah, Abdulrahman M. Alqahtani, Jalal S.Alsaad, Mai M. Alshammari, Ali H.A. Alsinan, Mohammad Amer, Kirsty Elisabeth Andrews, Aylar Ansarian, Michel Daniel Arnephy, Claus Nico Bader, Peter Robert Barr, Kynan Peter Bazley, Derryn Anne Bicknell, Adnan Luqman Bilgrami, James Andrew Blackett, Maxim George Bloomfield, Irene Eleanor Braithwaite, Elizabeth Clare Briggs, Hilary Margaret Burbidge, Kathy Elizabeth Burt, Ella May Calder, Katie Eleanor Carter, Daisy Sisi Chan, Georgina Tzu-Ching Chan, Raymond Man Wah Chan, Benjamin Lik Jin Chang, Animesh Chatterjee, Erin Yi-Wen Chen, Hung-Kai Chen, Ko-Hsuan Chen, Kong Leong Chin, Gloria Jean Dainty, Philippa Anne Davey (Brown), Andrew James Davidson, Dilantha Thushara De Alwis, Ingrid Johanna Cath De Ruiter, Andrew John Dodgshun,

Nicola Gail Dodson, Sarah Michelle Donald, Nicholas Martin Douglas (Travelling Scholar 2006), Duane John English, Marie-Michelle Theres Ernesta, Sally Jane Eyers, Nancy Magdy Fayez Iskander, Patricia Fogarty, Michael Edward Foss, Romilla Mary Franks, Jamish Gandhi, Robert John George, Andrew Maurice Gilkison, Hui Fern Goh, Dinesh Priyantha Gooneratne, Judith Mary Gregan, Yu Mi Ha, Rasita Bint Haji Abdul Rahman, Mohammad el Haji Mohd. Ismail, Matilda Elizabeth Hamilton, Avneet Kaur Hansra, Jessica Anne Hardyment, Sophie Elizabeth Amy Hart, Georgina Hawkins, Norafizan Binti Hazipin, Daniel Hernandez, Jennifer Ging Huong Hii, Andrew George Darvel Hill, Philippa Lee Peng Ho, Timothy Oliver Hodgson, Christopher James Hopkins, Joshua James Howe, Erica Ting-Yi Hsu, Judy Chien-Chun Huang, Jeremy Alexander Hudson, Julia Elizabeth Hudson, James Douglas Hulleman, Elizabeth Anne Insull, Christopher Andrew Angu Irwin, Abbey Sara Jebb, James Walter Johnston, Deborah Kerei Johnstone, Laura Rachel Menzies Joyce, Tejaswi Kandula, Penelope Jean Kane, Justin Fook Siong Keasberry, Rawiri Keenan, Kate Elizabeth Kerr, Jung-Hyun Kim, Joanne Karen Knappstein, Carl Philip Knox, Dong-Hwan Ignatius Ko, Archana Koirala, Shaw Hua Kueh, Amanda Kirstin Mei-Lin Kusel, Melanie Lauti, Kathryn Jane Law, Maria Christina Lea, Peter Jun Woo Lee, Tommy Sen Lee, Robyn Fay Lester, Rachel Anne Liang, Anthony Tien Hoe Lim, Anthony Yen-Yiu Lin, Chou-Jui Lin, Sung-Ya Lin,Felicia Tien-See Ling, Brendan Paul Little, Mark Gregory Longman, Ngov Jasen Ly, Andrea Marie McDonald, Natasha Louise McKay, Monique Deanne MacKenzie, Bhaveen Kaur Marne, George Anthony Marshall, Joshua Martin, Julia Anne Helen Matheson, John Hugh Molloy, James Edward Moore, Prathyusha Nakka, Mumraiz Salik Naqshband, Leanne Neill, Lincoln Maurice Nicholls, David Mark O'Byrne, Karen Margaret Oldfield (Hall), Cathryn Elizabeth O'Sullivan,Harshad Patel, Mansi Patel,Timothy Martin Platt, Sumit Raniga, Nicholas Clifford Reid, Stephen Phillip Reid, Benjamin Michael Revell, Edrich Joseph Rodrigues, Kate Alexandra Elizabeth Romeril, Aimee Elizabeth Rondel, Melyssa Claire Roy, Magdalena Malgorzata Sakowska, Faeg M.W. Sawaf, Ross Dominic Scott-Weekly, Aparna Seethepalli (Raniga), Amanda Jane Shelton (Yardley), Karen Sheng, Philippa Mary Shirley, Claire Alicia Simpson, Matthew James Stephens, Anne Louise Stevenson, Phillippa Mere Stuart, Linda Mei-Yi Sung, Katayoun Taghavi, Ghassan Talab, Alvin Boon Tee Tan, Emma June Taylor, Julia Kate Taylor, Dennis Eng Keat Teh, Aveline Ai Ping Teo, Shyh Poh Teo, Rebecca Jane Thomas, Deidre Maree Thomson, Steven Francis Thrupp, James Andrew John Tietjens, Francis Sie Hui Ting,Chiong Hui Tiong, Samuel James Toner, Benjamin James Trist, Jennifer Jia-Ying Tsai, Wen-Hsun Tsai, Vishesh Turaga, Angus Richard Turnbull, Erin Lise Turner, Yu-Chieh Tzeng, Thomas James Upton, Kerryn Louise Van Rij (Settle), Simon Philip Van Rij, Xaviour James Walker, Hayley Marie Waller, Richard Michael Walsh, Eloise Claire Watson, Amanda Patricia Willis, Rebekah Jean Wilson (Thompson), Sarah Lee Rik Wirihana-Tawake, Christopher Aaron Hau Gw Wong, Donny Ik Ming Wong, Ngai Man Annie Wong, Verity Helen Wood, Zoe Victoria Woodward, Sharon Hsin-Jung Wu, Gretchen Elizabeth Fran Yates, Eileen Youn, Kirsten Michelle Young, Yixun Zhang,

The Travelling Scholarship in Medicine

Established in 1909, the scholarship has been awarded annually to the top student in the graduating class of the MB ChB degree. In 1989 it was renamed the Rita Gardner Travelling Scholarship and generously funded from a trust set up by Dr Gillies in honour of her sister Rita Gardner (née Gillies), an Otago medical graduate.

1909 Thomas William James Johnson (MD 1911)
1910 Michael Herbert Watt (MD 1912)
1911 William Philip Johnston (MD 1915)
1912 Thaddeus Julian
1913 William Sowerby (MD 1916)
1914 Roland Arthur Hertslet Fulton
1915 Donald Stuart Milne
1916 Mary Francesca Compere Dowling
1917 James Alfred Jenkins (Ch.M. 1924)
1918 Arthur John Cottrell
1919 Louis Amos Bennett (MD 1921)
1920 Cyril Arnold King
1921 Maurice Bevan Brown
1922 Charles Ritchie Burns (MD 1926)
1923 Robert Stevenson Aitken (Rhodes Scholar 1924) (MD 1939)
1924 John Alexander Douglas Iverach
1925 Alice Campbell Rose (Tallerman)
1925 James Fitzsimons
1926 Archibald Durward
1927 Lindsay Sangster Rogers
1927 Alfred Bramwell Cook (MD 1944)
1928 Jack Carl Rudolph Hindenach (MD 1931)
1929 Eric Vener Maxwell
1930 Norman Lowther Edson
1931 Thomas Russell Cumming Fraser (MD 1946)
1932 James Verney Cable (MD 1937)
1933 Robert John McGill
1934 Allenson Gordon Rutter
1935 George Edward Moloney
1935 Bruce Walton Grieve
1936 Harold Basil Alexander
1937 William Maxwell Manchester
1938 Kenneth Robert Stallworthy
1939 Jean Mary Sandel
1940 William Wybrow Hallwright
1941 Reginald Henry Hamlin
1941 Mervyn William Arthur Gatman
1942 Keith Remington Lothian
1943 Windsor John Weston (MD 1979)
1944 Walter Victor Macfarlane
1945 John Cuthbert Parr
1946 Hugh Alexander Fleming (MD 1952)
1947 Helen Rarity Young (McCreanor) (MD 1972)
1948 John Desmond Hunter (MD 1962)
1949 Robert Mervyn Mitchell (ChM 1957)
1950 John William Saunders
1951 Christopher Morgan Stubbs
1952 Leslie Credis Stewart
1953 John Ludbrook (ChM 1961) (MD 1973)
1954 Albert William Liley
1955 Allan John Taylor
1955 David George Palmer (MD 1961)
1956 Ralph David Huston Stewart (MD 1968)
1958 Peter Ronald Garrod
1959 Peter Barrie Herdson
1960 Alister James Scott
1961 John Verrall Allison
1962 Maureen Joan Lester (Peskett)
1963 Bramah Nand Singh (MD 1975)
1964 Graeme John Taylor (MD 1990)
1965 Ian MacMurray Holdaway (MD 1973)

1966 Mary Anthea Wright (Ellis)
1967 Elizabeth Celia Purves
1968 Robert Beaglehole (MD 1977)
1969 Bruce James Spittle
1970 Anthony Ridgway Coates
1971 Lorraine Joyce Beard
1972 David Christopher Graham Skegg
    (Rhodes Scholar 1972)
1973 Alastair John Corbett (MD 1987)
1974 Richard John Mackay
1975 Derek Nigel John Hart (Rhodes Scholar 1975)
1976 Jennifer Pauline Pilgrim
1977 Bridget Anne Robinson (MD 1987)
1978 Stephen Richard Munn
1979 David Schroeder
1980 Peter John Browett
1981 Peter Bruce Bethwaite
1982 Gordon Livingstone Patrick
1983 Ian Colin Stuart Kennedy (MD 1993)
1984 Michael John Burt
1985 Christopher Morice Ward
1986 Anthony Campbell White
1987 Arthur Richard Kitching
1988 Terrie Eleanor Inder (Foster) (MD 1997)
1989 Janine Maria Bailey
1990 Stephen Peter Robertson
1991 Katherine Louise Bate
1992 John David Danesh (Rhodes Scholar 1992)
1993 David Neil Hailes
1994 Philippa Jane Depree
1995 Nicola Jane Dalbeth (Moore) (MD 2005)
1996 Kim Margrethe McFadden
1997 Rebecca Grainger
1998 Leanne Cameron
1999 Jake Shortt
2000 Heidi Christian Walker
2001 Julie Marie Fitzjohn
2002 Matthew Jacob Kelly
2003 Georgia Frances Stefanko
2004 Andrew John McNally
2005 Jesse Gale and Julie Clare McDonald
2006 Nicholas Martin Douglas

The Rhodes Scholarship

Otago medical graduates have featured strongly in the award of this prestigious scholarship, first offered in 1904 and held for two to three years at Oxford University.

A few, whose names are asterisked, began their medical degrees at Otago but completed in the United Kingdom.

Arthur Espie Porritt (1923)*
Robert Stevenson Aitken (1924)
Wilton Ernest Henley (1929)*
John Edward Lovelock (1931)*
John Derek Kingsley North (1950)
Graham Harry Jeffries (1952)
Kenneth Alfred Kingsley North (1954)
James Julian Bennett Jack (1960)*
Murray Grenfell Jamieson (1970)
David Christopher Graham Skegg (1972)
Anthony Evan Gerald Raine (1973)
Derek Nigel John Hart (1975)
John Alexander Matheson (1975)
Nancy Jennifer Sturman (1983)
David Edward Kirk (1985)
Ceri Lee Evans (1988)
Prudence Anna Elizabeth Scott (1990)
John David Danesh (1992)
Jennifer Helen Martin (1993)
Thomas Marcel Douglas (2003)
Nicholas Martin Douglas (2006)
Julia Anne Helen Matheson (2008)

NOTES

PART I

Scott's Medical School, 1875-1914

CHAPTER 1

The Southernmost Medical School: An Injudicious Enterprise?

1. Roy Porter, *The Greatest Benefit to Mankind*, p. 305, pp. 370–2, 377–81.

2. Gardner also stresses interprovincial rivalry as a motive for Macandrew's actions. Foiled by Canterbury in his bid to 'corner higher education in New Zealand', by making the University of Otago a colonial and not merely a provincial university, he offset this by pushing through a colonial medical school. W.J. Gardner, *Colonial Cap and Gown*, p. 29. Canterbury politicians Tancred and Rolleston had led the opposition to Otago becoming a New Zealand University. In 1874, the University of New Zealand was set up as an examining body to which Otago University reluctantly affiliated. W.P. Morrell, *The University of Otago, a Centennial History*, pp. 16–36.

3. Morrell, pp. 4–7.

4. University of Otago Ordinance, 3 June 1869.

5. Macandrew to University Council, 10 November 1869, cited in G.E. Thompson, *A History of the University of Otago, 1869–1919*, Otago University Council, Dunedin, p. 25.

6. Macandrew to Colonial Secretary, July 1871, cited in Thompson, p. 99. Otago eventually secured this reserve in 1874. Thompson, p. 99; Morrell, p. 10. The professors were Sale, Shand, Macgregor and Black. Thompson, Ch. VIII. The University was formally opened on 5 July 1871.

7. Thompson, pp. 99–100.

8. Morrell, pp. 42–3.

9. Provincial Council Records, Session XXX, 1872. Report of Select Committee on the Establishment of Legal and Medical Classes, 1872, cited in Thompson,

p. 100. The committee and its findings are discussed in Thompson, pp. 100–1, and Carmalt Jones, p. 48–51. Its membership was Hon Sir G. McLean, Dr Webster (Chair), Mr Barton and Mr Macassey.

10. Thompson, pp. 100–1.

11. Provincial Council records, cited in D.W. Carmalt Jones, *Annals of the University of Otago Medical School*, A.H. and A.W. Reed, Wellington and Dunedin, 1945, pp. 49–50.

12. *Otago Daily Times*, cited in Carmalt Jones p. 50. The paper later came to cautious support of a two-year course.

13. Gardner, p. 30. By 1876 there were 58 medical students at Melbourne, 24 of them in their first year. By 1880 there would be 137, half the total student population. G. Blainey, *A Centenary History of the University of Melbourne*, p. 32.

14. Gardner, p. 30.

15. OU Inwards correspondence, AG-180-27/04, Hocken Collections, University of Otago (hereafter HC).

16. OU Council Minutes, 9 December 1873, AG-180-1/01 (HC).

17. Hislop to Auld, 17 December 1869, OU Letter Book (Outward Letters), vol. 1, 1869–78, p. 12. AG-180-27/01 (HC).

18. Stuart to Auld, 21 January 1874 OU Letter Book (Outward Letters), vol. 1, 1869–78, p. 359.

19. Blainey, pp. 25–6; K. Russell, *The Melbourne Medical School, 1862–1962* (1977), p. 36.

20. More than 100 Canadians had completed their MD at Edinburgh before 1867. Edinburgh graduates also played a leading role in setting up medical Schools in Montreal, Quebec, Kingston and Halifax. D. Guthrie, *The Medical School at Edinburgh*, pp. 21–2.

21. Vice-Chancellor, University of Otago to Principal, University of Edinburgh, 21 January 1874, Edinburgh University Special Collections: Otago Medical School. Edinburgh University Court Draft Minutes and Related Papers, 1872–1875.

22. Edinburgh Special Collections relating to Otago.

Medical Faculty Minutes, 24 March 1874, p. 275. Minutes of Senatus, vol. IV, 1872–1875, 28 March 1874, p. 221.

23 Carmalt Jones, p. 52. Notable were F.F.M. Moir of Aberdeen and D.J. Cunningham of Edinburgh. The latter, who was then a final year student, went on to become professor in Dublin and Edinburgh.

24 Coughtrey to Black, OU Inwards correspondence, 1874–1915. AG-180-27/04 (HC).

25 Carmalt Jones p. 68.

26 Millen Coughtrey, 'The Introductory Address in the Faculty of Medicine of Otago University', May 31, 1875.

27 OU Council Minutes, 18 August 1874, AG-180-1/01 (HC); Carmalt Jones, p. 56.

28 Stuart to Dean of the Faculty of Medicine, 2 August 1875, Edinburgh Special Collection relating to Otago University Medical School, p. 611.

29 Carmalt Jones, p. 62. The whole issue of recognition is discussed, pp. 60–3.

30 Carmalt Jones, pp. 63–6; Thompson, Appendix C, p. 285 gives the overall numbers of students. Saul Solomon, who left the course, in time became Crown Prosecutor. Carmalt Jones, p. 63. Low went to Edinburgh, graduating in 1881. Since he was the first student who began his course at Otago, it is good to report that the 1879–80 Edinburgh Calendar lists him as gaining first class in Practical Chemistry and Materia Medica, and second class in Anatomy. In 1880–1 he gained a first class certificate in General Pathology, in which he came first equal in the class with 84 per cent and also gained a first class certificate of merit in Medical Jurisprudence. Low returned to New Zealand and practised in Gore. Edinbugh Calendars, 1879–80 and 1880–81; Carmalt Jones, Appendix IV, Early Students, p. 272.

31 Colquhoun in *NZMJ* vol. 1, no. 1; Carmalt Jones, pp. 65–7. There were 270 practitioners and fifty other medical men in the colony at this time. Dr Hocken was President of the Dunedin branch, which referred to itself as the New Zealand Medical Association.

32 Coughtrey in *NZMJ*, vol. 1, no. 2, December 1887, pp. 139–45. In his aims for the future of the School Coughtrey was reinforcing the Medical School's policy.

33 'New Zealand Scenery and Public Buildings. Leading Businesses of Dunedin: Being a Series of Illustrations and Descriptive Letterpress', *Otago Daily Times and Witness*, Dunedin 1895, pp. 56–7. I am grateful to Emeritus Professor Keith Jeffery for drawing my attention to this booklet and to the hospital, which was situated in Forbury Road, near the street that bears Coughtrey's name, and is no longer standing. It is not mentioned in Coughtrey's obituary in the *Otago Witness* of 21 October 1908 or in Carmalt Jones' *Annals*.

34 Carmalt Jones, p. 68.

35 Coughtrey to Council, 21 December 1876; Carmalt Jones, p. 67. The Council refused Coughtrey's offer of six to nine months' notice. Council Minutes, 21 December 1876. On 20 December 1876, Macandrew wrote to the Council urging them to forestall Coughtrey's resignation. Macandrew to Council, cited in Carmalt Jones, p. 69; The letter affirmed Macandrew's belief that a Medical School attached to the University was 'quite attainable'.

36 Hocken and Gillies were appointed on 9 June 1876. Both obtained individual recognition, as required, from the University of Glasgow, and Gillies from Aberdeen, but the Royal College of Surgeons and the Royal College of Physicians did not recognise individuals, only fully established medical schools. Thompson, pp. 105–6.

37 *ODT* 22 December 1876, cited in Carmalt Jones, p. 66; Carmalt Jones, p. 64.

38 Thompson, p. 142. On the other hand, Erik Olssen, in his *History of Otago*, pp. 73–4, points out the advantages in population and amenities gained in Otago during Vogel's Premiership in the decade after 1869.

39 J. Angus, *The Otago Hospital Board and its Predecessors*, p. 71. Committee administration lasted from 1877 to 1886. The first committee consisted of C.S. Reeves, A.C. Strode (Chairman), J. Fulton, R. Gillies and R. Wilson. They represented Dunedin's commercial and legal élite. Angus comments that the period from 1877 to 1900 was characterised by a decline in the importance of the resident medical staff, p. 78.

40 Chancellor to Governor, 30 April 1877. Annual Report, University of Otago, 1877, AJHR, H1B.

41 Canterbury College Annual Report for 1877 includes on the estimates reserves to finance a medical school. AJHR, 1877, H1C.

42 OU Council Minutes, 13 February 1877; Thompson, p. 106. An immediate result of the decision was to promote Captain Hutton from Lecturer in Zoology and Geology to Professor of Natural Science.

CHAPTER 2

An Outpost of Edinburgh

1 Chapman to Auld, Otago Office, Edinburgh 15 February 1877, cited in Carmalt Jones, p. 70. The agents were to sound out D.J. Cunningham before looking further but Cunningham was not interested unless he received a salary of £800 and the right to consulting-practice. Thompson, p. 106.

2 Carmalt Jones, pp. 70–1. The thesis, for which he won a gold medal, was on the nervous system of the dog.

3 L.E. Barnett, 'The Evolution of the Dunedin Hospital

and Medical School: a Brief History', *Proceedings of the Otago Medical School*, no. 12, 1935, p. 7, reprinted from the *Australian and New Zealand Journal of Surgery*, April 1934.

4   Indian, Colonial and Foreign Universities and Colleges, University of Edinburgh Calendar, 1878, p. 179. Professor Black was recognised on 13 October 1873, and Professors Scott and Hutton on 26 October 1877, p. 184.

5   1877 prospectus. Students proceeding to Edinburgh faced examinations in chemistry and anatomy on their arrival.

6   Thompson, p. 96. On 13 August 1877, the Professorial Board reported the winner of an architectural competition to design the buildings. For the sale of the old University buildings and the site of the new ones, see Thompson, pp. 85–91. For the Professorial Board's recommendations, see Thompson, pp. 92–3.

7   Even after a series of economies, the new University buildings cost more than £31,000, instead of the estimated £17,000. The Chemical and Anatomical Division cost £6844.18.0. Thompson, pp. 96–7. Morrell, p. 50. Scott's recommendations are in Hercus and Bell, p. 18.

8   Carmalt Jones, p. 74. Science subjects were taken as part of a BA degree until the BSc was introduced in the late 1880s.

9   Carmalt Jones, pp. 74–5. Brown's appointment, a part-time one at £200, in May 1878, was conditional on recognition from Edinburgh, which arrived in August 1879. Like McGregor, who was his brother-in-law, Brown took an MA at Aberdeen before studying at Edinburgh. Both graduated in 1870. K. Jeffery, 'Surgery in Victorian Dunedin', *Otago Settlers News*, December 2004, pp. 1–2.

10 Cited in D.J. Le Cren, *The Rich and Macandrew Families, 1280–1993*, p. 87. The letter is in the possession of the family. Herbert Macandrew (1859–1917) graduated from Edinburgh in 1883, worked for a time there and elsewhere in Britain, and returned to take up a position at Seaview Hospital, Hokitika. He remained there all his professional life.

11 Brookfield family documents, Hocken Collections; Edinburgh University Calendar, 1884, Appendix, p. 35. Will graduated in 1884 and returned to New Zealand, where he practised at Green Island, and later established the private psychiatric hospital, Ashburn Hall.

12 H.M. Inglis, *Otago University Review* (hereafter OUR), 1889.

13 Sir James Elliott, *Scalpel and Sword*, p. 63.

14 D. Colquhoun, 'Dr Scott: an Appreciation', in OUR, XXVIII, 1914, pp. 5–6; Hercus and Bell, p. 17; for students' opinions see, for example, 'A Student's Testimony'. OUR, XXVIII, 1914, p. 7.

15 Barnett, in Carmalt Jones, p. 85.

16 Scott in *Southern People*, p. 446. The Scotts later moved to a house designed by architect J.A. Burnside, in Garfield Avenue and, after his wife's death, Scott lived for a time at the Dunedin Club. Sir John Scott, family information. Helen Scott was born in Christchurch, but her family returned to England.

17 Hodgkins, cited in Scott entry, *Southern People*, p. 446.

18 Carmalt Jones, p. 146, summing up tributes paid to Scott in the University Council, Faculty and Professorial Board.

19 Louis Barnett, reminiscence written for Carmalt Jones and cited p. 84. There is a collection of Scott's diagrams in the Hocken Collections, Dunedin.

20 Hercus and Bell, p. 18; Barnett, cited in Carmalt Jones, p. 85.

21 Fieke Neuman, 'Pots and Pieces: the Anatomy Museum of the Otago Medical School and How it Came to Be', in *Museums Journal* 23 (1), 1993, pp. 17–22.

22 Scott to Council, 4 October 1881, cited in Carmalt Jones, pp. 76–7.

23 Scott to Council, 18 September 1882, cited in Carmalt Jones, p. 78. In the event, Midwifery was advertised at £200 and Medical Jurisprudence and Public Health at £100; request from OU Council to NZU Senate 7 March 1883. Carmalt Jones, p. 80.

24 Hunter, Compendium of Historical Data. p. 17.

25 Carmalt Jones, pp. 86–7; Hercus and Bell, pp. 262–4. Colquhoun's assistants included Drs John Macdonald in materia medica, Truby King in mental diseases and, later, Frank Fitchett and Marshall Macdonald in clinical teaching and Ernest Williams in paediatrics; Obituary, Daniel Colquhoun, *NZMJ*, vol. 34, February 1935, pp 136–7; *Southern People*, p. 99.

26 Carmalt Jones, pp. 87–8; Hercus and Bell p 318–9; Batchelor, Ferdinand Campion, (1850–1915) *Southern People*, p. 31.

27 Carmalt Jones, p. 89; Hercus and Bell, p. 278.

28 Hercus and Bell, pp. 21–2. Dr E.D. Mackellar, the first choice for Pathology, did not take up the position, which Roberts filled, temporarily, for 1884. Hercus and Bell, pp. 241–2, are dismissive of Roberts' training to teach Pathology, and later Bacteriology, but note that the value of his services must be assessed in relation to the conditions of the day, and that he gave of his best.

29 Hercus and Bell, p. 22: Obituary, Dr Isaiah de Zouche, *NZMJ* 8, 1895, pp. 84–5. Dr de Zouche, born and educated in Dublin, of Huguenot stock – he insisted his family always spoke French in the morning – had to give up his work in the early 1890s. He died in 1894, aged 55, in the United States, where he had gone to consult Dr Weir Mitchell, specialist in 'neurotic affections'.

30 A.W. Beasley, 'Barnett, Louis Edward, 1865–1946',

in DNZB 3, p. 32; George Griffiths, 'Barnett, Louis Edward (1865–1946)', in *Southern People*, p. 25; Hercus and Bell, pp. 288–92. H.W. Maunsell, who was appointed when Brown retired in 1889, stayed only two years before going overseas. Brown obligingly filled in again until 1894. Former students mentioned were surgeons McIndoe, Porritt, Read and Robb, all of whom were later knighted.

CHAPTER 3

The Medical School and the Dunedin Hospital, 1890s–1914

[1] The competition to design a new hospital was won by Dunedin architect David Ross. The Provincial Council decided to proceed instead with a lunatic asylum on the Arthur Street reserve. Scandals of the 1850s and 1860s at the earlier Moray Place hospital relating to dirt, poor management and the death of a man refused admission to the hospital without proper examination, led to scathing criticism by a Royal Commission in 1864. Angus, pp. 29–34, 81. University of Otago Calendar, 1878.

[2] Sir Lindo Ferguson, 'Landmark Passes', *Digest*, vol. 1, no. 1, October 1934, pp. 1–4. For the state of the Hospital in the 1880s, see also Angus, p. 83. Ferguson attributed the development of the Hospital into a modern institution to the presence of the Medical School.

[3] Ferguson, 'Autobiographical Notes', p. 28. Hercus and Bell cite this on p. 338, as part of a longer extract from the 'Autobiographical Notes', pp. 336–9. Ferguson adds that, thirty-six years after this operation, a woman came up to him in London's Cavendish Square and identified herself as having been that child.

[4] Ferguson, 'Landmark Passes', p. 4.

[5] Angus, pp. 82–4. The wardsmen were poorly paid and housed and several had to be dismissed for drunkenness; Carmalt Jones, pp. 87, 100–1.

[6] Angus, p. 85. The theatre cost £1516

[7] Angus, pp. 85–9. The Royal Commission, which was appointed at the request of both parties, consisted of Sir James Hector and E.H. Carew; Carmalt Jones, pp. 100–1; Evidence and Report of Royal Commission, in AJHR 1891. There was a sharp drop in medical student numbers after conditions at the Hospital were made public. Scott to Chancellor, 26 December 1893, cited in Carmalt Jones, p. 109.

[8] Angus, pp. 89, 95. The original building cost £2354, the 1903 extensions £1312 and the 1908 modifications another £3000.

[9] Angus, p. 89. The suggested site for a new hospital was near the main University buildings, between the botanic gardens and Dundas Street, Valedictory tribute to Sir Lindo Ferguson, NZMJ, vol. 36, 1937, p. 132. The article is not attributed, but Hercus and Bell, p. 62, state that Carmalt Jones was the writer. The pavilion was named after Mrs Robert Campbell, an early benefactor, and the wards were named Miller and Houghton, after two Chairmen of Trustees. Angus, p. 90.

[10] Angus, p. 93. George Griffiths, 'Barnett, Louis Edward. 1865–1946', *Southern People*, p. 25. Hercus and Bell, p. 254.

[11] Angus, pp. 98–100, 105.

[12] Angus, pp. 90–1. The pavilion was named after the premier of New Zealand and the wards were named Plunket and Dominion.

[13] Angus, pp. 106, 145. The block cost £16,000 in all. The former nurses' home fulfilled a variety of useful roles from outpatients for tuberculosis treatment, to staff quarters and accommodation for medical students working at the Hospital under a government scheme.

CHAPTER 4

Crisis and Expansion: Breaking out of the Financial Straitjacket, 1890s–1914

[1] Carmalt Jones p. 98. The Faculty met for the first time on 28 April 1891. Dr Coughtrey was the first Sub-Dean.

[2] Carmalt Jones, pp. 112–3. Of the six candidates, there was agreement that one had passed, two failed and three were in dispute. The seven person committee, chaired by Hon William Rolleston, included Rev J.C. Andrew, who was Vice-Chairman of the Senate of NZU, Dr Macgregor, Inspector General of Hospitals and Asylums, and Professor Scott. See Hercus and Bell, pp. 30–5, for its report.

[3] Thompson, p. 142. For a full discussion of the effect of the depression on the University, see Thompson pp. 142–6.

[4] Morrell, pp. 59–86.

[5] Scott to Council, 28 June 1898 and 1 May 1901, AJHR, 1902, E-7 pp. 8–9.

[6] Morrell, p. 87; Thompson, p. 149.

[7] Morrell, pp. 87–9.

[8] Thompson, pp. 152–3. Thompson, Ch. XXI, deals in detail with the whole 'Appeal to the People'.

[9] Seddon, in the *Otago Daily Times*, 24 December 1903; Morrell, p. 90.

[10] John Malcolm, 'An Inaugural Message', *Critic*, 6 April 1944, p. 1.

[11] 'The Bonny Wee Doctor', Otago University Capping Programme 1905.

[12] Sir Patrick Eisdell Moore, *So Old So Quick*, pp. 76–7; Thompson, p. 169; Hercus and Bell, pp. 232–5; Carmalt Jones, pp. 121–2, 146.

[13] Moore's cartoon, which hangs in the Sayers building at the medical school, appeared in the 1940 *Digest*; Moore, p. 77.

[14] James R. Robinson, 'Malcolm, John, 1873–1954',

DNZB 4, Wellington 1998, pp. 329–30.

15. James R. Robinson, 'Malcolm, John, 1873–1954', DNZB 4 Wellington, 1998, pp. 329–30. The medals were for Practical Chemistry, Physics, Practical Botany, Practical Anatomy and Public Health, and the awards were for Experimental Physics, Anatomy and Physiology, Pathology, Medical Jurisprudence and Public Health; Ian Carr and Douglass Taylor, 'Physiology in the Otago Medical School. The John Malcolm Letters', Linda Bryder and Derek Dow, eds, *New Countries and Old Medicine*, pp. 231–4; Carmalt Jones, p. 122.

16. 'Harry Manson', *Digest*, 1947, pp. 20–2.

17. Carmalt Jones p. 118; p. 130; Hercus and Bell, pp. 321–2; Carmalt Jones pp. 234–5; G. Bell, *Surgeon's Saga*, pp. 195–8.

18. Hercus and Bell, p. 27.

19. A.E.J. Fitchett, Fitchett family entry, *Southern People*, p. 165, Russell Chisholm, typescript.

20. Hercus and Bell, p. 251; pp. 241–2.

21. Hercus, 'Medical Research', p. 5. In 1964, Hercus and Bell maintained that Scott's research was still the 'most substantial work on the subject'. p. 177.

22. Carr and Taylor, pp. 233–4. Fitchett's thesis was entitled 'A Contribution to our Knowledge of the Physiological Action of Tutin'. Hercus and Bell, p. 186 Robinson, DNZB 4, pp. 329–30.

23. Hercus, 'Medical Research', p. 6. In 1919, Drennan addressed the New Zealand Institute on 'The Prevalence of Goitre in New Zealand and its Influence on the Coming Generation'. Carmalt Jones, p. 177.

24. Honor Anderson, 'Hydatids: a Disease of Human Carelessness'. MA in History, University of Otago, 1997, pp. 2, 8–9.

25. Hercus, 'Medical Research', p. 6.

26. Carmalt Jones, pp. 95–6.

27. Carmalt Jones, p. 125; Thompson, Appendix C, p. 185.

CHAPTER 5

Medical Students

1. Carmalt Jones, pp. 80–1. Jones based his figures on examination lists.

2. Carmalt Jones, p. 91; OUR August 1888, report of formation of OUMSA for the 'superintendence of the library and the general welfare of the medical students', p. 23. 'Medicus', letter to editor on a second examination to save those who fail having to repeat the whole year, pp. 30–2. On adding a surgery qualification, CM, to the degree, p. 69. Report of a meeting on 29 September 1888 at which it was agreed to petition Senate to add CM to the medical degree, pp. 84–5. Elworthy, *Ritual Song of Defiance*, p. 25.

3. Elworthy, pp. 19–27. The first public capping was in the University library in 1879, the debating club began in 1878, the *Review* in 1888. The first rugby match against Canterbury College was in 1886. See Elworthy, p. 161, for a list of OUSA presidents. The seven medical student presidents 1890–1914 were: A. Hendry 1891 (Hendry held an Arts degree and is listed as an Arts student), M.W. Ross, 1894, P. Buck (Te Rangi Hiroa) 1903, T.W.J. Johnson, 1909, H. Short, 1912, P.J. Jory 1914. The other presidents were all Arts students.

4. For Otago students at Edinburgh see, for example, OUR 1889, p. 21, where their examination results are carefully listed.

5. University of Edinburgh Calendar 1885. Truby King was appointed to the Medical School as Lecturer on Insanity in 1888. Jeffcoat also returned to the Medical School. In 1892, he was appointed honorary physician to the Gynaecology Department of the Hospital, at first in Batchelor's absence in 1892–3, and then working with him. Jeffcoat died in 1897, Carmalt Jones, p. 112. Lindsay returned to practise at Akaroa, Carmalt Jones, p. 262.

6. H.D. Erlam, 'Dr William Ledingham Christie, New Zealand's First Medical Graduate', *NZMJ*, January 1961, pp. 1–6.

7. Thompson, p. 109.

8. Caroline Freeman was the first woman to graduate from Otago, *ODT* 27 August 1885; OU Council minutes, 9 August 1881; P. Sargison, Emily Siedeberg, DNZB 3; 'Women Doctors' by Dunedin Medico, and 'Medical Notes' by Chiron, OUR, vol. 4, 1891, p. 192.

9. For Edinburgh events see Catriona Blake, *The Charge of the Parasols*, esp, 'The Riot at Surgeons' Hall', pp. 125–8. Russell, Ch. 6, 'The Ladies Enter the Course', p. 174. Sydney Medical School admitted women in 1886 and Melbourne in 1887; Dorothy Page, 'Dissecting a Community: Women Medical Students at the University of Otago, 1891–1924', in Brookes and Page, eds, *Communities of Women*, pp. 112–5; The comment was made by Doris Gordon, *Backblocks Baby Doctor*, p. 53. See Page, pp. 180–1 for list of women medical graduates from Otago, 1891–1924.

10. OUR, vol. IV, no. 1, June 1891, pp. 1–2.

11. Page, p. 117; Baker McLaglan, pp. 42, 48. The unnamed lecturer was Frank Ogston.

12. Goodlet and Siedeberg cited in Carmalt Jones, pp. 103–4.

13. Gordon, p. 51; W.A. Anderson, *Doctor in the Mountains*, p. 46.

14. Page, pp. 117–8; Erik Olssen discusses the episode in 'Truby King and the Plunket Society: an Analysis of a Prescriptive Ideology', *New Zealand Journal of History*, vol. 15, no. 1, April 1981, pp. 3–23.

15. Baker McLaglan, p. 69.

16. M.P.K. Sorrenson, 'Buck, Peter Henry 1877–1951' in DNZB 3, pp. 72–4; Irwin K. Jackson, 'Wi Repa,

Tutere, 1877–1945', in DNZB 3, pp. 563–4; Wi Repa's oratorical powers were noted in a letter by John Malcolm (information, Douglass Taylor); letter from Sir Peter Buck to *Digest*, 19 July, 1951.

17 Jackson; Carmalt Jones, p. 116.

18 Hugh Tohill, 'University of Otago Rugby and its Grounds', in Heslop ed. *The History of Logan Park*, p. 68; Elworthy, p. 20, also describes the rugby match, which he claims lasted 'for many hours of play over three days'. Professor Sale (Classics), who was an ex-pupil of Rugby School, was one of the players; G. Griffiths, 'Otago University at Cricket', in Heslop, pp. 28, 30. Sale was the star of the cricket match too, taking eight wickets. He was a long-serving patron of both rugby and cricket at the University, Griffiths, p. 31.

19 Griffiths, pp. 28, 33–5. The club ground was the Oval, the team colour light blue.

20 Griffiths, pp. 36, 38. Seven men from the 1913 tournament team went overseas and, of these, three were killed. Griffiths, p. 38.

21 Rex Thomson, 'Rugby at the University of Otago: Humble Beginnings for New Zealand's Premier Club', *International Journal of the History of Sport*, 14, 2, August 1997, pp. 174–86. Of these early players, Barnett would complete his medical training in Edinburgh and return to teach in the Medical School, ultimately as Professor of Surgery. Burns completed in Edinburgh, was a surgeon to the New Zealand contingent in the Boer War and served in World War I, before becoming Senior Medical Officer in Samoa. Sidney Gibbs completed at Edinburgh, where he captained the Australasian Football Club, before practising in Nelson, and representing his province in rugby. Robert Hogg, who trained fully at Otago, served in World War I as head of the surgical division at No. 1 New Zealand Hospital. He later rose to be President of the British Medical Association and was knighted in 1937. Tohill, pp. 68–72. From 1887 the club was also able to field a second (B) team, which won the second grade competition in 1896.

22 Tohill, pp. 68–72. The University club tried and failed to get access to the Museum reserve. Travel to Tahuna had to be by trap or train.

23 Sir James Elliott, *Scalpel and Sword*, pp. 48–53; Elliott graduated from Edinburgh in 1902. For his later distinguished career see Rex Wright-St. Clair, 'Elliott, James Sands, 1880–1959' in DNZB 3, p. 151.

24 Morrell, pp. 197–8, 201. I am grateful to Alison Clarke for unpublished data on Knox College student numbers; OUR, June 1918, p. 61. Most of the Knox students were studying for the Presbyterian ministry.

25 Page, pp. 123, 125–6. The first St Margaret's graduates were Doris Jolly (later Gordon) and Francie Dowling.

26 Carmalt Jones refers briefly to OUMSA, in his chapter on 1905–1914, as an active body that kept a close watch on the financial interests of its members and several times achieved a reduction in fees. p. 144. Minutes of OUMSA, vol. 1. 1905–1915.

27 Elworthy, pp. 36–7.

28 Elworthy p. 37.

29 OUMSA Rules of the Association, OUMSA file, HC. The Rules are not dated but reference to the need for OUMSA elections to precede those of the OUSA suggests a date between 1902 and 1905; OUMSA AGM, 8 June 1905.

30 OUMSA records, Faculty of Medicine, Dean's Department, 95-157-26/1, HC. Committee Minutes 31 October 1905; Annual Report, 1905–6; General Meeting 8 August 1908; farewell to Dr Scott 31 October 1908; AGM 5 February 1910; Committee 13 June 10; 27 February 1914; AGM 13 March 1915; Annual Report 1915. Nichol was killed in September 1913 during excavations for squash courts at Knox College.

PART II

The Ferguson Era, 1914–1937

CHAPTER 6

A Statesman at the Helm

1 Morrell, p. 117.

2 Thompson, Appendix C, p. 285, p. 179; Morrell, p. 117. Proposals were for an extension to the anatomy, physiology and chemistry block, and/or an entire new building for bacteriology and pathology.

3 Sir Gordon Bell, *Surgeon's Saga*, p. 156; the story appears elsewhere, with minor variations of wording, e.g. in Ferguson, Henry Lindo, *Southern People*, p. 159.

4 Bell, p. 155–6.

5 Carmalt Jones in *NZMJ* vol. 36, February 1937, p. 134.

6 Hercus and Bell, p. 65.

7 Medical Faculty Minutes, 30 November 1936, vol. 4, 1919–1943, p. 265. The Minute was moved by Professor Fitchett and seconded by Professor Carmalt Jones.

8 Carmalt Jones in *NZMJ*, 1937, p. 134; Hercus and Bell, p. 63.

9 Carmalt Jones in *NZMJ* vol. 36, February 1937, pp. 131–2. The Oculist to the Queen in Ireland was Charles Fitzgerald. The Arts degree was a prerequisite to medical study. Ferguson did not complete his medical degree until some years later.

10 Lindo Ferguson, 'Autobiographical Notes', written for Sir Hugh Devine, for the Archives of the Royal

Australasian College of Surgeons, Melbourne, 1945, pp. 21–6. (J.D Hunter Collection, HC). The practice handled 80–100 patients a day, as well as private ones. The overall estimate of patient numbers is Ferguson's own. In New Zealand, Ferguson's mother and brother settled in Wellington; Obituary *NZMJ* vol. 47, 1948; 'Henry Lindo Ferguson,' in J. Thomson ed., *Southern People*, p. 160.

11 Ferguson, 'Autobiographical Notes', pp. 27–32. He used the word 'whirlwind' more than once to describe Batchelor's activities; Carmalt Jones, 'Retirement of Sir Lindo Ferguson', *NZMJ* vol. 36, Feb., 1937, pp. 131–2.

12 Minutes, Otago University Professorial Board, 14 March 1914, AG-180-15/05 (HC). The appointment was confirmed by Council on 16 March. Hercus and Bell, p. 44; Hercus and Bell, p. 335. Batchelor died in 1915.

13 Morrell, p. 115. Sale retired in 1908, Black in 1910, Shand and Salmond in 1913. Shand and Black died in 1913.

14 'Colquhoun, Daniel (1849–1935)', *Southern People*, p. 99; Carmalt Jones, pp. 86–7, 145, 147, 150; Ferguson, 'Autobiographical Notes', pp. 32, 38. It was probably at this time that he moved from Moata in High Street to the splendid 'Wychwood' in Belmont Lane.

15 Morrell, Ch. VI, 'The Dominance of the Special Schools, 1914–1945', pp. 117–62.

16 Ferguson, 'Autobiographical Notes', pp. 43, 34; John Malcolm records in a letter that Ferguson earned £3000 a year from his practice (information from Emeritus Professor Douglass Taylor).

17 Hercus and Bell, p. 63. Champtaloup was Sub-Dean from 1914 until 1919, Drennan from 1920 to 1924, and Hercus from 1924 to 1936.

18 Carmalt Jones, p. 244. Miss G.M. Thomson remained to serve Hercus, retiring, after 28 years in the job, in 1948. 'Single-handed', he wrote, 'she maintained the School's records, attended to all the Dean's correspondence, controlled his interviews and generally supervised the running of the School's business'. Hercus and Bell, p. 66.

19 Carmalt Jones, p. 107; Bell, p. 123; H.L. Ferguson to Chancellor, University of Otago, Report of the Faculty of Medicine for the year 1925, Annual Reports 1924–1929, p. 22, AG-180-6/4 (HC).

20 The Lindo Ferguson bequest to the Dunedin Public Art Gallery comprised: Carlo Maratti (1625–1713) 'Joseph and Child', Sir George Clausen (d. 1944) 'Summer Evening', Lady Elizabeth Butler, (1850–1933) 'Outside Antwerp', James Nairn, (1904) 'New Brighton Head', Cumbrae Stewart, 'The Fortune Teller' and 'Silence and Shadow' described as a 'typical American desert' (Information from Dunedin Public Art Gallery).

21 Ferguson in *Southern People*, p. 160. Mary Ferguson served on the Hospital Board from 1913 to 1919,

polling top most of this time. She said that her husband had opposed her standing because money matters were involved, implying that he thought such matters were above a woman's head. It was reported in the press that she resigned because she was being kept out of financial decision-making. Angus, pp. 133–4.

22 J. Richards, 'Dr Elaine Gurr, Honorary Fellow of the Royal New Zealand College of General Practitioners', in M.D. Maxwell, ed. *Women Doctors in New Zealand: an Historical Perspective*, p. 124; L.K. Gluckman, 'Augusta Klippel, 1898–1989', Maxwell, p. 135.

23 Randall Elliott to John Hunter, September 1992.

24 OU Council Minutes, 16 July 1935, 19 November 1935, Report of the Committee on Retiring Age; 10 December 1935. Women had to retire at 60, with the possibility of extension after annual review to 65. Ferguson, Autobiographical Notes, pp. 40–2.

25 *NZMJ* vol. 36,1937, p. 133; Ferguson, in *Southern People*.

CHAPTER 7

World War I and its Aftermath

1 Ferguson, 'Autobiographical Notes', 1945, pp. 34–5.

2 Hercus and Bell, p. 296; Carmalt Jones p. 154; E. O'Neill, cited in Captain K.R. Treanor, *The Staff and the Serpent. The Story of the Royal New Zealand Army Medical Corps*, pp. 13–14. The pills were numbered and the large black number 9 pills were frequently prescribed. It was rumoured that if they ran out, patients would be given a 6 plus a 3, or a 5 plus a 4 instead,

3 A.E.J. Fitchett, 'Fitchett, Frank Williamson, 1870–1951', *Southern People*, p. 163; Carmalt Jones, p. 169.

4 Ian Church, 'Falconer, Alexander Robertson, 1874–1955', *Southern People*, p. 155. Falconer was Medical Superintendent of Dunedin Hospital from 1910 to 1927.

5 Carmalt Jones, pp. 117–8. Carmalt Jones rightly points out that the war does not feature in the University records; Treanor, pp. 13–5, lists twenty-one NZ medical officers who took part in the South African war. They included seven who subsequently held senior NZMC appointments.

6 Hercus and Bell, Ch. 15, 'Military Training', pp. 201–6; C. Hercus 'The Otago University Medical Corps', *Digest*, vol. II, no. 3, October 1942, pp. 10–11; Treanor, p. 19. The New Zealand Medical Corps was gazetted on 7 May 1908.

7 Report of University of Otago Medical School, AJHR 1915, E 7, Higher Education; D.S. Milne, cited in P. Cotter, 'A Tribute. The Contribution of the Otago University Medical School and its students in World War One', *NZMJ, 15 April 2005*. Cotter

lists the students. They deferred completing the Obstetrics and Gynaecology experience necessary before registration. All returned, except Webb, who was killed in a shipboard accident.

8   Report of University of Otago Medical School, AJHR 1915, E7, Higher Education; C. Hercus, 'OUMC', p. 12.
9   Christine Daniell, *A Doctor at War, A Life in Letters, 1914–43*, based on the diaries and letters of her father, Dr Montgomery Spencer. pp. 11–75, passim. (Spencer cited, pp. 10–11.); 'ANZAC Anecdotes', OUR 1915, cited in Cotter; Carmalt Jones, p. 154.
10 Morrell, p. 119; OUC Minutes, 15 February 1916. AG-180-1/06 (HC).
11 Report of Medical School, AJHR 1916, E 7, p. 27.
12 Carmalt Jones, pp. 162–3; Hercus and Bell, p. 202; Hercus, 'The Otago University Medical Corps', *Digest* vol. II, no. 3, October 1942, p. 13. The officers were Majors Malcolm, Ritchie and Gowland and Lieutenant Stanton Hicks; J.H Scott, 'The Otago Medical Company', *NZMJ*, March 1960, pp. 124–7.
13 Carmalt Jones, pp. 161–2, details the financial provisions of the scheme.
14 Carmalt Jones, pp. 148–54. Barnett was expected back in March 1917. Macdonald worked with a distinguished team of French neurologists.
15 Ferguson to Chancellor, April 1916, cited in Carmalt Jones, p. 158.
16 Carmalt Jones, p. 159. Stanley Batchelor was the son of Ferdinand Batchelor; Morrell, p. 118.
17 Morrell, p. 120; Report of Medical School for 1917. Ferguson also correctly predicted that placing women graduates would prove difficult. The School roll consisted of 182 men and 43 women.
18 Carmalt Jones, p. 176; Dr R.S.A. Graham, cited in Geoffrey Rice, *Black November*, p. 176.
19 Morrell, pp. 119–20.
20 F.J.Austin, 'Hercus, Charles Ernest, 1888–1971', *Southern People*, p. 222; Hercus and Bell, pp. 87–8; Ian McGibbon, 'Medical Treatment', in *The Oxford Companion to New Zealand Military History*. pp. 314–5.
21 Hercus and Bell, p. 266.
22 G. Griffiths, 'Barnett, Louis Edward (1865–1946)', *Southern People*, p. 25; Carmalt Jones, p. 154.
23 Gordon Bell, *Surgeon's Saga*, pp. 113–6; Hercus and Bell, pp. 242–3.
24 Bell, p. 113; McGibbon, p. 315.
25 Carmalt Jones, pp. 207–8. Carmalt Jones put the failure to establish the brief lecture course down to a 'series of accidents'; Hercus and Bell, p. 80. Even in 1953, when planning was under way for the 1955–59 quinquennium, it was not possible to get funding for a full-time chair of psychiatry and, when Hercus and Bell wrote in the early 1960s, 'mental diseases' were still taught by the superintendent and staff of Seacliff mental hospital. Hercus and Bell, p. 277.
26 Reginald Pound, *Gillies, Surgeon Extraordinary*.

Michael Joseph London and Whitcombe and Tombs New Zealand, 1964; Richard Battle, 'Gillies, Sir Harold Delf (1882–1960)', *Oxford Dictionary of National Biography*, vol. 22, 2004; M. Harvey Brown, 'Pickerill, Henry Percy, 1879–1956', DNZB 3, pp. 399–400 and personal information. 'Woodside' had been the home of Judge Chapman.
27 David Renfrew White, 'James Renfrew White (1888–1961)', *Southern People*, p. 543.
28 Hercus and Bell, pp. 203, 206. Both Thompson, Appendix B, and Carmalt Jones, Appendix V, list the names.
29 Scott, p. 125; Hercus and Bell, p. 203; Hercus, p. 13. The amount made available was £8000, which more than covered the cost of the building.
30 Hercus, 'OUMC', pp. 13–4.
31 Scott, p. 126; Hercus and Bell, p. 203. Colonels Gabites and O'Neill briefly held the command before Hercus's appointment.
32 Scott, pp. 126–7. The Defence Department terminated the unit because, since 1916, only 19 per cent of the unit had obtained certificates. Fulton and Iverach had served as officers under Hercus; Hercus, p. 14; Hercus and Bell, p. 204.

CHAPTER 8

'A Monument in Bricks and Mortar'

1   Medical Faculty Minutes, vol. 4, 1919–1937, 30 November 1936; Carmalt Jones, p. 152; Hercus and Bell, p. 59.
2   Carmalt Jones, pp. 142–3; Thompson, pp. 179–80.
3   Ferguson, 'Autobiographical Notes', p. 36. Ferguson says that at that time he had 'got absolute refusal' from the Otago University Council for funding for 'all sorts of things'. Carmalt Jones, p. 142, says that the Hospital Board 'for some curious reason', had been requested to take out the option on the Great King Street land in 1913.
4   'New Medical School', reprinted from the *Otago Daily Times*, March 1914. An anonymous donor, later identified as W. Dawson, gave £2000.
5   Ferguson, 'Autobiographical Notes', p. 36. Ferguson also faced opposition on the professorial board from arts staff, who objected to his demands for more staff and better salaries than they were able to get; Hercus and Bell, p. 46; Carmalt Jones, pp. 142–3, 152, 159, 163; Morrell, p. 120, incorrectly attributes the building to Anscombe.
6   'The University of Otago. Descriptive Syllabus of the Medical School, 1916', p. 25.
7   'Descriptive Syllabus', p. 27. The epidiascope was described as 'an electric arc lantern by means of which images of specimens, lantern slides, photographs etc., which are being discussed by the lecturer, can be thrown on the screen.' It was simply noted of Bacteriology that it would occupy a set of

class rooms and laboratories in the new building, p. 28.

8   'New Medical School. Official Opening Ceremony', *ODT*, 3 April 1917.

9   'The Medical School', *ODT*, 17 July 1919.

10 'The Medical School', *ODT*, 6 August 1919. As a member of the University Council, Ferguson received the deputation rather than participating in it; Carmalt Jones pp. 179–80. The grant to purchase the northern part of the block was £6925, but the cost of the properties to the corner (known as Fogo's Corner) was £8225. There was also difficulty over the purchase because a right-of-way had to be closed, and the Public Works Act had to be invoked.

11 Hercus and Bell, p. 48.

12 *NZMJ* vol. 36, Feb 1937, p. 134.

13 Carmalt Jones, pp. 194–5.

14 'New Medical School Foundation Stone Laid', *ODT*, 19 June 1925. As well as Thompson's history of the University, the casket Hercus deposited contained the 1925 University calendar, that day's *ODT* (18 June 1925), the previous evening's *Star* (17 June 1925) and coins of the realm.

15 'Medical School. Forecast of Development', *Evening Star*, 27 June 1925 reproduces the whole report; 'The Medical School', *ODT*, 27 June 1925 has a summary and comment.

16 Hardwicke Knight and Niel Wales, *Buildings of Dunedin: an Illustrated Guide to New Zealand's Victorian City*, p. 73; Hercus and Bell, p. 48.

17 Carmalt Jones, p. 179, succinctly sums up the elements of the Ferguson plan.

18 Hercus and Bell, pp. 318–21; Angus, pp. 198–9.

19 Ferguson, Annual Reports, 1928, 1929. £10,000 of the £50,000 was for purchase of the site, and £40,000 for the building.

20 Ferguson, Annual Report, 1930; Angus, p. 200; *ODT*, 17 March 1937, 'A Cinderella Medical School hampered', a report of Ferguson's address to the Council.

21 Ferguson, Annual Report, 1933.

22 Ferguson, Annual Reports, 1931–1936.

23 Annual Report 1936; Angus, pp. 198–201; Dawson, p. 189. He points out that when a further 18 beds had to be added 17 years later, the cost was far greater.

24 Angus, p. 197.

25 'A Cinderella: Medical School hampered,' *ODT*, 18 March 1937. As well as buildings, Ferguson referred briefly to the increase in the School's endowments and the need for more staff.

26 *NZMJ* 1948. The author's name is not attached to the obituary but it was almost certainly written by Carmalt Jones.

CHAPTER 9

Expansion and Modernisation

1   Hercus and Bell, pp. 50–2; Carmalt Jones, p. 150.

2   Ferguson, report to Reichel commission on the University of New Zealand, July 1925, cited in Hercus and Bell, pp. 54–6; Ferguson to Gregg, Rockefeller Foundation, in Carmalt Jones, p. 196. The budget at that stage was £17,000.

3   Annual Report, 1925 notes with satisfaction Cairney's promotion to Associate Professor, preceding his departure for America on a Rockefeller Fellowship. Annual Report 1929 regrets the School's failure to retain Cairney, after this special training, AG-180-6/04 (HC); Paul Sorrell, 'Henry Percy Pickerill, 1879–1956', *Southern People*, pp. 388–9; David Renfrew White, 'James Renfrew White, 1888–1961', *Southern People*, p. 343; John Borrie, 'Marion King Bennie Whyte, 1895–1983', *Southern People*, pp. 545–6; Annual report 1936; University of Otago Calendars 1914, pp. 3–6, 1937, pp. xiii–xiv.

4   Bell, pp. 54–5.

5   Ferguson, 'Autobiographical Notes', pp. 32, 39, 42. In 1925, he also arranged for a show of American pictures for the 1925–6 Dunedin and South Seas Exhibition. Some were purchased by the Dunedin Art Gallery: 'Being President of the Gallery', Ferguson commented with heavy irony, 'and having nothing else to do, it fell to my lot to raise the funds for their purchase', p. 39; Carmalt Jones, p. 150; Annual Reports, 1925, 1929, AG-180-6/04 (HC); Bernard Dawson, 'Without Varnish: a Simple Story. An Autobiography in the Third Person', Ch. 10, pp. 153–72; Annual report, 1936.

6   Annual Reports, 1928, 1929, 1930, 1931; Hercus and Bell, pp. 59–60, 196–8.

7   H.B. Turbott, Medical Research in New Zealand. Report of Medical Research Council, A-J H 31 B December 1959; Hercus, 'Medical Research', p. 4; Derek A. Dow, *Safeguarding the Public Health: A History of the New Zealand Department of Health*, 'Introduction'; Carmalt Jones, p. 91.

8   Hercus, obituary in *NZMJ* 73, April 1971 p. 232; Hercus gave the Cawthron lecture in 1929 on 'Goitre in the Light of Recent Research', Cawthron Institute, 1930; Derek Dow, 'Hercus, Charles Ernest' in DBZB 4, Department of Internal Affairs and Auckland University Press, Wellington, 1998, p. 235.

9   Carmalt Jones, p. 176. Mrs D. Johnson worked in the Physiological laboratories, publishing a number of papers on the nutritional value of New Zealand fish.

10 Carr and Taylor, in *New Countries and Old Medicine*, pp. 233–4; Robinson, Malcolm in DNZB 4, pp. 329–30. The rats were later destroyed in a fire in the department, but were able to be replaced from the Wallaceville Laboratory.

11 Hercus, 'Medical Research', p. 4.

12 Hercus, 'Medical Research', p. 7; Hercus and Bell, pp. 179–80; E.R. Nye ed. Introduction, *Medical Research in Otago, 1922–1997*, p. 5; Annual Reports of the Otago Medical School, 1922–1936.

13 Annual Reports, 1925–1931.

14 Carmalt Jones, pp. 186–7; P.A. Cragg, Introduction, in E. Nye ed., *Medical Research in Otago, 1922–1997*, p. 2; Annual reports, 1925–1931.

15 Carmalt Jones, pp. 180–1. The Deans' 1920 meeting was the last of the triennial Inter-Colonial Medical Congresses, which were replaced by triennial Australasian Medical Congresses of the BMA; Hercus and Bell, p. 102.

16 Hercus and Bell, p. 127. The three northern centres became Branch Faculties in 1938.

17 Chisholm, 'The Otago Medical School 50 Years Ago', unpublished memoir, written for Geoffrey Brinkman 1980; David Richmond, obituary, 'Frederick Russell Chisholm', *NZMJ* August 1990, p. 384. Years later, during the war, Chisholm met Gowland and Cairney again. Gowland was Chief of Medical Services and Cairney Superintendent in Chief of the Wellington Hospital Board. He thought they still worked as brilliantly together as they had in anatomy classes.

18 D. Denny-Brown, obituary, William Percy Gowland, *NZMJ* 1965, pp. 661–2.

19 W.E. Adams, obituary, 'William Percy Gowland', *NZMJ* vol. 64, 1965, pp. 660–1; D. Denny-Brown, *NZMJ* vol. 64, 1965, pp. 661–2; Patrick Moore, *So Old so Quick*, p. 76. Moore recounts one of Gowland's stories and student response it received, pp. 75–7.

20 Professor W.E. Adams, *NZMJ* vol. 64, 1965, p. 660. Gowland's first demonstrator was Dr M.H. Watt, later Director-General of Health; his first technician was A.E. Kidd, who had worked in the Zoology department at Liverpool. The first class was made up of approximately half junior and half senior students; Hercus and Bell, pp. 228–9; Derek Dow, 'Cairney, John, 1898–1966', DNZB 5, pp. 85–6.

21 Adams in *NZMJ* 1965, p. 661; Hercus and Bell state that Gowland 'emphasised the strong integration between histology, embryology and topographical anatomy and reduced the amount of didactic teaching, particularly in the thorax and abdomen, by his emphasis on embryology', p. 228.

22 Derek A. Dow, 'Watt, Michael Herbert 1887–1967', DNZB 4, p. 556. Watt was the Travelling Scholar of 1910 and was the second student from the Medical School to gain the Diploma of Public Health. He was Director General of Health 1930–1947; Hercus and Bell, p. 233, call the lack of graduate assistants the 'besetting dragon' of physiology in these years. Other assistants were Dr R.D. Milligan, Dr W.S. Fogg and Dr N. Edson.

23 Muriel Bell, Obituary, 'Emeritus Professor John Malcolm, CMG, MD, FRSE', *Digest*, 1954, p. 70. Earlier women MDs from Otago were Margaret Cruickshank (1903) and Grace Stevenson (1922).

24 David Cole, unpublished memoir, p. 13; Moore, pp. 77–8.

25 Notes, *Digest*, 1940, p. 61.

26 I am grateful for information from Brian Barraclough who has been researching Carmalt Jones' life; Chisholm, 'The Otago Medical School 50 years ago'; Hercus and Bell, pp. 265–7.

27 Chisholm, 'The Otago Medical School Fifty Years Ago'; Begg, p. 43; Frank Williamson Fitchett (1870–1951), family entry under A.R. Fitchett, *Southern People*, p. 163; Obituary, *NZMJ* February 1951, pp. 48–51; Hercus and Bell, p. 269.

28 Obituary, Sir Francis Gordon Bell, *NZMJ* April 1970, pp. 243–5; Hercus and Bell, pp. 293–4; A.W. Beasley, 'Bell, Francis Gordon, 1887–1970', DNZB 5, p. 50; John Heslop, Appreciation delivered at the Annual General Meeting of the Otago Medical Research Society, *NZMJ* April 1970, pp. 245–6; Gordon Bell, *Surgeon's Saga* Chapter 10, especially pp. 152–7, contains an attractive picture of the Medical School and the Hospital as he found them in 1925.

29 Hercus and Bell, pp. 295–8, give pen portraits of the men.

30 'James Renfrew White (1888–1961)', *Southern People*, p. 543. Hercus and Bell, who describe him as a born teacher, also make the curious comment that towards the end of his career his teaching was 'marred by eccentricities', p. 309; Oral information, B. Heslop and E. Nye. The original Eefie White was a south Dunedin rag and bone man, information, Lawrence Wright.

31 Bell, *Surgeon's Saga*, p. 157; Hercus and Bell, pp. 311–2.

32 Dr J.I. Clayton, *The History of Anaesthesia in Dunedin Hospital*, pp. 41, 45–6. In the Appendix, pp. 164–76, Clayton lists the anaesthetists at Dunedin Hospital, going backwards from 2005 to 1906. Russell Ritchie was the first, serving from 1906–9; John Borrie, 'Whyte, Marion King Binnie (1895–1983)', *Southern People*, pp. 545–6.

33 Hercus and Bell, pp. 243–4; Chisholm; Obituary, Drennan, *NZMJ* 1984; OUR XXXV, July 1922, pp. 9–11; Descriptive Syllabus, p. 27; Eric D'Ath replaced Drennan in 1928, Hercus and Bell, p. 246.

34 Ferguson to Gregg, cited in Carmalt Jones, pp. 195–200.

35 J.F. Gwynne, Obituary, Emeritus Professor Eric Frederick D'Ath, *NZMJ* vol. 90, 1979, pp. 307–8; Citation for honorary DSc, Otago, 1975. D'Ath died in 1979, after a protracted illness; Sir David Hay, *Heart Sounds: a life at the forefront of health care*, p. 118, summed D'Ath up as 'an autocratic Otago graduate who loved the morgue and the courtroom … had no higher qualifications, published little if at all, but successfully administered a large laboratory …'.

36 G. Bell, *Surgeon's Saga*, pp. 156–7.

37 Doris Gordon, *Back-Blocks Baby-Doctor*, pp. 177–98, gives a full account of the nation-wide fund-raising campaign, which brought in well above its £25,000 target; Dawson, cited in Hercus and Bell, pp. 324–5, 327–30; Carmalt Jones, p. 235; Sir Bernard Dawson 'Without Varnish' an unpublished autobiography, pp. 187–9; Obituary, Sir Joseph Bernard Dawson, *NZMJ* October 1965, pp. 525–7.

CHAPTER 10

The Clinical Club and the Monro Collection

1 J.D. Hunter, 'The Clinical Club of Dunedin (1915–1939), from a Minute Book of the 1928–1939 period', in R. Wright-St Clair, ed., *Proceedings of the First New Zealand Conference on the History of New Zealand and Australian Medicine*, Waikato Postgraduate Medical Society Inc., Hamilton, 1987, pp. 177–84; J.D. Hunter, 'The Clinical Club (1915–1939) "Medical Giants in their dressing Gowns"', Otago Medical School Alumnus Association Newsletter, 24, 1999/2000, pp. 35–8. When Hunter wrote, he believed that only the minutes of 1928–39 had survived, but the earlier volumes have now come to light. Champtaloup was appointed Professor of Bacteriology and Public Health in 1911, Drennan, Pathology in 1915, Gowland, Anatomy in 1914, Malcolm, Physiology in 1905, Fitchett, Physician to Dunedin Hospital 1905 (promoted to Professor of Clinical Medicine 1920), Stanley Batchelor, Consultant and Lecturer in Surgery, 1906 and Ritchie, Consultant and Lecturer in Obstetrics, 1910.

2 Hunter, in *Proceedings* 1987, p. 177; Fitchett described Champtaloup's purpose in a minute passed by the club on the occasion of his death in 1921, cited in Hercus and Bell, p. 362.

3 Hercus and Bell, pp. 166–7. Scott bequeathed his own volumes of the *Journal of Physiology* and *Brain*.

4 Minutes of the Clinical Club, 1928–1939. 85th meeting of 26th October 1928, Otago Medical School; Hunter, 'The Clinical Club, 1915–1939', Alumnus Association Newsletter, 1999–2000, pp. 35–8. Hunter includes the report of this meeting. It also appears in *Digest*, 1969, pp. 105–6; Hercus and Bell, pp. 361–3. This appendix reproduces the minute passed in 1921 to mark the death of Champtaloup.

5 Hercus and Bell, pp. 169–70; Ferguson to Gregg, Rockefeller Foundation, 1923.

6 R. Wright-St Clair, 'The Monros and their Books', *Digest*, 1963, pp.27–8. Dr Wright St-Clair has published a full-length account in *Doctors Monro: a Medical Saga*, Wellcome, London, 1964.

7 D.W. Taylor, *The Monro Collection in the Medical Library of the University of Otago*, Otago University Press, Dunedin, 1979; *The Monro Collection in the Medical School Library of the University of Otago*, Medical School, Dunedin 1975, pp. 5–6; Hercus and Bell, p. 173, credit Dr Charles Monro Hector, the son of Sir James, who was researching poliomyelitis at the Otago Medical School in 1927, with the suggestion of giving the collection to the School. However, in a paper on 'The Books and Manuscripts of Alexander Monro primus in the medical Library of the University of Otago' delivered at the University of Edinburgh in 1976, Douglass Taylor draws attention to Fitchett's letter and the correspondence of 1927–1929; When the collection was catalogued by the General Assembly Library, it was stated, incorrectly, to have been donated by Lady Hector. *The Early Days of the Edinburgh Medical School*, p. 66; David Monro's diary is cited in Wright St-Clair, *Digest*, p. 29. Sir David Monro also inherited the Monro anatomical museum, which he gave to Edinburgh University. Sir James Hector was Director of the New Zealand Geological Survey, and the first Chancellor of the University of New Zealand.

8 D.W. Taylor, *The Monro Collection*, pp. 8–10.

9 W.J. Mullin, 'Memo for Professor Adams from W.J. Mullin, MB (NZ) 1890', handwritten communication, c. 1954; Hercus and Bell, p. 173; W.J. Mullin, 'The Monro Family and the Monro Collection of Books and MSS', *NZMJ* 1936, vol. 35, pp. 221–9; Taylor notes that Monro secundus did not claim to have discovered the foramen (or more correctly the plural foramina) but maintained he had described it more accurately than any predecessor (personal communication).

CHAPTER 11

Medical Students Between the Wars

1 'Semicolon Bijjj', OUR, June 1893, p. 53; P. McIntyre, 'The Varsity review', *Critic*, 1 May 1930, p. 32.

2 'Ray', 'Public Enemy No. 1: The Superior Medicals', *Critic*, 5 June 1936, p. 7.

3 W. Anderson, *Doctor in the Mountains* (1964), Ch. 3; p. 42; R. Burns Watson, *The Doctor Must Get Through* (1971), p. 21.

4 Francis Bennett, *A Canterbury Tale*, pp. 54, 108–9. The friends were a formidable group: John Cairney, R.S. Aitken, Jack Hinton and J.D. Iverach all later became professors. Aitken became Otago University's first executive Vice-Chancellor. John Cairney, later a Director General of Health, was the coach.

5 Sir Patrick Eisdell Moore, *So Old So Quick*, pp. 67–71.

6 Ellis Dick, typescript, 'Reflections of an Undergraduate at Otago Medical School, 1936–1940'; Fred Fastier, *Recollections of an Old Scarfie*, p. 33.

Maunsell wrote up his exploits for *Critic* not long before he was killed in action in World War II, Fastier, p. 33.

7   Dorothy Page, 'Dissecting a Community: Women Medical Students at the University of Otago, 1891–1924', in Brookes and Page, eds, *Communities of Women*, pp. 123, 125–6; an example of student humour at the expense of women medical students is 'Scenes of Medical Life', *Review*, June 1920, pp. 21–3; Elworthy, p. 50.

8   Eva Ng, 'Pih-Chang, Kathleen, (1903–1991)', *Southern People*, p. 389. Francis Chang died in 1978.

9   Thomas Brons and Sean Ellison, 'Ellison, Edward Pohau, 1884–1963', in DNZB 4, pp. 158–9; I am grateful to Bruce Young of Wilfrid Laurier University, Ontario, Canada, for making unpublished material about Potaka available to me. His 'Louis Hauiti Potaka: a Biographical Essay', 2005, is available on the internet.

10 Nicola Mutch, 'Distant Education', an interview with Dr Annie Stuart, *Otago Magazine*, October 2007, pp. 22–4. Mutyala Satynand's son is the present Governor-General of New Zealand.

11 Elworthy, pp. 28–9. List of presidents, appendix, p. 162; 'Officers of OUSA from Our faculty', *Te Korero*, September 1922, p. 79. Iverach, who won the travelling scholarship in 1924, became a much admired teacher at the Medical School. Gwynne, p. 21, describes him as 'perhaps the most impressive and memorable teacher we had – the great physician'; When Porritt won a Rhodes Scholarship the next year, *Te Korero* commented, 'We expect great things of him.' May 1923; Denny-Brown became professor of neurology at Harvard University; J.A.D. Iverach, *Digest*, 1955, p. 7. Even the caustic Gowland was impressed with Iverach's class, which also included the future plastic surgeon, Archibald McIndoe, and the future professor of pathology at Otago, Eric D'Ath. They were not, he told them, the worst class in anatomy he had ever taught, but they were just like it.

12 Bennett, pp. 109–10. *Critic* replaced *Te Korero* (1923–5) which Bennett calls a 'dismal rag'. He describes how he and his study mate usually filled it up with 'imaginative froth' a few hours before it went to press, p. 109.

13 Tohill, pp. 76–8. Sir John Stallworthy was received an honorary degree on the centenary of the medical school and gave the graduation address on that occasion. The main instigator of the grandstand project was Stallworthy's predecessor as OUSA president, P.S. de Q. Cabot, 1925–27. For Lovelock, see Roger Robinson, 'Lovelock, John Edward, 1910–1949', in DNZB 4, pp. 291–3.

14 'Arts student', in *Critic*, 1 May 1930, p. 34; Elworthy, pp. 58–60, 65. The student sent down for the Allen Hall episode was F.B. Edmundson. The authorities were not in a mood to tolerate disorder after a riotous graduation ceremony in 1930 and the chaos of the 1931 capping ball, held in the Otago Early Settlers Museum. Not only was the ballroom awash with alcohol, but students extended their drunken activities to the nearby Leviathan Hotel. Elworthy, p. 55. Dan Davin refers to the 'Leviathan scandal' in his novel *Not Here Not Now*, p. 224; Ellis Dick, 'Reflections of an Undergraduate, Otago Medical School, 1936–1940', typescript. Dick notes that Fookes' unusually long training made him a good GP. It was Dick who described the parachute incident.

15 See Frank Rogers, 'Roberts, Murray Beresford, 1919–1974', DNZB 5, pp. 443–4, for other medical impersonations; 'Con Man to the End', *Evening Star*, 6 August 1974 reported Roberts' death at 56 in a Parakura hotel. The previous week he had been posing as a Supreme Court judge; Patrick Moore, pp. 74–5, describes how Roberts took his anatomy exam paper out of the room in the general bustle at the beginning of the exam, wrote it with benefit of references and slipped back into the room in the confusion when papers were being handed in.

16 *Medical Digest*, vol. 1, no. 1, October 1934, passim.

17 *Medical Digest*, vol. 1, 1934, vol. 1, no. 2, 1935, 1936; Michael Dunn, *The Drawings of Russell Clark*, pp. 7–17. Dr D.T. Stewart, one of the founders of *Digest*, acknowledged Clark's contribution. In Dunedin Clark worked for the publishing company McIndoes and held art classes.

18 *Medical Digest*, 1935. There was also an article by A.M. Dunne, on Maori medicine.

19 Professor C.E. Hercus, in *Digest*, 1954.

CHAPTER 12

The Dean's Assessment

1   Ferguson, Annual Report, 1936. AG-180-7/01 (HC).

PART III

Research and Expansion: The Hercus Era, 1937–1958

CHAPTER 13

World War II

1   Morrell p. 153. The recommendation was to acquire all or part of the block bounded by Leith, St David, Clyde and Union Streets for a hall of residence, new departments of zoology and botany, and a purpose-built library.

2   Hercus and Bell, pp. 66–9; *Critic*, 2 July, 1937. The conversazione took place on 23 June.

3   Annual Report, 1939, Otago Medical School (OMS).

4   Annual Report of Medical Faculty, 1939 (OMS).

5   *ODT,* 18 December 1939.

6   *Dominion*, Wellington, 17 January 1940. The Hamilton speaker was Mr Ziman. The same report appeared in the *ODT,* 18 December 1940.

7   Annual Report of Medical Faculty for 1939, amended version.

8   'Oration by Dr Carmalt Jones', *ODT*, 10 May 1939.

9   Neil Begg, *The Intervening Years*, p. 48.

10 Annual Report of Medical School, 1939, p. 3; Annual Reports of Medical School, 1940 and 1942. In the 1942 report, the departments most in need of further accommodation were listed as Pathology, Preventive Medicine and Medical Research, p. 2.

11 Annual Report of Medical School, 1940. Horace Smirk was appointed. The 1944 appointments were Professor Eccles (Physiology) and professor Adams (Anatomy). There were a number of appointments at a more junior level, e.g. in Annual Report, 1942, p. 2.

12 Annual Report 1940. Staff on active service were Drs M.R.F. Fitchett, H.W. Fitzgerald, J.R. Fulton, E.R. Harty, D.P. Kennedy, G.R. Kirk, J.A. Meade, N. North, A. Perry, N.C. Speight and S.L. Wilson; The 1942 Annual Report noted military distinctions to staff and ex-students and the deaths on active service of Major Wyn Irwin, W.L.R. Gilmour and Dr Florence Craig. Military awards to former staff and students and casualties among them form a part of all the reports until the end of the war.

13 'A State of War exists', *Critic*, 20 September 1939, p. 4.

14 *Critic*, 4 July 1940, p. 2.

15 *Critic*, 18 July 1940, p. 1. The first ballot was announced in the *ODT* on 5 December 1940, the second on 5 March 1941. Newspaper items for this period come from the Medical School cutting book, 1934–45. 95-157-22/3 (HC).

16 'Medical Students. Military Obligations', *ODT*, 14 March 1941; *ODT*, 4 February 1941.

17 Letter to the Editor, *ODT*, 23 July 1941.

18 G. Brinkman, interview with D. Page, December 2002.

19 Hercus, *Digest*, II. 3 October 1942, p. 15.

20 Hercus and Bell, p. 205.

21 'Position of Medicals. Dr Hercus Explains', *Critic*, 18 July 1940.

22 Annual Report of Medical School, 1941; Editorial, *ODT*, 16 July 1941. The intake was limited after consultation with the Government.

23 Annual Reports, Medical School, 1939, 1940, 1941. In addition to the 83 who gained places by examination, the entrants to second year were made up of two who had passed earlier, 11 second

years who were re-admitted, and the four who gained highest marks in the Special Examination of February 1941. Nine others who passed the Special were granted preference for 1942. Annual Report, 1941.

24 *ODT*, 14 February 1940, 'Alien Doctors'. The ban was moved by Dr J. Fitzgerald, on the grounds that New Zealand doctors returning after the war should not have their position prejudiced by foreigners; E.H. Caswell, '"An overdose of refugees": refugee medical practitioners in New Zealand c. 1930–c. 1950', BA Hons History, University of Otago, 2005, deals with European Jews escaping Nazi persecution, most of whom arrived in New Zealand early in World War II. Chapter 3, 'The relationship of the refugee medical practitioners and the medical profession', covers the question of access to requalifying and the various bodies involved in granting this.

25 Editorial, 'Medical Refugees', *ODT*, 16 February 1940.

26 Sir Carrick Robertson, cited in 'Alien Doctors Practising', *ODT*, 29 May 1940.

27 'Refugee Doctors', *ODT*, 19 June 1940. Dr Fitzgerald was reported as expressing his opinion in Council that all Germans were the same; Letters on refugee aliens 21 June 1940, 22 June 1940 (six letters), 14 June 1940.

28 'RSA Allegations', *ODT*, 19 June 1940 and Editorial, 'Subversive Activities', *Evening Star*, 17 July 1940; 'Aliens Come First', *New Zealand Truth*, 31 July 1940. The article also raised the issue of foreign doctors practising in New Zealand while New Zealand doctors were serving overseas; 'Limitation of Medical Students. Official Explanation', *Truth*, 7 August 1940.

29 'Refugee Doctors. Building up Practices', *ODT*, 20 January 1942. Married men were called up by ballot in January 1942, *ODT* 21 January 1942; E.H. Caswell, 'An Overdose of Refugees'.

30 'Refugee Doctors', Report of Senate, *ODT*, 22 January 1942; De la Mare, 'Refugee Doctors', *ODT* 24 January 1942; 'Refugee Doctors. Dr Newlands Replies to Critic', *ODT* 42 January 1942. Dr Newlands had been lecturer in Surgery at Otago from 1911 until 1936, Annual Report, 1944.

31 'Refugee Doctors. Admission as Students', *ODT*, 19 January 1943; Editorial, 'The Refugee Doctor', 20 January 1943; report of OU Council, *ODT*, 17 February 1943. Dr Fitzgerald was the member concerned.

32 *ODT*, 21 January 1943. The Minister of Health was Mr Nordmeyer.

33 R.G. Osborne, in Report from Wellington, *ODT*, 1 August 1940.

34 'The Medical School', Editorial, *ODT*, 16 July, 1941. In the replacement of house surgeons with senior medical students, Auckland hospital was allocated five students, Wellington four, Palmerston North

two and Dunedin, Invercargill and Waikato, one each.

35 Hercus and Bell, p. 71.
36 *ODT*, report from Wellington, 30 August 1941. *ODT*, Editorial, 1 September 1941.
37 'National Council of Women (Dunedin)', *ODT*, 9 October 1941.
38 'Medical School: Admissions Increased', *ODT*, 24 February 1943; 'Medical Training: Output of Doctors', *ODT*, 16 March 1943; 'Medical School. Reported Plan for Auckland', *ODT*, 6/9/43; 'Medical School: Staffing Difficulties', *ODT*, 3 December 1943. Hercus's own view as that a second medical school would not be necessary until the New Zealand population reached 5 million; 'Refusal of Admissions. Perturbation in Auckland', *ODT* 12 February 1944. The MP for Remuera expressed his 'outrage' at the exclusion of Auckland students.
39 Hercus and Bell, p. 73. The Dean and Dr H.D. Purves had prepared a forecast for the *NZMJ* of 1943 of New Zealand's needs for medical practitioners. They argued that 100 graduates per annum were sufficient to provide one doctor per 1120 head of population and that no increase would be required until 1987. Hercus still adhered to this view in 1964.
40 'Medical School Staffing Difficulties', *ODT*, 3 December 1943.
41 Hercus and Bell, pp. 73–5.
42 Hercus and Bell, pp. 71–2; 193–4. The building was completed in 1948.
43 *ODT*, 'Medical School Record Enrolments,' 17 February 1944; Annual Report of Medical School, 1944.
44 Hercus and Bell, p. 206; *Digest*, 1946, pp. 59–62. Miss Thomson was the Dean's secretary. Her war file includes a small but moving collection of letters written by Singapore friends of the Craig sisters, to their parents Dr and Mrs Craig of Sydney. She also kept a newspaper clipping book about the exploits of the graduates serving in the forces, including their decorations; A.B.M. 'Heroism in the East', *Digest*, 1942, pp. 63–4.
45 Lindsay Rogers, *Guerrilla Surgeon*; The *Time* article, cited in *ODT* 1944, is in the Medical School cutting book, 1934–45.
46 J. Borrie, *Despite Captivity.*
47 Neil Begg, *The Intervening Years* ,p. 51.
48 Christine Daniell, *A Doctor at War. A Life in Letters, 1914–1943.*
49 Treanor, Chs. 9–13 passim, Freyberg cited p. 78; Begg, p. 73.
50 Begg, p. 61; R. Battle, revised H.C.G. Mathew, 'McIndoe, Sir Archibald Hector (1900–1960)', *Oxford Dictionary of National Biography*, vol. 35, 2004.
51 John Heslop, 'Surgery in Dunedin', Stanley Livingstone Wilson, *Otago Medical School Alumnus Association Newsletter*, 2000/01, p. 46.
52 Treanor, for Lt Col N.C. Speight, pp. 62, 103–4; Lt Col V.T. Pearse, p. 64; Brian McMahon, interview.
53 Lawrence Wright, interview; 'Tribute to John Borrie, Honorary Curator for Historic Artefacts', *Alumnus Newsletter*, 1999/2000, p. 18; John Heslop, 'Sir Michael Woodruff KBE FRS MD FRCS FRCS (E)', in *Alumnus Newsletter*, 2000/01; Hercus and Bell, pp. 193–4.
54 Dow, Derek A., 'Hercus, Charles Ernest 1888–1971', DNZB 4, pp. 235–6; Obituary, *NZMJ* April 1971, pp. 231–4.

CHAPTER 14

Research and Expansion Under Hercus

1   Hercus and Bell, pp. 92–3.
2   F.N. Fastier, 'Sir Horace Smirk: Professor Emeritus', *NZMJ* 67, March 1968, p. 258.
3   C.E. Hercus, 'New Zealand and Medical Research', reprinted from *New Zealand Science Review* 8 (1950), p. 1.
4   Hercus, 'Medical Research', p. 2.
5   Medical School Annual Report, 1938.
6   Medical School Annual Reports, 1938, 1939; Derek Dow, *Safeguarding the Public Health: a History of the New Zealand Department of Health*; Watt, an outstanding public health administrator, was an Otago medical graduate of 1910 and the second person to win the travelling scholarship. Derek A. Dow, 'Watt, Michael Herbert, 1887–1967', DNZB 4, p. 556.
7   N. Edson, cited in Hercus and Bell, p. 239. Edson became Professor of Biochemistry in 1949.
8   Medical School report, 1939; H.D. Purves, Muriel Bell and Duncan Adams, Obituary, 'Walter Edwin Griesbach'. *NZMJ*, September, 1968, pp. 187–8. Griesbach was also a concert-standard pianist (Douglass Taylor); Daphne Purves, 'Purves, Herbert Dudley, 1908–1993', *Southern People*. p. 403; J. Hubbard, 'Herbert Dudley Purves', Obituary, in *Proceedings of the Royal Society of New Zealand*, 1993. The Thyroid Research Department went through several name changes, to become the Endocrinology Research Unit and eventually, in 1971, the Neuroendocrinology Group.
9   Moore, p. 83; Digest 1940, cited in F. Fastier, 'Sir Horace Smirk: Professor Emeritus', *NZMJ*, vol. 67, 429, Special Issue March 1968, p. 258; University orator, citation for Hon DSc, 1975.
10 Fastier, p. 262.
11 Obituary, Sir Horace Smirk, *NZMJ*, vol. 104, 1991, pp. 271–2; A.W. Beasley, 'Smirk, Frederick Horace, 1902–1991', DNZB 5, pp. 480–1.
12 I.H. Page MD, 'Sir Horace Smirk: a View from the World Around', *NZMJ* 'Special Issue,' March 1968, p. 257; A.W. Beasley, 'Smirk, Frederick Horace, 1902–1991', DNZB 5, pp. 480–1.

13 Hercus and Bell p. 181, pp. 273–5; Hercus, 'Medical Research', p. 6; Fastier in *NZMJ* 1968 p. 258.

14 Annual Report, 1942; Hercus and Bell, p. 181.

15 Philippa Mein Smith, 'Bell, Muriel Emma, 1898–1974', DNZB 4, pp. 47–8. Bell is frequently referred to as the first woman to be awarded an MD from Otago university, but this honour belongs to Margaret Cruickshank, 1903; Marion F. Robinson, 'Bell, Muriel Emma (1898–1974)', *Southern People*, pp. 41–3; Obituary, Muriel Emma Bell, *NZMJ* 26 June 1974, pp. 1082–3; Diana Brown, 'Between Lab and Kitchen: the Unconventional Career of Dr Muriel Bell', MA in History, University of Otago, 2006.

16 Hercus and Bell, pp. 74–5; There were 312 students in the department, of whom 229 were medical students who spent two years on anatomy and physiology, p. 229.

17 David Cole, unpublished memoir. The unfortunate student was Rex Wright St Clair; David Cole, as Dean of the Auckland Medical School, at the centenary assembly for the conferment of honorary degrees. He conveyed greetings from the Medical Schools of Australasia, and also spoke on behalf of former students of the Otago Medical School. Cutting book, Centenary 1975, OMS.

18 Hercus and Bell, pp. 235–6; D. Cole, memoir.

19 Gavin Glasgow, unpublished lecture on J.C. Eccles, 1997.

20 McIntyre, cited in Hercus and Bell, p. 236; Hercus and Bell, p. 236.

21 Prof. J.C. Eccles, 'Research and the Medical School', *Digest*, 2, no. 5, October 1944, pp. 3–8. The article welcoming Professor Eccles, 'Ring in the New', appeared on pages 36–7.

22 Sir John Scott, 'Sir John Carew Eccles, 1903–1997', Obituary, Royal Society of New Zealand, 1999 Academy Yearbook.

23 Hercus and Bell, p. 238.

24 Hercus and Bell, pp. 234–7.

25 Scott, p. 3. The Nobel prize was shared with A.L. Hodgkin and A.F. Huxley.

26 Annual Report 1925; Hercus and Bell, pp. 140–2.; David Cole unpublished memoir, 'Some Recollections of Being a Medical Student in the 1940s', pp. 22–4. The other BMedSc students in 1945 were Mary Hannafin, Deryck Gallagher and Marianne Fillenz. Fillenz was the only one to remain in research, at Oxford. The MMedSc could be taken in any of eight areas: anatomy, physiology, biochemistry, pathology, microbiology, pharmacology, clinical science, preventive and social medicine. The student was required to work in the discipline already selected for the BMedSc.

27 Medical School Annual Report, 1947.

28 Hercus, 'Medical Research', p. 8.

29 Annual Report, 1944.

30 *Evening Star*, 20 July 1944; J. Uglow, Edith Summerskill, in *Macmillan Dictionary of Women's Biography*.

31 Annual Report, 1948.

32 Annual Reports, 1946, 1947, 1948; Commemorative brochure, 'University of Otago Medical School. Opening of South Block, 8 September, 1948, by Hon T.D. McCombs, MSc, M.P., Minister of Education'. Professor Hercus's speech on this occasion detailed the history of the building and reaffirmed his commitment to research; Hercus and Bell, pp. 76–7; *NZMJ*, July 1969, p. 43.

33 Hercus and Bell, pp. 97–8. The GMC's 1947 recommendations include the first changes.

34 Hercus and Bell, p. 103. The committee membership was the Chancellor and Vice-Chancellor of NZU, Sir Hugh Acland, Messrs Cocker, Herron, Johnstone, Schroder, Stout, and Dean Hercus. Two minority reports advocated sending all sixth year students to a single centre other than Dunedin. Hercus and Bell, p. 103.

35 Hunter, p. 18; Hercus and Bell, p. 106. In 1964, Hercus and Bell believed the course had already failed and it was, in fact, abandoned in 1969. The six term curriculum in medical sciences had been in operation since 1923.

36 Hercus and Bell, pp. 104–5, 130–1.

37 'We want Psychology: plea that a Diploma of Psychological Medicine should be part of one's study before coming out to enter general practice', *Digest* 1936, pp. 20–1; J.A. Iverach, 'Proprietary Medicine', *Digest* 1936, pp. 34–8; A.M. Gunn, 'Maori Medicine', *Digest* 1936, pp. 39–43; N.L. Edson, 'Examinations at Otago University and Elsewhere', *Digest* 1937, pp. 14–8; W.P. Gowland, 'Some European Anatomical Departments', *Digest* 1942, pp. 29–39.

38 J.L. Malcolm', *Digest* 1947, pp. 42–4. Malcolm claimed that only the Department of Obstetrics and Gynaecology was using visual aids effectively. Much of this issue was given over to National Health Services in New Zealand and Overseas; Editorial, *Digest*, 1948; Chandler M.C. Brookes, 'Letter from Brooklyn', *Digest*, 1949, pp. 6–8.

39 R.S. Aitken, 'Medicine in the University', *Digest*, 1950, pp. 3–12.

40 Ian Rutherford, 'An Ounce of Practice …', *Digest*, 1955, pp. 45–9; D.S., 'A New System of Medical Education at an American University', *Digest*, 1955, pp. 51–6; Editorial, 'Medical Education – Progress is Possible', *Digest*, 1957. The journal editors, John Steiner and Richard Mark, referred to medical education as a 'hardy annual'; Editorial, *Digest*, 1959. The editors were Brian Muir and Earle Wilson.

41 Student figures from Morrell, Appendix, p. 245.

42 Peter J. Morris, 'Sir Michael Woodruff, 1911–2001', Annual Report of the Royal Society of New Zealand, incorporating the 2001 Yearbook; Hercus and Bell, pp. 306–8. Sir Gordon Bell filled in between Woodruff's departure and Fraenkel's arrival;

Morrell, p. 185; 'New Professor of Surgery', *Critic*, 13 March 1958.

[43] Hercus and Bell, p. 333; L. Wright, interview with D. Page. Hercus wrote more than one letter offering the position, his tone becoming increasingly insistent.

[44] Hunter, Compendium, pp. 10–11. Sandy (J.M.B.) Smith, Obituary, John Arthur Reginald Miles, CBE MA MD *Cantab* FRSNZ FRACP, 1913–2004, Royal Society of New Zealand 2004 Academy Yearbook, rsnz.org/directory/yearbook/2004/miles.

[45] Obituary, Associate-Professor John Borrie, *ODT*, 12 August 2006; Hunter, Compendium; F. Fastier, interview with D. Page.

[46] Medical Research Council booklet, c. 1956.

[47] Obituary, Franz Bielschowsky, *NZMJ* June 1965, pp. 338–9.

[48] J. Hubbard, Obituary, H.D. Purves, RSNZ, 1993. Daphne Purves, 'Purves, Herbert Dudley (1908–1993)', *Southern People*, p. 403.

[49] Fastier, *NZMJ*, pp. 261–2; E.G. McQueen and F. Fastier, 'Smirk, Frederick Horace (1902–1991)', *Southern People*, pp. 462–3.

[50] Marion F. Robinson, 'Bell, Muriel Emma, 1898–1974', *Southern People*, pp. 41–2; Mein Smith, DNZB 4, pp. 47–8. Citation for honorary degree, 1968. Bell was the second woman to receive an honorary degree from Otago University, a year after her friend Elizabeth Gregory was awarded an honorary LLD. Until 2006 , when Dr Beryl Howie was awarded an honorary DSc, she was the only woman medical graduate to be honoured in this way. University of Otago Calendar, 2007, p. 131.

CHAPTER 15

Medical Students in the Mid-Twentieth Century

[1] 'I Hereby Nominate', *Critic*, 18 September 1941, p. 2.

[2] Prior, pp. 90–1. David Cole, unpublished memoir. I am grateful to Professor Cole for making this available to me.

[3] Information, Alison Clarke; 'OUSA Closes Down on Capping Frolics', *Critic*, 19 March 1942, p. 3; Elworthy, Appendix, p. 162. Student presidents were: H.H. Francis, 1942, J.A.M. Boyd, 1943 and D.W. McGregor 1944 and 1945; p. 67.

[4] Prior, p. 96.

[5] Griffiths, p. 44; Cole, pp. 6–7, remembers slightly different figures, and the window-breaking as part of the same game.

[6] Cole, p. 7. Mara's success in the Drinking Horn was the more surprising in that he was a non-drinker.

[7] *Critic*, 25 June 1942, p. 2.

[8] 'Lebensraum' and 'Med', *Critic*, 21 April 1943, p. 6.

[9] Barbara Heslop, 'Postgraduate Training – the Eternal Tug of War for Women and How It has

Got Tougher', in Jill McIlraith, ed., *The Goods Train Doctors: Stories of Women Doctors in New Zealand, 1920–1993*, pp. 9–17. She first attended a fifth year dinner in the 1980s, as guest speaker;

[10] Heslop, p. 9; Karin Beatson, 'Rina Moore (1923–1975)', in Charlotte Macdonald, Mermeri Penfold and Bridget Williams, eds, *The Book of New Zealand Women, Ko Kui Ma Te Kaupapa*, pp. 455–7.

[11] Elworthy, p. 76; J.F. Gwynne, 'The Medical School Then and Now', *Medical Digest*, 1975, pp. 20–3. Gwynne deplored the casual dress of 1975, but thought little could be done about it when some staff lectured in polo-necked jerseys, T-shirts and jeans.

[12] 'Pamela', 'The Medical Student, or "How to Avoid Solecisms in Good Society"', *Critic*, 4 May 1954. The medical student should have the same nonchalant attitude to study. In a subsequent issue, Pamela considered 'The Medical Student at a Party', *Critic*, 3 June 1954. Both pieces were part of a witty series, by Arts student Diana Mahy, on the characteristics of students from various faculties.

[13] 'The Microscope', 'As Others See Us', *Digest*, September 1950, p. 30.

[14] Elworthy, Appendix, pp. 162–3. Presidents were: M.W Hursthouse, 1949, J.E. McCoy, 1950 and 1951, L.H. Wright, 1952, K.A.K. North, 1953, W.N. Smith (later Adams Smith), 1955 and 1956, K.E.W. Melvin, 1957, A.R. Brown, 1960 and J.C. Cullen, 1961; pp. 85–6. Representation on the Council was by a graduate, not currently a student, of not less than two years standing. The Union Building committee, established in 1948, was initially chaired by Professor Hercus.

[15] 'Elder statesman', interview with Dr W.N. Adams Smith, *Critic*, 9 August 1962, p. 1.

[16] 'New President of OUSA', *Critic*, 30 June 1960, p. 1.

[17] David Cole, unpublished memoir, pp. 26–39.

[18] 'Med. Stranglehold on Capping', *Critic*, 5 May 1959.

[19] John Heslop to D. Page, January 2007.

[20] Lindsay Knight, Profile of Ron Elvidge, All Black Player Profiles, New Zealand Rugby Museum. Elvidge had a collar bone injury and a facial gash that required stitches. He returned to the field because the team had lost another player to injury; Cole, p. 4.

[21] J.F. Gwynne, 'The Medical School Then and Now (1945 and 1975)', *Medical Digest* 1975, p. 20. Oddly, he makes no comment on women students in 1975.

[22] Heslop to Page, January 2007. Heslop herself first attended a fifth year dinner in the 1980s, when she was guest speaker. 'Eefie' White was an orthopaedic surgeon, with a fine reputation as a teacher, and a recognised eccentric.

[23] 'Hospital doctor dies from bullet wounds. Young woman doctor to face murder charge', *Otago Daily Times*, 13 December 1954; *ODT*, 14 December 1954 and from 9 February 1955 to 19

February 1955. Whittingham was released in May 1957. She at once went to Australia, where she became a highly respected immunologist; *ODT*, 13 October 1955, reported the application for Whittingham's name to be struck off the medical roll; Beverley Howells, 'A Crime of the Times' *ODT*, 23–24 September 2006. At that time the case was the subject of a play, 'My Heart is bathed in Blood', by Michelanne Forster, performed at the Fortune Theatre, Dunedin; Charlotte Amodeo, 'The Murder Trial of Senga Florence Whittingham: an Examination into the Nature of Gender Relations in the 1950s', 490 Dissertation, History, University of Otago, 2001; Obituary, Bill Saunders, *Digest*, 1955, pp. 68–9.

24 OUMSA President's Report, 1961; Susi Williams (nee Lemchen, graduated 1957), 'Sober Suits and Low Heels – And Don't Dare be Pregnant', pp. 6–8. Susi Lemchen was the women's rep on the OUMSA. Glenys Arthur (nee Smart, graduated 1960) 'Swimming Against the Tide', pp. 25–30, Robyn Hewland, 'From Hats and Brandy Snaps to Sexual Abuse', pp. 46–50, all in Jill McIlraith. ed., *The Goods Train Doctors. Stories of women doctors in New Zealand, 1920–1993*.

CHAPTER 16

A Formidable Dean: Charles Hercus in the School and the University

1 Morrell, pp. 162–3, 185. Student enrolments in 1937, when Hercus became Dean, totalled 1376 (well above the 1203, itself a record, when he first joined the staff in 1922) and they rose to 1450 in 1939. In 1946, the total was 2440. This figure was not surpassed until 1959, when there were 2543 enrolments, but the number did not sink below 2000 over this period and was usually well above it. Morrell, Appendix, pp. 244–5.

2 Morrell, pp. 157–8. In 1944, the Chancellor, Mr Morrell, who had devoted his retirement years to university business, became ill. The Vice-Chancellor, Rev D.C. Herron, who was also a parish minister, had to step in. He became Chancellor when Morrell resigned in February 1945.

3 Morrell, p. 169. The sense of a new order was reinforced at the same time by the retirement of Mr Chapman, registrar for the previous 37 years, and the appointment of the assistant registrar, Mr J.W. Hayward, to succeed him; Medical School Annual Report, 1948.

4 Hercus and Bell, p. 210. Mr Carl Smith was the Visitor.

5 R.S. Aitken, 'Medicine in the University', in *Digest* 3, 5 September 1950, pp. 3–12.

6 Morrell, p. 178; Interview, Jock Hayward, OU Registrar 1948–1974 with John Hunter, 22 November 1991.

7 Morrell, pp. 170–1. The formula was based on student numbers and staff-student ratio.

8 UGC Report, 16 December 1949, Minutes and Proceedings of NZU Senate, 1950, p. 53; Hercus and Bell, pp. 192, 194.

9 See Hercus and Bell, pp. 194–5, for detail, including a table of grants from 1950 to 1958.

10 Morrell, pp. 172–3. The Dental School had recently displaced a new library and new biology block from the top place on Otago's list; Hercus and Bell, p. 194. The South Block cost £385,000.

11 Morrell, pp. 179–80. The bequest, for £38,000, came from Mr H.C. Le Cren Russell. The task of formally opening the building fell to the same Minister, Mr Algie, who had refused permission for it to go ahead. Morrell, pp. 179–80.

12 Hercus and Bell, p. 306; Hayward, interview with Hunter, 1991. The building was later demolished to make way for the Sayers building.

13 Angus, pp. 227–9. By the time the decision was taken the OHB was chaired by Dr Moody.

14 Angus, pp. 232–4, discusses the long-term plan in some detail. The consultant architect, P.G. Stephenson, from Australia, had experience in hospital architecture. The intention was to have a hospital of 400–500 beds, the eventual hospital had 180; Hercus and Bell, pp. 314, 345.

15 Hercus and Bell, pp. 198–200

16 Morrell, pp. 165–6. There were 172 dental students in 1946; Sir John Walsh, obituary in *ODT*, 30 August 2003; Derek Dow, 'Hercus, Charles Edward', DNZB 4; Obituary in *NZMJ* April 1971, pp. 231–4.

17 Morrell, pp. 159, 164; Report of Dr Hercus on Physical Education, 12 February 1940, Committee Reports, 1939–1941.

18 Obituary in *NZMJ* April 1971, p. 232; Hercus and Bell, pp. 259–60; Morrell, p. 168; Annual Report, Department of Preventive Medicine, 1946.

19 Hercus and Bell, p. 260.

20 Morrell, p. 173. Construction of the new student union building did not commence until 1958; p. 187.

21 Medical School Annual Report, 1958 (OMS). The Report also included material relating to the year's activities, such as visitors to the School, staff changes and lists of scholarship and prize winners. Attached to it were a sheaf of annual reports, many of them much longer than the Dean's six and a half pages, from the departments of Physiology, Biochemistry, Microbiology, Medicine including Thoracic, Ear, Nose and Throat, Obstetrics and Gynaecology and Preventive and Social Medicine, the Library, the Photographer and Artist, the Animal Department and the Postgraduate Committee.

PART IV

The Medical School in a Changing Environment, 1959-1981

CHAPTER 17

From Crisis to Christie, 1959–69

1   Obituary, Sir Charles Hercus, *NZMJ* 73, April 1971, p. 233.
2   Minutes of Medical Faculty, 31 May 1957; C.E. Hercus, 'The Future of the Deanship', Sir Charles himself was an elected member of the University Council.
3   Minutes of Medical Faculty, 20 September 1957, Special Faculty on the Future of the Deanship; Miles, 'Memorandum on Easing the Burden of the Office of Dean of the Medical School'. Submissions, Bell, Borrie; Submission, Fastier, Ironside, R.D. Batt, Brock, 'A Case for the Status Quo in Electing a Dean'; Submission, Morris Watt.
4   Medical Faculty, 28 February 1958. A precis of faculty deliberations on the deanship between September 1957 and March 1958, which summarised the divergent views, gave credit to the detailed work of the Smirk committee in achieving this unanimity. Faculty, 26 March 1958.
5   Sir Edward Sayers, Obituary, *NZMJ* 12 June 1985, p. 458; Soper, cited in 'Auckland Physician New Medical Dean', *ODT*, 13 March 1958. In Faculty, on 10 September 1958, Smirk gave notice of motion that Dr Sayers, the incoming Dean of the Otago Medical School, be appointed Professor of Therapeutics. This was hastily amended that Senate be requested to establish a Chair of Therapeutics.
6   J.D. Hunter, interview with D. Page; Annual Reports, Faculty of Medicine, 1959, 1960; Faculty of Medicine Minutes, 1960–9; All students had four half-terms in medicine and surgery and one half-term each in psychological medicine, paediatrics, neurosurgery clinical work and preventive and social medicine. Hunter, Compendium, p. 18; Annual Report, 1963.
7   Annual Report, Faculty of Medicine, 1959; Annual Report, Department of Medicine, 1959.
8   Hunter, 'Of Deans and their Deeds', *Alumnus Association Newsletter 1999/2000*, p. 10.
9   Annual Report, 1963.
10 J. Hunter, interview with D. Page; Annual Reports, Faculty of Medicine, 1962, 1963; Graeme C. Smith, Obituary, Wallace Ironside MB ChB, DipPsyMed, FAPsyA, FRANZCP, FRCPsych, FRACP, *Australian Health Review: Medical Journal of Australia*, 17 June 2002, 176 (12), p. 593.
11 Interview James and Marion Robinson, 19 July 2001; Professor C.W. Dixon, Valedictory Minute, Faculty of Medicine, Dunedin Division, 6 December 1976;

Department of Preventive and Social Medicine, Annual Report, 1959. Dixon had served as Medical Officer of Health in Whangarei.
12 Annual Reports, Faculty of Medicine, 1960, 1961, 1962, 1963.
13 Obituary, Sir Edward Sayers, *NZMJ* vol. 98, 1985, pp. 458–9; A.W. Beasley, 'Sayers, Edward George. 1902–1985', DNZB 5, pp. 460–1.
14 Hugh Parton, *The University of New Zealand*, pp. 218–9. In addition to enjoying a distinguished academic career spanning thirty years in the London School of Economics, Sir David Hughes Parry was widely experienced at the highest level in academic government, including terms as Vice-Chancellor and member of the British University Grants Committee; John Gould, *The University Grants Committee, 1961–1986: a History*.
15 Parton, p. 234; Gould, p. 10.
16 Morrell, p. 224. The comment seems to have rankled with both Gould, p. 236, and Parton, p. 248, each of whom quotes Morrell to illustrate university resentment of the UGC. Gould considers Otago's view to be not fully representative. Parton comments, 'The opinion that if autonomy is not absolute it is not autonomy at all dies as hard in academic circles as elsewhere.'
17 Gould, pp. 13–14, 16. The search for a chairman began about May 1960 and, by July, Llewellyn was known to have been selected, probably on the recommendation of the Parry committee. Born in 1915 and educated at the University of Birmingham, he lectured at Birkbeck College during World War II and came to Auckland as Professor of Chemistry in 1947. He was Vice-Chancellor at Canterbury from 1956–61. Parton, p. 158.
18 Chairman UGC to Vice-Chancellor, 18 December 1962, Otago University correspondence, Grants Committee file. In 1925, the Reichel Tate Commission recommended separate funding for the special schools.
19 Morrell, p. 226. Note on meetings of UGC with representatives of the University of Otago, 13–15 November 1963.
20 Morrell, p. 227; Ryburn to Llewellyn, 28 October 1964.
21 Morrell, pp. 227–8; Robin Williams to J.D. Hunter, 1998.
22 Williams to Hunter, 1998.
23 Gould, p. 237; Otago University Report to the Minister of Education, 1965, AJHR 1965, vol. II, E 1, Higher Education, p. 345.
24 Morrell, pp. 236–7.
25 J.D. Hunter, 'Of Deans and their Deeds', pp. 10–11; Williams to Hunter, 1998.
26 Llewellyn returned to the UK as Vice-Chancellor of the University of Exeter. Parton, p. 258; Danks had been on the UGC since 1960. Gould, p. 243.
27 Beacham, cited in Morrell, p. 234. Otago's grant

had increased by 62 per cent, compared with a 95 per cent increase for the other metropolitan universities.

28 Williams to Hunter, 1998; Morrell, p. 234; In his 1965 report to the Minister of Education Beacham queried whether quinquennial grants were suited to a country with so brittle an economy as New Zealand and whether the secrecy surrounding them was helpful. 'One of the causes of our present troubles may be that we have adopted a method of university financing and control better suited to the Britain of yesterday than the New Zealand of today.' Otago University Annual Report to Minister of Education, 1965, p. 2, AJHR 1965, E 1.

29 G. Petersen, 'Biochemistry', in E. Nye ed., *Medical Research in Otago, 1922–1997*, p. 29. Petersen says that the intention, apparently driven by a lobby in the University outside the Medical School, was to separate the department's teaching of Science students from its teaching of medical students. Biochemistry would teach Science students and second year medical students in a stand alone building and Clinical Biochemistry would remain on the Medical School campus and teach third year medical students; Hunter, 'Deans and their Deeds', p. 11; Compendium.

30 J.D. Hunter, interview with D. Page.

31 *ODT*, 29 September 1966.

32 *ODT*, 30 September 1966.

33 Williams to Hunter, 1998. Williams also discussed the idea with Christie's colleague David Bates.

34 *NZMJ* October 1967, p. 696.

35 Editorial, 'Medical Education,' *NZMJ*, October 1967, pp. 689–90.

36 E. Sayers, *NZMJ*, November 1967, pp. 821–4.

37 *NZMJ*, November 1967; North, p. 824; Irvine, pp. 824–5.

38 Editorial, 'Medical School Future', *ODT*, 19 September 1967.

39 *NZMJ*, December 1967, p. 887. At this stage, it was expected that Christie would arrive on 14 January and work through until the end of March, presenting his report to the University of Otago two weeks before he left the country.

40 A. Clarke, interview with D. Page, George Rolleston was the Sub-Dean of the Christchurch Branch Faculty.

41 Editorial, *Digest*, 1960, p. 5. The editor was Geoffrey Clarke; E.G. Sayers, 'Medical Education in the United States', *Digest*, 1960, pp. 6–10; J.E. Caughey, 'Medicine in a Changing World', pp. 11–18, and H.E.W. Robertson, 'The Changing Status of the GP and his Education, pp. 27–30, also address aspects of medical education; John Hunter, 'Any Questions?' *Digest*, 1960, pp. 39–40.

42 Editorial. *Digest*, 1961, pp. 5–10; Comment, *Digest*, 1962, p. 5; C.W. Dixon, 'Vocational Choice in Medical Education', *Digest*, 1965, pp. 11–18;

Students' Report, Medical Education Section, *Digest* 1967, pp. 19–36. In the clinical course, medicine and surgery were criticised as being little better than 'miniature lectures, plus a patient'. Psychiatry came out better, and it was thought pathology needed more time. Obstetrics and gynaecology lectures were considered amusing and the Queen Mary weeks enjoyable. Pharmacology is said to have allowed students to gain their own knowledge.

43 W.D. Trotter, 'The Selection of Students and the Pre-clinical Curriculum', Digest, 1967, pp. 37–41. The selection process gave preferential entry to Scholarship holders, so long as they passed Intermediate, and it allowed some flexibility in the choice of first year subjects, to students who had achieved very high grades in the key sciences at school; Dr Howie, 'Tilting at a Windmill', *Digest*, 1967, pp. 47–8; Dr Emery, 'Medical Education – Whither Otago?', *Digest*, 1967, pp. 60–3; G. Fraenkel, 'Some Problems of Medical Education at Otago', *Digest*, 1967, pp. 43–6. Professor Fraenkel maintained that his own area, surgery, should be postgraduate only.

44 Information from Douglass Taylor, 2 May 2007. The committee consisted of Douglass Taylor (convener), Alan Clarke, Robin Irvine, Merv Smith, Bill Trotter, and coopted members Ted Hawkhead (the University Liaison Officer) and Jim Gwynne. The committee began work in July and made its preliminary report before Christmas.

45 Christie Report, p. 3

46 Christie Report, p. 8.

47 Christie Report, pp. 11–13. Christie referred to evidence of the Royal College of London before the CMG on final examinations.

48 Christie Report, pp. 13–14. Christie believed that at least five full-time physicians and five registrars were needed urgently, even if the student intake was reduced to sixty.

49 Christie report, pp. 15–17.

50 R.V. Christie, MBChB, Edin., DSc Dub. and London, M.S. *Report on the Medical School*, University of Otago, Dunedin , 1968.

51 Williams to Hunter, 1998; J.D. Hunter, 'The Otago Medical School Revisited', *NZMJ*, 1998, p. 272.

52 'Report on the Otago Medical School', *NZMJ*, May 1968, pp. 559–66.

53 Editorial, 'Medical Education in Crisis', *NZMJ*, May 1968, pp. 558–9.

54 Editorial, *Digest*, 1968, p. 6. The editor was A.H. Townsend. OUMSA had already produced an informal supplement on medical education in 1968 (Medical School).

55 'Medical School's Future in Jeopardy', and 'Start to Talks on Medical School', *ODT*, 3 May 1968; *ODT*, interview with Dr Williams, 25 May 1968.

56 K. Eunson, 'Caginess Greets Christie report', *ODT*, 4 May 1968; 'Pressure Necessary in Medical Cause',

ODT, 27 May 1968; 'Christie Report Assured of urgent Treatment', ODT, 4 July 1968. Mr Kinsella, Minister of Education, was responding to an Opposition question.

57 'Extra $100,000 for Medical School', ODT, 26 October 1968; ODT, 13 December 1968, model of the new library.

58 J.D. Hunter, 'The Otago Medical School Revisited', NZMJ, July 1998, pp. 272–3; Williams to Hunter, 1998.

59 Williams to Hunter, 1998; 'University Future Depends on Facilities it Provides', ODT, 3 October 1967. In the late 1960s, the University achieved a new library and Arts block and the conversion of the Clock Tower building to house the Registry.

60 Hunter in NZMJ 1998; Angus, pp. 169, 217–9. The Joint Relations Committee dated from 1926. It was made up of two representatives from each of the Hospital Board and the University Council, plus the Dean of the Medical School and the Hospital Superintendent. Harry Gibson was Chairman of the Hospital Board at the time of the Christie review. The University representatives were Professor Bill Adams, Dr Robin Irvine, Dr Jock Hayward, Dr Robin Williams and Mr W. Hilliker; Irvine Report, p. 2.

61 R.O.H. Irvine, 'The Future of the Medical School. A Report on the Future of the Medical School, with Particular Reference to the Implementation of Proposals made in the Christie Report', typescript letter to Vice-Chancellor, 1 May 1969.

62 Irvine Report, pp. 1–3. The main curriculum changes were: statistics and behavioural sciences were introduced into the second and third years of the course. Most of the teaching of anatomy was now at second year and the second-year examination covered anatomy, physiology (including statistics) and biochemistry. Third year comprised a course based on a combined physiological, anatomical, and clinical approach to teaching of the central nervous system and a course in human behaviour, comprising human growth and development, introductory psychology and introductory psychological medicine. Applied physiology would be taught in relation to a course in general pathology and microbiology. There would be clinical demonstrations throughout the year. Departments allocated one new staff member were biochemistry, pharmacology, pharmacy, psychological medicine, paediatrics and child health, obstetrics and gynaecology, preventive and social medicine, clinical biochemistry.

63 Irvine Report, pp. 3–6.

64 C.A. Gibson, 'Irvine, Robin Orlando Hamilton, 1929–1996', Southern People, p. 247; 'Sir Robin Orlando Hamilton Irvine', Alumnus Bulletin, 1993–4, p. 6.

65 Irvine Report, pp. 7–19.

CHAPTER 18

Building a 'Three-Legged Stool': The Christchurch and Wellington Schools

1 J. Hunter, 'The Otago Medical School Revisited', NZMJ, July 1998, p. 272.

2 Michael King, The Penguin History of New Zealand, p. 463.

3 Obituary, William Adams, NZMJ vol. 77, June 1973, pp. 406–9. Several former colleagues contributed to this warm tribute; J.D. Hunter, 'Deans and their Deeds', Alumnus Association Newsletter, 1999/2000, pp. 12–14; Valedictory Minute, Faculty of Medicine, 1 June 1973. Hercus and Bell, pp. 228, 230.

4 Hunter, Compendium, pp. 11–13; Calendars, University of Otago, 1968–76.

5 Irvine Report, pp. 4–5. The fifth year exam was to include medicine, surgery, obstetrics and gynaecology, paediatrics, psychological medicine, pathology, microbiology, clinical pharmacology, and preventive and social medicine.

6 Hunter, p. 19; O'Donnell, information.

7 P. Hutchison, 'Medical Education at Otago', Digest, 1969, p. 25; G.J. Fraenkel, 'Thoughts on the Medical School at Otago', Digest, 1970, pp. 66–7. In a private letter to John Hunter years later, Fraenkel wrote that the decision to increase student numbers was a 'prescription for disaster' and one of his reasons for leaving Otago. Fraenkel to Hunter, 31 July 1991, Hunter papers; Editorial, 'Medical Student or Schoolboy?', Digest, 1971, p. 5. The editors were S. Rowley and R. Somervile.

8 Professor R.O.H. Irvine, Clinical Dean, 'Trends in Medical Education', Digest, 1972, pp. 27–30. Other contributors on the theme included Professor W.D. Trotter, 'Preclinical curriculum: an evaluation', p. 31, Professor J. Blennerhassett. 'Clinical Science', pp. 32–3, Professor A.M. Clarke, 'Clinical Teaching', pp. 34–8; Professor J. Loewenthal (Sydney), 'The Crisis in Medical Education', pp. 47–8 and Don McIver, 'Teaching Teaching', p. 43.

9 Editorial, ODT 27 December 1971, claimed the OHB had been working towards the Heart Surgery Unit for twenty years; Throughout August there was extensive press coverage, notably: 'Will both Dunedin and Christchurch Go Ahead?', ODT 24 August 1972; 'Otago Presents Case for Next Heart Unit', ODT 29 August 1972; G. Parry, My Dunedin, pp. 81–2. Parry, who would take up a position the next year as Assistant Registrar (Information) at the University, describes his own role in setting the campaign in motion and his close collaboration with John Hunter, meeting every couple of days to 'manufacture bullets for the Hospital Board to fire, or to prepare arguments in rebuttal of the Canterbury claims'. Doubtless party politics played their part. Holyoake was no longer Prime Minister, having stepped down early in 1972 in favour of John

Marshall. The National party would not have wanted to alienate its strong support base in Christchurch with an election due in November – which Labour won. David Hay, *Heart Sounds*, p. 100; 'Cardiac Unit Given Go Ahead', *ODT* 3 November 1972; 'Prof. Pat Molloy Appointed Director', *ODT* 11 November 1972; 'Open Heart Surgical Unit Ready', *ODT*, 28 June 1973.

[10] 'Child Psychiatry Pioneer Killed', *ODT* 2 February 1974. The Lewis family were part of a group of eight Otago people among the 16 New Zealanders killed in the accident.

[11] 'Distress at Loss of Paediatrician', *Evening Star*, 6 August 1973; 'Resignation Withdrawn', *ODT* 22 November 1973; 'Taking Maternity Beds Last Straw', *Evening Star* 27, November 1974; 'Resignation of Dr Malcolm regretted', *Evening Star*, 29 November 1974; 'Dr Malcolm's Resignation Accepted with Regret', *ODT* 29 November 1974; Various Letters to the Editor, *Evening Star*, 'Paediatrics', 3 December 1974.

[12] 'Successor named to Present Dean', *Evening Star*, 5 November 1970

[13] 'Key Education Post University to Lose Vice-Chancellor', *ODT* 4 July 1971; *ODT* 7 November 1971; *NZMJ* April 1973, p. 262. The assistant deans were Professor J. Watt, clinical affairs, Dr R. Medlicott, postgraduate affairs, Dr D.W. Taylor curriculum and students affairs.

[14] J. Hunter, interview with D. Page.

[15] Sayers report, 1959 and 1963. In 1963, he did express his pleasure at the Wellcome building and the conversion of the old dental school for pharmacy and pharmacology; A. Beacham, Annual Report, University of Otago, 1964. In 1965, the University gained a new library/arts building which enabled the conversion of the clock tower building to administration, but there was nothing of direct benefit to the Medical School.

[16] Irvine, pp. 10–11.

[17] Gould, p. 105; p. 87, pp. 88–91; *ODT*, 'University Halt', 2 July 1977.

[18] 'The Dunedin Hospital Ward Block with its Medical School Facilities', booklet to commemorate the opening, Dunedin 1980.

[19] Booklet to commemorate the opening of the Dunedin Hospital Ward Block, 1980.

[20] Bates Report, p. 2.

[21] Christopher Moore, George Rolleston, John Riminton, Andrew Hornblow, *A Vision Realised. Christchurch School of Medicine, University of Otago, 1972–1997*, pp. 1–4. Chapters 2 and 3 of this history provide a more detailed account of the origins of the Christchurch School. The first Christchurch Sub-Dean was the Medical Superintendent, Dr A.D. Nelson (1937–1950), followed by Dr M.K. Gray (1950–58) and Dr J.F. Landreth (1958–62).

[22] Moore et al., pp. 5–7.

[23] Moore et al., pp. 9–12; Faculty Minutes, 7 August 1968.

[24] 'The Christchurch Clinical School', *NZMJ* October, 1973, pp. 316–8. Moore et al., pp. 14–15.

[25] Moore et al, pp. 14–15. The working party, consisting of Rolleston, Shannon, Beaven and Cotter, worked with the sub-dean and clinical dean Robin Irvine, to produce the report; pp. 15–16, 18–21. Riminton had developed his administrative and diplomatic skills as manager of a Sri Lankan tea estate.

[26] Moore et al., pp. 22, 24.

[27] 'News from Divisions: Canterbury', *NZMJ* September 1971, p. 203; 'News from Divisions: Canterbury', *NZMJ* December 1971, p. 405; Moore et al., pp. 30–1; 'Aickin, Professor Donald Russell', *New Zealand Who's Who Aotearoa*, p. 10; Obituary, 'Frederick Thomas Shannon', *NZMJ* vol. 112, 1999, pp. 390–1; Valedictory Minute, Christchurch Staff Assembly, 1990.

[28] 'News from Divisions: Canterbury', *NZMJ* September 1971, p. 203; Helen Angus, Obituary, Roy McGiven, *NZMJ* vol. 100, 1987, pp. 509–10.

[29] Moore et al, pp. 29–32; p. 113.

[30] 'The Christchurch Clinical School', *NZMJ* 10 October 1973, pp. 316–18. Speakers at the opening were Dr Leslie Averill, Chairman of the North Canterbury Hospital Board and the Christchurch Clinical School Council, the very Rev. Dr J.S. Somerville, Pro-Chancellor, University of Otago, the Rt Honourable Mr Norman Kirk, Prime Minister and the Dean of the Christchurch Clinical School, Professor George Rolleston; Moore et al, p. 33.

[31] Obituary, George Rolleston, *NZMJ* vol. 114, 2001, p. 533; Christchurch *Press* August 2001; Moore et al, Ch. 3 'Setting the Course'.

[32] T.V. O'Donnell, 'A University Department of Medicine in Wellington', *NZMJ* February 1975, p. 142. O'Donnell cites Hercus to WHB, 1937.

[33] O'Donnell, p. 142; Hercus and Bell, pp. 128–30; Jo Mercer was Sub-Dean until 1962, when he was succeeded by John Keeling (1963–1965) and Guy Hallwright (1966–1972); Rachel Barrowman, *Victoria University of Wellington, 1899–1999: A History*, p. 191.

[34] B.M. Corkill, 'The Wellington School of Medicine – Origins', undated typescript, p. 4. Hunter Collection, HL; T.V. O'Donnell, 'A University Department of Medicine in Wellington', *NZMJ* February 1975, p. 142. J. Hunter, 'The "Branch Faculties" (1938–1972)', in Compendium, p. 35.,Corkill and O'Donnell date the Wellington Medical Unit from 1959. Dr Prior left to head a new Epidemiology Unit; Ian Prior, *Elespie and Ian: Memoir of a Marriage*, Ch. 6, 'Medicine', pp. 100–18, passim. Prior says the unit had 15 beds, p. 103.

[35] Mercer to WHB, 8 November 1965, in Corkill. The letter was considered briefly at the November meeting of the Board and in more detail at its

meeting on 9 December 1965.

36 Corkill, pp. 6– 10.

37 Corkill, pp. 10–11; 'Government delays New Medical School', *ODT* 21 February 1973, notes that a third medical school had been a 'principal plank' of Labour's election manifesto the previous year.

38 Irvine Report, p. 12; Corkill, pp. 10–12.

39 Corkill, pp. 14–16; Barrowman, p. 192.

40 *ODT* 28 July 1970; *ODT* 1 December 1970, *Evening Star* 1 December 1970; *ODT* 13 February 1971.

41 *ODT* 5 March 1971; *ODT* 8 March 1971.The Minister Hon Brian Talboys suggested a School for 130 students would cost about $12 million. North said this was too high.

42 *ODT* 1 September 1970; *ODT* 15 September 1970; Professor Sir Charles Illingworth, *ODT*, 5 March 1971; Articles on the Hospital plans include *Evening Star* 1 April 1971, 'Plans Approved', and 'Modern Medical Complex Should be Ready in 1977'; *ODT* 3 April 1971, 'Immediate Action on Medical Block'.

43 'Dean of clinical school Announced', *Evening Star*, 1 October 1971; *NZMJ* March 1977, p. 241.

44 Corkill, p. 16; Obituary, Graham Francis Hall, *NZMJ* July 1979, pp. 27–8.

45 Obituary, Graham Francis Hall, *NZMJ* 11 July 1979, pp. 27–8; *NZMJ* October 1971, 'Wellington', p. 270; *Evening Star* 1 October 1971, 'Dean of Clinical School Announced'; Corkill, 'Origins of Wellington Clinical School'; O'Donnell, 'Collated material of interest during the development of the Wellington Clinical School, 1971–January 1992.'

46 'News from Divisions: Wellington', *NZMJ* 23 March 1977, p. 241; Corkill, pp. 16. The architects selected were the Auckland firm, Cutter and Pickner. The Board's former architects threatened to sue. The firm employed in Dunedin, Stephenson and Turner, was not acceptable because of disputes dating back to the 1930s.

47 Peter Holst to D. Page, 2006; Interview, T. O'Donnell with D. Page, 2003; T.V. O'Donnell, 'Founding Dean and Initial Heads of Departments', Thomas V. O'Donnell, B Med Sc (NZ) 1946, MB ChB (NZ) 1949, MD (NZ) 1959, FRACP 1963, FRCP (Lond) 1972, Historical Note, Wellington School of Medicine and Health Sciences.

48 O'Donnell, William E Stehbens, MBBS (Syd) 1951, MD (Syd) 1962, D Phil (Ox0n) 1969, FRACP 1961, FRC Path. 1961, Historical Note; Stehbens, Professor William Ellis, MBBS, MD, DPhil, FRCPA, FACPath, *New Zealand Who's Who Aotearoa*, p. 624. Stehben's Chair was funded half by the Wellington Hospital Board and a quarter each by the University and the Wellington Division of the Cancer Society, now the Malaghan Institute for Medical Research. Public fundraising had been undertaken for the Institute prior to the planning of the School.

49 O'Donnell, Richard J. Seddon, MB ChB (NZ) 1954, MRCOG (1961) F (1972), FRNZCOG 1982, FRACOG 1989; Jeffray Weston, ED 1972, MB ChB, 1950, FRCP(Lond) 1974, FRACP 1967, DCG 1957;William H. Isbister, MB ChB (Manc) 1958, MD (Manc) 1964, FRCS (Edin) 1966, FRCS 1975; F. John Roberts, MBBS (Lond) 1956, DPH (Durham) 1960, MD (Bristol) 1974, MRCP (Edin) FRC Psych 1979, FRACP 1978, FRANZCP 1979; Kenneth W. Newell, MB ChB (NZ) 1948, DPH (Lond) Ph D (Tulane), Historical Note.

50 Thomas V. O'Donnell, 'The Development of the Wellington School of Medicine, A Personal View', typescript, Hunter Collection. HC. pp. 2–7. Peter Holst joined the department as senior lecturer, and future Dean Eru Pomare also joined at this time. T.V. O'Donnell, ed., 'Collated Material of Interest during the Development of the Wellington Clinical School, later Wellington Clinical School of Medicine, subsequently Wellington School of Medicine of the University of Otago' (hereafter 'Collated Material'), pp. 2, 4. Hospital Board members of the School Council included two members elected by the Board's senior clinical staff. In May 1976, its constitution was amended to allow for the addition of two academic staff (initially O'Donnell and Roberts) and the Vice-Chancellor of Victoria University.

51 O'Donnell, 'Development of the Wellington School,' pp. 3–5; T.V O'Donnell ed., 'Collated Material', pp. 1–10 passim. In October 1975, a joint sub-committee of Council was set up to investigate problems between the Clinical Department of Pathology and the Hospital Laboratory Services, p. 3. Two resignations (Drs Steele and Thomson) from pathology were recorded in August 1977, p. 10; Medicine benefited by being established in the area previously occupied by the University Medical Unit.

CHAPTER 19

Interlude: A Year to Celebrate, 1975

1 G. Parry, *Otago Medical School, 1875–1975. An Historical Sketch.*

2 J. Hunter, Foreword, in G. Parry, *Otago Medical School, 1875–1975. An Historical Sketch.* The 4623rd student was a woman, who graduated on 13 December 1974.

3 Gordon Parry, 'A Place of Honour after Early Struggle', *ODT* 6 February 1975.

4 *ODT* 17 February 1975.

5 R. Irvine, 'Medical Education in a University Setting', *NZMJ*, 12 February 1975, pp. 130–2.

6 *ODT* 15 February 1975; *Evening Star*, 11 February 1975. Woodruff had been Professor of Surgery between 1953 and 1956, and McIntyre, Professor of Physiology between 1951 and 1961.

7 *ODT* 19 February 1975; *ODT* 22 February 1975.

8 'Medical School's Messages, Gifts', *ODT* 19 February 1975; *ODT* 15 February 1975; *ODT* 17 February 1975; *ODT* 21 February 1975. The first account gives a number of 300 wives in attendance, the second 400; Otago Medical School centenary, 1975, scrapbook, Otago Medical School.

9 'Medical Science at Decisive Point', *ODT* 18 February 1975.

10 What follows is based on Professor E.A. Horsman (English Dept), citations for honorary degrees, Medical School Centenary Assembly, February 1975, typescripts, University Registry. All quotations are from these documents. A small amount of supplementary material comes from the *NZMJ* obituaries and other sources cited below.

11 Obituary, Sir Charles Burns, *NZMJ* vol. 98, 1985, pp. 405–7; A.W. Beasley, 'Burns, Charles Ritchie 1898–1985', DNZB 5, pp. 77–8.

12 K. Ibbertson, Obituary, 'Fraser, Thomas Russell Cumming', in Sarah Jane Gillies and Ian Mc Donald eds., *Lives of the Fellows of the Royal College of Physicians*.

13 Obituary, Sir John Stallworthy, *NZMJ* vol. 107, 1994, p. 23.

14 Obituary, Stanley Wilson, *NZMJ* vol. 103, 1990, pp. 332–3; John Heslop, 'Surgery in Dunedin, 1925–1957', in Alumnus Association Newsletter, 2000/01, pp. 46–8.

15 Editorial, 'Medical Education: Essays for the Otago Medical School Centenary 1875–1975', *NZMJ* vol. 81, 12 February 1975.

16 R.O.H. Irvine, 'Medical Education in a University Setting', pp. 130–2; R. Aickin, 'The Making of an Obstetrician', pp. 92–5; D. Beaven, J.S. Dodge, J.A. Kilpatrick, G.F.S. Spears, 'Education and Diabetes: Attitudes, Opinion and Needs of New Zealand Doctors', pp. 95–100; F. Shannon, 'Paediatric Teaching in Retrospect and Prospect', pp. 168–71. Also from Christchurch, E.A. Espiner, Associate Professor in the Medical Unit at Princess Margaret Hospital, contributed 'Clinical Departments and Medical Education: a Pivotal Role in Need of Broader Base', pp. 124–6, *NZMJ* 12 February 1975.

17 T.V. O'Donnell, 'A University Department of Medicine in Wellington', pp. 142–6; E.M. Nanson, 'Medical Education 100 Years After', pp. 134–9; J.B. Carman, 'What Did Happen to Anatomy at Auckland? The Teaching of Anatomy in a Fully Integrated Preclinical Course', pp. 108–14; Sir Douglas Robb, 'Medical Education', pp. 154–9. Sir Douglas had died by the time the commemorative issue appeared; J.D.K. North, 'Topic Teaching in Clinical Medicine', pp. 139–41; P.J. Scott, 'The Community Challenge to Medical Education in NZ: Preparation for Partnership or Servant-Master Status?', pp. 163–8; also from Auckland, Professor J.D. Sinclair, Department of Physiology, contributed, 'Physiology in a Human Biology Course for Medical Students', pp. 171–7, *NZMJ* 12 February 1975.

18 N.C. Begg, 'Child Health and Sickness', pp. 100–5; J. Hiddlestone, 'Prospects for Medical Education in New Zealand', pp. 129–30; G. Brinkman, 'Evaluation and Continuing Medical Education', pp. 105–7; R.E. Wright-St Clair, 'The Historical Background to New Zealand Medicine', pp. 181–4; A.M. Clarke, 'The Medical Student and the Problem of Relevance', pp. 114–9, *NZMJ* 12 February 1975.

19 L.W. Cox, 'Trends in Medical Education in Australia', pp. 119–22; J. Ludbrook, 'Medical Schools in the Year 2000: Trade Schools or Centres of Academic Excellence?', pp. 133–4; D. Denny-Brown, 'On Medical Education', pp. 122–4; D.G. Potts, 'Techniques, Structure and System', pp. 146–9. Sir John Stallworthy, 'Gaudeamus', pp. 177–81, all in *NZMJ* 12 February 1975.

20 *NZMJ* July 1973, p. 84; 'Wider Role for Medical Schools', *ODT* 22 May 1975.

21 Otago Medical School Centenary, 1975, scrapbook; *Evening Star* 22 February 1975; Alumnus Association Newsletter, 1976, Hocken MS 1537 773; Alumnus Association Newsletters, 1976–98.

22 'Otago Medical School Alumnus Association'. 1985. The writer gave Brinkman the credit for these initiatives. The afternoon tea was arranged by Dr Sneyd and a group of volunteers.

23 Interview with Hunter, 'Open day at Medical School. First time in fifteen years', *ODT* 29 November 1975; 'Keeping up with constant change', *Evening Star*, 29 November 1975; Medical School Open Day, public notice, *ODT* 4 December 1975; Report and picture of Prof. Alan Clarke showing Sir John and Lady Walsh modern equipment used in experimental animal surgery, *ODT* 5 December 1875; 'Visitors Fascinated', with picture of two young high school boys inspecting display of the latest electron scanning microscope, *Evening Star*, 5 December 1975.

24 F.O. Simpson, 'Medicine: Hypertension and Related Subjects', in Nye ed., *Medical Research in Otago 1922–1997*, pp. 99–100; F.O. Simpson et al, 'The Milton Survey: Part 1. General Methods, Height, Weight and 24 Hour Excretion of Sodium, Potassium, Calcium, Magnesium and Creatinine', *NZMJ* vol. 87, June 1978, pp. 379–82; 'Medical Survey in Milton – a Multi-purpose Survey', *ODT* 4 May 1975; '1000 Participating in Medical Survey', *ODT* 9 May 1975; 'Milton Survey Unique', *Evening Star*, 28 July 1975.

25 R. Laverty, Convener, Staff Centennial Celebrations Committee, 'To present and past staff', OMS Centenary scrapbook; Report in *NZMJ* 24 December 1975, p. 429.

26 Alumnus Association Newsletter, 1976. Richard Acland's grandfather was Christchurch surgeon Sir Hugh Acland.

CHAPTER 20

Times of Tension, 1975–1981

1 Gould, pp. 232–3. The 1965 proposal was for a large increase in funding. Treasury queried the 1970 proposal and suggested a lower overall figure, but did not press the point; Information, T O'Donnell.

2 J. Hunter, interview with D. Page; J. Clayton, *Anaesthesia at Dunedin Hospital*, pp. 111–2. Baker stayed seventeen years, before leaving to become Nuffield Professor of Anaesthetics in the University of Sydney. Information on John Parr Prize in Ophthalmology, Dunedin School of Medicine. Parr's textbook, *Introduction to Ophthalmology*, is still used. He contributed substantially to the planning of the new Dunedin Hospital.

3 G. Brinkman, interview with D. Page, 13/8/03. It was not only Dunedin that was affected. Tom O'Donnell points out that the University was not funding registrar posts at Christchurch or Wellington either.

4 J. Hunter, Compendium p. 14; *New Zealand Who's Who Aotearoa*, Heap, Professor Stuart Westbourne MBBS, FRACR, FRCR, p. 292. Heap moved to Auckland in 1986; Skegg, Professor David Christopher Graham, OBE, NZ 1990 medal, BMedSc, MB ChB, DPhil, MCCMNZ, FRSNZ, p. 605; Faculty Board Minutes, 11 December 1980; 2 September 1981.

5 The original decision in favour of maintaining full neurological services in Dunedin was taken on the advice of a meeting of the Hospital Advisory Council's subcommittee on neurosurgery, chaired by Sir Randal Elliott, with representatives of the OHB, the North Canterbury Hospital Board, the Otago Medical School and the Christchurch Clinical School, on 15 November 1977. The recommendation was for two specialist neurologists in Dunedin and one in Christchurch, to work in collaboration. Major articles in the *ODT* were, for example, 'Dirty Politics Accusation', 31 January 1980; '"No Scanner" Decision Stuns Otago People', 13 February 1980; 'Loss of Unit "Dreadful"', 15 February 1980 and editorials, on 13, 15 and 16 February; Minutes of a Meeting of the Executive of the General Medical Staff, attended by OHB Chair Mrs Dorothy Fraser, 20 February 1980; Minutes of the Special meeting of the General Medical Staff of the Dunedin Hospital, 27 February 1980; Minister of Health, Mr G.F. Gair, claimed that medical students would not be hurt by the scanner decision. Submission to the Rt Hon R.D. Muldoon concerning (I) The Future Role of the Otago Neurosurgical Unit (II) The Acquisition of a Body Scanner by the Otago Hospital Board; Faculty Board Minutes,12 March 1980.

6 'Otago Southland body scanner now in action', *ODT*, 6 August 1981; 'Body scanner in full use', 22 October 1981; Faculty Board Minutes, 11 December 1980, 2 September 1981; Information, Martin Pollock.

7 Moore et al, p. 35.

8 Moore et al, pp. 26–9.

9 Moore et al, pp. 33–5.

10 O'Donnell ed., 'Collated Material', pp. 6–7; Corkill, p. 29.

11 Corkill, p. 27; O'Donnell, ed., 'Collated Material', pp. 7–8; The MRC wrote twice to the School Council, in March and April 1977, referring especially to surgery and pathology. Stehbens wrote to Johnson personally and the Professors of Psychological Medicine, Surgery and Pathology wrote to the Council.

12 A.W. Beasley, Obituary, Ralph Hudson Johnson, *NZMJ* vol. 106, 1993, pp. 439–40; *New Zealand Who's Who Aotearoa*, 1996 edition, Obituaries. In Memoriam, 'Johnson, Dr Ralph Hudson', pp. 744–5; Information, Tom O'Donnell, Linda Holloway.

13 O'Donnell, ed., 'Collated Material', pp. 10–11; Barrowman, p. 192.

14 O'Donnell ed., 'Collated material', p. 13; Permanent accommodation for Psychological Medicine was blocked by an owner's refusal to move from a house in the location of a proposed extension to the Psychiatric ward. Senior lecturer Paul Davidson was made acting Head of the Department, on Roberts' departure; P. Holst to D. Page, 7 July 2006; D.R., 'Wellington Clinical School Report', *Digest*, 1978, p. 8. The marae visit was organised by Dr Ian Prior, 'Collated Material', p. 8; 'Wellington', *NZMJ* 26 December 1979, p. 512; O'Donnell, 'Collated Material', p. 17. The Board was responding to a submission by the Vice-Chancellor to the Department of Health, on 30 April 1981, requesting representation from each Clinical School to the relevant Hospital Board; 'Intake of Medical Students Cut', *NZMJ* 26 September 1979, p. 259.

15 J. Hunter, 'The Future of the Medical School (Dunedin Division)', pp. 1–2. The document was discussed on 5 December 1977; 'A Basis for Medical Manpower Cuts', *NZMJ* 27 June 1979, pp. 480–1.The Department of Health's advisory committee was made up almost entirely of representatives of various sections of the medical profession. The recommended 25 per cent cut in student intake was a relatively gentle solution to the problem of medical oversupply. Another scenario combined an immediate 25 per cent cut, with a further reduction of 20 entrants in 1982 and restricted the immigration of doctors to 50 a year. This, it was claimed, would still provide more than 400 doctors beyond what the current 2 per cent growth factor suggested was affordable. p. 480.

16 Geoffrey Brinkman, 'Planning for the Future', 1978 (prepared in conjunction with an ad hoc advisory committee). This document was discussed in Faculty on 8 June 1978; University of Otago Report, 1980, AJHR.

17 David Bates, 'Report on the University of Otago Medical School', 28 October 1981, pp. 1–4.

18 Bates, pp. 5–12, passim; Emeritus Professor J.D. Hunter, Honorary Archivist to the Faculty, 'Annual Report', 1997; Alumnus Association Newsletter, 1997/8, p. 2.

CHAPTER 21

Student Life: A Change of Direction

1 OUMSA Minute Books and Annual Reports, 1956–1972; For the 1958 ball, OUMSA Exec., 7/4/58; Drinking Horn, President's Annual Report 1960; farewell to Prof. Schofield, President's Report, 1961.

2 OUMSA Minute Books and Annual Reports, 1956–72; President's Reports 1960–1970; Secretary's Reports, 1961 1963, 1964.

3 OUMSA Secretary's Report 1961, President's Report, 1962, 1968. Jim Tull, the OUMSA Treasurer, had the idea of taking over the medical book exchange and persuaded the Executive to move from requesting a modest £300 for renovations to a much higher figure. The renovations began over the 1961–2 vacation. Secretary's Report, 1961; Secretary's Report, 1966.

4 Roger Wilson, 'Introversion amongst Medical Students', *Digest* 1975, p. 29.

5 Elworthy, pp. 96, 108, 114–21. In 1968, the OUSA had complained to the Governor General Lord Porritt, himself a former OUSA vice-president (1923), about the proposed regulations.

6 The sole medical student president was Ayesha Verrall, 2001; Elworthy, Ch. 4, 1964–90, 'Our model society has cracked at the seams', pp. 97–138 passim; The President's honorarium is currently $20,000 and students take a year out to fill the position. OUSA office, 2006.

7 Special general meeting, 28/6/68, OUMSA Minutes and Annual Reports, 1960–72. Five further motions expressed approval of specific parts of the Christie report, urging improvements in the 'grossly inadequate' teaching facilities and staff/student ratio, improvement in the patient/clinical student ratio and strongly supporting the concept of a second clinical school. A further general meeting, on 5/7/68, endorsed these views; Special general meetings re white coats, 4/8/65, 9/5/66 and 14/7/67. At another special general meeting on 17/4/67, the Executive reported on steps it had taken to protest government cuts in allowances to the Otago Hospital Board, and a telegram it had sent to the Minister of Health; Students on faculty, Minutes 3/7/69; Education Committee, Minutes, 2/10/67. The committee had two representatives from each class and four from executive; S. Wilson, 'Student Power at Otago University Medical School', *Digest* 1970, pp. 78–81.

8 W.E. Adams to P.D. Gluckman, 20 July 1970. The canteen was not operational until 1974.

9 P. McGeorge, report on OUSA Union Fees, in OUMSA Minutes 3/10/68. The OUMSA asked for a reduction of $6 for the $21 fee, to put towards rising costs of the canteen, coffee bar and common room; Minutes, 23/5/69, with the OUSA representative present. Relations were better in 1978, when the OUSA paid $8000 to the OUMSA for upgrading the medical canteen.

10 John MacDougall, report to executive, 6/7/72, OUMSA Secretary's file 1970–72.

11 Russell Tregonning, Annual Report 1967. The AMSA began in 1960. In 1968, John Hawk was a delegate to the AMSA Council. Noel Digby, Annual Report 1972; John Chrisp, 'Convention Otago 1975: AMSA in Action', *Digest* 1975, p. 38.

12 A. Neil Graham, 'Quo Vadis NZMSA?', *Digest* 1975, p. 40. Graham states that the NSMSA had joined the International Federation of Medical Students' Associations, the 50th association to do so. If it happened, this evidently lapsed.

13 Bob Smith, 'International Sportsmen', *Digest* 1960. For Gill, see also *Critic*, 30 June 1960, p. 1.

14 OUMSA, Secretary's Report, 1966; 'Dave Gerrard', inductee of Sports Hall of Fame. Gerrard continues to serve on a number of national and international sporting bodies. His contribution to sports administration culminated in his role as chef de mission of the New Zealand team at the 1996 Olympic Games.

15 J.F. Gwynne, 'The Nichol Cup and Medical School Rugby', *Digest*, 1976, pp. 55–6. The Nichol cup had a chequered career. In the 1964 *Digest*, A.J. Aynsford, 'The Rutherford Nichol Cup', wrote that it had been competed for from 1915 to 1928 and, thereafter, only in 1941, 1949, 1951 and 1952, until the competition was resurrected in 1964, p 121. In the 1976 *Digest*, J.F. Gwynne maintained that it had been competed for annually, but sometimes between medical and dental students. Some time after 1976 it seems to have disappeared. The Phys Ed School opened in 1948.

16 Griffiths, pp. 45, 48.

17 Lt. Col. C.P.M. Geary, 'Information Paper on the University Medical Unit', typescript, 1979, p. 3. From 1951 to 1957, camps were held at Sutton, near Middlemarch and, in 1958–9, at Tekapo. 'OUMC Notes', *Digest*, 1966, pp. 79–80; J.D. Adams, 'OUMC Notes', *Digest*, 1967, pp. 121–2. The achievements of the OUMC at the 1967 camp included fielding a rugby team that defeated the regular force team on two occasions and taking out honours in the drinking horn.

18 Lt. Col. C.P.M. Geary, pp. 5–6.

19 'UMU', *Digest* 1977, pp. 39–40.

20 President's Reports, 1971, 1972, 1973–4, 1978; OUMSA Executive Minutes, 15 September 1981;

W.E. Adams to Editor, *Litterhoea*, 15 October 1971; President's Report, 1972–3; OUMSA Executive Minutes 18 September 1979. Early copies of *Borborygmi* are hard to find, but there are a few in the medical library.

PART V

Decades of Challenge and Opportunity, 1980–2000

CHAPTER 22

The 1980s: Economic and Political Pressures

1 'Letter from the Dean', Alumnus Association Bulletin, 1980, pp. 10–12.

2 'Letter from the Dean', Alumnus Association Bulletin, 1982, p. 8.

3 G. Rice, *Oxford History of New Zealand* (2nd edition), p. 485.

4 Interview, G. Brinkman with D. Page; *ODT* December 1985.

5 Philippa Mein Smith, 'Gurr, Eily Elaine, 1896–1996', DNZB 5, pp. 200–1; 'Eily Elaine Gurr 1896–1996', M.D. Maxwell, ed., *Women Doctors in New Zealand: an Historical Perspective, 1921–1986*, pp. 123–6.

6 Dean's Reports, Alumnus Association Bulletins, 1980–85; Skegg, in Campbell et al, interview; Alumnus Association Bulletin 1982, p. 8; 1983, p. 7.

7 'Letter from the Dean', 1982, p. 8; 1983, p. 8.

8 'Report to the Alumnae' (sic), Alumnus Association Bulletin 1984; 'Campbell, Professor (Archibald) John, MD, FRACP', *New Zealand Who's Who Aotearoa*, 1996, p. 103.

9 'Report to the Alumnae', Alumnus Association Bulletin 1985 (pages not numbered).

10 Barrowman, pp. 194–5. The professor was Michael Clinton, from the South-West Thames Regional Health Authority, London. Despite the promising start, the project proved short-lived and foundered in 1993; Brinkman, 'Report to the Alumnae', 1985.

11 O'Donnell timeline, p. 25 and additional information; Barrowman, p. 354; Faculty of Medicine, Valedictory Minute, April 1986.

12 Moore et al, pp. 35–7. Shannon to Hunter, cited by Hunter in a valedictory minute to Professor Shannon at the Christchurch School of Medicine Assembly, 1990. (HC, MS 1537/58).

13 Moore et al, pp. 39–40.

14 J. Hunter, comments on his role as Dean, 20 March 1996, Hunter Collection, Christchurch School of Medicine; Moore et al, pp. 40–3.

15 Faculty paper for meeting 18 July 1985; *Critic*, 16 July 1985, pp. 8–9. The article included other University crises, such as the possible need to restrict entry to second year Law and Commerce because there was not enough money for staff salaries; 'Increased Intake', *ODT* 2 August 1985; 'Doctor Shortage', *ODT* 3 August 1985; Some of Brinkman's former colleagues believed he had been influential in negotiating the increased student intake, but he denied this in interview, Campbell et al, 2001; Brinkman, interview with D. Page.

16 Interview, G. Brinkman with D. Page. Dunedin members predominated on the Faculty Board, the main liaison committee for the three Schools.

17 Brinkman, valedictory minute, Faculty Board, Minutes, 13 December 1985; Brinkman, valedictory minute, Divisional Board Minutes, 12 December 1985.

18 Carmalt Jones, p. 244; Hercus and Bell, pp. 54, 66; *ODT* 10 December 1985; Information, Fred Fastier.

19 Rice, pp. 486–7.

20 Barrowman, pp. 354–5, gives a succinct account of the changes; Information, John Hunter.

21 Otago University Medical Faculty Board Minutes, 9 April 1986; Stewart, in Campbell et al, Interview; Moore et al, p. 44; T.V. O'Donnell, Timeline, April 1985; O'Donnell to Page, 2 May 2007. O'Donnell was initially part of the elected three-person committee, with Eru Pomare and John Hutton, but withdrew when his colleagues informed him that a majority consensus of staff surveyed indicated that Johnson's reappointment was not likely to be recommended and that he was recommended to take over. He had favoured Johnson's reappointment.

22 Stewart in Campbell et al, Interview; Stewart, Interview, 9 June 2006.

23 Moore et al, pp. 45, 47–8. Professor Laurie Geffen and Administrator John Blandford were the Flinders facilitators.

24 Tom O'Donnell, Interview, 18 September 2003. Karen Poutasi was Chief Executive.

25 Hunter, 'News from the Dean of Faculty', Alumnus Association Bulletin, 1986, pp. 4–5.

26 Hunter, Alumnus Association Newsletter, 1989, p. 2

27 Hunter, Information for the Review Committee of the Medical Council of New Zealand, 1988, p 4.

28 Hunter, 1988, p. 37.

29 Otago Faculty of Medicine – Dean's Report, 1990, p. 3.

30 Alumnus Association Bulletin, 2000/01, pp. 23–6.

CHAPTER 23

The 1990s: A Decade of Upheaval and Expansion

1. D. Stewart, interview with D. Page, 22 November 2000.

2. Rice, p. 491; Barrowman, pp. 354–6. That the UGC's $26 million assets were absorbed into the general government accounts was an added grievance.

3. Rice, p. 495; Brandon Adams, president of the OUMSA in 1999, organised a well-supported medical students' fees protest in June of that year. *Enema*, 1999, 'Student Protest'.

4. R. Gauld, 'New Zealand', in R. Gauld, ed., *Comparative Health Policy in the Asia-Pacific*, p. 201.

5. Gauld, *Revolving Doors*, p. 203; Rice, pp. 489, 493.

6. D. Stewart, interview with D. Page, 22 November 2000. Recent examples of the Medical School's success in negotiating non-governmental funding were the gift of the Elaine Gurr Chair in General Practice, in 1983, and the complex financial arrangements put in place to fund a Chair in Biomedical Ethics, 1990.

7. D. Stewart, 'The New Health System in New Zealand', University of Otago Faculty of Medicine, data base for AMC, 1994, pp. 257, 265.

8. 'Medical School costs CHE $1m', *ODT* 19 August 1993; 'Medical School cuts possible', *ODT* 1 March 1994.

9. Accreditation of the Undergraduate Course in Medicine, Faculty of Medicine, University of Otago. Report of the Accreditation Committee, 1994, (Hereafter Accreditation Report, 1994). List of persons interviewed, Appendix 3, pp. 1–9. List of members of committee, Appendix 1. Other members were Dr Adrian Bower, University of Queensland, Prof. Mark Harris, University of New South Wales, Prof. David Healy, Monash University, Prof Ross Kalucy, Flinders University, and Prof. Caroline McMillen, University of Adelaide.

10. Database, 1994, pp. 282, 257, 265, 269–271, 275, 177–8.

11. Accreditation Report, 1994, pp. 6, 54, 56.

12. Annual Reports, 1994, Otago, G. Mortimer, Christchurch, A. Hornblow, Wellington, L. Holloway; Interview, G. Mortimer.

13. Gauld, 'New Zealand', p. 205; Gauld, *Revolving Doors*, pp. 122–3; D. Skegg, 'Health Commission successor needed', *ODT* 28 June 1995.

14. Moore et al, pp. 54–5. Ian Frame was the CEO and Dr Brent Layton, an economist, the Chair of the Board. He went on to chair the Lyttelton Port Company. 'Crisis in Christchurch', *Sunday Star-Times*, 5 April 1998. Dr Robin Stent was the Health and Disability Commissioner; when Jane Parfitt became CEO of Healthlink South, in August 1997,

a spirit of genuine cooperation ensued. Moore et al, p. 56.

15. 'Medical School staff resign', *ODT* 28 April 1996. The other staff were Drs Barrie Berkeley and Alex Dempster. Blennerhassett returned shortly afterwards to work in the Dunedin Hospital Laboratories; 'Another top pathologist to leave Medical School', *ODT* 30 May 1996; 'Professor fires parting salvo', *ODT* 26 June 1996.

16. 'University and CHE differ over joint staff', *ODT* 22 April 1997. The salary increase had been negotiated in 1996 by the Association of Salaried Medical Specialists.

17. 'Unhealthy Signs', *ODT* 13 Ma ch 1997.

18. 'Inefficiency in delivering medical teaching', *ODT* 26 April 1997; J Campbell, 'Simplistic and inaccurate', *ODT* 26 April 1997; D. Cole and L.J. Simpson, 'Two medical schools "essential" in New Zealand', *ODT* 28 April 1997.

19. Snively Report, pp. 47–48, 52. The Dunedin School was also found to be bearing a direct net cost for library services and for smaller items, such as administrative costs for joint clinical staff.

20. 'Not an easy four years at CHE: Ayling', *ODT* 18 June 1998; 'Three managers resign from CHE', *ODT* 29 July 1998.

21. Interview David Stewart, 2006; Faculty Newsletter, April 1998

22. Ross Black, *Pulse*, HCO News Magazine, 1 December 1998, pp. 2–3; 'Healthcare Otago ahead of budget', *ODT* 9 July 1999. The budget had been for a $26 million deficit. A staff briefing, on 16 July, confirmed that HCO had broken even.

23. Gauld, in *International Political Science Review*, 2003, pp. 204–6; Minister of Health to HHS Chairs, 15 May 1998.

24. University of Otago Faculty of Medicine Accreditation Database, 1999, pp. 54–5. Details the School's appreciation of its strengths and weaknesses.

25. Accreditation Report, 1994, Introduction, p. 2. The alternative to a limited review was a full review aiming at ten years' accreditation; 'Settings for Clinical Teaching', p. 25.

26. Accreditation Report 1999, pp. 25–7.

27. Robin Gauld, 'One Country, Four Systems: Comparing Changing Health Policies in New Zealand', *International Political Science Review*, 2003, pp. 208–12. The DHBs had seven elected and four government-appointed members, including two Maori members either elected or appointed. The first elections were in 2001.

28. Accreditation Report, 2004, Interaction with Health Sector, p. 42.

29. D. Stewart, 'Report from Dean of Faculty', Alumnus Association Bulletin, 1991, p. 6; Interview, G. Mortimer and G. Petersen, 2006. The superannuation transfer added more than a million dollars to the

medical school budget; Dr J.I. Clayton, *The History of Anaesthesia at Dunedin Hospital*, p. 111. Baker went to the prestigious C. Nuffield Chair of Anaesthesia at Sydney; pp. 141–2. At strength, the department had a professor, two full-time senior lecturers, six full-time hospital staff as well as six visiting anaesthetists and a dozen registrars, p. 141.

30 T. O'Donnell, 'Collated Material Relating to the Wellington School of Medicine'; In his 'Report from Dean of Faculty', in the 1991 Alumnus Association Bulletin, David Stewart includes the Vice-Chancellor's tribute at the Senate meeting of November 1991 to each of the retiring professors, pp. 6–8.

31 'Professors voice pride and concern', *Dominion*, 10 December 1991.

32 'Medical School not under closure threat – professor', *ODT* 10 April 1992. The article referred to the 1991 Annual Report and asserted that the improved management system of the new CHEs would create positive opportunities for the School.

33 Annual Reports, Otago Medical School, 1992, 1993; 'Maverick off to greener pastures', *ODT* 6 May 1992. This was hardly a literal description, since Murdoch was going to a position in the United Arab Republic.

34 Although Peter Buck was the first Maori medical graduate at Otago, Maui Pomare was the first Maori to graduate in medicine. He graduated from the American Medical Missionary College in 1899. Graham Butterworth, 'Pomare, Maui Wiremu Piti Naera 1875/76?–1930', DNZB 3.

35 Richard Beasley, *NZMJ* 14 July 1995; Information, Prof John Nacey, Dean, Wellington School of Medicine and Health Sciences; Prof Linda Holloway, formerly PVC Health Sciences, University of Otago.; Dr I.M. St George, Obituary, Eru Pomare, Alumnus Association Newsletter, 1995, p. 10.

36 Annual Reports, Wellington School, 1992, 1993, 1994.

37 Obituary, Eru Woodbine Pomare, *NZMJ* 14 July 1995, p. 282. Annual Report, Wellington School, 1996. Dr Ken Thompson, Chairman (later President) of the Medical Council of New Zealand gave the Nordmeyer lecture. The Mayor of Wellington was Mark Blumsky; 'Holloway Away', Otago Bulletin, 21 April 2006, p. 3; Interview, L. Holloway with D. Page.

38 University of Otago, Christchurch, Obituary, Emeritus Professor Alan Maxwell Clarke, 1932–2007.

39 Moore et al, pp 51–2. Educated at Victoria, Canterbury and Monash Universities, Professor Hornblow was the first Christchurch Dean who had not studied at Otago; Interview, A. Hornblow with D. Page, 27 August 2002. Four appointments were made in Psychological Medicine, in preparation for the new Diploma in Mental Health, due to begin in 1994.

40 Interview, A. Hornblow with D. Page, 27 August 2002.

41 Moore et al, pp. 91–130.

42 Interview, with D. Page, 27 August 2002.

43 Database for AMC, 1994, p. 215.

44 Accreditation Report 1999, pp. 29–30; Accreditation Report 2004, p. 31. By this time, it was clear that there were problems in attracting junior academic staff and the team noted with concern the high proportion of senior staff.

45 Accreditation Report 1999, p. 5, 'Otago Faculty of Medicine, Dean's report'.

46 J.D. Hunter, 'Otago Faculty of Medicine – Dean's report', Alumnus Association Bulletin, 1990; R.D.H. Stewart, 'Report from Dean of Faculty', Alumnus Association Bulletin, 1991, p. 9.

47 Accreditation database, 1999, pp. 46–7, 57. The committee on restructuring was advised by Professor John Hamilton, then Dean of the School of Medicine at the University of Newcastle, New South Wales; G. Mortimer, Annual Report, Dunedin School of Medicine, 1996; 'Otago Medical Faculty Restructuring Outlined', *ODT* 12 April 1995; Accreditation Report 1999, pp. 5–6; Interview, D. Jones with D. Page, 2006.

48 'New Dean for the Dunedin School of Medicine', Alumnus Association Newsletter, 1997–8, p. 10; W.J. Gillespie, 'What's New in the Dunedin School of Medicine?', Alumnus Association Newsletter, 1999/2000 pp. 25–6; Accreditation Report, 1999, p. 5.

49 Accreditation Report, 1999, p. 7.

CHAPTER 24

New Ways of Teaching and Learning

1 Peter L. Schwartz, Christopher J, Heath, Anthony G. Egan, *The Art of the Possible: Ideas from a Traditional Medical School Engaged in Curricular Revision*, pp. 26–8, 30. See all of Chapter 2, pp. 21–32, for detail on the curriculum and teaching methods at the Otago Medical School in 1985.

2 Schwartz et al, pp. 12, 36–7. The 1984 conference was organised by teachers from the Schools of Medicine, Dentistry, Physiotherapy and Nursing; C. Heath, interview with D. Page, December 2004. Heath was Assistant Dean for Curricular Affairs and then Associate Dean for Undergraduate Studies.

3 C. Heath, interview with D. Page, December 2004.

4 Chris Heath, ed. *The Lincoln Conference* (22–24 February 1985).

5 Discussion, Campbell, Heath, Skegg, Stewart, with D. Page, 22 February 2001.

6 *Lincoln Conference*, pp. 94–8.

7 'National Conference on the Role of the Doctor in New Zealand; Implications for Medical Education', Palmerston North, 7–11 October 1985, issued by conference participants. See Schwartz et al, *Art of the Possible*, Ch. 4, pp. 45–53.

8 'Role of the Doctor Conference', p. 14. Peter Schwartz thought these recommendations quite unrealistic. Interview with D. Page, 2006.

9 'Role of the Doctor Conference', pp. 14–23.

10 Schwartz et al, p. 53.

11 E.W. Pomare, 'Maori Health: new concepts and initiatives', *NZMJ*, 11 June 1986, pp. 410–1. In 1980, Pomare had published Maori Standards of Health, containing accurate data for the previous two decades. Obituary, Eru Woodbine Pomare, *NZMJ* vol. 108, July 1995, p. 282.

12 J. Herd, *Cracks in a Glass Ceiling .New Zealand Women, 1975-2004*, pp. 57–61. Interview, Cartwright, cited p. 58.

13 'Problem Based self-directed Learning at the University of Otago Medical School?', discussion paper, July 1987.

14 Tom Fiddes, convener, 'Introduction', The Teschemakers Workshop, 18–20 April 1986, p. 2; list of participants, pp. 19–20. Representatives were nominated by the three divisional curriculum committees and by heads of department.

15 Teschemakers, 1986, p. 10.

16 P. Schwartz, 'Forward from the retreat', in Peter Schwartz, Stewart Mennin and Graham Webb, eds., *PBL: case studies, experience and practice*, pp. 60–7. Schwartz was astonished at the sweeping decision. Chris Heath also thought it had jumped ahead of what the curriculum committees expected or thought possible. Interview with D. Page, Dec. 2004.

17 'Implications of the Proposals of the Teschemakers Workshop', April 1986. A report prepared by the FBCC for the Faculty Board on 6 August 1986. Board Minutes, Hocken MS 1760–20. The plan is in the appendix to the document. Terms of reference for the working parties, and their members, are in 'Problem-Based Self-directed Learning', July 1987, Appendix A.

18 FBCC, 1987, p. 29.

19 'Problem-based Self-directed Learning at the University of Otago Medical School?', pp. 10–11. The MEDU was set up on Faculty decision on 12 December 1986. It worked until early 1991.

20 'Problem-based Self-directed Learning at the University of Otago Medical School? – a discussion paper', July 1987.

21 'Problem-based and Self-directed learning?', Appendix E.

22 Schwartz et al, p. 81. By this time, self-directed courses had been introduced in anatomy (briefly), second year biochemistry, third year clinical biochemistry and third year pathology; Schwartz et al, Ch. 12, pp. 153–64, passim; p. 175; p. 196. A loss of momentum, evident among the committees in 1989, was exacerbated when all Faculty committees and working parties were disbanded for some months, during the restructuring of the University administration; Hunter, p. 20.

23 'Goals and General Objectives for the Undergraduate Curriculum of the Faculty of Medicine, University of Otago, June 1989', cited in full in Schwartz et al, *Art of the Possible*, pp. 90–1. For development of the document, pp. 88–9. The committee met monthly between mid 1987 and the end of 1988. The 1978 Goals are reproduced on pp. 86–7.

24 Schwartz et al, pp. 191–203; p. 209.

25 Schwartz et al, pp. 179–81. See Appendix VII, pp. 279–80 for a description of the course in 1990, taken from a paper, presented by Lewis, B. Welsh and Mellsop, to the ANZME conference 1991.

26 Schwartz et al, pp. 181–2; Moore et al, pp. 45–6. In 1998, a new curriculum committee, without heads of department, persuaded the Assembly of Faculty to give up the course. Under the new scheme, pathology was the only subject with whole-class teaching and most of this was self-directed.

27 Tom Fiddes, Introduction, University of Otago Dunedin Division, Faculty of Medicine, The Teschemakers Workshop, 1987.

28 Ibid., passim. For a summary see, pp. 32–3. The students feared that the proposed course would be more difficult than the existing one; Participants, pp. 34–35.

29 Schwartz et al, pp. 184–7.

30 Medical Council of New Zealand, (MCNZ) *The education of medical undergraduates in New Zealand. Report of the review Committee set up by the Medical Council of New Zealand*. Wellington, 1988 para. 82.

31 MCNZ accreditation report 1988, recommendations 13 and 14.

32 General and Intermediate Objectives to be achieved by the end of Sixth Year, Faculty of Medicine, University of Otago, Faculty Board Curriculum Committee, 1988–95. Typescript, HC MS 1760/20.

33 MB ChB 2nd/3rd year curriculum review working party, Faculty Curriculum Committee 1992.

34 MB ChB 2nd/3rd year curriculum working party, working paper. Discussion in Minutes of FCC, 9 December 1992 (The FBCC became the FCC in 1989).

35 Accreditation Database for AMC, 1999, Section 6, p. 280.

36 John Campbell, Alumnus Association Bulletin, 1998/9, p. 4; Accreditation Database, 1999; The Structure of the new 2nd and 3rd years of the Medical Course, Section 6, pp. 281–2. The committee was a senior one, chaired by the Dunedin Dean and including the Dean of the School of Medical Sciences.

37 Accreditation Database, 1999, pp. 281–2.
38 Report of the second and third year review group, 31 March 1999, Faculty Curriculum Evaluation and Assessment Committee. The review group was convened by associate dean for preclinical education, Dave Loten.
39 AMC Accreditation Report, 1999, Comment on the Curriculum, Second and Third Years, pp. 12–13; AMC Accreditation Report, 2004, Section 2.3.1, pp. 16–17.
40 Peter L. Schwartz, MD, Ernest G. Loten MB ChB, PhD, and Andrew Miller, MB ChB, 'Curriculum Reform at the University of Otago Medical School', *Academic Medicine*, vol. 74. No 6/June 1999, pp. 673–9; Andrew P. Miller, Peter L. Schwartz and Ernest Loten, Department of Pathology, University of Otago Medical School, Dunedin, New Zealand, '"Systems Integration": a middle way between problem-based learning and traditional courses', *Medical Teacher*, vol. 22, no. 1, 2000, pp. 51–8.
41 Campbell, p. 4; Accreditation Database, 1999, pp. 272–3; Accreditation Report, 2004, Students, Admission Policy, p. 25. The top 120 of the Health Science First Year were offered places; UMAJ 2007 Information Booklet, ACER, Camberwell, Australia, 2007.
42 Accreditation Database, 1999, Section 6, 4th–6th year, pp. 352–3.
43 Report of the 4th and 5th year review group to the Dunedin School of Medicine Curriculum Committee, June, 2001. Emeritus Professor Keith Jeffery convened the nine-person group, which included the Director of the Medical Teaching Support Unit, the Associate Dean for Preclinical Education and student representatives of 4th, 5th and 6th years.
44 Michelle Simmons, 'Fourth Year Report', in *Otago Med Enema 99*.
45 John Campbell, interview with D. Page; Accreditation Report, 2004, p. 60, David Jones, interview with D. Page, 2006; Joy Rudland, interview with D. Page, 2006.

CHAPTER 25

The Research Culture

1 'Vice-Chancellor's comment', *University of Otago Magazine*, 16 February 2007, p. 5.
2 Eccles was Professor of Physiology from 1944–50, Woodruff, Professor of Surgery 1953–6. Smirk was Professor of Medicine 1940–1962 then, until his retirement in 1967, he held a specially created Chair of Experimental Medicine; E.R. Nye ed., *Medical Research in Otago, 1922–1997*, as portrayed by 75 years of the Proceedings of the University of Otago Medical School (hereafter, *Medical Research*).
3 F.O. Simpson, 'Medicine and Related Subjects', *Medical Research*, p. 93. Among the hundreds of papers on hypertension and related areas published in the period, Simpson has counted 130 over the 75 years of the *Proceedings*; p. 96. Simpson notes overseas professors A.E. Doyle, medicine, Melbourne, P. Bolli, cardiovascular epidemiology, Winnipeg, and J.A. Millar, clinical pharmacology, Perth; p. 99.
4 J.R. Robinson, 'Physiology', *Medical Research*, pp. 61–4.
5 B.F. Heslop, 'Surgery. Transplantation Research in Dunedin', *Medical Research*, pp. 154–5. Andre van Rij, 'Surgical Research in Dunedin', *Medical Research*, p. 145; For the temporary building see Hercus and Bell, pp. 78–9. It was demolished to make way for the Sayers building.
6 Annual Reports, Medical Research Council of New Zealand, 1952 to 1989, in AJHR Welfare and Justice, E 11. In 1956, the MRC disbursed £49,895, the bulk of the funding going to endocrine research (22 per cent), clinical medicine (17 per cent), microbiology (16 per cent), nutrition (12 per cent) and the rest being more or less evenly divided among the other committees, 1956 Report. In 1964, hydatid research received 16 per cent, 1964 Report; J. Hunter, 'Medical Research', Information for the Review Committee, 1988, p. 36.
7 Heslop, p. 157; Simpson, *Medical Research*, p. 93.
8 Simpson, p. 93; Annual Report MRC, 1977.
9 J.V. Hodge, Director's Report, MRC 1977. Other grants for long-term projects were made to researchers at the Auckland Medical School.
10 J.V. Hodge, Director's Report, MRC 1981; 1986 and 1987 reports; A. McRobie, 'The Politics of Volatility', in G. Rice, ed. *The Oxford History of New Zealand*, 2nd edition, pp. 397, 406. In 1981, New Zealand inflation reached a record high of 15.4 per cent, unemployment was above 70,000 and the projected budget deficit for the coming year was more than $2 billion. The government changed in 1984, from Muldoon's National to a Labour Government led by Lange and influenced by Finance Minister Roger Douglas. The world stock market crash occurred in 1987.
11 MRC Report, 1988; HRC Report, 1990.
12 Interview, D. Page with G. Petersen, 2006; 'Medical Researchers receive $3 million', *ODT* 5 July 1991; Annual Reports, 1993, 1994. See Database for Review, 1994, pp. 219–22.
13 J. Hunter, Information for Review Committee 1988, p. 36; Sir David Hay, *Heart Sounds*, Ch. XV, pp. 109–20. The NHF of Australia derived from the example of the American Heart Association, which had become a community organisation in 1948. Proceeds from the sale of Sir David Hay's autobiography have gone towards the Heart Foundation.
14 H.B. Turbott, 'Medical Research in New Zealand',

report of MRC, 1959, AJHR H 31B, p. 7; Moore et al, pp. 62–6, 69. The Medical Expos were organised by Philippa Tait, the School's and Foundation's publicity and liaison officer; Hunter, Faculty of Medicine, information for Review 1988, p. 36; Database for AMC Review 1994, pp. 221–2.

15 Victoria University Research Funding website: Marsden Fund and PGSF, 2007.

16 J.W.G. Tiller, 'Research Report', *Digest*, 1966, pp. 64–77.

17 E.R. Nye, 'Research in the Otago Medical School', typescript, not dated.

18 P.A. Cragg, Foreword, *Medical Research in Otago*, p. 1. Before 1951, the *Proceedings* consisted of reprints of staff articles from other journals. D.P.L. Green's chapter on the School of Medical Sciences covers anatomy and structural biology, biochemistry, microbiology, pharmacology and physiology. R.J. Olds' chapter on the Dunedin School of Medicine covers anaesthesia and intensive care, biomedical ethics, general practice, medicine and its sub-specialties, obstetrics and gynaecology, orthopaedic surgery, paediatrics and child health, pathology, psychological medicine, surgery, and preventive and social medicine, pp. 163–76.

19 Cragg, p. 2; Hercus and Bell, pp. 130–1. In 1948, following a recommendation of the NZU Senate committee on medical education, the Medical School had been funded to provide a tutor-registrar in each Branch Faculty, the salaries to be shared by the University and the Hospital Board, pp. 103–4. The new annual grant was £3000 to each Branch Faculty.

20 Catherine Gunn, 'Rhodes 1950, Derek North', *University of Otago Magazine*, October 2002, p 18; North, Professor John Derek Kingsley, CBE, MB ChB, DPhil, FRCP, FRACP, *Who's Who Aotearoa New Zealand*, 1996; Ian Prior, *Elespie and Ian*, pp. 103, 105.

21 Moore et al, pp. 62–3. The endocrinology group included Fred Shannon, George Rolleston and George Uttley. In pathology, Denis Stewart brought in Gunz, Carrell, Winterbourn and Fitzgerald. Beaven, Don, MB ChB, FRCP (Lond), FRCP (Edin), FRACP, FACP (Hon), *Who's Who in Aotearoa New Zealand*, 1996.

22 J. Hunter, Information for Review, 1988, p. 36.

23 *Research Strengths. University of Otago*, 2000. Introduction, p. 2; *Research Themes at the University of Otago: A Review: 1997–1999*, p. 4.

24 *Research Strengths*, University of Otago, New Zealand, 2000, pp. 5–14. *He Kitenga*, 2004. University of Otago Research Highlights, pp. 67, 70.

25 *Research Themes at the University of Otago: A Review: 1997–1999*, pp. 4–5.

26 'Asthma and Respiratory Disorders', *Research Themes Review 1997–1999*, pp. 11–18; 'Respiratory Disorders', *Research Strengths*, p. 74. 'Asthma epidemiology', *Research Strengths*, p. 28.

27 *Research Themes Review*, pp. 19–26.

28 *Research Themes*, pp. 59–63. The external reviewer, Professor Roger Dean, Director of the Heart Research Institute, Sydney, urged the provision of funding to train clinicians in basic oxidative research methods and to train basic scientists to understand problems from the point of view of clinicians; 'Professor Christine Winterbourn: a career of curiosity', *He Kitenga* 2004, pp. 4–5; *Research Report*, 1998, p. 57.

29 *Research Strengths*, pp. 24–88. Contestable funding sources were not specified in the self review, but in *Research Strengths* these were listed as the Health Research Council, National Heart Foundation and Canterbury Medical Research Foundation, p. 6; 'Affective Disorders', *Research Strengths*, p. 24; 'Health in Mind', *University of Otago Magazine*, June 2006, pp. 5–7.

30 'Sleep, Wake and Shiftwork', *Research Strengths*, p. 76; 'Socio-Economic Inequalities in Health', p. 78. 'Research into Housing Insulation and Health', *University of Otago Magazine*, October 2002, p. 6; 'Urban excellence', *University of Otago Magazine*, February 2007, p. 29.

31 'Hauora Maori', *Research Strengths*, p. 49. Dr Reid moved to Auckland in 2005.

32 Department of Human Nutrition, University of Otago, website; University of Otago Magazine, October 2004, p. 25; *He Kitenga*, Research Highlights, 2006, p. 20.

33 *Research Strengths*, pp. 33; 'Completing the Jigsaw', *Research Report* 1998, pp. 28-31.

34 *Research Strengths*, p. 73; 'Solid Endeavour; stellar results', *He Kitenga*, Research Highlights, 2006, pp. 6–7; 'Completing the Jigsaw', *Research Report* 1998, p. 29.

35 'Bioethics', *Research Strengths*, p. 30; R.J. Olds, 'Dunedin School of Medicine', in Nye ed., pp. 169–70.

36 Nigel Zega, 'Real-life Research', *University of Otago Magazine*, February 2007, pp. 6–11.

37 Obituary, 'Frederick Thomas Shannon', *NZMJ* vol. 112, 1999, pp. 390–1; Zega; Christchurch Health and Development Study, http://www.chmeds.ac.nz/research/chds

38 *Research Strengths*, p. 42; Zega; 'Otago's remarkable 32 year research project', *ODT* 16–17 July 2005.

39 *Research Strengths*, p. 33; 'University of Otago Welcomes New Chancellor and Vice-Chancellor', *University of Otago Magazine*, February 2004, p. 5.

CHAPTER 26

A Rich Diversity: Medical Students in the Late Twentieth Century

1   Elworthy, pp. 131–8. Phyllis Comerford was the first woman president of the OUSA.

2   University of Otago registry statistics; Erihana Ryan, 'The price of being visible', Rosy Fenwicke ed., *In Practice*, p. 77; Sandy Smith to D. Page, 20 February 2007.

3   Tai Sopoaga, Maori and Pacific Island Report, 1987; Susan Wetere, OUMSA newsletter 1988. Pomare was Professor of Medicine at the Wellington School at this stage.

4   Francie Robbins, 'Te Oranga Ki Otakou, 1999. Maori Medical Students', *Enema*, 1999; Arihia Waaka, 'Maori Report. Te Oranga ki Otakou: Maori Medical Students Association', *Enema* 2006, p. 18; 'Gizzy 06', *Enema* 2006, p. 40; Shekhar Sehgal, 'PIHPSA Report', *Enema*, 2006, p. 19; Xaviour Walker to NZMSA colleagues, re. Maori and Pacific Island Medical Student Recruitment and Retention, 18 April 2006; Walker, report to NZMSA AGM August 2006, p. 7.

5   'A Word on Malaysia', *Enema* 1998. Photo *ODT* Dec 2006.

6   Humerus, 'the Med Revue 1997', *Enema*, 1997.

7   Francie Robbins, 'Cultural Night 1999', *Enema*, 1999.

8   Jacqui Hall, 'Otago Medical Students' Association', Accreditation Database, 1994, p. 170; Reports in *Enema*, 1997, 1998, 1999; William Perry, 'President's Report', pp. 6–7; Fiona Loan, 'Medieval', pp. 8–9.

9   Sneyd to Brinkman, June 1983, and subsequent reports in Faculty of Medicine, OUMSA 1979–1988. The house manager at the Town Hall told the Dean he thought student behaviour at the ball had been better than the previous year, but agreed there was room for improvement. The cream had been blown through brandy snaps.

10 University Proctor to Brinkman, 2 August 1985; Keith Hunter (Chemistry), Social Convener to Brinkman, 16 October 1985.

11 W. Perry, in *Enema* 2006, pp. 7–8. Celia Keane, 'Art Extravaganza', *Enema* 2006, pp. 26–7; Lesley Nichol, interview in *Enema* 1999.

12 The Otago Medical Students' Association (Incorporated) Constitution, 2004; Information from 2006 OUMSA president Will Perry and 2006 NZMSA president Xaviour Walker.

13 A. Verrall to D. Page, 27 April 2006.

14 A. Verrall to D. Page, 27 April 2006: Brandon Adams, 'Student Protest', in *Enema* 1999.

15 President's Reports, 1971, 1972, 1973–4, 1978; OUMSA Executive Minutes, 15 September 1981; W.E. Adams to Editor, *Litterhoea*, 15 October 1971;

President's Report, 1972–3; OUMSA Executive Minutes 18 September 1979; *Borborygmi '88*; OUMSA Executive Minutes 15 March 1999.

16 *Enema*, 1997, 1999; *New Zealand Medical Student Journal, Te Hautakaa o ngaa Akongaa Rongoaa*, March 2004, p. 1. The publication committee was chaired by Ayesha Verrall; *NZMSJ*, 1 May 2006, Editorial, p. 4.

17 Michael Goodwin, 'Christchurch Medical Students' Association', Accreditation Database, 1994, pp. 171–2; Paul Butel, 'Wellington Medical Students' Association', Accreditation Database, 1994, p. 173. The descriptions provided for the 1999 accreditation visit are almost identical to those of 1994. Christchurch, pp. 466–7; Wellington, p. 469.

18 Interview, B. McMahon with D. Page, August 2006

19 Information provided by Lt Col Andrew Dunn, MNZM, ED, RNZAMC to D. Page, 30 November 2006.

20 Dunn to Page, 30 November 2006; Vanessa Weenink is another recent graduate (2002) who took a Medical Corps cadetship, served in Afghanistan and East Timor and then, as MO at Waiouru, combined medical duties with marriage and motherhood. Information, Brian McMahon.

21 For student fees, loans etc, see e.g. NZMSA Bulletin, February 2005; President's report to NZMSA AGM 12–13 August 2006; Chris Jackson, 'NZMSA', in *Enema* 1999; Nicola Mutch, 'ACE – Coming up Trumps?', *NZMSJ*, March 2004; Premjit Gill, 'Advanced Choice of Employment: Friend or Foe?', *NZMSJ* October 2005; Xaviour Walker, President's report to AGM, NZMSA, 2006. Almost 10 per cent of the remaining students were matched with their second or third choice.

22 AMSA Convention Report, *Enema*, 2006, pp. 24–5; Xaviour Walker, 'New Zealand medical students join the world', *NZMSJ*, October 2006, pp. 22–3.

POSTSCRIPT

CHAPTER 27

Made at Otago: Some of the Graduates

1   University of Otago Calendar, 2007. The University of Otago began to award honorary degrees in 1962 when it ceased to be part of the University of New Zealand; Diana Beaglehole, 'Porritt, Arthur Espie (1900–1994)', DNZB 4, pp. 417–8.

2   Aitken, Robert Stevenson, RACP History of Medicine Library, College Roll, 1901–97, internet; C.A. Gibson, 'Robin Orlando Irvine (1929–1996)', *Southern People*, p. 247.

3   Ratu Sir Kamisese Mara, and Sir Peter Tapsell, Wikipedia. Tapsell, the first Speaker who was not a member of the governing party, was selected Speaker

because the newly elected National Government did not want to lose its one-vote majority by selecting a Speaker from its own ranks.

4   Otago University Bulletin, 20 May 2005; Nicola Mutch, 'Born Leader', *University of Otago Magazine*, October 2005, pp. 16–18.

5   Professor Alan Musgrave, Oration for Paratene Ngata, August 2004; 'Honorary doctorate for Maori doctor', *ODT* 13 August 2004. In 1984, Ngata played a leading role, together with Eru Pomare and Mason Durie, in the Hui Whakaoranga, described as one of the most important Maori health initiatives since the days of Apirana Ngata and Sir Peter Buck.

6   James Ng, *Windows on a Chinese Past*, vol. 1, 1993; vol. 2, 1995; vol. 3, 1999; vol. 4, 1993, Otago Heritage Books.

7   Obituary, William Percy Gowland, *NZMJ* vol. 64, 1965, pp. 660–3; J.R. Robinson, Obituary, Muriel Emma Bell, *NZMJ* June 1974, 1082–3; J.I. Hubbard, 'Herbert Dudley Purves, 1908–1993', *Proceedings of the Royal Society of New Zealand*, 1991–1995; The recipients of honorary degrees in 1975 were Sir Charles Burns, Professor Eric D'Ath, Professor Russell Fraser, Sir Edward Sayers, Sir Horace Smirk, Sir John Stallworthy and Dr Stanley Wilson.

8   Boston City Hospital website. Denny-Brown was appointed to the Chair at Harvard in 1939, but was called up for active service in Britain when war began. The President of Harvard requested Churchill to release him to take up his post in 1941; Ian McDonald, Graduation Address, Dunedin, December 2000.

9   Carroll du Chateau, interview with Murray Brennan, ' Wielding a Blade with the World's best', *New Zealand Herald*, 27 December 2004; Sloan Kettering website, including tributes to Brennan at his retirement in 2006.

10 University of Otago, Oration for the honorary degree of DSc, James Julian Bennett Jack, 1999. Jack's mountaineering exploits as a student included climbing several peaks at the head of the Tasman Glacier and, with David Herron, making the first traverse from Hackel Peak to Mount Annan.

11 Public orator's presentation of candidates for the honorary degree of Doctor of Science, Ian McDonald and George Petersen, December 2000, in Alumnus Newsletter, 2000/2001, pp. 14–19. Ian McDonald died suddenly at the end of 2006.

12 'Fred Hollows (1929–1993)', Te Ara Encyclopedia; Newsletter of Retina New Zealand Inc, a member of Retina International, May 2006, no. 29, website Hollows Foundation.

13 'Making miracles happen', *University of Sydney Gazette*, October 2003, pp. 7–9; 'ANZAC Couple Bring Hope to Outcasts of Ethiopia', *ODT* 15 December 1984, an article written when the Hamlins had been awarded the ANZAC peace prize. Reg Hamlin, who had trained as a teacher before studying medicine, won the Medical School's travelling scholarship in 1941, as well as the Batchelor medal for obstetrics and the Colquhoun prize in systematic medicine. He took his Fellowship before going to Ethiopia. In 2003, Dr Catherine Hamlin, then aged 79, was still working at the hospital.

14 University orator's address, Graduation Ceremony, 20 May 2006. A six-storey building at the College is named for Dr Howie.

15 'Rhodes: the man, the vision, the scholars', *University of Otago Magazine*, October 2002, pp. 12–14. Profiles of eight Otago Rhodes scholars follow, including medical students Derek North (1950), Ken North (1954) and David Skegg (1972), pp. 15–23; A number of the scholars have appeared in the narrative. Otago medical graduates also won Rhodes scholarships in 2003, 2006, and 2007. See the appendix for the full list to that date.

16 A.H. McLintock ed., *The Encyclopaedia of New Zealand*, 1966. The list is made up of Dudley Ashcroft (ENT surgeon), John Barron (plastic surgeon), Cedric Britton, (allergist and haematologist), Sylvia Chapman (Hon Registrar of the College of General Practitioners, London), Patrick Clarkson (plastic surgeon), Archibald Durward (professor of anatomy), Murray Falconer (neurosurgeon), Geoffrey Flavell (thoracic surgeon), Harold Foreman (superintendent, Sully Hospital Glamorgan), Duncan Forrest (paediatric surgeon), Russell Fraser (professor of endocrinology), Anthony Green (radiologist), William Hawkesworth (obstetrician and gynaecologist), J.C.R. Hindenach (orthopaedic surgeon), Douglas Jolly (orthopaedic surgeon), Norman Jory (aural surgeon), Philip Jory (aural surgeon), Sir Robert Macintosh (professor of anaesthetics, University of Oxford), Lawrence Malcolm (regius professor of physiology, University of Aberdeen), George Maloney (surgeon), Arthur Rainsford Mowlem (plastic surgeon), James Murdoch (obstetrician and gynaecologist), K.I. Nissen (orthopaedic surgeon), Sir Arthur Porritt (sergeant-surgeon to Her Majesty the Queen), A.G Rutter (surgeon), Murray Stewart (radiotherapist). The inclusion of plastic surgeons Arthur Rainsford Mowlem and John Barron is a reminder of the role that Otago graduates, working with Sir Harold Gillies (who was born in Dunedin, but did his medical studies at Cambridge University) and Sir Archibald McIndoe, played in this field in Britain before and during World War II.

17 *Encyclopaedia of New Zealand*, 1966. Others on the list who served on the staff at the Otago Medical School were Durward, Malcolm and Maloney; Hercus and Bell, pp. 312–3; Ian Church, 'Alexander Robert Falconer 1874–1955', in *Southern People*: Australian Academy of Science, Biographical

Memoirs of Deceased Fellows, Walter Victor McFarlane, 1913–1982.

18   Professor C. Katona, presentation of Professor Eugene Paykel for the Honorary Fellowship of the Royal College of Psychiatrists, July 2001. *Psychiatric Bulletin 2001*, 25 (12) 491; Professor R.W. Carrell, FRS, FRSNZ, Royal Society of New Zealand website, http://www.rsnz.org/members/fellows. Professor Carrell retired in 2003, but continues research in the Institute of Medical Research of Cambridge University.

19   Catherine Gunn, 'Rhodes 1950, interview with Derek North MB ChB (1951), D Phil Oxon, FRACP (1957), FRCP London (1962), CBE', *University of Otago Magazine*, October 2002; Sir John Scott, Obituary Sir William Liley 1929–1983; University of Auckland, Obstetrics and Gynaecology website, Sir Graham Liggins, emeritus professor of obstetrics and gynaecology; Harvey White, 'Sir Brian Gerald Barratt-Boyes' *NZMJ* vol. 119, no. 1232, 21 April 2006; In 1995, Sir Brian was selected to feature on a postage stamp ($1.20) in a series of Famous New Zealanders. He was the representative for Science, Medicine and Education, alongside Richard Hadlee (Sport) and Barry Crump (Fine Arts and Literature).

20   Derek A. Dow, 'Michael Herbert Watt, 1887–1967', DNZB 4, p. 556. Michael Watt's son, James, became the first professor of paediatrics at Otago.

21   Derek A. Dow, 'Cairney, John 1989–1966', DNZB 5, pp, 85–6. T.R. Ritchie held the post, briefly, between Watt and Cairney.

22   Derek. A. Dow, 'Turbott, Harold Bertram, 1899–1988', DNZB 5, pp. 526–8. Dow claims that Turbott's management of staff and radical restructuring of his department was divisive.

23   Jill McIraith ed., *The Goods Train Doctors. Stories of Women Doctors in New Zealand, 1920–1993*; M.D. Maxwell ed., *Women Doctors in New Zealand: an Historical Perspective, 1921–1986*; Rosy Fenwicke ed., *In Practice: the Lives of New Zealand Women Doctors in the 21st Century*.

24   Hercus and Bell, pp. 161–2; Geoffrey W. Rice, *Black November. The 1918 Influenza Pandemic in New Zealand*, p. 157.

25   Hercus and Bell, Ch. 11, 'Women of the Otago Medical School', pp. 159–65; Margaret Tennant, 'Paterson, Ada Gertrude, 1880–1937', in DNZB 3, pp. 387–8; Michael Belgrave, 'A Subtle Containment: Women in New Zealand Medicine, 1893–1945', *New Zealand Journal of History*, vol. 22, 1, April 1988, pp. 50–51; p. 48.

26   Hercus and Bell, pp. 160–3. Their list of women graduates before 1914 includes: Emily Siedeberg, Margaret Cruickshank, Constance Frost, Alice Woodward, Daisy Platts, Eleanor Baker, Winifrede Bathgate, Violet Ridley, Jane Kinder, Ada Paterson, Ina Dugleby and Catharine Will. There are two

omissions from the list: Jessie Maddison (1902) and Agatha Adams (1904); Dorothy Page, 'Dissecting a Community', Women Medical Students at the University of Otago 1891–1924', in *Communities of Women*, ed Barbara Brookes and Dorothy Page, pp. 111–27, and the list of graduates in Appendix B, pp. 180–1; Obituary, Doris Gordon, *NZMJ* vol. 15, 1956, p. 326; Linda Bryder, 'Gordon, Doris Clifton, 1890–1956', in DNZB 4, pp. 201–2.

27   Philippa Mein Smith, 'Bell, Emma Muriel, 1898–1974', DNZB 4, pp. 47–8; Whyte, Dr J.I. Clayton, *The History of Anaesthesia in Dunedin Hospital*, pp. 45–6; J. Borrie, Obituary, 'Marion King Bennie Whyte', *NZMJ* vol. 96, no. 741, October 1983, p. 773. A.C. Begg, Obituary, 'Ruth Marjorie Cruickshank Barclay', *NZMJ* vol. 88, no. 626, December 1978, pp. 302–3.

28   Harvey Brown, Pickerill, 'Cecily Mary Wise, 1903–1988', DNZB 4, pp. 406–7; Harvey Brown, *Pickerill, Pioneer in Plastic Surgery, Dental Education and Dental Research*, pp. 211–2, 216–20.

29   Sir Charles Burns, Obituary, 'Alice Campbell Rose (Tallerman)', *NZMJ* vol. 59, September 1960, pp. 440–1; Obituary, 'Jean Sandel', *NZMJ* vol. 81, April 1960, pp. 359–60 ; Victor Hadlow, Sandel, Jean Mary, 1916–1974, DNZB 5, p. 459. Hercus and Bell, p. 163, are mistaken in associating her with the Hutt Hospital; Linda Bryder, 'Helen Muriel Deem, 1900–1955', DNZB, 5, pp. 143–4; Obituary, *NZMJ* December 1955, 1394–5.

30   Valedictory Minute, Dr Dorothy Marian Stewart, Medical Faculty Minutes, 12 December 1969; Dorothy Marian Stewart, obituary, *ODT* 7–8 June 2003. It is indicative of assumptions about women that the obituary refers to Zoe Robertson as the wife of the Ashburton Hospital superintendent, not as a doctor in her own right. Stewart took early retirement to live on her farm near Waitati. A skilled horsewoman, she bred her own hunters and at least one successful race horse. She died aged 94.

31   Esther Irving, 'Chapman, Sylvia Gytha de Lancey, 1896–1995', DNZB 5, pp. 95–6; Radcliffe-Taylor, *Dictionary of Australian Biography*; Bronwyn Labrum, 'Todd, Kathleen Mary Gertrude, 1898–1968', DNZB 5, p. 252; Sir Charles Burns and Prof. W. Ironside, Obituary, 'Kathleen Todd', *NZMJ* September 1968, pp. 191–3.

32   Fay Hercock, 'Alice Bush, 1914–1974', *The Book of New Zealand Women, Ko Kui Ma Te Kaupapa*, ed. Charlotte Macdonald, Merimeri Penfold and Bridget Williams; Fay Hercock, *Alice. The Making of a Women Doctor, 1914–1984*; Linda Bryder, 'Bush, Alice Mary, 1914–1974', DNZB 5, pp. 83–4.

33   Marples, Dr Mary Joyce, 'Loutit, Professor Margaret Wyn', in *Who's Who in Aotearoa New Zealand*, 1996.

34   Barbara Heslop, 'Postgraduate Training: the

Eternal Tug of War for Women and How It Has Got Tougher', in Jill McIlraith ed., *The Goods Train Doctors: Stories of Women Doctors in New Zealand, 1920–1993*, p. 9; Andre van Rij, 'Surgical Research in Dunedin', in E. Nye ed., *Medical Research in Otago, 1922–1997*, p. 145.

35 Barbara F. Heslop MD, FRCPath, Associate Professor, Department of Surgery, Robin Molloy BA, Scientific Officer, Department of Preventive and Social Medicine, Hendrika J. Waal-Manning BMedSc, MB ChB, Medical Research Officer, Department of Medicine, Ngaire M. Walsh BSc, MD, Lecturer in Anatomy, University of Otago Medical School, Dunedin, 'Women in Medicine in New Zealand', *NZMJ* vol. 77, no. 491, April 1973, pp. 219–29.

36 Barbara F. Heslop, Professor in Surgery (Experimental Surgery), University of Otago Medical School, Dunedin, 'For Better or Worse? Women doctors at the end of the decade', *NZMJ* vol. 100, no. 820, March 1987, pp. 176–9. The article is reprinted in Maxwell, *Women Doctors in New Zealand*, pp. 217–28; Heslop, 'Postgraduate Training', pp. 14–15.

37 Valedictory Minute, Associate Professor Dame Norma Restieaux.

38 University of Otago Calendar, 2000.

39 'Students Attend First Medical Leadership Development Seminar', *Otago Bulletin*, 11 August 2006, p. 9; information, Xaviour Walker.

CHAPTER 28

Medical School at the Millennium

1 J.C. Beaglehole, *The University of New Zealand: an historical study*, p. 383.

2 The New Zealand University Calendar, 1940, p. xiv; University of Otago Calendar, 2000, pp. 27–62.

3 Figures from OSMS; Interview, David Jones.

SELECT BIBLIOGRAPHY

Abbreviations used in this index

AUP	Auckland University Press
AJHR	*Australian Journal of Historical Research*
DNZB	*Dictionary of New Zealand Biography*
IA Dept	Department of Internal Affairs
HC	Hocken Collections
IPSR	*International Political Studies Review*

MSS	Manuscripts
NZJH	*New Zealand Journal of History*
NZMJ	*New Zealand Medical Journal*
ODT	*Otago Daily Times*
OUR	*Otago University Review*

The Hocken Collections, Dunedin, is the principal repository for Otago Medical School records, published and unpublished. Some of the more recent material in both categories is held at the Medical School. The Hocken Collections also houses Government documents, notably the *Appendices to the Journals of the House of Representatives (AJHR)*, which contain material relating to the Medical School. This includes annual reports from the University of Otago, the University Grants Committee and the Medical Research Council and Health Research Council, as well as reports of various commissions.

Primary Sources

PUBLISHED

Calendars, University of Edinburgh, 1878; 1879–1880; 1880–1881.

Calendars, University of Otago, 1877–2007.

Coughtrey, Millen, 'The Introductory Address in the Faculty of Medicine of Otago University', May 31, 1875, Mackay, Risk, Munro & Co, Dunedin.

Christie, R.V., 'Report on the Medical School', University of Otago, Dunedin 1968.

'Dunedin Hospital Ward Block with its Medical School Facilities' (brochure to commemorate the opening) Dunedin, 1980.

Descriptive Syllabus of the Medical School, University of Otago, Wilkie and Co., Dunedin, 1916.

Health Research Council of New Zealand, Annual Reports, 1990–2000, *AJHR*

He Kitenga. University of Otago Research Highlights, 2004, 2006, Marketing and Communications, University of Otago.

Hunter, J.D., *Compendium of Historical Data* (1873–1992), compiled by the Honorary Archivist of the Faculty, Otago Medical School Alumnus Association, Dunedin, 1993.

Medical Research Council of New Zealand, Annual Reports, 1951–1989, *AJHR*.

The New Zealand Medical Research Council, pamphlet, Medical Research Council, McIndoe, Dunedin, ?1956.

Province of Otago, N.Z., Report of the University Council, 1875–6. (includes correspondence with British medical schools concerning recognition).

Research Strengths, University of Otago New Zealand, 2000, Marketing and Communications, University of Otago.

Research Themes at the University of Otago: a Review: 1997–1999, Marketing and Communications, University of Otago, 2 vols, 2000.

Tihei Mauri Ora! The Maori Health Commission, No 2, October 1999, Maori Health Commission, Wellington, 1999.

UMAT Information Booklet 2007 (Undergraduate Medicine and Health Sciences Admission Test) Australian Council of Educational Research, 2007.

'University of Otago Medical School, Opening of South Block, September 8, 1948', memento published by University of Otago Council, 1948.

University of Otago, Annual Reports, 1878–1992 *AJHR*.

University Grants Committee, Annual Reports 1961–1986, *AJHR*.

PERIODICALS/ NEWSPAPERS
Selected issues only

Alumnus Association Bulletin, (Otago Medical School Alumnus Association) 1976–2004.

Critic, (OUSA) 1925–2000.

Enema, (OUMSA) 1993–2006.

Medical Digest, (OUMSA) 1934–1978.

New Zealand Medical Journal, (New Zealand Medical Association) 1887–2007.

New Zealand Medical Student Journal, (NZMSA*)*
2004–2006.
Otago Daily Times (mainly Medical School Cuttings
Books, 1903–2000).
University of Otago Magazine, Marketing and
Communications, 2002–2007.
Otago Bulletin (newsletter for University staff)
2002–2007.
Te Korero (OUSA), 1922–1924.

Primary Sources

UNPUBLISHED

Most unpublished papers relating to the Otago
Medical School, such as Annual Reports, Minutes
of the Faculty of Medicine and its Committees and
correspondence, are to be found with the Otago
University records in the Hocken Collections, mainly
in the 'Faculty of Medicine, Dean's Department,
1887–1991'. Recent material, some student records,
and duplicates of some earlier material are held
at the Medical School or the Medical Library. The
Hunter Collection consists of less formal material
gathered by Emeritus Professor Hunter as Honorary
Archivist between 1991 and 1996, typically through
correspondence with staff or former staff of the
School. It is divided into General File Notes and
Departmental File Notes and access to some of it is
restricted.

Annual Reports, Faculty of Medicine, University of
Otago, (especially 1924–1959) in 'Annual Reports
of Faculties, Otago University, Records of Registry
and Central Administration'.
Annual Reports from Medical School, University of
Otago, to Australian Medical Council, 1996–2002.
Australian Medical Council, Accreditation of the
Undergraduate Course in Medicine, Faculty of
Medicine University of Otago. Report by the
Accreditation Committee, August 1994.
Australian Medical Council, Accreditation of the
Undergraduate Course in Medicine, Faculty of
Medicine, University of Otago, Report by the
Accreditation Committee, March 1999.
Australian Medical Council. Accreditation of
University of Otago Medical School, Report to the
Medical School by the Accreditation Committee,
October 2004.
Bates, David V., 'Report on the University of Otago
Medical School', 1981.
Brinkman, Geoffrey, 'Future of the Medical School',
for discussion by Dunedin Division, July 1985.
Brinkman, Geoffrey, with senior academic staff.
'Planning for the Future', report, 1978.
Christchurch Clinical School, 1969–1984, Faculty of
Medicine, Dean's Department.
Christie Report: Materials relating to the compilation,

Faculty of Medicine, Dean's Department.
Coughtrey, Millen, papers 1867–1876. Includes letter
books 1874–1881.
Dunedin School of Medicine, Year 4/5 Curriculum
Objectives, 2001.
Edinburgh University Special Collections: Otago
Medical School, Medical Faculty Minutes and
related papers, 1872–1875; Minutes of Senatus, vol.
IV, 1872–1875.
Fiddes, Tom, ed., 'The Teschemakers Workshop,
18–20 April 1986', University of Otago, Faculty of
Medicine 1986.
Fogelberg, G., 'Otago Medical School. Proposed
Future Organisation Structure' presented by Vice-
Chancellor to School Assembly, 11 April 1995.
Heath, Chris, 'The Lincoln Conference, 22–24
February 1985', University of Otago Faculty of
Medicine, 1985.
Heath, Chris (Planning Committee Convenor)
'National Conference on the Role of the Doctor in
New Zealand: Implications for Medical Education'
Palmerston North, 7–11 October 1985. Summary
Report'.
Hercus, Sir Charles Ernest, papers, 1890–1961.
Hercus, C.E. 'Report of Dr Hercus on Physical
Education', 12 February 1940, Otago University
Committee Reports, vol. 8, 1939–1941.
Hunter Collection, 'University of Otago Medical
School', 5 boxes of notes and correspondence.
Hunter, J.D., 'Faculty of Medicine, Undergraduate
Medical Course. Information for the Review
Committee of the Medical Council of New
Zealand', May 1988.
Hunter, J.D., 'Final Report from the Royal Australasian
College of Physicians, 1981, to the W.K. Kellogg
Foundation'. Royal Australasian College of
Physicians, Sydney.
Hunter, John, 'Future of the Medical School (Dunedin
Division)', 1977.
Irvine, R.O.H., 'University of Otago. The Future of
the Medical School. A Report on the Future of the
Medical School With Particular Reference to the
Implementation of Proposals Made in The Christie
Report, 1969'.
Jeffery, Keith (Convenor) Report of the 4th and 5th
Year Review Group to the Dunedin School of
Medicine Curriculum Committee, June 2001.
Loten, E.G., Memo: 'Overview of the New 2nd and
3rd Year Curriculum', 24 August 1998.
Loten E.G. (Convenor), Report of the second and
third year review group, 31 March 1999.
Officer Training Corps (Medical), 1909–1922.
Otago Medical School Alumnus Association,
1975–2007.
Otago Medical School, Faculty Board Curriculum
Committee, 'General and Intermediate Objectives
to be achieved by the end of sixth year', 1992.
Otago Provincial Council, Proceedings and Corres-

pondence, 1869–1876.

Otago University Medical Students' Association records, Executive Minutes and Presidents' Annual Reports, 1905–2007.

Otago University Professorial Board, Minutes and other papers relating to meetings, 1875–1961, Records of Registry and Central Administration.

Sayers, Sir Edward George, papers,

Sayers, Sir Edward George, correspondence with Vice-Chancellor. 1964–1967.

Scott, John Halliday, papers, 1870–1909.

Scott, Prof. J.H. Letter Book, 1891–1905

Siedeberg-McKinnon, Dr Emily, papers, 1905–1959.

Snively, Suzanne (Coopers and Lybrand), 'Snively Report, Healthcare Otago Limited and Dunedin School of Medicine: Value of Joint Relationship', 1997.

Staff Establishment, Memorandum to Clinical Heads of Departments, 1985. Submissions from chairmen of the clinical departments, for discussion on 10 June, to set priorities.

University of Otago Council: Minutes and Committee Reports, 1873–2005.

University of Otago, Faculty of Medicine, Minutes and Reports, 1891–2007 (Note, vol. 4, June 1919–June 1943, is missing).

University of Otago Faculty of Medicine, Database for Australian Medical Council, 1994.

University of Otago, Faculty of Medicine, Accreditation Database, 1999 (6 vols).

University of Otago, Faculty of Medicine, Accreditation Database, 2004.

University of Otago, orations for medical recipients of honorary degrees 1968–2006 (Registry).

Wellington Clinical School, Minutes and Planning Committee, 1968–1975, (Dean's Department).

INTERVIEWS
All interviews conducted by D. Page

Dr John Adams (11 August 2006)

Emeritus Professor Don Beaven, Christchurch School (26 March 2004)

Associate Professor John Borrie (30 January 2001; 9 May 2001)

Emeritus Professor Geoffrey Brinkman (21 November 2002; tape sent by post)

Professor John Campbell (1 August 2001; 4 April 2004)

Professors John Campbell; Chris Heath; David Skegg; David Stewart, in discussion (22 November 2000)

Emeritus Professor Alan Clarke, Christchurch (12 November 2003)

Professor David Cole, formerly Dean, Auckland Medical School (7 June 2002)

Emeritus Professor Frederick Fastier (17 January 2001)

Professor Chris Heath (15 December 2004)

Emeritus Professor Barbara Heslop (17 July 2001) and in discussion with Mr John Heslop (13 December 2005)

Emeritus Professor Linda Holloway (10 July 2006)

Professor Andrew Hornblow, Christchurch School (27 August 2002)

Emeritus Professor John Hunter (2 November 2001; 8 November 2001; 11 February 2002; 27 July 2002)

Professor David Jones (1 August 2006; 11 August 2006)

Professor Peter Joyce, Christchurch School (16 June 2006)

Brigadier Brian McMahon (31 August 2006)

Dr Donald Malcolm (14 February 2001)

Emeritus Professor Graham Mortimer and Emeritus Professor George Petersen, in discussion (15 May 2006)

Professor John Nacey, Wellington School (27 July 2006)

Emeritus Professor Thomas O'Donnell, Wellington School (18 September 2003)

Emeritus Professor James Robinson, with Professor Marion Robinson (19 July 2001)

Associate Professor Peter Schwartz (8 December 2004; 18 December 2006)

Emeritus Professor David Stewart (22 November 2000; 9 June 2006)

Dr Hugh Stringer (16 July 2001)

Emeritus Professor William Trotter 12 July 2001)

Emeritus Professor Lawrence Wright (14 February 2001; 20 February 2001; 28 June 2001; 20 December 2006)

Dr Rex Wright St-Clair (7 June 2002; 19 September 2002)

Among others consulted were:

Dr Pat Cotter

Lt Col Andrew Dunn

Dr Colin Geary

Dr Peter Holst

Mr Gregor Macaulay

Dr Will Perry

Ms Joy Rudland

Emeritus Professor Douglass Taylor

Mr David Thomson

Dr Ayesha Verrall

Dr Xaviour Walker

Secondary sources

BOOKS

Anderson, R.G.W. and Simpson, A.D.C., eds, *The Early Years of the Edinburgh Medical School*, Royal Scottish Museum, Edinburgh, 1976.

Anderson, W.A., *Doctor in the Mountains*, A.H. and A.W. Reed, Wellington, 1964.

Angus, John, *A History of the Otago Hospital Board and its Predecessors*, Otago Hospital Board, Dunedin, 1984.

Bade, James N., ed., *Out of the Shadow of War. The German Connection with New Zealand in the Twentieth Century*, Oxford University Press NZ, 1998.

Begg, Neil, *The Intervening Years: a New Zealand account of the years between the last two visits of Halley's Comet*, John McIndoe, Dunedin, 1992.

Bell, Sir Gordon, *Surgeon's Saga*, A.H. and A.W. Reed, Wellington, 1968.

Bennett, Francis, *A Canterbury Tale. The Autobiography of Dr Francis Bennett*, Oxford University Press, Wellington, 1980.

Blainey, Geoffrey, *A Centenary History of the University of Melbourne*, University Press, Melbourne, 1957.

Borrie John, *Despite Captivity: a doctor's life as prisoner of war*, Kimber, London, 1975.

Borrie, John, *Art and Observables in the Otago Medical School*, University of Otago Medical School, Dunedin, 1975.

Bowerbank, Fred Thompson, *A Doctor's Story*, Harry H. Tombs, Wingfield Press, Wellington, 1958.

Brown, Harvey, *Pickerill, Pioneer in Plastic Surgery, Dental Education and Dental Research*, Otago University Press, Dunedin, 2007.

Bryder, Linda, ed., *A Healthy Country: essays on the social history of medicine in New Zealand*, Bridget Williams Books, Wellington, 1981.

Bryder, Linda and Dow, Derek, eds, *New Countries and Old Medicine: proceedings of an International Conference on the History of Medicine and Health, Auckland, New Zealand, 1994.* Pyramid Press, Auckland, 1995.

Bryder, Linda, *A Voice for Mothers: the Plunket Society and infant welfare, 1907–2000*, Auckland University Press, Auckland, 2003.

Chambers, Ron, *Justice and Jellybeans: from Ulster policeman to Otago University proctor*, Missing Stocks Press, Dunedin 2006.

Clayton, J.I., *The History of Anaesthesia in Dunedin Hospital*, Department of Anaesthesia and Intensive Care, Dunedin Hospital and Otago Medical School, Dunedin, 2006.

Daniell, Christine, *A Doctor at War: a Life in Letters, 1914–1943*, Fraser Books, Masterton, 2001.

Dictionary of New Zealand Biography, vol. 1, 1769–1869, Allen and Unwin and the Department of Internal Affairs (I.A. Dept), Wellington, 1990; vol. 2, 1870–1900, Bridget Williams Books and I.A. Dept, Wellington, 1993; vol. 3, 1901–1920, AUP, Auckland and I.A. Dept., Wellington, 1996; vol. 4, 1921–1940, AUP, Auckland and I.A. Dept, Wellington, 1998; vol. 5, 1941–1960, AUP Auckland and I.A. Dept, Wellington, 2000.

Dow, Derek A., *Annotated Bibliography for the History of Medicine in New Zealand*, Hocken Library, University of Otago, Dunedin, 1994.

Dow, Derek A., *Maori Health and Government Policy, 1840–1940*, Victoria University Press with Historical Branch, Department of Internal Affairs, Wellington, 1999.

Dow, Derek A., *Safeguarding the Public Health: a History of the New Zealand Department of Health*, Victoria University Press in association with the Ministry of Health and with the assistance of the Historical Branch, Department of Internal Affairs, Wellington, 1995.

Dunn, Michael, *The Drawings of Russell Clark*, Collins Auckland, 1976

Durham, Gillian, Salmond, Clare and Eberly, Julie, *Women and Men in Medicine: the Career Experiences*, Health Services Research and Development Unit, Department of Health, Wellington, 1989.

Durie, Mason, *Whaiora. Maori Health Development* Oxford University Press. Auckland, 2nd edition, 1998.

Elliott, Sir James, *Scalpel and Sword*, A.H and A.W. Reed, Dunedin and Wellington, 1936.

Elworthy, Sam, *Ritual Song of Defiance: a Social History of Students at the University of Otago*, Otago University Students' Association, Dunedin, 1990.

Erlam, Harry D., *A Notable Result: an historical essay on the beginnings and the first fifteen years of the School of Medicine, University of Auckland*, School of Medicine, University of Auckland, Auckland, 1983.

Fastier, F.N., *Recollections of an Old Scarfie*, Amidine Publications, Dunedin, 2004.

Fenwicke, Rosy, ed., *in practice: the lives of New Zealand women doctors in the 21st century.* Random House, Auckland, 2004.

Fulton, Robert, *Medical Practice in Otago and Southland in the Early Days, Otago Daily Times and Witness*, Dunedin, 1922.

Gauld, R., ed., *Comparative Health Policy in the Asia-Pacific*, Berkshire, England, Open University Press, 2005.

Gauld, Robin, ed., *Continuity amid Chaos: Health Care Management and Delivery in New Zealand*, University of Otago Press, Dunedin, 2003.

Gauld, Robin, *Revolving Doors: New Zealand's Health Reforms*, Institute of Policy Studies and Health

Services Research Centre, Victoria University of Wellington, Wellington, 2001.

Gordon, Doris C., *Backblocks Baby-doctor: An autobiography.* Whitcombe and Tombs, Christchurch and Faber and Faber, London, 1955.

Gordon, Doris, *Doctor Down Under*, Whitcombe and Tombs, Christchurch and Faber, London, 1957.

Gould, John, *The University Grants Committee, 1961–1986: a History.* University Grants Committee, Wellington, 1988.

Guthrie, Douglas, *The Medical School of Edinburgh*, British Medical Association, Edinburgh, 1959.

Hay, Sir David, *Heart Sounds. A life at the forefront of health care*, Steele Roberts Ltd., Wellington, 2005.

Hercock, Fay, *Alice: the making of a woman doctor, 1914–1974*, AUP, Auckland 1999.

Hercus, Sir Charles and Bell, Sir Gordon, *The Otago Medical School under the First Three Deans*, E. and S. Livingstone, London, 1964

Herd, Joyce, *Cracks in a Glass Ceiling: New Zealand Women 1975–2004*, New Zealand Federation of Graduate Women, Otago Branch, Dunedin, 2005.

Heslop, John, ed., *The History of Logan Park, The evolution of a sporting complex*, University Oval Development Committee, Dunedin, 2003.

Hocken, A.G. 'Dr T.M. Hocken: a Gentleman of His Time', Hocken lecture 1986, Hocken Library, University of Otago, Dunedin.

Hodge, Merton, *The Wind and the Rain*, A play in three acts, Victor Gollanz, London, 1934.

Jones, D.W. Carmalt, *Annals of the University of Otago Medical School*, A.H. and A.W. Reed. Wellington and Dunedin, 1945.

King, Mary, *Truby King – the Man*, George Allen and Unwin, London, 1948.

Myers, Bernard, *The Reminiscences of a Physician*, Reed, Wellington, 1949.

King, Michael, *The Penguin History of New Zealand*, Penguin Books Auckland, 2003.

Knight, Hardwicke and Wales, Niel, *Buildings of Dunedin: an Illustrated Architectural Guide to New Zealand's Victorian City*, John McIndoe, Dunedin, 1988.

Macdonald, Charlotte, Penfold, Merimeri and Williams, Bridget, eds, *The Book of New Zealand Women, Ko Kui Ma Te Kaupapa*, Bridget Williams Books, Wellington, 1991.

McGibbon Ian, ed., *The Oxford Companion to New Zealand Military History*, Oxford University Press, Auckland, 2000.

McIlraith, Jill, ed., *The Goods Train Doctors: stories of women doctors in New Zealand, 1920–1993*, New Zealand Medical Women's Association, Dunedin, 1994.

McLeave, Hugh, *McIndoe, Plastic Surgeon*, Frederick Muller Ltd, London 1961.

Maxwell, Margaret D., ed., *Women Doctors in New Zealand: an Historical Perspective, 1921–1986*,

IMS (NZ) Auckland, 1990.

Moody, Winifred, *The Dynamic Doctor – Arthur Moody of Otago*, Richards, Collins, Auckland, 1978.

Moore, Christopher, Rolleston, George, Riminton, John and Hornblow, Andrew, *A Vision Realised: the Christchurch School of Medicine, University of Otago, 1972–1997*, Christchurch School of Medicine, Christchurch, 1998.

Moore, Sir Patrick Eisdell, *So Old So Quick*, David Ling Publishing Ltd, Auckland, 2004.

Morrell, W.P., *The University of Otago. A centennial history*, John McIndoe Ltd, Dunedin, 1969.

Morrison, Elizabeth J., *In Memory. Dr Margaret Cruickshank*, Whitcombe and Tombs Ltd, Christchurch, ?1923.

Nye, E.R., ed., *Medical Research in Otago, 1922–1997, as portrayed by 75 years of the Proceedings of the University of Otago Medical School*, Otago Medical School Research Society, Dunedin, 1998.

Parry, Gordon, *Otago Medical School, 1875–1975. An historical sketch.* John McIndoe, Dunedin, 1975.

Parton, Hugh, *The University of New Zealand*, Auckland University Press/Oxford University Press, for the University Grants committee, Auckland 1979.

Porter, Roy, *The Greatest Benefit to Mankind: a Medical History of Humanity from Antiquity to the Present*, Harper Collins, London, 1997.

Pound, Reginald, *Gillies, Surgeon Extraordinary*, Michael Joseph, London and Whitcombe and Tombs, New Zealand, 1964.

Prior, Ian, *Elespie and Ian: memoir of a marriage*, Steele Roberts, Wellington 2006.

Rice, Geoffrey W., *Black November. The 1918 Influenza Pandemic in New Zealand*, revised and enlarged second edition, Canterbury University Press, 2005.

Rice, Geoffrey W., ed., *The Oxford History of New Zealand*, 2nd edition, Oxford University Press, Auckland, 1992.

Robb, Sir Douglas, *Medical Odyssey. An Autobiography*, Collins, Auckland, 1967.

Rogers, Lindsay, *Guerrilla Surgeon*, Collins, London, 1957.

Russell, Kenneth F., *The Melbourne Medical School, 1862–1962*, Melbourne University Press, Melbourne, 1977.

Sargison, P.A., *Notable Women in New Zealand Health*, Longman Paul, Auckland, 1993.

Schofield, G.H., ed., *A Dictionary of New Zealand Biography*, Department of Internal Affairs, Wellington, 1940.

Schwartz, Peter L., Heath, Christopher J., Egan, Anthony G., *The Art of the Possible: Ideas from a Traditional Medical School Engaged in Curricular Revision*, University of Otago Press, Dunedin, 1994.

Schwartz, Peter, Mennin, Stewart and Webb, Graham, eds, *PBL: Case Studies, Experience and Practice*,

Kegan Page Ltd, London, 2001.

Scott, David, ed., *The Story of Auckland Hospital, 1847–1977*, Medical Historical Library Committee of the Royal Australasian College of Physicians in New Zealand, Auckland, 1977.

Scott, John H., *Without Parade or Fuss. A biographical memoir of John Halliday Scott, M.D.*, John Scott, Administration Services, Christchurch, 1996.

Shackleton, Michael, *Operation Vietnam. A New Zealand Surgical First*, University of Otago Press, Dunedin, 2004.

Stout, T. Duncan M., *New Zealand Medical Services in Middle East and Italy*, War History Branch, Department of Internal Affairs, Wellington, 1956.

Taylor, Douglass W., *The Monro Collection in the Medical Library of the University of Otago*, University of Otago Press, Dunedin, 1979.

Thompson, G.E., *History of the Otago University, 1869–1919*, J. Wilkie, Dunedin, 1919.

Watson, R. Burns, *The Doctor Must get Through: 50 Years a General-Practitioner-Surgeon*, A.H. and A.W. Reed, Wellington, 1971.

Winton, Ronald, *Why the Pomegranate? A History of the Royal Australasian College of Physicians*, Royal Australasian College of Physicians, Sydney, 1988.

Wright-St. Clair, R.E., *A History of the New Zealand Medical Association: the first 100 years*, Butterworth, Wellington, 1987.

Wright-St Clair, R.E., ed., *Proceedings of the First New Zealand Conference on the History of New Zealand and Australian Medicine, Waikato Hospital, 1987*. Waikato Postgraduate Medical Society, Waikato Hospital, Hamilton, 1987.

ARTICLES

Belgrave, Michael, 'A Subtle Containment: Women in New Zealand Medicine, 1893–1941', *New Zealand Journal of History*, vol. 22.1, April 1988, pp. 44–55.

Bolitho, D.G., 'Some Financial and Medico-Political Aspects of the New Zealand Medical Profession's Reaction to the Introduction of Social Security', *NZJH*, vol. 18.1, April 1984, pp. 34–49.

Carr, Ian and Taylor, Douglass, 'Physiology in the Otago Medical School: the John Malcolm Letters', in Linda Bryder and Derek Dow, eds, *New Countries and Old Medicine*, Pyramid Press, Auckland 1995, pp. 231–234.

Cotter, Pat, 'A Tribute. The Contribution of the Otago University Medical SDchool and its Students in World War One', *NZMJ*, vol. 118, no. 1213, 15 April 2005.

Entin, M.A., 'Edinburgh Medical College at the End of the Eighteenth Century and the Training of North American Doctors', *Proceedings of the Royal College of Physicians, Edinburgh*, 1988, 28: pp. 218–228.

Erlam, H.D., 'Dr William Ledingham Christie, New Zealand's First Medical Graduate', *NZMJ*, January 1961, pp. 1–6.

Fraenkel, G.J. 'The Medical School of the University of Otago at Dunedin', *British Journal of Surgery*, vol. 52, no. 11, November 1965, pp. 835–841.

Hercus, Sir Charles Ernest, 'New Zealand and Medical Research'. The second Hudson Lecture, delivered to the Wellington Branch of the Royal Society of New Zealand, 23 August 1950, *N.Z. Science Review*, 8, 1950, pp. 105–112.

Hercus, Professor C.E. and H.D. Purves, 'New Zealand's Requirement for Doctors', *NZMJ*, vol. XLII, no. 229 June 1943, pp. 89–96.

Hercus, C.E. 'Women and National Survival', Wilding Memorial Lecture, 1940, Canterbury University College, Whitcombe and Tombs, 1940.

Heslop, Barbara F., 'Where are Tomorrow's Specialists?' *NZMJ*, 13 October 1995, pp. 407–410.

Heslop, Barbara, Robin Molloy, Hendrika Waal-Manning and Ngaire Walsh, 'Women in Medicine in New Zealand', *NZMJ*, vol. 77, no. 491, April 1973, pp. 219–229.

Hocken, A.G. 'Hocken the Coroner: the Dismissal', R.E. Wright-St Clair ed., *Proceedings of the First New Zealand Conference on the History of New Zealand and Australian Medicine*, Waikato Postgraduate Medical Society, Hamilton, 1987.

Hunter, J.D., 'The Clinical Club of Dunedin (1915–1939)', R.E. Wright-St Clair, ed., *Proceedings of the First Conference on the History of New Zealand and Australian Medicine*, Waikato Postgraduate Medical Society, Hamilton, 1987.

Miller, Andrew P. MB ChB, Haden, Patricia, MS., Schwartz, Peter L. MD, and Loten, Ernest G., MB ChB, PhD, 'Pilot studies of In-course Assessment for a Revised Medical Curriculum: II. Computer-based, Individual', *Academic Medicine*, vol. 72, no. 12, December 1997, pp. 1113–1115.

Miller, Andrew P., Schwartz, Peter L. and Loten, Ernest G., Department of Pathology, University of Otago Medical School, Dunedin, New Zealand, '"Systems Integration": a middle way between problem-based learning and traditional courses', *Medical Teacher*, vol. 22, no. 1, 2000, pp. 51–58.

Mullin, W.J., 'The Monro Family and the Monro Collection of Books and MSS', *NZMJ*, vol. 35, 1936, pp. 221–229.

Neuman, Fieke, 'Pots and Pieces: the Anatomy Museum of the Otago Medical School and How It Came To Be', New Zealand Museums Journal, 23 (1) 1993, pp. 17–22.

Page, Dorothy, 'Dissecting a Community: Women Medical Students at the University of Otago, 1891–1924, in Barbara Brookes and Dorothy Page, eds, *Communities of Women: Historical Perspectives*, University of Otago Press, Dunedin, 2002, pp. 111–127.

Page Dorothy, 'The First Lady Graduates: Women with Degrees from Otago University, 1885–1900', in Barbara Brookes, Charlotte Macdonald and Margaret Tennant, eds, *Women in History 2: Essays on Women in New Zealand*, Bridget Williams Books, 1992, pp. 98–128.

Schwartz, Peter L., MD, Loten, Ernest. G., MB ChB, Ph D, and Miller, Andrew P., MB ChB, 'Curriculum Reform at the University of Otago Medical School', *Academic Medicine*, vol. 74, no. 6, June 1999, pp. 673–680.

Schwartz, Peter L. MD, Loten, Ernest G., MB ChB, PhD, and Miller, Andrew P., MB ChB, 'Pilot Studies of In-course Assessment for a Revised Medical Curriculum: I, Paper-based, Whole Class', *Academic Medicine*, vol. 72, no. 12, December 1997, pp. 1109–1112.

Simpson, F.O. et al., 'The Milton Survey: Part 1, General methods, Height, Weight and 24-hour Excretion of Sodium, Potassium, Calcium, Magnesium and Creatinine', *NZMJ*, vol. 87, no. 613, 14 June 1978, pp. 379–382.

Taylor, D.W. 'The Books and Manuscripts of Alexander Monro *primus* in the Medical School of the University of Otago', in R.G.W. Anderson and A.D.C, Simpson, eds, *The Early Years of the Edinburgh Medical School*, Royal Scottish Museum, Edinburgh, 1976.

Taylor, D.W. 'The Monro Collection: a New Zealand Archive', in R. E. Wright-St Clair ed., *Proceedings of the First New Zealand Conference on the History of New Zealand and Australian Medicine*, Waikato Postgraduate Medical Society, Hamilton, 1987.

Wright-St Clair, R.E., 'The Monros and their Books', *Digest*, 1963, pp. 27–32.

Wright-St Clair, Rex E., 'Sir David Monro, MD (1813–1877) of New Zealand: his antecedents and his descendants' *Journal of Medical Biography* 2004; 12, pp. 32–37.

Secondary Sources

UNPUBLISHED

Amodeo, Charlotte, 'The Murder Trial of Senga Whittingham: an Examination into the Nature of Gender Relations in the 1950s', 490 Dissertation in History, University of Otago, 2001.

Anderson, Honor', Hydatids: a Disease of Human Carelessness. A History of Human Hydatid Disease in New Zealand', MA in History, University of Otago, 1997.

Brown, Diana, 'Between Lab and Kitchen: the Unconventional Career of Dr Muriel Bell', MA in History, University of Otago, 2006.

Brown, Diana, '"Stepping Stone to Cretinism": Goitre in New Zealand 1920–1950'. BA Hons, History, University of Otago, 2000.

Caswell, E.H., "An overdose of refugees": refugee medical practitioners in New Zealand, c. 1930– c. 1950, BA Hons History, University of Otago, 2005.

Corkill, B.M., 'The Wellington School of Medicine: Origins', typescript, n.d., Hunter Collection.

Dawson, Sir Joseph Bernard, 'Without Varnish: a Simple Story' (an autobiography in the third person), c. 1952.

Dooley, Sharon, 'Ivory Tower Idyll: students at the University of Otago in the Depression', Long essay, BA Hons History, University of Otago, 1983.

Hunter, J.D., 'The Christie Review', Hunter Collection, 1994.

Jeffery, Keith, 'Surgical Beginnings' Dunedin and the Edinburgh Connection, Sir Gordon Bell Memorial Lecture, 6 September 2000.

Jeffery, Keith 'Back to the Future'. Dunedin's Medical Heritage and its Relevance Today', Ritchie Memorial Lecture, 1999.

Jeffery, Keith,' Surgery in Victorian Dunedin', lecture to Otago Settlers Association, September 2004.

Macdonald, April, 'The Chemotherapy Revolution? Tuberculosis in New Zealand 1940–1960', BA Hons History, University of Otago, 2000.

O'Donnell, T.V., 'Collated Material of Interest During the Development of the Wellington Clinical School, Later Wellington School of Medicine, Subsequently Wellington School of Medicine of the University of Otago, 1971– January 1992', Hunter Collection.

O'Donnell, T.V., 'The Development of the Wellington School of Medicine: a Personal View', Hunter Collection.

Rolleston, George, 'The Genesis of the Christchurch School', Hunter Collection, 1992.

Treanor, Captain K.R., (RNZAMC, retired.) *The Staff, the Serpent and the Sword. The Story of the Royal New Zealand Army Medical Corps*, 2nd edition, Christchurch, 1995.

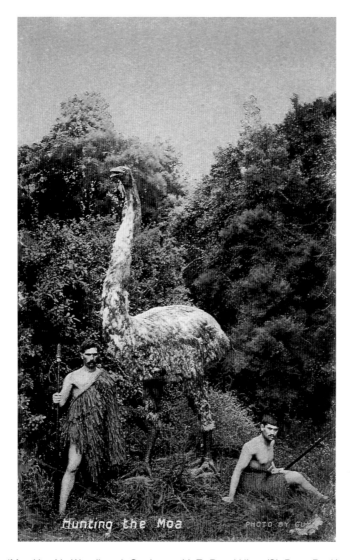

Hunting the Moa

'Moa Hunt' in Woodhaugh Gardens, with Te Rangi Hiroa (Sir Peter Buck),
left, and Tutere Wi Repa. A popular postcard of the day.

John Broughton collection.

INDEX

A number in **bold** indicates an illustration. **C** in bold
indicates an illustration in the colour section.
An en dash (–) between two numbers indicates
continuous treatment of a topic, a tilde (~) only
that a topic is referred to on each page in the range.

abbreviations 14
Abnormal Structure and Function course 254, 258
Acland, Richard Hugh 207
accreditation of Medical School: AMC 237, 240, 241,
    245, 250~52, 261, 262; MCNZ 236, 240, 260
Adam, Bill 244
Adam, Hugh 140
Adam, Ken 191
Adams, Albert **124**
Adams, Brandon 283, 285
Adams, D.D. (Duncan) 128, 140, 266
Adams, R.N. 53
Adams, William Edgar (Bill) **C**, 131, 133, 144, 181,
    186, **188**, 205, **207**, 222, 231, 301; Acting Dean
    169; biographical sketch 182; Dean 161, 177, 181;
    death 184; on Gowland 89; professorship 121;
    research 182; teaching methods 131
Aickin, Donald R. 191, 204, **235**
Aisinan, Ali **281**
Aitken, Robert S. **152**, 277, 289; on medical
    education 137, 151–2; Vice-Chancellor 151, 152
Alexander, Edward William 19
Alldred, Alan 182
Allen Hall 105, 130
Allen, James 76
Allen, Sydney 70
Alqahtani, Abdulrahman **281**
Alshammari, Mai 281, **281**
Alumnus Association 204–5; Dean's reports 205,
    225, 226, 234, 236, 253
anaesthesia 17, 93, 295
Anaesthesia (and Intensive Care) 155, 247, 253, 300;
    Christchurch 191; lectureship in 84, 93; professors
    208; splits from Surgery 208

Anatomy **135**, 300; and Structural Biology 251;
    Christie Report 173; dissection room 50, **50**;
    Gowland period 87–9; library 89; Museum **C,** 31,
    80; professors 83, 87–8, 89, 121, 131, 182; research
    269; splits from Physiology 41; student numbers
    89; technical assistants 50
Anatomy Act 21, 22
Anatomy and Physiology 31; Chair established
    19–20; department splits 41; first students 27, 27,
    28; professors 21, 25; technical assistants 31
Anderson, J.W. **47**
Anderson, W.A. (Bill) 50, 102
Andrew and Auld (Edinburgh) 19~21, 25
Angus, John 35–6, 82, **154**; *History of the Otago
    Hospital Board* 35
Annand, A. 266
Anscombe, Edmund 78
antibiotics 124
arteriosclerosis 98
Arthur, Glenys 150
aseptic principle 17, 33
Ashburn Hall 66
Asthma and Respiratory Foundation 268, 272, 273
asthma research 249, 271–2
Auckland Hospital: sixth-year clinical training 87
Auckland Hospital Board 120
Auckland Medical School 87, 132, 156, 169, 188,
    193, 197, 204, 236, 265, 284; Christie Report 176;
    medical students' association 219; *NZMJ* support
    170, 203; opens 176, 183, 194; origins 77, 118, 120,
    136, 189; Otago graduates on staff 293; student
    intake 180, 181, 214; Trainee Intern programme
    211; *see also* Branch Faculties
Australasian and New Zealand Association for
    Medical Education (now the Association for Health
    Professional Education) 255
Australian Medical Council (AMC): accreditation of
    Med. School 237, 240, 241, 245, 250~52, 261, 262
Australian Medical Students' Association (AMSA)
    219, 220, 285–6

Averill, L.C.L. **188**
Aviation Medicine 251, 285
Axford, Ian 229
Ayling, John 242, 244, **244**

Bachelor of Medical Laboratory Science (BMedLabSc) 237, 260
Bachelor of Medical Science (BMedSc) 127, 133, 156, 237
Bachelor of Physiotherapy 260
Bacteriology (and Public Health) 44, 75, 87, 300; accommodation 75, 78, 134; department splits 155; professors 44, 83, 93, 95, 125; salaries 85, 111
Baird, Margaret 265
Baker, A.B. (Barry) 208, **235**, 247
Baker, Eleanor 49–50, 52, 85
Bamforth, Aileen 130
Barbezat, G.O. **235**
Barclay, Marjorie 84, 295
Barker, Coralee **244**
Barnett, Louis 31, 37, 45, 54, 85, 92, 97, **110**, 111; biographical sketch 33; donations 33, 83, 85, 86, 92, 105; military service 66, 70, 71; MRC committee 127; on Scott 25, 29, 31; professorship 33, 44; siting of new building 77; surgical hygiene 33
Barnett, Ralph 33, 154
Barratt-Boyes, Brian 293
Barry, John 220
Batchelor, Ferdinand 32, 34, 38, 63, 75, 83; lack of maternity cases 80; military service 66, 71; on hospital conditions 35, 36; opposes women doctors 50, 52; OUMSA president 56; professorship 44, 63
Batchelor Hospital 80, 81
Batchelor, Stanley 70, 92; Clinical Club 97, **98**, 99
Bates, David 169, 187, 215, 225
Bates Report (1981) 215–16, 229, 230
Baxter, Helena 53
Bayley, Catherine **51**
Beacham, Arthur 167, 168, 186
Beaglehole, J.C. 299
Bealey, Helen 29
Beasley, A.W. **147**
Beasley, Richard 247
Beaven, D.W. (Don) 191, **201**, 204, 235, 266; professorship 191; research 188, 191, 270
Begg, A.M. 86
Begg, J.A. **121**
Begg, Neil 91, 116, 124, 204; *The Intervening Years* 122
Belgrave, Michael 295
Bell, Gordon 92, 108, **129**, 138, 151; Clinical Club 97, 98; military service 71; on BMedSc 133; on Ferguson 61, 62, 64, 74, 84, 231; on Fitchett 91; on Hercus 126; on Malcolm 42; on medical education 136; on Miss Thomson 231; on Murray Falconer 292; on R.S. Aitken 151; on Scott 29; on women

graduates 294–5, 296; *Otago Medical School ... first three Deans* 43, 62, 92, 125; professorship 61, 71, 83, 92, 93; *Surgeon's Saga* 71; teaching methods 92
Bell, J.A.T. **47**
Bell, Muriel 83, 89–90, 131, **141**, 294; Department of Health 117, 131; honorary degree 141, 290; *Lecture Notes on Normal Nutrition* 141; Milk Board 141; MRC appointment 127; nutritional work 131, 141; on Griesbach 127
Benevolent Institute 80
Benham, William Blaxland 111
Bennett, Francis 103, 105
Bennett, L.A. **188**
Bielschowsky, Franz 139–40
Bielschowsky, Marianne 139, 140
Biochemistry 78, 155, 251, 300; buildings 177, 178, 186, 238, 302; Christie Report 173; Clinical Biochemistry splits off 168; professors 127, 132, 168, 297
Bioethics Research Centre 242, 253, 260, 275, 300; *Medical Ethics* 275
Biomedical Ethics 242
Black, David **47**
Black, James 19, 21, 26, 27
Black, Ross 244
Blackman, Gary 264
Blennerhassett, John B. 182, **235**, 242
Blundell, Denis 204
Booth, L.H. **69**
Borborygmi 222, 283
Borrie, Alex **124**
Borrie, John 122, 124, 138–9, 205; *Despite Captivity* 122; John Borrie History Hall 139
Borrie, W.H. **44**, **47**
Boswell, Ross 250
Botany 27, 31
Bowerbank, F.T. 108
Branch Faculties 87, 115, 136, 155, 156, 161, 162, 170, 171, 178, 203, 270; Auckland 162, 165, 188, 189, 193; Christchurch 188–9, 193; Clinical Dean's role 178; established 188; Medical Units 270; post-war staffing 136, 156; research 270, 301; Wellington 188, 193, 194; *see also* Christchurch Clinical School; Wellington Clinical School
Brennan, Murray 290
Brinkman, Geoffrey **C**, 117, 118, 204, 210, 214, 225~32; biographical sketch 226; Dean 161, 209, 225; Lincoln conference (1985) 228, 255
British Empire Cancer Campaign 86, 140, 154
British Empire Science Conference (1946) 133
British Medical Association: Auckland Branch 119; New Zealand Branch 87; Otago Branch 63, 77, 98
Brock, Lawrence 132
Brookes, Chandler M.C. 137
Brown, Harvey 72
Brown, William 28, 29, 48, 53
Brunton, Warwick 281

Buck, Peter (Te Rangi Hiroa) 52, **52**, 53, 56, 104, 290, 301
Buckfield, Patricia **205**, 276
Budge, Margaret **239**
buildings *see* Dunedin Hospital buildings; Otago Medical School buildings
Burnham Military Camp 117, 122, 221
Burns, Charles Ritchie 107, 200, 202, 295
Burns, Thomas 54
Burns, W. 19
bursaries 69–70, 121, 178
Bush, Alice 296, 297
Butler, Eddie **103**
Byrd Antarctic Expedition 98, 104

Cairney, John 88, 89, 193, 294
Cairns, Hugh 134
Cameron, Andrew 64–5, 75
Campbell, Alistair 242–3
Campbell, Anne 285
Campbell, John **C,** 243, 244, 249, 252; Dean of Faculty 251, 263; 'New Pathway' proposal 263; professorship 227
Cancer Genetics Laboratory 275
cancer research 86, 139, 140, 274–5; MRC committee 95
Cancer Society 140, 268, 273
Canterbury College 24
Canterbury Health 241, 242
Canterbury Medical Research Foundation 268
Canterbury Medical Students Association (CMSA) 284
Capital Coast Health 241
Capping 102, 105; chorus 148; concert 104; inclusion of women 148; Knox farce 148; post-war resumption 146, 148; procession 105, 148; Selwyn ballet 148; sexism 104, 278; Sextet **103**, 148; wartime suspension 143
Cardiac Surgery 247
cardiovascular research 271, 272
Carmalt Jones, Dudley W. 53, 90–91, **91**, 97, 100, 107, 117, 128, 231; *Annals ... Otago Medical School* 25, 41, 43, 91; bookplate **128**; military service 71; on bursaries 69; on Champtaloup (poem) 94; on Colquhoun 32; on Coughtrey 21; on Ferguson 61–2, 63, 74, 77; on outbreak of WWII 116; on thyroid research 45; *Proceedings ... Otago Medical School* 86; professorship 71, 83, 90
Carman, J.B. 204
Carney Centre for Pharmacogenomics 273
Carrell, Robin 273, 293
Carswell, W.E. 111
Cartwright Inquiry 257
Cartwright, Silvia 257
centenary celebrations 131, 181, 184, 199–207, **201**
Centre for Urban Health and Development 273
cervical cancer 257
Chadwick, Vincent S. 227

Chaffer, Harold 154
Chamberlain, C.W.S. 85
Champtaloup, Sydney 64, 66, 70, 75, 83, **94**, 94–5; Clinical Club 97; death 94, 98; new building campaign 75, 76, 84, 94; professorship 44, 83, 93; research 45, 85, 93
Chang, Kathleen (née Pih) 104, **104**
Changi prison camp (Singapore) 124
Chapman, Sylvia 295–6
Chemistry 20, 21, 26, 31
Chetwynd, Jane 250
Child Cancer Foundation 282
child development research 266, 273, 274, 275–7
Children's Health Service 294–5
Chinese medical students 104
Chisholm, Russell 87; teachers evaluated 88, 90, 91, 94
cholesterol research 98, 141, 163, 207
Christchurch Child Development Study *see* Christchurch Health and Development Study
Christchurch Clinical School 177, 179~81, 183, 199, 225, 228, 251, **252**, 253, 300, 302; accreditation 245; administrative structure 191; Bates Report 215; building programme 184, 186, **190**, **211**, 302; Council 191; Deans 185, 190, 229, 232, 249, 273; departments 191; Detailed Planning Committee 189, 190; funding 208, 210–11, 229, 233; health reforms 241; Health Science degrees 250; mace **233**; 'Mission Conference' 234; opening 192; origins 169, 187–8, **188**; relations with Dunedin 209, 229, 234, 250; relations with Hospital & CHEs 229, 234, 241, 242, 245; renamings 229, 233, 253; research 266, 270, 271, 272–3; research funding 268; student intake 189, 190, 229; teaching methods 211; trainee intern programme 211–12; *see also* Branch Faculties
Christchurch Consultation Liaison Psychiatry Service 191
Christchurch Health and Development Study 191, 210, 266, 273, 275–6
Christchurch Hospital 189, 270; clinical school buildings 189, 210; population-based funding 230; sixth-year clinical training 87
Christchurch School of Medicine (and Health Sciences) *see* the earlier name Christchurch Clinical School
Christchurch Women's Hospital 189, 191
Christie, Grant **239**
Christie Report (1968) 171–7, 178, 182~7, 218–19, 230, 302; Clinical School advocated 175, 189; clinical training 173–5; Dean's role 175; medical education 172–5; political response 177; preclinical curriculum 173
Christie, R.L. **69**
Christie, Ronald 169~71, 176, 181, 189, 194, 215; honorary degree 207; *see also* Christie Report
Christie, Ross 206
Christie, William Ledingham 46–7, **47**, 48

Church, Robert 68
Clark, Helen 232, 266
Clark, Russell **44**; *Medical Digest* drawings **89**, **107**, 107–8
Clarke, Alan M. **C**, 204, **206**, **233**, 234, **235**, 249, 259, 268; Christie Report 171–2; Dean 232; professorship 182; Spinal Injuries Unit Director (Burwood) 249
Clinical Biochemistry 168, 171, 258, 300
Clinical Club 61, 94, 97–8, **98**, 99
clinical medicine 28, 32, 56, 179, 193, 259; research 85, 131, 139
Clinical Medicine and Therapeutics 90
clinical pathology 162, 193
clinical pharmacology 204, 216, 260
Clinical Pharmacology 198, 264
Clinical Schools *see* Christchurch Clinical School; Wellington Clinical School
Clinical Society 108, 148, 217
clinical training 17, 19, 23, 27–8, 31, 41, 111, 246; Christie Report 173–5; curriculum 211; deficiencies 166, 170; facilities 36, 38, 40; increased 162; initial class 34; sixth-years to Christchurch etc. 87; staff 43
Closs, J. **27**, 28, 53
Cole, David 131, 133, 142, 230, 293; Capping Controller 148
Coleman, Patricia Dorothy 165
Coll, Barry 212
Colquhoun, Daniel 32, 39, 40, 66, 70, 85, 90, **110**; founds *NZMJ* 64; goitre research 45; library 98; new building campaign 75; on hospital conditions 35, 36; on Scott 29; professorship 44
Conference on the Role of the Doctor (1985) 255–7
Cook Island medical students 289
Cook Islands 104, 133, 289
Coombs, Jack 132
Cooper, Nic **244**
Corbett, Elizabeth 179
Corkill, Brian 193, 213; development of Wellington Clinical School 193~8
Coronary Care Club 222
CORSO 296
Cotter, Pat 191
Cotton, Marguerite: Hercus (portrait) **115**; *Physiology* (art work) **90**
Coughtrey, Millen 21, 22, 23, 24, 207
Cox, L.W. 204
Craig, Florence 122
Craig, Tessa 122
Crane, Julian 271
Crawshaw, J.H. 99
cricket 53, 105, 220; Knox vs Selwyn 143–4; Tournament 148; University club 53
Critic 105, 106, 115, 142, 145, 148, 230; first woman editor 144; founding 105; on medical students 102, 145, 148; on World War II 117; student 'types' **106**

Crooks, Terry 258
Crown Health Enterprises (CHEs) 238, 242, 245; management style 242; relations with Med. School 240, 241
Cruickshank, Margaret 48, 49, **49**, **50**, 294, 295
CT scanner 210
Cullen, John 146, 220
curriculum *see* medical education

Danks, Alan 168, 175, 177, 181, 189
D'Ath, Eric 95, 97, **129**, 164; honorary degree 200; professorship 83, 95
Davis, Thomas 289
Davies, Tony 220
Dawson, J.B. (Bernard) 81, 84, 97, 108, **129**, 134, 138, 295; MRC committee 127; professorship 83, 96
Dean's Department 155, 162
Dean's role 161–2, 209, 232, 251, 253; Bates Report 216; Brinkman's views 230; Christie Report 175; Clinical Dean 178, 181, 184; Dean of Faculty 230, 232; staffing 167, 175
Dean's Secretary 64, 231
Deck, John Field 19
Deem, Helen (née Easterfield) 141, 295
Delahunt, Brett 249
Denny-Brown, Derek 88, 89, 105, 204; honorary degree 290
Dental School 45, 125, 151, 152–4, 164, 186, 217, 251, **252**, 271; canteen 217; Dean/Director 71, 92, 154, **252**, 295; funding 166, 246; MRC committee 139; subsumed in Health Sciences 234; siting of 77; staff 72, 177
dental students 83, 125, 143, 156; involvement in student affairs 142; military service 67, 69, 73, 118; sports 283
dentistry 87, 154, 253, 271
Department of Health 38, 85, 125, 131, 157, 168, 171, 175, 176, 228, 238, 239, 267; Children's Health Service 294–5; Division of School Hygiene 294; medical manpower 214; establishment of clinical schools 189; iodised salt 140; Maori Hygiene Division 52; maternity training 80, 81; *see also* Medical Research Council; Ministry of Health
Department of Public Health 85, 111, 293
Dews, Ted 186, 189, 196
diabetes research 191, 206, 207, 246, 274
Digest see Medical Digest
Diploma in Health Science 250
Diploma in Public Health 228
District Health Boards (DHBs) 246
Dixon, Cyril W. 164, 209, 266
doctor's role 255–7
Dodd, Roger 196
Dominion 247
Dow, Derek 294
Dowell, Anthony 249
Drennan, Murray 64, 84, 93, 94–5, 100; Clinical Club 97, 98, **98**, 99; military service 70, 71; on

Champtaloup 94; professorship 44, 70, 71, 83; research 45, 85, 86; teaching methods 93–4
Drinking Horn 144, 147, 217
Dunedin Child Development Study *see* Dunedin Multidisciplinary Health and Development Research Unit
Dunedin Club 65, 90, 200
Dunedin Goitre Clinic 98
Dunedin Heart Unit Trust 268
Dunedin Hospital 21, 22, 24, 175, 209; 19th-century conditions 34–6; building programme 36–7, 38, 154; Christie Report 174; Clinical Department 92; 'clinical material' supply 40, 87, 174, 178, 228; CT scanner 210; Medical Superintendents 66, 187; relations with Medical School 36, 37–8; Superintendents 19, 24; teaching hospital 34, 157, 174, 177, 195; x-ray plant 37; *see also* Queen Mary Maternity Hospital, Wakari Hospital
Dunedin Hospital buildings 302; Campbell Pavilion 36, **37**; 'Exhibition' Building 34, **35**, 82; Gt King St Building (1936) 79, 82; King Edward VII Memorial Block 38, **38**; laboratories 37; maternity hospital siting 81; new ward block 177, 178, 187; Nightingale Ward **38**; nurses' homes 36, 38, 82, 154; operating theatres 36, 37; ophthalmic ward 36; Queen Mary Maternity Hospital 81, **82**, 96; Victoria Jubilee Pavilion 37; Wakari Hospital **153**, 153–4; Ward Pavilion 38
Dunedin Hospital Trustees 35, 36, 38, 56
Dunedin Multidisciplinary Health and Development Study 266, 274, 275–7
Dunedin Public Art Gallery 65
Dunedin Savings Bank 40
Dunedin School of Medicine *see* Otago Medical School 1980–2000
Dunn, Andrew 285
Dunn, Anna (née Wyeth) 285

ear, nose and throat 63, 79, 82, 136, 292
Ear, Nose and Throat 111
Eccles, J.C. (Jack, later Sir John) 131–2, **132**, 264, 265, 269, 292, 301; Nobel Prize 133; professorship 121; research 132–3
Eccles, Michael 275
Edgar Centre for Diabetes Research 274, 300
Edinburgh Medical School 94, 100; *see also* University of Edinburgh
Edson, Norman 78, 127, 137, 168; professorship 132
Egan, Tony 254
Elliott, James 28, 55
Elliott, Randall 65
Ellison, Edward 104
Elvidge, Ron 148, **148**
Elworthy, Sam 56, 145, 278
Emery, G.M. 172
Enema 263, 279, 280, 283–4
endocrinology 139, 140, 163, 173, 188, 202, 266, 270~72

epidemiology 216, 254, 266, 270, 272~4
ethics *see* medical ethics
Eunson, Keith 176
Evans, Donald 275
Evening Star 205, 207; fundraising for University 40
eye, diseases of 33, 63, 82, 136, 138, 291

Faculty of Dentistry 234
Faculty of Medicine 120, **235**, 236, 279; administrative structure 211, 251–2, **252**, 253; Bates Report 215, 225; Branch Faculties 115; Christie Report 171, 172, 175, 181; Clinical Schools 180, 188, 230, 236; curriculum committees 175, 178, 183, 257, 262; Dean's role 161–2, 175; established 39; Faculty Board 209, 211, 253, 258, 260, 261; Ferguson 62, 63, 64, 74; inter-School relations 209, 229, 230; library committee 100; OUSA representative 52–3; refugee doctor question 119; research culture 126; siting of buildings 77, 81; six-year course 87; student representation 219; Sub-Dean 23; subsumed in Health Sciences 234; teaching responsibilities 83
Falconer, Alexander Robertson 38, 53, 66, 67, 292
Falconer, Murray 131, 133, 292
Family Planning Association 296
Fastier, Frederick (Fred) 126, 141, 209, 264, 270; professorship 139, 164, 208
Ferguson, Henry Lindo (Sir Lindo) **C,** 36, 37, 61, **62**, 97, 107, **110**, 161, **207**, 208, 231, 299; appointed Dean 63, 64; appointed lecturer 33; biographical sketch 63; building programme 74–82; character & style 61–2, 65; deanship reviewed 109–11; donations 86; income 64, 65; knighthood 65; library purchases 100; marriage 63, 65; maternity hospital planning 80–81; on Hercus's teaching methods 95; on hospital conditions 34–5; on medical salaries 111; professorship 44, 63, 82; travels 63, 84; World War I 66, 67, 69, 70; *see also* Otago Medical School 1914–1937 (Ferguson)
Ferguson, Mary Emmeline (née Butterworth) 63, 65
Fergusson, David 273, 276, **276**
Fijian medical students 104–5
Fitchett, Frank 44, 84, 91, 117, 128, **128**; character & style 91; Clinical Club 97, 98, **98**, 99; military service 66; professorship 83, 90; research 45
Fitzgerald, G.P **69**
Fitzgerald, J. 54
Fitzgerald, W. 54
Fitzgerald, Walden 124
Fletcher Construction 190
Fletcher Development 187
Florey, Howard 133
fluoridation 141, 154
Focken, C.M. **44**
Fookes, 'Hatch' 105
Fraenkel, Gustav 138, 169, 172, 182, 183
Fraser, Peter 81, 127
Fraser, Robin **235**, 250

Fraser, Thomas Russell Cumming 200–2
free radicals research 272–3
Freyberg, Bernard 122
Fulton, Noel H. 86
Fulton, R.A.H. 73
Funder, J.W. 272

Gallipoli 66, 68, **68**, 71
Gander, Philippa 273, 297
Gardner, Jim 17, 19
Gauld, Robin 238, 245, 246
General Medical Council (GMC) 22, 134, 137, 236, 240; medical training recommendations 31, 41, 87, 118, 136; obstetric training requirements 80, 96
General Practice 251; Christchurch 250, 251; professors 227, 247, 249, 250; Wellington 251
genetic research 271
Geriatric Medicine 227
Gerrard, Dave 220
Gibbs, J.M. **235**
Gibbs, Sidney 54
Gibbs Taskforce on Hospitals and Related Services (1988) 238
Gibson, R.D. **235**
Gill, Michael 220
Gillespie, W.J. (Bill) **C, 235**, 250, 253
Gillies, Harold 71, 124
Gillies, John 24
Gillies, Mrs J. **186**
Glasgow, Gavin 133
Glasgow, W.T. **69**
Glendining, Mary 90, 154
Gluckman, Peter 240
goitre research 45, 85, 98, 125, 127, 139, 140
Goodenough Committee 134, 136
Goodlet, 'Wullie' 50
Gordon, Doris (née Jolly) 96, **96**, 295
Gould, John 166, 167, 186, 208
Goulding, Ailsa 297
Govan, Lawrence **233**
Gowland, W.P. (Percy) 42, 43, **89**, 106, 107, **129**, 182, 293, 294, 301; BMedSc introduction 133; character & style 87–9; Clinical Club 97, 98, **98**, 99; honorary degree 88, 290; military service 73; professorship 70, 83; publications 89; resignation 120–21, **121**; Rockefeller Fellowship 84; teaching methods 88–9, **121**
graduates *see* medical graduates
grant applications 265, 269
Graves' disease 140
Green, Lindsay 220
Gregg, J.L. **47**
Gregory, Elizabeth 141
Griesbach, Walter 127–8, 140
Griffiths, G. 143, 220
Grimwood, Keith 249
Grove, Jane Lumsden 165
Guilford, Parry 275

Guinea Pig Club 124
Gurr, Elaine 65, 227
Guthrie, Margaret (née Hoodless, later Wray) 296
Gwynne, James F. 145, 149, 218, 220
Gynaecology *see* Obstetrics and Gynaecology

Hall, Graham Francis (Frank) **C,** 195~8, 212; Graham Francis Hall Prize 196
Hall, Robert (Robinson?) **103**
Hamlin, Catherine 291
Hamlin, Reg 291
Harris, Wolff 41, 154
Hauora Maori 274
Hawke Report (1988) 232, 238
Hawley, T.G. 204
Hay, David 184, 267–8
Hayward, J.W. **188**
He Kainga Oranga 273
He Kitenga 271
Health and Disability Commissioner 242
Health and Hospital Services (HHS) 245
Health Charter 266
Health Funding Authority (HFA) 245, 246
Health Research Council (HRC) 237, 248, 266, 267; funding by 249, 267, 272, 273, 277
health system: and Maori 256, 257; and women 256, 257; booking/scoring system 243, 246; first Labour Government 111, 120; population-based funding 226, 230, 231, 234, 243
health system restructuring 226, 232, 238–9, 245, 246; effect on clinical staff 239–40, 241; protests **242**; 're-reforms' 245
Healthcare Otago 245; clinical staff costs 243; relations with Medical School 239–40, 241, 242, 243–4, 245, 246; senior staff 242, **244**
Healthlink South 241, 242
Heap, Stuart 209
heart disease research 131, 139, 141, 163, 207, 267, 270~73
Heath, Chris 254, 255, **256**, 263
Hector, Charles Monro 86, 100
Hector, James 100
Henderson, Isobel **124**
Henderson, R.S.F. 69
Hendry, Alexander 46
Hercus, Charles **C,** 55, 68, 82, 84, **95**, 108, 111, **115**, 117, 120, **129**, 134, 136, 151, 161, 164, 175, 193, 207, 231; acting Vice-Chancellor 152; biographical sketch 125; building programme 121, 134, 153; Clinical Club 97, **98**, 99; Dean 65, 151–7, 299; death 183; fostering of research 126, 128, 131, 264, 270, 300; honours 125, 289; military service 67, 71~3, 108; MRC appointment 127; on Aitken 151; on BMedSc 133; on Ferguson 62, 74, 231; on Fitchett 91; on Malcolm 42; on medical education 136, 155, 156; on Murray Falconer 292; on role of Dean 161–2; on Scott 29; on women graduates 294–5, 296; *Otago Medical School ... first three*

Deans 43, 92, 125; Preventive and Social Medicine 138; professorship 71, 83, 95; public health commitment 125, 133, 154, 155; refugee doctors 116, 119; relations with UGC 153; research 85, 86, 125; secretaries 231; Sir Charles Hercus Medal 125, 277; Sub-Dean 64, 65, 77, 111, 115; teaching methods 95, 155; University Councillor 157; wider university influence 154–5; *see also* Otago Medical School 1937–1958 (Hercus)

Heslop, Barbara F. (née Cupitt) 265, 296, 297; as medical student 144–5; sexism at Med. School 149; survey of women doctors 296–7

Heslop, John 92

Hewitson, W.H. 102

Hewland, Robyn 150

Hiddlestone, John 204

Higher Education Development Centre (HEDC) 258, 263

Hill, Diana 297

Hill, Mabel **128**

Hillary, Edmund 220

histology 27, 43, 80, 88, 89, 127

Hobson, Audrey **124**

Hocken, T.M. 19, 24, 57

Hodge, Jim 265

Hodgkins, Frances 29

Holgate, Stephen 272

Holloway, Linda **C**, 247, 248, 249, 257, 297

Hollows, Fred 291

Holyoake, Keith 184, 195, 214

Home Science School 45, 141, 165

home science students 83, 144, 156

Hornblow, Andrew R. **C, 235**, 241, 249–50

Hospital Boards *see* Otago Hospital Board; North Canterbury Hospital Board; Wellington Hospital Board

Howden-Chapman, Philippa 273, **274**

Howden, Mary **124**

Howie, Beryl 291–2, 296

Howie, J.B. 172, 266

Hubbard, John I. 140, 182, 265

Hulme, Edward 19, 21, 24, 34

'Humerus' (revue) 280, 281, **282**, 283

Hunter, Irwin 54

Hunter, John D. **C,** 167, 172, 182, 184, 199, 207, 214, 231, 234, **235**, 239, 264; accreditation review 236, 265, 267; Alumnus Association 204; Assistant Vice-Chancellor Health Sciences 234, 239; biographical sketch 185; Christie Report 169, 177, 181; Clinical Schools 169, 181, 184, 189; Dean 161, 182, 199, 229; Dean of Faculty 232, 233, 236, 239; difficulties of deanship 208, 209; General Practice Chair 227; NHF Coronary Committee 267; *ODT* 'crisis' interview 168–9, 171; on Adams 182; on research 271, 277; on role of Dean 167; on the Clinical Club 97–8; professorship 163; research 163; research funding 265, 267; Teschemakers workshop (1986) 257; Travelling Scholarship 185

Hutt Valley Health Corporation 241

Hutton, F.W. 20, 26, 27

Hutton, J.D. **235**, 249

hydatids research 45, 86, 125, 127, 156

hypertension research 131, 141, 163, 264, 265, 270

immunological research 138, 271, 272

Immunology Group 265

Immunopathology Research Unit 266

influenza pandemic (1918) 70, 85

Inter-Colonial Medical Conference (Dunedin, 1896) 63

Intermediate course 31, 70, 87, 173; at Dunedin only 227, 262, 301; entry to Med. School 118, 178, 252, 262, 301; student numbers 118, 121

International Federation of Medical Students' Associations (IFMSA) 286, 301

International Student Conference 145

iodised salt 85, 140, 154

Ironside, Wallace 138, 163–4

Irvine Report (1969) 177–8, 180, 194

Irvine, Robin Orlando Hamilton 171, 186, **188**, 221, 264, 277; biographical sketch 179; Clinical Dean 177, 179, 181; Clinical Schools 189, 194; Dean 184; honorary degree 289; Medical School centenary 199; on medical education 183; professorship 179; Vice-Chancellorship 179

Irwin, Mark 220

Isbister, William H. 197, 198, 212, **235**

Iverach, J.A.D. 73, 105

Jack, Julian 290–91

Jackson, Chris 285

James, Colin 181

Jamieson, D.G. **186**

Jeffcoat, F.H. 46

Jefferson, Alfred 31

Jeffery, A.K. (Keith) **235**, 263

Jellett, Henry 96

Jenkins, James Alfred 93

John Borrie History Hall 139

Johnson, Gillian 213

Johnson, Ralph Hudson **C,** 228, 229, 232–3; biographical sketch 213; Dean 198, 212

Joint Relations Committees 154, 180, 188, 189, 195; discontinued 240; membership 245; re-established 232, 241

Jones, David **C,** 252

Jones, D.W. Carmalt *see* Carmalt Jones, Dudley W.

Jones, Isabella Rea 125

Joyce, Peter R. **235**, 250, 273

Kennedy, Douglas 106, 175

Kennedy, Martin 273

Kennedy, T.H. 140

Kilpatrick, J.A. **201**

King, F. Truby 33, 39, 44~6, 56; sexism 50, 52

King, Michael 181

Kirk, David 283
Kirk, Norman 181, 192
Kirklin, John 293
Knight, Hardwicke 78
Knox College 55~7, 68, 102, 103; Executive (1945)
    143; inter-college cricket 143–4; Knox farce 148;
    medical student predominance 142; Misogynists'
    Society 104
Kronfeldt, Moe **103**

Labour Government: first 108, 110, 111, 120, 293,
    294; fourth 246, 285; third 226, 232, 238, 255
landladies 55, 103
language tuition: English 280; Maori 279
Larkins, Richard 240
Laverty, Richard 209, **235**, 264
Law, Susan **244**
Leslie, Blair **239**
Lewis, Peter 184
libraries 55~7, 76, 78, 94, 134, 137, 168, 170, 175,
    176, 240, 258, 260; anatomy 89; bequests 89, 100;
    bookplate **128**; Christchurch 189, 211; Christie
    Report 175; Dewey classification 100; Dean's
    Department 155; funding 85, 98, 100, 154, 195;
    inadequacies 43, 82, 120, 156, 164, 185–6; Irvine
    Report 178; Medical Library established 64, 98,
    100; military camp library 73; Monro Collection
    98, 100–101, 205; new building 109, 177, 178, 180,
    186, **186**, 195; Selwyn College **55**; Wellington 196,
    198, 212, 234
Liggins, Graham 293
Liley, William 293
Lincoln College 234, 271; curriculum conference
    (1985) 228, 255
Lindsay, P.A. 46
Lister, Joseph 17
Litterhoea 222
Llewellyn, F.J. 166~8, 177
Logan Park 105, 218
Loten, David 261, 262
Lottery Board 267, 272
Loutit, John 209
Loutit, Margaret 296
Lovelock, Jack 105
Low, Charles 22, 53
Lubbe, Wilhelm 267
Ludbrook, J. 204
Lyness, Jean 148

Macandrew, Herbert **27**, 28
Macandrew, James 17~19, **18**, 24, 28
Macbeth, W.A.A.G. (Bill) 191, **235**, 250
Macdonald, John 32, 39
Macdonald, W. Marshall 43, 70
mace, presentations 230, 233
MacGregor, Duncan 19
Macknight, A.D.C. (Tony) 209, 266
MacMahon, Brian 284

Madraiwiwi, Ratu Dovi 104–5
Magill, Elizabeth 23
Malaghan Institute of Medical Research 197, 272
Malaghan Research Trust 268
Malaysian medical students 279–80, 301
Malcolm, Donald 184
Malcolm, J.L. 137
Malcolm, John 43, 64, 87, 98, 109, 120, **121**, **129**, 299;
    Acting Dean 75; biographical sketch 41, 42, **42**;
    Clinical Club 97, 98, **98**, 99; military service 67,
    69, 73; MRC committee 127; nutrition research
    45, 85; professorship 41; teaching methods 90
Malcolm, L.A. **235**
Mann, Jim 274, **274**
Manson, Harry 43, **43**
Maori and the health system 256, 257
Maori health 246, 251, 261–2, 266, 270, 274, 279;
    cardiovascular health 267
Maori Health Research Unit (Te Hotu Manawa Maori)
    248, 267
Maori medical students 52–3, 104, 145, 278, 279, 286,
    289, 290, 301
Maori medicine 137
Maori Research Centre (Te Manawa Hauora) 249
Mara, Ratu Kamisese 144, 289
marae visits 214, 279, **279**
Marama Hall 72, 72–3
Marples, Mary (Molly) 296
Marsden Fund 268–9, 272, 273
Marshall, A. McPhee 93
Martin, Tangi (Richmond) **143**
Mason and Wales 76
Master in Health Science 250
Master of Medical Science (MMedSc) 133
materia medica 31, 32, 44, 74, 76
maternity hospitals: Batchelor Hospital 80, 81;
    planning for 80–81; Queen Mary Maternity
    Hospital 81, **82**, 96, 115, 184, **205**, 276, 302;
    Redroofs 80; St Helen's Maternity Hospital **48**, 80,
    81, 227
Mathewson, Ena 182
Maunsell, James 103
Maunsell, Terry 103
McAra, W. **47**
McBrearty, J.W. **47**
McCredie, Margaret 297
McDonald, Ian 290, 291
McFarlane, Victor 292, 293
McGiven, Roy 191, 250
McIndoe, Archibald (Archie) **103**, 124
McIntyre, Archibald (Archie) 131, 132, 164, 200, 264,
    265
McIntyre, Peter 102, **106**
McKay, D.W. 169
McKellar, Sheila 231, **231**
McMillan, D.G. (Gervan) 108, 120, 154, 293
McQueen, E.G. (Garth) 264, , 266, 270
McQuilkan, Winifred 196

McVey, Duncan 220
Medical and Surgical Sciences 253, 300
medical ball **108**, 143, 148, 217, 281, 282, 284
Medical Council of New Zealand (MCNZ) 116;
  accreditation of Med. School 236, 240, 260;
  refugee doctor policy 119
Medical Debating Society 108
Medical Digest 34, 107–8, 143, 150, 176, 214, 217,
  219, 283; artwork **43**, **90**, **107**, **115**, **142**, **163**;
  caricatures **62**, **89**, **91**, **95**, **121**, **129**, **147**; ceases
  publication 183–4, 222; Eccles on research 132;
  editors 103; first issue 107; Marguerite Cotton
  90, **115**; medical education 137, 172, 183; military
  service 68, 122, 221, 222; post-war medical
  students 145, 146, **147**; Med. School staff 43, 62,
  90, 130; research 269; Russell Clark **62**, **89**, **107**,
  107–8; sportsmen 220
medical education 156, 162, 178, 199–200; Aitken's
  views 151–2; Christie Report 172–5; clinical
  courses 259–60, 262; communication skills 254,
  256, 258, 261, 262; computerised assessment
  254, 261, 301; conferences & workshops 162,
  228, 255–7, 257~61; continuous assessment
  178, 183, 211, 218, 259; course integration 228,
  253, 258, 261~3; curriculum 26, 27–8, 31–2,
  136, 178, 254–63; early courses 26, 27–8, 31–2;
  Goodenough Committee 134, 136; lengthened/
  shortened courses 118, 178; Maori component
  262, 279, **279**; *Medical Digest* articles 137;
  medical ethics 228, 255, 261, 262; new GMC
  recommendations 136; *NZMJ* Med. School
  centenary issue 203–4; organ system-based
  courses 254, 261; Preliminary Examination 22;
  Problem-Based Learning ; research/teaching
  balance 172; Royal Commission (UK) 176, 178;
  six-year course 87; student evaluations 263; *see
  also* clinical training; Intermediate course; teaching
  methods; trainee interns
Medical Education Trust 204
medical ethics 228, 255, 261, 262, 275; Bioethics
  Centre 275
medical graduates: distinguished 289–97; military
  service 52, 122; women 294–7
Medical History Society 108, 148, 217
Medical Jurisprudence (and Public Health) 31~3, 87,
  94; professors **44**, 83
medical manpower 109, 110, 120, 136, 181, 214, 230;
  Maori doctors 279; Pacific Island doctors 279;
  rural doctors 285; specialists 137; WWI shortage
  69, 70; WWII shortage 120
medical register 17, 109, 156; women 48, 49, 297
Medical Research Council (MRC) 42, 127, 130, 154,
  162, 178, 212, 266, 268, 300; capital equipment
  fund 266, 267; committees 95, 127, 139, 266;
  established 294; funding by 127, 131, 265–6, 268;
  funding of 127, 139, 265, 266; Pacific Island health
  research 133
Medical Research Foundations 267, 268, 272;

Canterbury 268; Otago 268; Wellington 268
Medical Research in Otago, 1922–1997 264, 270
medical schools 87; Canada 17, 254; Edinburgh 94,
  100; Melbourne 17, 19, 20, 22, 48; Netherlands
  254; Newcastle (Australia) 254; Sydney 48, 85;
  see also Otago Medical School; University of
  Edinburgh
Medical Society 45
medical student activities 282; Cultural Night
  280–81; Drinking Horn 144, 147, 217; 'Humerus'
  (Med Revue) 222, 280, 281, **282**, 283; Med Camp
  222, 281; medical ball **108**, 143, 148, 217, 281,
  282, 284; medical dinners 53, 56, 57, 104, 149;
  orientation 281, **282**; publications 283–4; *see also*
  Otago University Medical Students' Association;
  sports
medical students 46–57, **47**, **51**, 102–8, 145–50,
  217–22, **218**, 278–86; accommodation 55–6,
  70, 103; apathy 217, 219; bursars 69–70, 121;
  Chinese 104; Christie Report 219; Cook Island
  289; daily timetable 46, 280; drinking 102, 105,
  145; Edinburgh experience 28; élitist background
  69; ethnic composition 262, 279, 301; Faculty
  representative 219; Fijian 104–5, 144, 289;
  financial requirements 48; first 22, 27, 28, 46; full
  cost recovery 237, 279; interwar period 102–8;
  language difficulties 280; late 20th century
  278–86; leadership in student affairs 145–6, 148;
  lifestyle 150; loss of seniors from Dunedin 222;
  Malaysian 279–80; Maori 52–3, 104, 145, 278,
  279, 286, 289, 290, 301; military service 57, 67,
  67–9, **68**, **69**, 70, 117–18, 143, **143**, 221–2, 285;
  Muslim 280; numbers of 40, 45, 46, 61, 76, 83, 109,
  116, 118, 121, 137, 142, 156; Pacific Island 279,
  301; post-war 145–50, 217–22; pre-WWI 46–57;
  proportion of women 227, 278, 296, 301; returned
  servicemen 121, 137; role in student affairs 46;
  Saudi Arabian 280, **281**; sexism 144, 149, 150;
  social life 57; stereotypes 102–4, **106**, 280; student
  loan scheme 238; wartime 'shirking' 66, 69, 117;
  women 48–52, 53, 56, 103–4, 144, 145, 148~50,
  278, 301, 302; *see also* medical graduates
Medical Students' Association *see* Otago University
  Medical Students' Association
Medicine 31, 130, 155, 156, 178, 179, 253, 297, 300;
  accommodation 162–3, 185, 198; Christchurch
  191; Christie Report 173, 178; early appointments
  32; Milton medical survey 206; professors 44,
  83, 90, 128, 163, 182–3, 191, 197, 232, 247, 264;
  research 269; split into Clinical & Sytematic 90;
  Wellington 197, 198, 247, 264
Melbourne Medical School 17, 19, 20, 22, 48
Mellsop, Graham W. **235**, 249
mental health 31, 33; research 273
Mental Health Clinical Research Unit 273
Mercer, John (Jo) 193
Microbiology 155, 251, 296, 300; accommodation
  186, 209, 302; Chrisite Report 173; professors 138,

209; research 269

midwifery 31, 32, 44, 74, 108, **149**, 227; Ethiopia 291; training 80–81

Midwifery 83

Miles, John A.R. 138, 209, 266, 269

military medicine 284–5; hospitals **123**; medical student cadetships 285; women 285; WWI 71–2; WWII 122, **123**, 124

military service: by Med. School graduates 52, 71, 122; by Med. School staff 66, 70, 71–2, 73, 117; by Med. School students 57, **67**, 67–9, **68**, **69**, 70, 117–18, 143, **143**, 221–2, 285; South African War 23, 66–7; WWI 52, 57, 66, 67–9, 70; WWII 117–18, 122, 124

Miller, Andrew 262

Milton medical survey **206**, 206–7

Ministry of Health 240, 245, 270; role re-asserted 246; *see also* Department of Health

Molloy, Pat 163, 184, 247

Monheimer, Benno 107

Monro, Alexander (I, II, III) 100, 101

Monro Collection 61, 100–101, 205

Monro, Sir David 100

Monroe, C.A. **235**

Montgomery, Diana 148

Moore, Patrick Eisdell 42, 88, 103, **129**, 299

Morison, Ian 275

Morrell, W.P. 40, 61, 64, 65, 70, 151, 167; on UGC 153, 166

Mortimer, Graham **C**, **235**, 240, 247, 251, 253

MRC *see* Medical Research Council

Mulder, Roger 273

Muldoon, Robert 181, 226

Mullen, Paul E. **235**, 247

Mullin, W.J. 101, **110**, 299

Murdoch, J. Campbell 227, **235**, 247

Murray, J.A. **27**, 28

museums: Anatomy 31, 80; materia medica 76; medical history 139, 205; Pathology 76, 93

Nacey, John Norman **C**

Nanson, E.M. 204

National Council of Women 120

National Heart Foundation (NHF) 267–8, 273; committees 267

National Poisons Centre 270

National Women's Hospital 257

Natural History 20, 26, 31

Neil, James Hardie 53

Neurological Foundation 268, 273

Neurological Unit 210

Neurology 155

neurophysiological research 264–5

Neurophysiology 182, 265, 300

Neurosurgery 292, 300

New Zealand Medical Association 24, 63, 199; founded 22; teaching standards 39

New Zealand Medical Corps (NZMC) 67, 69, 73, 124

New Zealand Medical Council *see* Medical Council of New Zealand

New Zealand Medical Journal (*NZMJ*) 32, 86, 89, 101, 155, 169, 293, 296; Christie Report 176; doctor glut 214; founded 64; Maori health 257; Med. School centenary 199, 203–4; Med. School problems 170, 176; on Ferguson 82; on Hercus 161; on Smirk 130

New Zealand Medical Student Journal 284

New Zealand Medical Students' Association (NZMSA) 219–20, 279, 284~6; Advanced Choice of Employment scheme 285; AMSA Conference 286; Medical Leadership Development Seminar 285, 298

New Zealand Obstetrical Society 85, 96

New Zealand University Endowment Act (1868) 18

New Zealand University Students' Association (NZUSA) 146

Newell, Kenneth 197

Newlands, William 70, 92, 111, 119

Ng, James 290

Ngata, Apirana 52

Ngata, Paratene 290

NHF *see* National Heart Foundation

Nichol, Lesley 283

Nichol, Rutherford 57

Nicholls, Lincoln **286**

Nicholson, Helen 297

Nightingale, Florence 17

Nisbet, Norman 265

Nobel Prize 133

Nordmeyer, Arnold 197

North, C. 111

North Canterbury Hospital Board 210; cardiac surgery unit row 184; Christchurch Clinical School established 189, 190–91; relations with University of Otago 192

North, J.D.K. (Derek) 204, 270, 293

North, Ken 193~6

North, N.H. 171

nurses' homes 36, 38, 82, 154

nursing 17, 228

nursing students 156

Nursing (Wellington) 228

nutrition research 131, 139, 274; iodised salt 85, 140, 154

Nye, Ted 206, 264; 'Research at the Otago Medical School' 269

obstetric research 127

obstetric training 80–81, **149**

Obstetrical Society *see* New Zealand Obstetrical Society

Obstetrics and Gynaecology 178, 184, 253, 295; accommodation 153, 198; Christchurch 191, 250; Christie Report 174; early appointments 32; initial difficulties 96; professors 43, 44, 81, 83, 96, 124, 138, 191, 250; Wellington 198, 247, 249

O'Donnell, Thomas V. (Tom) **C**, 204, 234, **235**, 247, **248**, 264; Dean 232; professorship 197

Officers' Training Corps (OTC) 67, 69, 72, 73, 125

Ogston, Frank 32–3, 39, 44, 83

Olds, R.J. 275

O'Neill, Eugene 66, 92

Ophthalmology 33, 63, 82, 111, 155, 253, 300; professors 44, 208

Orientation Week 281, **282**

orthopaedic surgery 72, 83, 92–3

Orthopaedic Surgery 182, 250, 253, 265, 300; Christchurch 191, 250

O'Sullivan, A.W.T. **69**

Otago Boys' High School 54, 65

Otago Daily Times 19, 24, 162, 171, 187, 230, 245, 247; Auckland Medical School 120; Brinkman 226; cardiac surgery unit row 184; Christie Report 176; CT scanner 210; fundraising for University 40; health reforms **242**, 243, **244**, 245; Med. School centenary 199; Med. School status 168–9; military service of students 117; refugee doctor question 119; relations with Med. School 184; research funding 267; siting of Med. School buildings 77; third medical school 195; World War I 67

Otago Hospital Board 111, 171, 176; cardiac surgery unit row 184; maternity funding 81; population-based funding 209–10, 230; University representation 157, 175, 177; women members 65

Otago Medical School: honorary degrees (DSc) 290–91; honorary degrees (LLD) 289–90; summary of changes 299–302; Taieri farm for animal breeding 154, 156, 164; *see also* Branch Faculties; Christchurch Clinical School; Wellington Clinical School; *see also* names of individual departments

Otago Medical School 1875–1914 (Scott) 17–57; admission of women 48–50, 52; Dean's position established 39; degree completion in Britain 20–21, 25, 26, 28–9, 46, 47–8; early appointments 19, 21, 31, 32–3, 43; Faculty of Medicine established 39; first endowed chair 41; founding 17, 18–24, 25, 27; full medical course 31–2, 40, 47, 48; government funding 41, 45; honorary medical staff 23, 28, 31–3, 35, 36; initial courses 26, 27–8, 31–2; library 98; 'national' character of School 41, 45; recognition by Senate 31; recognition in UK 19, 21–22, 24, 25–6; relations with Hospital 36, 37–8; research 44–5; salaries 39; South African War 66–7; student numbers 27, 40, 45, 46, 109; teaching standards 39

Otago Medical School 1914–1937 (Ferguson) 61–111; accommodation needs 74, 75; appointments 83; budget 78, 84–5; building programme 74–82; clinical training outside Dunedin 87, 111; Dean's salary 65; degree completion in Britain 69, 109; donations 84, 86, 90; effects of the Depression 85, 87, 96, 111, 302; endowed chairs 85; funding by government 61, 74, 90; library 98, 100–101;

'national' character of School 77; research 84, 85–6; research funding 85, 86; salaries 83, 85, 111; six-year course 87; special funds 85, 86; staff growth 84; staff travel 84; student numbers 61, 76, 83, **86**, 109, 111; Sub-Deans 64; teaching evaluated 88, 90, 91, 94; women on staff 83, 84, 89, 90, 295; World War I 66–73, 302

Otago Medical School 1937–1958 (Hercus) 115–57; building programme 121, 134, 153; Dean's Department 155; donations 156; endowed chairs 154; entry criteria 118; funding 121, 136, 152~4, 156; open days 115; overcrowding 116, 120–21, 122; refugee doctor question 116, 118–20; research 126–34, 138, 139–41, 156; research funding 127, 131, 154; salaries 137–8, 152–3, 156; staff expansion 126, 128, 137–9, 155–6; student intake 118, 120, 136; student numbers 116, 118, 121, 137, 156; Taieri farm for animal breeding 154, 156; women on staff 295; World War II 115–25, 302

Otago Medical School 1958–1981 161–222; artists 186; autonomy 161, 166; building programme 184, 186–7; centenary celebrations 131, 181, 184, 199–207, 201; Clinical Dean 177, 178, 181, 184; curriculum committees 162, 178, 183, 219; Deans 161, 162, 177, 181, 199, 207, 208, 209; Dean's role 161–2, 175, 178; entry criteria 178; funding 167, 169, 170, 175, 178, 208; library grant 195; 'national' character of School 167; open days 164, 205, **205**, **206**; relations with ODT 184; research 171; salaries 174, 177; staff morale 168; staff numbers 178, 199; staff/student ratio 168, 170, 178; staffing committee 167; student intake **174**, 175, 177, 180, 181, 199, 214, 215; student representation on committees 219; Taieri farm for animal breeding 164; *see also* Christie Report; Irvine Report

Otago Medical School 1980–2000 225–286; accreditation 236, 237, 240, 241, 245, 250~53, 260~62, 265; administrative structure 251–2, 252, 253; attitudes to women 278; autonomy of Clinical Schools 237; bequests 227; 'clinical material' availability 228; clinical/preclinical split of schools 251–2; clinical staff costs 243; cost centres 246, 252, 300; curriculum committees 227, 254, 257, 258, 261, 262; Dean of Faculty 230, 232, 251; Deans 225, 232, 239, 240, 247, 251~3, 263; Dunedin School of Medicine 237, 251, 252; entry criteria 252, 262, 301; funding 225, 237; funding by population 226, 230, 231, 234, 243; funding by student numbers 237; funding division among Schools 233; gavel 230; health reforms 239–40, 240–41; inter-School relations 225, 228, 229, 234, 250; Otago School of Medical Sciences 237, 251–2, 252–3, 300; relations with Healthcare Otago 239–40, 241, 242, 243–4, 245, 246; renamings of Schools 229, 233, 251, 253; research 264–5, 269–70, 271–3, 274–5; research funding 237, 265~8, 271~3, 275; research/teaching balance 259; salaries 243, 251; sexism 278; staff/student ratio 228; staffing levels 236, 246; strategic plan 234, 236; student intake 225, 230, 262, 279, 300; University of Otago Medical School 251; women on staff 251, 297

Otago Medical School Alumnus Association *see* Alumnus Association

Otago Medical School buildings 41, 74, 153; Adams building 186, 265, 302; Biochemistry Building 186, 238, 265, 302; costs 84; government funding 74, 77; Hercus Building (South Block) 121, **134**, 139, 153, 156, 238, 265, 302; Irvine Report 180; Knox Church Sunday School 185; library 186, **186**; Lindo Ferguson Building 76–80, 79, 82, 302; Marama Hall 72, 72–3; Microbiology Building 186, 265, 302; new hospital ward block 187; Sayers Building 186, 265, 302; Scott Building 70, 74–6, 74, **75**, 82, 121; siting 75, 76–7; Stock Exchange **20**, 26; University of Otago wing (1879) **26**; Wellcome Research Institute 130, 163, **163**

Otago Medical Society 108

Otago Polytechnic 260

Otago Provincial Council 18, 24

Otago School of Medical Sciences *see* Otago Medical School 1980–2000

Otago University Cricket Club 53

Otago University Medical Company/Corps (OUMC) 42, 71~3, 108, 116~118, 122, 125, 221, 284–5; becomes University Medical Unit 221

Otago University Medical Students' Association (OUMSA) 52, 56–7, 105, 117, 148, 183, 217–18, 219, 281, 283~5; affiliation to OUSA 283; corporate sponsorship 283; Education Committee 219; ethnic representatives 279, 283; exclusion of women 56, 104; facilities 217; fees protests 56; formation 46; Intellectual Affairs 105, 106, 183, 219; OUSA fees 219; publications 222; relations with Auckland 219; relations with Australia 219; relations with OUSA 56; student loan protest 283; *see also* Medical Digest; medical student activities

Otago University Review 28, 46, 48, 53, 55; Gallipoli 68; Lindo Ferguson building 78; on medical students 102; sexism 49, 104; tribute to Champtaloup 94

Otago University Students' Association (OUSA) 52, 105, 145; buildings 146, 218; compulsory fees 105; exclusion of women 56; formation 46; Health Sciences representative 283; incorporated society 146; Lady Vice President 104; Logan Park 105; medical student involvement 105, 142, 146, 218; president's role 218; representation on University Council 146; University Book Shop 218; woman president 278, 283

Otakou Marae 279

OUMC *see* Otago University Medical Company/Corps

oxidative stress research 271, 272–3

Pacific Island health 266, 270, 279; research 133, 139

Pacific Island Health Professional Students' Association 279

Paediatrics (and Child Health) 155, 171, 178, 184, 247, 253, 300; accommodation 198; Christchurch 191, 210, 250; professors 164, 191, 249, 250; Wellington 198, 247, 249

Paewai, Nitama 143, **143**

Palmer, David G. 247, 264

Parker, S.T. **69**

Parr, James 77, 78

Parr, John 208

Parry committee 164–6

Parry, David Hughes 164

Parry, Gordon *An Historical Sketch* 199

Parton, Hugh 167

Pasifika Medical Association 279

Paterson, Ada 294

Paterson, James 68

Pathology 31, 76, 171, 242, 251, 253; accommodation 134; Christchurch 191, 250, 297; Clinical Pathologist position 93; museum 76, 93; professors 44, 70, 71, 83, 93, 95, 164, 182, 197, 249, 250, 297; teaching methods 93–4; Wellington 197, 247, 249

Patient, Doctor and Society course 261

Paul, Charlotte 257, 297

Paykel, Eugene 293

Pearse, Victor 124

penicillin 124

Perpetual Trustees 227

Petersen, George B. 168, **235**, 267, 291

Pharmac 246

pharmacogenomics 273

Pharmacology (and Pharmacy) 251, 300; accommodation 164, 170, 173, 178, 186, 251, 265; Christie Report 173; professors 139, 208, 209, 264, 270; research 269, 271

pharmacy 21, 228, 246, 253

Physical Education School 154, 155; Milton medical survey 206

physical education 93, 155, **286**

Physical Education School 154, 155, 206

physical education students 156, 220

Physiology 76, **135**, 155, 251, 300; Christie Report 173, 178; endowed chair 41; Neurophysiology 182, 265, 300; professors 41, 45, 121, 131, 132, 164, 182, 209, 264; research 269; self-directed learning 258; splits from Anatomy 41; staffing 43, 178; student numbers 74; under Malcolm 89–90

Physiotherapy 237, 238, 251~3; Bachelor of Physiotherapy 260

Physiotherapy School 45, 154

physiotherapy students 83, 93

Pickerill, Cecily (née Clarkson) 295

Pickerill, Percy 71–2, 83, 92, 93, 295

Pih-Chang, Kathleen 104, **104**

plastic surgery 71–2, 83, 92, **103**, 124, 174, 300

Plunket, Lord 38

Plunket Society 45, 141, 204, 295
poliomyelitis 86
Pollock, Martin 210
Pomare, Eru Woodbine **C**, **235**, 241, **248**, 249, 257, 267, 279; biographical sketch 248; Dean 247
Pomare, Maui 248, 279
Popper, Karl 132
population-based funding 209–10, 226, 230, 231, 234, 243
Porritt, Arthur 105, 107, 289
Porter, Roy 17
Potaka, Louis 104
Potts, D.G. 204
Poulton, Richie 276, **277**
Preliminary Examination 22
Press CHEs and Med. School 242
Preventive (and Social) Medicine 78, 117, 134, **135**, 162, 171, 251, 253, 297, 300; accommodation 134, 186, 210; Christchurch 191, 210; Christie Report 174; department established 155; Milton medical survey 206; National Poisons Centre 270; professors 138, 164, 191, 209, 297; research 269–70, 274–7
preventive medicine 71, 78
Princess Margaret Hospital 188, 189, 270
Prior, Ian 142, 143, **143**, 193, 197, 270
Proceedings of the Otago Medical Research Society 156
Proceedings of the University of Otago Medical School 86, 264, 270
psychiatry 71, 128, 184, 216
Psychiatry 138, 155, 157, 162, 171, 300
Psychological Medicine 178, 247; Christchurch 245, 250, 273; Christie Report 174; professors 164, 191, 197, 247, 250, 297; research 273; Wellington 197, 213, 247, 249
Public Good Science Fund 237, 269
public health 45, 125, 141, 154; Maori 257, 266; research 155, 266, 271, 273–4
Public Health: accommodation 78; Christchurch 250; professors 71, 250; salaries 111; student theses 95, 125; Wellington 249, 273, 297; *see also* Bacteriology (and Public Health); Medical Jurisprudence (and Public Health); Preventive (and Social) Medicine
Public Health Commission 239, 241, 243
Purves, H.D. (Dick) 128, 140, **140**, 200, 290

Qualifications Authority 238
Queen Mary Maternity Hospital 81, **82**, 96, 115, 184, 205, 276, 302
Quilliam, Peter **103**

Radcliffe-Taylor, Marion 296
radiology 162, 295
Radiology 209; Christchurch 190, 192; professors 190, 192, 209
Ramsay, J. **91**
Rayns, D.G. 264

Redroofs 80
Redshaw, Nelson **206**
Reeve, Anthony 275
refugee doctor controversy 116, 118–20
Regional Health Authorities (RHAs) 238, 241, 243, 245
Reid, Matthew **239**
Reid, Papaarangi 249, 267, 274
research: 'blue skies' 269; Government priorities 266; post-1958 171, 264–5, 269–70, 271–3, 274–5; research themes 271–3; under Ferguson 84, 85–6; under Hercus 126–34, 138, 139–41, 156; under Scott 44–5
research funding: grant applications 265, 269; post-Hercus 237, 265~8, 271~3, 275; under Ferguson 85, 86; under Hercus 127, 131, 154
Research Management Plans 271
Restieaux, Norma 163, **268**, 297
Returned Servicemen's Association (RSA) 119
Rheumatology 264
Rhodes Scholarships 292; Aitken 151, 292; Eccles 131, 289; Jack 290; Kirk 283; Lovelock 105; North 270, 293; Porritt 107, 289, 292; Skegg 209
Richards, Mark 267, 272
Richardson, John 24
Riley, F. Ratcliffe 38, 43, 97, 107; attacks advertising hoardings 43, **44**; professorship 43, 83
Riminton, John 189
Ritchie, Russell 73; Clinical Club 97, **98**, 99
Roake, Justin 250
Robb, Douglas 70, 204, 293
Robbins, Francie 279
Roberts, John 197, 213
Roberts, M.S. **235**
Roberts, Murray Beresford 106
Roberts, Sir John 85, 86
Roberts, W.S. 32, 39, 66, **110**; professorship 44
Robertson, Zoe Cuff (later Mason) 295
Robinson, James R. 45, 161, 209, 264, 266, 269; professorship 164
Robinson, Marion 164
Robinson, R.G. 210
Rockefeller awards 84, 202
Rockefeller Foundation 95, 134
Rogers, Lindsay 122
Rolleston, George L. **C**, 172, **188**, 189, 210~12, 229, **233**, 266; biographical sketch 192; Dean 190, 192
Romans, Sarah 247, 297
Ropiha, Rina (later Moore) 144, **144**
Rose, Alice 104, 295, 296
Ross, Angus 199
Royal Army Medical Corps (RAMC) 67, 69~71
Rudland, Joy 263
rugby 53, 54, **54**, 57, 143, 148, **148**, 220, 283; Maori students 52, 53; Nichol Cup 57, 220, 283; University A 52, 54, 143
Russell bequest 154

Sale, G.S. 53, **54**
Salmon, Pam 265
Samoa 133
Sandel, Jean 295
Satyanand, Mutyala 105
Saudi Arabian medical students 280, **281**
Saunders, Bill 149, 150
Sayers, Edward **C**, 130, 162~4, 167~9, 175, 177,
181, 185, **207**, 231, 296; biographical sketch 165;
Dean 161, 162; defends Med. School in NZMJ
170–71, 176; honorary degree 200; NHF Scientific
Committee 267; on medical education 162, 172;
opposes Clinical Schools 189; Wellcome Research
Institute 162–3
Scales, Sid **174**
School Dental Service 85
School of Dentistry *see* Dental School
School of Home Science 45, 141, 165
School Medical Service 85
School of Physical Education 154, 155, 206
Schwartz, Kurt 191
Schwartz, Peter 254, 256, 262
Scott, John H. (Med. School secretary) 231
Scott, John Halliday **C**, 26, 27, 28, 32, 35, 43, 57, 64,
87, 109, 161, **207**, 299; Anatomy Museum 31;
biographical sketch 29; cricket 53; Dean 39; death
45, 57, 63, 64, 74, 88; draughtsmanship 29, **30**;
finances 39, 40; full medical course 31–2, 40, 47,
48; library 89, 98, 101; professorship 25; research
44–5; teaching 29, 31; women students 48–9
Scott, P.J. 204
Seacliff Hospital 33, 52
Second New Zealand General Hospital **123**
Seddon, Richard J. (Prof.) 197, **235**, 247
Seddon, Richard John (Premier) 41
Selwyn College 55–6, 102, 103; inter-college cricket
143–4; library **55**; Selwyn ballet 148
Senate of the University of New Zealand 106, 111,
119, 166, 167, 296; post-war medical education
review 136, 188; recognises Med. School 31;
refugee doctor question 116, 119–20; six-year
medical course 87; UGC appointments 152
Services Medical Team 221
Shannon, Fred T. 191, 204, 229, **235**, 250, 266;
professorship 191
Sherrington, Charles 131, 290
Sidey, T.K.S. **188**
Siedeberg, Emily 45, **48**, 48~50, 52, 295
Silva, Phil 276
Simpson, F.O. (Olaf) 206, 264
Simpson, James Young 17
Simpson, Vicky 42
Sir Charles Hercus Medal 277
Skegg, David C.G. 233, 264, 274, **277**; professorship
209; Public Health Commission 241; Vice-
Chancellor 277
Sleep/Wake Centre 273
Small, Joe 105

Smirk, Horace **129**, 130, **130**, 162, 169, 179, 197, 200,
226, 227; 'coat of arms' **163**; Dean's role 162; *High
Arterial Pressure* 141; hypertension research 131,
141, 163, 200, 269; professorship 128; Wellcome
Research Institute 163, 182, 264, 265
Smith, Bill 146
Smith, J.M.B. (Sandy) **235**, 278
Smithells, Philip 155
Sneyd, J.G.T. (Sam) 168
Sneyd, Rosalie 205
Snively Report 243–4
Snively, Suzanne 243
social security 293, 294, 302
Soper, Frederick 152, 162
Sopoaga, Tai 279
South African War 23, 66–7
South Pacific Commission 133
Southland Hospital 228
Speight, Norman 124
Spence, J.C. 134
Spencer, F. Montgomery (Montie) 68, 69, **69**, 122
sports 52~4, 143, 220; Easter Tournament 53, 148;
Ellen Hendry Cup 283; *see also* cricket; rugby
sports grounds 54, 105, 218
sports medicine 220
Sports Medicine 300
Springbok rugby tour (1981) 278
St Helen's Maternity Hospital **48**, 80, 81, 227
St John Ambulance 222
St Margaret's College 55, **55**, 56, 103–4
Stallworthy, John (Jack) 200, 202–3, 204; honorary
degree 200, **201**; OUSA president 105
Steenson, K.R. 86
Stehbens, William H. (Bill) 197, 198, 212, **235**, 247
Stewart, Downie 78
Stewart, Marian 295
Stewart, R.D.H. (David) **C**, 240, 244, 246, 247, 250,
251, 257; Assistant Vice-Chancellor Health
Sciences 237, 239; Dean 232, 233; Dean of Faculty
237; Healthcare Otago Board appointment 244;
professorship 182–3
Stout, Duncan 193
Stout, Robert 24
Student Health Service 155, 164
student loan scheme 238, 283, 285
Student Representative Council 278
Student Union building 146, 155
Study Right allowance 238
Sugrue, Bill 219
Summerskill, Edith 134
Sunderland, Sydney 148
surgery: aseptic principle 17, 33; steam sterilisation
37; use of rubber gloves 33, 37
Surgery 28, 31, 155, 178, 184, 186, 253, 300;
accommodation 153; Anaesthesia splits off 191,
208; Barnett endowment 92; Christchurch 191,
250; Christie Report 174, 178; clinical tutors
43; endowed Chair 154; orthopaedics 92–3;

Orthopaedics splits off 182; professors 44, 61, 83, 92, 124, 138, 182, 191, 197, 250, 265; staffing 92–3, 178; stomatology 92; under Bell 92; urology 93; Wellington 197
Surgical Dental Unit 93
Sykes, Margaret 292
Systematic Medicine 71, 90
Systems Integration course 261, 262

Tahuna Park 105
Taieri Air Force Station 156
Tapsell, Peter 289
Tate, Warren 275, **275**
Taylor, Douglass 42, 173; Monro Collection 100–101
Te Aute College 52, 104
Te Hotu Manawa Maori 248, 267
Te Manawa Hauora 249
Te Rangi Hiroa (Peter Buck) 52, 52, 53, 56, 104, 290, 301
teaching hospitals 115, 169, 174~6, 195, 241; costs 243; Dunedin 34, 157, 174, 177, 195; funding 225, 226, 231, 234, 236; ownership change 240; relations with Med. School 168, 245; Wellington 193, 195
teaching methods 87, 89, 90, 92, 93–4, 254, 301; case-based teaching 258, 260; computer-assisted learning 227, 254; problem-based learning 254, 255, 256, 257–8, 259, 260; self-directed learning 254, 255, 256, 257–8, 259~61, 263; small-group learning 254, 258; student theses 95, 125; *see also* medical education
Teele, David 250
The Lancet 17, 86
therapeutics 128, 162
Therapeutics 162, 165, 300; Clinical Medicine and 90
Thompson, G.E. 24
Thomson, James **44**
Thomson, Miss (G.M.) 64, 231
Thoracic Surgery 155, 300
Thorpe, Cutter, Pickmere and Douglas (architects) 189
thyroid research 45, 127–8, 139, 140
Tiller, J.W.G. 269
Tilyard, Murray 247
Todd, Kathleen 296
Toop, Les 250
Toxicology Research Unit 266
trainee interns 199, 211, 229, 240, 249, 254, 284; Advanced Choice of Employment scheme 285
transplantation research 265
Travelling Scholarships: Aitken 151; Fraser 202; Hunter 185; Jenkins 93; McFarlane 292; Rose 104, 295; Sandel 295; Stallworthy 202; Watt 295; women 104, 295
Travis Laboratory 127
Travis Trust 127, 131, 154; Fellows 127
Trentham Military Camp 122
Trotter, Ninian 54

Trotter, W.D. (Bill) **135**, 172, 182; Fee for Parts (poem) 144; professorship 182
Truth refugee doctor question 119
tuberculosis: Champtaloup's death 94; research 86, 94, 127, 133
Turbott, Harold 268, 294
Turnbull, Alec **201**

UGC *see* University Grants Committee
'unfortunate experiment' 257
University A (rugby team) 52, 54, 143
University Book Shop 218, 282
University Club 90
University Council (Otago) 40, 56, 86, 87, 115, 120, 128, 153, 154, 169; block-grant funding 166; Board of Discipline 106; Christie Report received 172; Clinical Schools plan 195; Coughtrey's appointment 21, 22, 24; Dean's membership 161, 162; domiciliary scheme 80; executive Vice-Chancellor 151; Ferguson's last meeting 82; grants to Branch Faculties 270; Hospital Board representation 157; Irvine Report supported 180; medical library approved 177; Medical School founding 18~22; members 24; OUSA representation 146; public appeal for funds 75; refugee doctor question 116, 118–19, 120; siting of buildings 75, 76–7, 81; six-year medical course 87; Visitor to the Medical School 151
University Cricket Club 105
University Endowment Act (1868) 18
University Grants Committee (UGC) 125, 152~4, 156, 194; chairmen 166, 168; Christie Report 171, 175~8; Clinical Schools 189, 194, 198, 230; disestablished 232, 237, 238; enhanced powers 165–6; funding by 166–7, 210; Med. School failings 167, 168, 170; third medical school 212–13; Treasury influence 181, 208
University Medical Unit (UMU) **221**, 221–2, 284; includes Auckland students 222; women 222
University of Edinburgh 20, 41, 44, 100; Otago degree completion 20–21, 25, 26, 28–9, 46~8, 66; recognition of Otago courses 22, 25–6
University of New Zealand: disestablished 165; *see also* Senate of the University of New Zealand
University of Otago 45, 55, 171; administrative changes 238; Assistant Vice-Chancellor Health Sciences 185, 234, 239, 251, 253; autonomy 166; Chancellor position 151; Chancellors 64, 65, 75, 76; Division of Health Sciences created 234; early financial difficulties 18, 22, 40–41; Faculty of Medicine established 39; founding 17–18; funding 152, 166, 238, 246; Medical School dominance 151, 155; post-war overcrowding 134; Pro Vice-Chancellor position 253; Professorial Board 42; research 264, 271, 273; retirement age 65, 155, 161; sports grounds 54, 105; staffing committee 167; Vice-Chancellor position 151, 232; Vice-Chancellors 137, 152, 152, 167, 168, 179, 277; *see*

also Otago Medical School; University Council (Otago)

University of Otago, Christchurch *see* the earlier name Christchurch Clinical School

University of Otago Magazine 271, 273, 276, 292

University of Otago Medical School *see* Otago Medical School

University of Otago, Wellington *see* the earlier name Wellington Clinical School

University Reserves Act (1904) 41

Upton, Simon 266–7

Urology 93, 300

Valintine, T.H.A. 74

van Rij, Andre M. **235**, 265

Veale, A.M.O. 264, 266

Verrall, Ayesha 283

Victoria University College 193~5; relations with Wellington Clinical School 212, 228, 229; third medical school 212

Victoria University Council 193

Virus Research Unit 266

vitamin deficiency 124

Voselegi 143

Waimate 48

Wakari Hospital 153, 153–4, 156, 157, 174

Wales, Neil 78

Walker, Xaviour 286

Walsh, John 154, **206**

Ward, Joseph 40

Watson, Robert Burns 103

Watt, James M. 164, 266

Watt, Michael 89, 127, 293–4

Wearing, Donovan **244**

Webster, G.M. 19

Wellcome Medical Research Institute 163, 165, 182, 184, 264, 269; Milton medical survey 206; professors 163, 227

Wellcome Trust 130, 170, 184

Wellington Cancer and Research Institute 197

Wellington Clinical School 179, 181, 198, 199, 204, 225, 251, 252, 253, 300, 302; accreditation 245; Bates Report 215–16; building programme 184, 186, **195**, 195–6, 197–8, 212~14, 302; clinical training 183; Council 195, 197; Deans 195, 196, 198, 212, 232, 247, 249; funding 208, 233, 247; health reforms 241; initial staff 183, 197; initial student intake 212, 213–14; Maori Health Research Unit 248; open days 249; origins 175, 180, 193–5, 203; relations with Dunedin 209, 228, 234; relations with Hospital 198, 234, 245; relations with Victoria University 212, 228, 229; renamings 229, 233, 253; research 271, 272, 273–4; research funding 268

Wellington Hospital: clinical training of students 194, 195; population-based funding 230; teaching hospital 193, 195

Wellington Hospital Board: Clinical School establishment 193~5; Dean's rights 214

Wellington Medical Students Association (WMSA) 284

Wellington School of Medicine *see* the earlier name Wellington Clinical School

Welsh, Peter 220

Westenra, F.G. **27**

Weston, H.J. (Jeffray) 197, **235**, 247

W.H. Travis Trust 127, 131

Whangaparaoa army camp 222

White, James Renfrew ('Eefie') 72, 83, 84, 92–3, 149

Whitehead, 'Algy' 103

Whittingham, Senga 149–50

Whyte, Marion 84, 93

Wi Repa, Tutere 52–3, 104

Will, William J. **27**, 28, 53

Williams, Ernest 97, 98, **98**, 99

Williams, Robin 168, 169, 175, 181, 184, 186, **188**; Christie Report 177; Vice-Chancellor 167, 168

Williams, Susi 150

Wilson, Don 253

Wilson, Roger 217

Wilson, Stanley Livingstone 124, 200, 203

Wilson, Sue 219

Wimsett, Norm 148

Winterbourn, Christine 272, **272**, 273, 297

Wise, Winifred 227

women: absence from senior positions 251; admission to Medical School 48; and health system 256, 257; discrimination against 50, 52, 104; Hospital Board 65; in medicine 294–7; medical students 48–52, 53, 56, 103–4, 144, 145, 148~50, 278, 301, 302; military service 222, 285; on teaching staff 83, 84, 89; OUSA vice presidency 104; 'unfortunate experiment' 257

Women's and Children's Health 253

Woodruff, Michael 138, 153, 200, 264, 265; professorship 124, 138

Woodside 'Jaw' Hospital 72

Woodward, Alice 53

World Health Organization 197, 256, 267, 277, 286, 291, 294

World War I 66–71, **67~9**

World War II 115–25, **123**, **143**

Wright, Lawrence 124, **124**, 138

Wright-St Clair, Rex 204

Wynn-Williams, Alun 164, 182

x-ray equipment 37

Young, James 100

Zoology 27

Zouche, Isaiah de 33